Dr … kens

PROGRESS IN CLINICAL AND BIOLOGICAL RESEARCH

Vol 1: **Erythrocyte Structure and Function,** George J. Brewer, *Editor*

Vol 2: **Preventability of Perinatal Injury,** Karlis Adamsons and Howard A. Fox, *Editors*

Vol 3: **Infections of the Fetus and the Newborn Infant,** Saul Krugman and Anne A. Gershon, *Editors*

Vol 4: **Conflicts in Childhood Cancer,** Lucius F. Sinks and John O. Godden, *Editors*

Vol 5: **Trace Components of Plasma: Isolation and Clinical Significance,** G.A. Jamieson and T.J. Greenwalt, *Editors*

Vol 6: **Prostatic Disease,** H. Marberger, H. Haschek, H.K.A. Schirmer, J.A.C. Colston, and E. Witkin, *Editors*

Vol 7: **Blood Pressure, Edema and Proteinuria in Pregnancy,** Emanuel A. Friedman, *Editor*

Vol 8: **Cell Surface Receptors,** Garth L. Nicolson, Michael A. Raftery, Martin Rodbell, and C. Fred Fox, *Editors*

Vol 9: **Membranes and Neoplasia: New Approaches and Strategies,** Vincent T. Marchesi, *Editor*

Vol 10: **Diabetes and Other Endocrine Disorders During Pregnancy and in the Newborn,** Maria I. New and Robert H. Fiser, *Editors*

Vol 11: **Clinical Uses of Frozen-Thawed Red Blood Cells,** John A. Griep, *Editor*

Vol 12: **Breast Cancer,** Albert C. W. Montague, Geary L. Stonesifer, Jr., and Edward F. Lewison, *Editors*

Vol 13: **The Granulocyte: Function and Clinical Utilization,** Tibor J. Greenwalt and G.A. Jamieson, *Editors*

Vol 14: **Zinc Metabolism: Current Aspects in Health and Disease,** George J. Brewer and Ananda S. Prasad, *Editors*

Vol 15: **Cellular Neurobiology,** Zach Hall, Regis Kelly, and C. Fred Fox, *Editors*

Vol 16: **HLA and Malignancy,** Gerald P. Murphy, *Editor*

Vol 17: **Cell Shape and Surface Architecture,** Jean Paul Revel, Ulf Henning, and C. Fred Fox, *Editors*

Vol 18: **Tay-Sachs Disease: Screening and Prevention,** Michael M. Kaback, *Editor*

Vol 19: **Blood Substitutes and Plasma Expanders,** G.A. Jamieson and T.J. Greenwalt, *Editors*

Vol 20: **Erythrocyte Membranes: Recent Clinical and Experimental Advances,** Walter C. Kruckeberg, John W. Eaton, and George J. Brewer, *Editors*

Vol 21: **The Red Cell,** George J. Brewer, *Editor*

Vol 22: **Molecular Aspects of Membrane Transport,** Dale Oxender and C. Fred Fox, *Editors*

Vol 23: **Cell Surface Carbohydrates and Biological Recognition,** Vincent T. Marchesi, Victor Ginsburg, Phillips W. Robbins, and C. Fred Fox, *Editors*

Vol 24: **Twin Research,** Proceedings of 2nd International Congress on Twin Studies
Walter E. Nance, *Editor*
Published in 3 Volumes:
Part A: Psychology and Methodology
Part B: Biology and Epidemiology
Part C: Clinical Studies

Vol 25: **Recent Advances in Clinical Oncology,** Tapan A. Hazra and Michael C. Beachley, *Editors*

Vol 26: **Origin and Natural History of Cell Lines,** Claudio Barigozzi, *Editor*

Vol 27: **Membrane Mechanisms of Drugs of Abuse,** Charles W. Sharp and Leo G. Abood, *Editors*

Vol 28: **The Blood Platelet in Transfusion Therapy,** G.A. Jamieson and Tibor J. Greenwalt, *Editors*

Vol 29: **Biomedical Applications of the Horseshoe Crab (Limulidae),** Elias Cohen, *Editor-in-Chief*

Vol 30: **Normal and Abnormal Red Cell Membranes,** Samuel E. Lux, Vincent T. Marchesi, and C. Fred Fox, *Editors*

Vol 31: **Transmembrane Signaling,** Mark Bitensky, R. John Collier, Donald F. Steiner, and C. Fred Fox, *Editors*

NORMAL AND ABNORMAL RED CELL MEMBRANES

NORMAL AND ABNORMAL RED CELL MEMBRANES

Proceedings of the ICN–UCLA Symposium
held at Keystone, Colorado
March 1978

Editors

SAMUEL E. LUX
The Children's Hospital Medical Center
Boston, Massachusetts

VINCENT T. MARCHESI
Yale University School of Medicine
New Haven, Connecticut

C. FRED FOX
University of California
Los Angeles, California

Alan R. Liss, Inc. • New York

Address all inquiries to the publisher:
Alan R. Liss, Inc., 150 Fifth Avenue, New York, NY 10011

Printed in the United States of America.

Library of Congress Cataloging in Publication Data

Normal and abnormal red cell membranes.

(Progress in clinical and biological research; vol. 30)
Includes bibliography and index.
1. Erythrocytes – Congresses. 2. Cell membranes – Congresses. 3. Membrane proteins – Congresses. 4. Erythrocyte disorders – Congresses. I. Lux, Samuel E. II. Marchesi, Vincent T. III. Fox, C. Fred. IV. ICN Pharmaceuticals, inc. V. California. University. University at Los Angeles. VI. Series
QP96.N67 612'.111 79-5017
ISBN 0-8451-0030-0

NOTE

Pages 1–436 of this volume are reprinted from Journal of Supramolecular Structure, Volumes 8, 9, and 10. The page numbers in the table of contents, author index, and subject index of this volume correspond to the page numbers at the foot of these pages.

IMPORTANT NOTICE

Most of the issues that were covered at the conference are treated in this proceedings volume. The table of contents does not necessarily follow the actual pattern of the plenary sessions, but rather, reflects the thrust of the meeting as it evolved from the combination of plenary and poster sessions culminating in the final collection of invited and submitted papers. The actual order of the articles appearing in this volume does not follow the order in which the articles are cited in the table of contents. Many articles were submitted jointly for consideration by Journal of Supramolecular Structure and for publication in these proceedings. These articles are included in the text in the order in which they were accepted for publication and then published in the Journal, and they are followed by invited papers which were submitted solely for publication in the proceedings. This procedure allows considerable savings in publication cost.

Contents

D. ABNORMALITIES OF THE MEMBRANE SKELETON

E. INTEGRAL MEMBRANE PROTEINS: TRANSPORT PROTEINS

Preface

The ICN-UCLA Conferences are a continuing series of medium-sized, interdisciplinary annual meetings devoted to topics of interest to biochemists, molecular and cellular biologists, and physicians involved in research. The major purpose of the present meeting was to bring together physicians and basic scientists interested in various aspects of the red cell membrane. A great deal has been learned about membrane structure in the past decade and particularly about the structure of the normal red cell membrane, but little of this knowledge has been applied to the analysis of pathologic red cells. Hopefully, the interactions fostered by this conference will stimulate this analysis.

The conference focused on three major subdivisions of the red cell membrane: the lipid bilayer, the peripheral membrane proteins (particularly the spectrin-actin membrane skeleton), and the integral membrane glycolipoproteins. Approximately equal time was given to discussion of normal and pathologic red cell membranes. The present volume includes papers from all of the plenary session speakers and selected contributions from the many poster session presentations. We believe they provide a good illustration of our current understanding of the red cell membrane.

The organizers acknowledge the generosity of the National Heart, Lung and Blood Institute of the National Institutes of Health whose contribution supported part of the expenses of many of the symposium participants. In addition, ICN Pharmaceuticals, Inc., contributed generously as usual to the general support of the conference series. Our special thanks go to Fran Stusser and Donna Vratari of the ICN-UCLA Symposia staff, whose prodding, patience and organizational discipline made this conference possible; to Loretta Harris for her invaluable secretarial skills; and to Kathryn John for her assistance in reporting the conference proceedings.

Samuel E. Lux
Vincent T. Marchesi

Journal of Supramolecular Structure 8:191–213 (1978)
Normal and Abnormal Red Cell Membranes 1–23

Topology of Amino-Phospholipids in the Red Cell Membrane

Guido V. Marinetti and Richard C. Crain

Department of Biochemistry, University of Rochester Medical Center, Rochester, New York 14642

The red cell membrane has an asymmetric arrangement of phospholipids. The amino-phospholipids are localized primarily on the inner surface of the membrane and the choline phospholipids are localized to a large extent on the outer surface of the membrane. Evidence is presented based on the use of covalent chemical probes in sequence that the red cell membrane contains heterogeneous domains of PE and PS and that the transport systems for Pi and K^+ are asymmetrically arranged. Certain amino groups of PE, PS, and/or protein localized on the outer membrane surface are involved in Pi transport and certain amino groups of PE, PS, and/or protein localized on the inner surface of the membrane are involved in K^+ transport.

Cross-linking studies with DFDNB show that the cross-linked PE-PE molecules are rich in plasmalogens. This suggests that clusters of plasmalogen forms of PE occur in the membrane. Both PE and PS are cross-linked to membrane protein. These PE and PS molecules contain 24–28% 16:0 and 18:0 fatty acids and 12% fatty aldehydes. PE and PS molecules are cross-linked to a spectrin-rich fraction. It is proposed that the binding of spectrin to membrane PE and PS may help anchor spectrin to the inner surface of the membrane and regulate shape changes in the cell.

K^+-valinomycin forms a complex with TNBS and converts it from a nonpenetrating probe to a penetrating probe. Valinomycin enhances K^+ leak and Pi leak in the red cells. SITS inhibits completely the valinomycin-induced Pi leak and inhibits partially the valinomycin induced K^+ leak. Valinomycin and IAA have additive effects on Pi leak. Ouabin has no effect on basal or valinomycin-induced Pi leak. These data suggest that Pi leak and K^+ leak occur by separate transport systems.

In summary, the amino-phospholipids in the red cell membrane are asymmetrically arranged; some occur in clusters and some are closely associated with membrane proteins. Amino-phospholipids also are believed to bind spectrin to the inner surface of the membrane and also may play a role in cation and anion leak.

Key words: **amino-phospholipids, chemical probes, red cell membrane, valinomycin, ion transport, membrane topology**

Abbreviations: TNBS, 2,4,6-trinitrobenzenesulfonic acid; FDNB, 1-fluoro-2.4-dinitrobenzene; MA, methylacetimidate; PE, phosphatidylethanolamine; PS, phosphatidylserine; DFDNB, 1,5-difluoro-2.4-dinitrobenzene; Pi, inorganic phosphate; TLC, thin layer chromatography; IAA, iodoacetate; BHT, butylated hydroxytoluene; DMA, dimethylacetal; DEGS, diethyleneglycolsuccinate; SITS, 4-acetamido-4′-isothiocyanostilbene-2,2′-disulfonic acid.

Received for publication March 5, 1978; accepted April 25, 1978.

Phospholipids are integral components of cell membranes, where it is generally agreed they are arranged in large part as a bilayer [1, 2]. The more detailed arrangement of phospholipids in cell membranes, such as asymmetry, clusters, and association with specific membrane proteins are relatively new ideas that are being explored. In previous studies evidence was provided for the asymmetric arrangement of amino-phospholipids in the red cell membrane using nonpenetrating chemical probes [3–7]. This work was supported by others using phospholipases [8] or phospholipid exchange proteins [9, 10]. We also provided data, using cross-linking probes, which indicated that PE and PS occurred as nonrandom clusters in the red cell membrane [11, 12]. Occurrence of lipid clusters in artificial membranes recently has been reported [13, 14].

In this paper we consider in more detail the topology of PE and PS in the red cell membrane. In particular it was our aim to examine the molecular species of PE which are localized on the outer surface of the membrane and compare it with the PE molecules localized on the inner surface. We also examined the molecular species of those PE molecules which are cross-linked to themselves by DFDNB and those PE and/or PS molecules which are cross-linked to membrane proteins.

We have found that valinomycin forms a complex with TNBS in the presence of K^+, Rb^+, or Cs^+ and that the complex permeates the red cell membrane, thereby converting TNBS from a nonpenetrating probe to a penetrating probe [15]. This allows one to use the same probe to examine the amino-phospholipids on both the outer and inner membrane surface and avoids comparison of data of whole cells to ghosts.

The effect of chemical probes and valinomycin on the labeling of PE and PS is compared to the effect of these probes on anion and cation leak in the red cell. Evidence is presented for an asymmetric arrangement of these transport systems in the red cell. This was established by the sequential use of penetrating and nonpenetrating probes. Evidence is also presented for different domains of PE and PS in the red cell membrane.

MATERIALS AND METHODS

Human red cells were obtained from the Red Cross Blood Bank and stored at 4°C until used. Cells were used within 1–2 weeks. The extraction of lipids and the TLC analysis of the dinitrophenyl, trinitrophenyl derivatives, and amidine derivatives of PE and PS were carried out as described previously [5, 6, 7, 11, 16]. Inorganic phosphate was measured as previously reported [6]. K^+ and Na^+ were measured by flame photometry using an Instruments Lab, Inc. Model 143 flame photometer. Cell counting was performed by means of a haemocytometer. Hematocrits were done on a MSE Microhaemocrit reader. Protein was assayed by the Lowry procedure [17].

Cross-Linking of Red Cell Lipids and Proteins at 0°C and 37°C With DFDNB

Human red cells were centrifuged for 10 min at 2,000 rpm and the plasma and buffy coat removed. The packed cells were washed twice with isotonic saline. Into each of nine tubes was pipetted 1 ml packed cells. Ghosts were prepared by a modification of the method of Dodge, Mitchell, and Hanahan [18] by lysis of cells at 21°C in 20 volumes of 10 mM Tris buffer (pH 7.4) containing 1 mM EDTA. The ghosts were spun down at 40,000g for 15 min and washed twice with lysing buffer. The ghosts were divided into three sets of three tubes. The first set was incubated at 37°C for 4 h in 20 ml 120 mM NaC1–40 mM $NaHCO_3$ buffer (pH 8.5) containing 100 μM DFDNB. The second set was incubated at 0°C for 16 h with the same buffer containing 100 μM DFDNB. The third set was incubated 16 h at 0°C in buffer not containing DFDNB. The reaction was stopped by centrifugation for 15 min at 40,000g. The ghosts were washed with isotonic saline. The lipids were extracted with chloroform-methanol containing 0.01% BHT by the method of Folch et al [19] and dried under nitrogen. The lipids were analyzed by TLC. The plates (Merck-Darmstadt silica gel 60, 0.25 mm) were developed in chloroform:methanol: acetic acid:water (65:25:2:4). FDNP-PE and PE-DNP-PE were scraped from the plates from DFDNB-treated red cells. PE was scraped from the plates from control cells. The PE bands were treated for 1 h at 80°C in 3 ml anhydrous methanol containing 1% conc. HCl. The samples were cooled and 3 ml of water were added, followed by 6 ml hexane containing 0.01% in BHT. The hexane layers were removed and washed with 0.1% Na_2CO_3. The washed hexane layers were dried with anhydrous Na_4SO_4. The resulting extracts containing fatty acid methyl esters and dimethylacetals of fatty aldehydes were stored under nitrogen until read for analysis.

The analysis of the fatty acid methyl esters and dimethylacetals of fatty aldehydes was carried out on a Hewlett-Packard 5830A gas chromatograph equipped with a 18850 computer terminal. A 10% DEGS on an acid-washed, dimethylchlorosilane-treated chromosorb W column (6 ft, glass, 2 mm ID) was used at 190°C. The flow rate of helium was 30 ml/min.

Reaction of Red Cells With TNBS

Human red blood cells were washed three times with isotonic NaCl. In each of three tubes were added 1.5 ml packed cells. The cells were reacted with 2 mM TNBS in 60 ml 40 mM $NaHCO_3$–120 mM NaCl buffer (pH 8.5) for 1 h. The cells were centrifuged and washed once with saline; ghosts were prepared and lipids extracted as described previously. The lipid extracts were dried under nitrogen, applied to TLC plates, and developed in chloroform:methanol:acetic acid:water (65:25:2:4). Unreacted PE (visualized by spraying with 5% rhodamine 6G in methanol) and TNP-PE were scraped and reacted with methanol-HC1 as described above.

Spectrin Preparation From Control and FDNB- and DFDNB-Treated Red Cells

Packed red cells (10 ml) were reacted with 0.5 mM FDNB or DFDNB in 190 ml of 120 mM NaC1–40 mM $NaHCO_3$ (pH 8.5) for 0.5 h at 23°C. Control cells were incubated in buffer alone. The cells were washed with the same buffer and lysed in 20 volumes of first 30mM $NaHCO_3$, then 15 mM $NaHCO_3$ pH 7.4. The spectrin plus soluble proteins were obtained by dialysis over night at 4°C against 0.2 mM EDTA (pH 7.4) [20]. The contents of the dialysis bags were centrifuged at 30,000 rpm for 30 min at 5°C. The supernatants contain the total soluble ghost proteins. Spectrin was isolated by precipitation at pH 5.3. Aliquots of the protein fraction were assayed for total protein and analyzed by SDS gel electrophoresis as described previously [21]. Aliquots also were reacted with antispectrin antibody. Antiserum to spectrin was supplied by Dr F. H. Kirkpatrick, University of Rochester (New York). Rabbit antiserum was prepared by subcutaneous injection of electrophoretically pure spectrin in Freund's adjuvant. The spectrin (bands 1 and 2) was purified by preparative SDS gel electrophoresis in an apparatus described by Ryan et al [22]. The antiserum had a single precipitin line by Orchterlony double diffusion. Cross-immunoelectrophoresis indicated that the antiserum was directed mainly against band 1 and had a lesser reaction against band 2.

RESULTS

The asymmetric arrangement of PE and PS in a variety of cell membranes as determined in different laboratories by chemical probes, phospholipases, or phospholipid exchange proteins is summarized in Table I. Several membranes have an asymmetric arrangement of PE and PS. In most cases these amino-phospholipids face the interior of the cell. There are some discrepancies in the findings from different laboratories indicating that the type of probe or experimental conditions used may lead to different results.

In the present work it was our aim to explore the topology of amino-phospholipids in the erythrocyte membrane in greater detail. In order to see whether the small number of PE molecules (5–10% of the total PE) on the outer surface of the red cell were different from those on the inner surface, the fatty acids and aldehydes of the TNP-PE and of the unreacted PE were analyzed. Since TNBS is not permeable under our conditions, the TNP-PE molecules are localized on the outer surface, whereas the unreacted PE molecules (these PE molecules in part are buried within the membrane) are localized on the inner surface of the membrane. The results in Table II show that the fatty acid and fatty aldehyde patterns are very similar. Therefore there appears to be no significant difference in the molecular species of the small number of PE molecules which are localized on the outer membrane surface compared to the bulk of the PE molecules localized on the inner membrane surface or buried within the membrane.

We next wished to see if the PE molecules which are cross-linked to themselves by DFDNB differed from the PE molecules which were not cross-linked. We also compared

TABLE I. Asymmetry of Amino-Phospholipids in Cell Membranes

	% on outer surface	
Membrane	PE	PS
Red cell[a]	2–20	0–2
Inner mitochondria[a]	30–70	–
Retinal rod disk[f]	60	25
Yeast[a]	20	0
E coli[a]	20	–
Platelet[b]	10–20	0–2
Endoplasmic ret.	90[c](50)[e]	85[c](50)[e]
Golgi	90[c](50)[e]	85[c](50)[e]
Lysosomal[c]	80	–
Nuclear membrane[c]	90	83
Inner mitochondria[c]	90	–
Influenza virus[d]	50	3
PM2 bacteriophage[d]	∿20	–
B megaterium[d]	31–35	–

[a] Data from References 5, 7, 25, 28 using chemical probes and References 8, 9, 24 using protein probes.

[b] Data from References 26, 27.

[c] Data from Reference 29.

[d] Data from References 37, 41.

[e] Data from Reference 40.

[f] Crain and Marinetti, unpublished data.

TABLE II. Fatty Acid and Fatty Aldehyde Composition of PE on the External and Internal Surfaces of the Red Cell Membrane*

	External surface	Internal surface
	TNP-PE	Unreacted PE
16:0 DMA	15 ± 4	10 ± 3
16:0	11 ± 3	13 ± 3
18:0 DMA	7 ± 1	12 ± 2
18:0	6 ± 1	8 ± 1
18:1 DMA	2 ± 0.3	4 ± 1
18:1	13 ± 1	12 ± 2
18:2	4 ± 1	3 ± 0.4
20:4	23 ± 4	18 ± 4
22:4	8 ± 1	7 ± 1
22:6	6 ± 1	4 ± 1
% Saturated fatty acids (16:0 + 18:0)	17 ± 3	21 ± 3
% Fatty aldehydes (16:0, 18:0, 18:1)	24 ± 4	26 ± 4
% Total saturation[a]	39 ± 5	43 ± 5

* Values (mean ± SD) represent the area percentage of each fatty acid or fatty aldehyde relative to the total area of all the peaks obtained by gas chromatography. Details are given in the text.

[a] Percentage total saturation is the percentage of 16:0 + 18:0 fatty acids plus 16:0 + 18:0 fatty aldehydes. DMA indicates the dimethylacetal derivatives of the respective fatty aldehydes.

the fatty acid and fatty aldehydes of the PE molecules cross-linked to themselves with the PE and PS molecules which are cross-linked to membrane protein. The results in Table III show that the 30% of total PE molecules which become cross-linked to themselves have a much higher content of fatty aldehydes, a higher total saturation, and a lower content of 16:0 and 18:0 fatty acids than the non-cross-linked FDNP-PE or the total PE. This indicates that the plasmalogen PE molecules exist as clusters, and in particular, the clusters are favored at 37° compared to 0°C.

It is also noteworthy that with increasing temperature, the amino-phospholipids (PE + PS) which become cross-linked to protein contain a somewhat higher content of saturated fatty acids. Since PE contains a very high content of plasmalogen (about 50%) and PS has very little plasmalogen, we can estimate the percent of PE and PS cross-linked to protein. These calculations show that 30–50% of the cross-linked phospholipids is PE. This varies with different batches of red cells.

Use of Chemical Probes in Sequence – Evidence for Heterogeneous Domains of PE and PS in the Membrane

Red cells were reacted with TNBS and MA singly and in sequence. The results in Table IV show that under these conditions of excess probe used singly and where available sites are saturated, only 10.7% of the total PE reacts with TNBS compared to the 84% which reacts with MA. More significant, however, is the observation that about 1% of the PE molecules are accessible to TNBS but not to MA. Therefore about 10% of the

TABLE III. Nature of Fatty Acids and Aldehydes of Cross-Linked PE to PE and of Amino-Phospholipids Cross-Linked to Proteins in the Red Cell Membrane*

	PE Cross-linked to PE[b]		FDNP-PE		Phospholipid Cross-linked to Protein[a]		Control PE	Control PS
	0°C	37°C	0°C	37°C	0°C	37°C		
% Saturated fatty acids (16:0 + 18:0)	6	8	18	19	24	28	21–24	48
% Fatty aldehydes (16:0, 18:0, 18:1)	52	64	28	32	12	12	22–26	0.4
% Total saturation[b]	49	61	41	46	34	38	39–43	48

* Values represent the area percentage of each fatty acid or fatty aldehyde relative to the total area of all the peaks obtained by gas chromatography. Details are given in the text.

[a] Cross-linked with 100 μM DFDNB for 16 h at 0°C or 4 h at 37°C. Experimental details are given in the text.

[b] Percentage total saturation is the percentage of 16:0 + 18:0 fatty acids plus 16:0 + 18:0 fatty aldehydes.

TABLE IV. Sequential Reaction of Red Cell Phosphatidylethanolamine With MA and TNBS*

Probe	TNBS	MA	MA then TNBS
Derivative	TNP-PE	MA-PE	TNP-PE
nmoles	45 ± 4.6	353 ± 24	3.8 ± 1.4
% reaction	10.7	84	0.9

* Packed cells (0.5 ml) were reacted once with 2 mM TNBS for 1 h, or twice with 20 mM MA for 0.5 h each time, or twice with 20 mM MA for 0.5 h followed by reaction with 2 mM TNBS for 1 h. The cells were reacted in 20 ml of 40 mM $NaHCO_3$ – 120 mM NaCl buffer (pH 8.5) at 22°C. The cells were washed and lysed, ghosts were prepared, and the lipids were extracted with chloroform-methanol and analyzed by TLC as described in the text. Values represent the mean ± SD of six analyses. The total PE in 0.5 ml of packed cells is 419 ± 8 nmoles.

PE molecules available to react with TNBS are not available to MA. These are believed to represent PE molecules in a more hydrophobic domain which are reached by the hydrophobic TNBS but not by the hydrophilic probe MA. If this domain is positively charged it also would be more available to TNBS, which is anionic, rather than to MA, which is cationic.

Similar studies were done with MA and FDNB. As seen in Tables V and VI, a significant number of PE and PS molecules are available to react with FDNB but not with MA. These findings also suggest heterogeneous domains of PE and PS in the membrane.

The significance of the above results using probes in sequence is apparent when one examines the effect of these probes on anion and cation leak in the red cell. These results are given in Table VI and Figures 1–3. MA has no effect on Pi leak in intact red cells under these experimental conditions. However, FDNB and TNBS markedly inhibit Pi leak. Moreover, pretreatment of cells with MA only very slightly prevents the FDNB effect on Pi leak and only moderately prevents the TNBS effect on Pi leak. Therefore, a certain population of PE or PS molecules may be involved in anion leak and these PE or PS molecules are accessible to FDNB and TNBS but not accessible to MA. Since TNBS

TABLE V. Sequential Reaction of Amino-Phospholipids of the Red Cell Membrane With FDNB and MA

Probe	FDNB[a]	MA[b]	MA then FDNB[c]
Derivative	DNP-PE	MA-PE	DNP-PE
nmoles	166 ± 3	435 ± 9	10 ± 1
% reaction	37	98	2
Derivative	DNP-PS	MA-PS	DNP-PS
nmoles	37 ± 1	85 ± 8	30 ± 1
% reaction	14	31	11

[a] Packed red cells (0.5 ml) were suspended in a total volume of 20 ml of buffer containing 120 mM NaCl–40 mM $NaHCO_3$ (pH 8.5) at 22°C and reacted with 2 mM FDNB for 1 h. Ghosts were prepared and the lipids extracted and analyzed by TLC as given in the text. Values are the mean ± SD of four analyses.

[b] The cells were reacted twice for 0.5 h with 20 mM MA under conditions described above.

[c] The cells were first reacted twice with 20 mM MA, washed, then reacted with 2 mM FDNB as described above.

TABLE VI. Sequential Reaction of Amino-Phospholipids of the Red Cell Membrane With FDNB and MA – Correlation With Pi and K+ Leak*

	Control	FDNB	MA then FDNB	TNBS	MA then TNBS	MA
			Labeling of PE and PS (nmoles)			
XNP-PE	–	307	120	28	6	–
XNP-PS	–	56	32	0	0	–
			Effect on Pi and K+ leak (nmoles/liter/10^{10} cells/h)			
Pi Leak	360	1	48	6	125	341
K+ Leak	1,170	7,000	7,660	1,350	890	1,120

* Packed cells (25 ml) were suspended in 170 ml of 120 mM NaCl–40 mM $NaHCO_3$ buffer (pH 8.5) and reacted twice with 20 mM MA at 23°C for 0.5 h. Control cells were incubated in buffer alone. Aliquots (7 ml) of cells were taken from each and these were incubated with 2 mM TNBS, 2 mM FDNB, or buffer alone at 23°C for 1 h. From each of these samples, 1-ml aliquots were removed, ghosts were prepared, and the lipids were analyzed by TLC. The remaining cells were centrifuged, suspended in the same buffer at pH 7.4, and incubated for 15, 30, and 60 min at 37°C. The cells were centrifuged and the supernatants analyzed for Pi and K+ as given in the text. XNP-PE or XNP-PS designates the DNP or TNP derivative of PE or PS.

does not penetrate the cell membrane and it inhibits Pi leak nearly as much as does FDNB, it is apparent that these amino groups which are involved in Pi leak are localized on the outer membrane surface.

When the effect of these probes on K^+ leak is examined, the observations are analogous but in the opposite direction to those seen with Pi leak. As seen in Table VI and in Figure 2, MA has no effect on K^+ leak but FDNB markedly enhances K^+ leak. However, pretreatment of cells with MA has no effect on the FDNB-enhanced K^+ leak. Therefore the PE molecules which react with FDNB after cells are pretreated with MA may be involved with K^+ leak. Amino groups on certain proteins may also be involved.

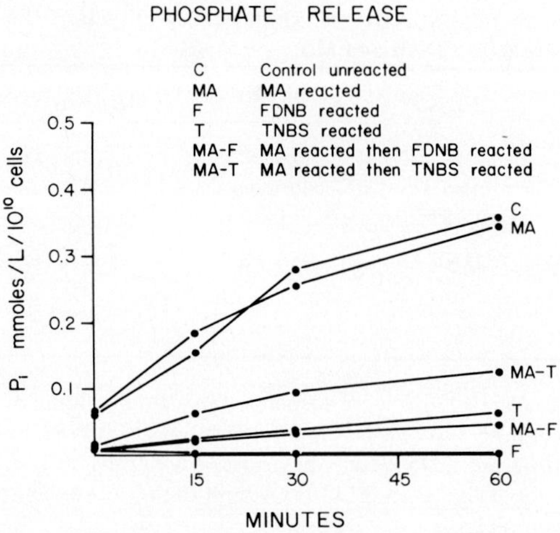

Fig 1. Effect of MA, FDNB, and TNBS alone and in combination on Pi leak in red cells. MA reaction: Packed cells (25 ml) were suspended in 170 ml of 120 mM NaCl–40 mM $NaHCO_3$ buffer (pH 8.5) containing 20 mM MA. The cells were reacted for 0.5 h at 23°C, spun down, and resuspended in fresh buffer containing 20 mM MA and reacted for another 0.5 h at 23°C. TNBS or FDNB reaction: packed cells (25 ml) were suspended in 170 ml of buffer containing either 2 mM TNBS or 2 mM FDNB and reacted for 1 h at 23°C. Sequential reaction of cells was done by first reacting cells with MA and then with either TNBS or FDNB as described above. Control cells were also used. These cells were incubated in buffer without probes for 2 h at 23°C. All cells were washed with buffer then 1-ml aliquots of packed cells were suspended in 120 mM NaCl–40 mM $NaHCO_3$ buffer (pH 7.4) and incubated for various times. The cells were spun down and aliquots were used for analysis of Pi or K^+ as given in the text. C) control cells; MA) cells reacted with MA; T) cells reacted with TNBS; F) cells reacted with FDNB; MA-T) cells reacted first with MA then with TNBS; MA-F) cells reacted first with MA then with FDNB.

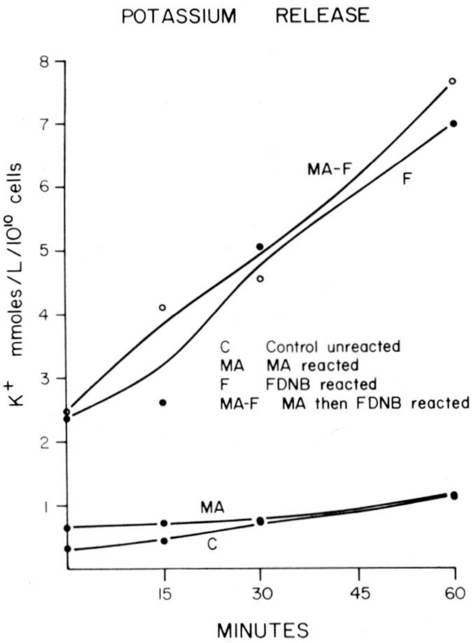

Fig 2. Effect of MA and FDNB alone and in combination on K^+ leak in red cells. Experimental conditions are given in Figure 1. Aliquots of the supernatants of control and treated cells were analyzed for K^+ as given in text. The symbols MA, F, C, and MA-F are explained in Figure 1.

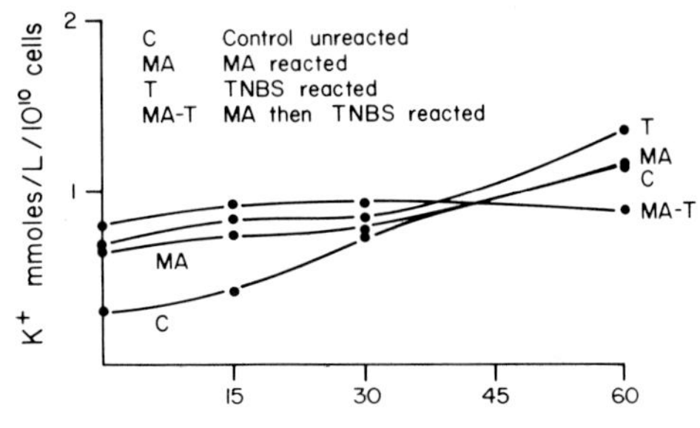

Fig 3. Effect of MA and TNBS alone and in combination on K^+ leak in red cells. Experimental conditions are given in Figure 1. Aliquots of the supernatants from control and treated cells were analyzed for K^+ as given in text. The symbols C, T, MA, and MA-T are explained in Figure 1.

As seen in Figure 3, TNBS has no significant effect on K^+ leak. Since TNBS is a nonpenetrating probe and FDNB is a penetrating probe, we conclude that a certain small population of amino groups* on either phospholipids or proteins located on the inner surface of the cell membrane play an important role in K^+ leak.

Effect of Valinomycin on the Labeling of PE and PS of the Red Cell Membrane by TNBS and FDNB

We have found recently that K^+-valinomycin forms a complex with trinitrophenol (picric acid) and that K^+-valinomycin converts TNBS from a nonpenetrating to a penetrating probe [15]. Valinomycin has no effect without K^+. We have carried out these studies in greater detail. As seen in Table VII, valinomycin in the presence of K^+ increases the extent of labeling of PE in intact red cells from 9% to 52% but has no effect on the labeling of PE by FDNB. K^+ valinomycin also enhances the labeling of PS from 0% to

TABLE VII. Effect of Valinomycin on the Labeling of PE and PS in Intact Red Cells by TNBS and FDNB*

	TNBS	TNBS + valinomycin	FDNB	FDNB + valinomycin
XNP-PE (nmoles)	34 ± 1	192 ± 35	184 ± 53	172 ± 37
% reaction	9.1	52	51	47
XNP-PS (nmoles)	0	20 ± 1	38 ± 20	43 ± 17
% reaction	0	11	18	19

* Packed red cells (0.5 ml) were reacted for 2 h in 20 ml of 120 mM NaCl–40 mM $NaHCO_3$ buffer (pH 8.5) at 23°C with 2 mM TNBS or 2 mM FDNB with and without 2 μM valinomycin. The cells were washed, ghosts prepared, and the lipids extracted and analyzed by TLC as explained in the text. XNP-PE and XNP-PS designate the DNP or TNP derivatives of PE and PS. The total PE in 0.5 ml of packed cells was 385 ± 75 nmoles and the total PS was 241 ± 47 nmoles. The percentage reaction is the percentage of total PE or PS which reacts with each probe. Values are the mean ± SD of these experiments from three different batches of red cells analyzed in duplicate.

*Since FDNB is not specific for amino groups, these may in part represent SH, imidazole, and tyrosine OH groups.

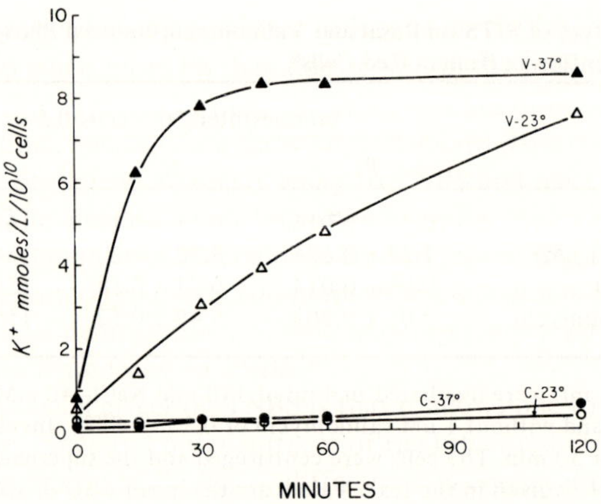

Fig 6. Effect of temperature on the basal and valinomycin-enhanced leak of K^+ on the red cell. The same cells given in Figure 4 were used for K^+ determinations of the supernatants after incubation. V) valinomycin; C) control.

TABLE IX. Effect of Valinomycin, Ouabain, and Iodoacetate on Pi Leak in Human Erythrocytes

	mmoles Pi/liter/10^{10} cells/h
Control	0.99 ± 0.03
+ Valinomycin	1.25 ± 0.03
+ IAA	1.12 ± 0.02
+ Ouabain	0.99 ± 0.07
+ Valinomycin and IAA	1.33 ± 0.05
+ Valinomycin and ouabain	1.28 ± 0.04
+ IAA and ouabain	1.17 ± 0.05

Packed red cells (1 ml) were incubated in 4 ml of 140 mM NaCl–40 mM $NaHCO_3$ buffer (pH 7.4) with and without 1 μM valinomycin or 1 μM SITS, 1 μM ouabain or 1 mM iodoacetate (IAA) for 1 h at 37°C. The cells were centrifuged and the supernatants analyzed for Pi as given in the text. Values are the mean ± SD of six analyses from two experiments done in triplicate.

valinomycin or IAA. Therefore, valinomycin and IAA exert independent effects on Pi leak and the leak is not related to the ouabain sensitive ATPase. Studies on the effect of ouabain on K^+ leak showed no significant effect of this agent, indicating that the valinomycin-induced K^+ leak is not mediated by its action on the ouabain-sensitive ATPase.

Effects of pH on the Labeling of PE and PS in Intact Cells by TNBS and FDNB

The effects of pH on the labeling of PE and PS by TNBS and FDNB are shown in Figure 7. The labeling of PE by FDNB reaches a plateau between pH 7.5 and 8.5 but above 8.5 there is a sharp increase in the labeling of PE. The labeling of PS by FDNB is nearly constant over the pH range 6–8.5 but undergoes a sharp rise at pH 9.0. Therefore some alteration has occurred at pH 9.0 which exposes PE and PS amino groups. This

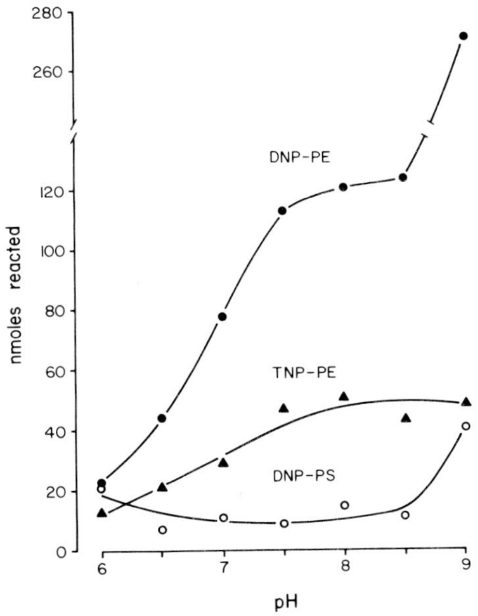

Fig 7. Effect of pH on the labeling of PE and PS in the red cell by TNBS and FDNB. Packed cells (1 ml) were suspended in 20 ml of Krebs-Ringer bicarbonate buffer adjusted to different pH values from 6 to 9. The cells were reacted for 0.5 h at 23°C with either 2 mM FDNB or 2 mM TNBS. The cells were washed, ghosts were prepared, and lipids were extracted and analyzed by TLC as given in text.

occurs under conditions where cell lysis is negligible. However, with TNBS the results are very different, since the labeling of PE reaches a plateau at pH 8.0 and does not increase at pH 9.0. Moreover, little or no PS is labeled with TNBS at all pH values. Therefore the pH effect in making more PE and PS molecules accessible to FDNB occurs on the inner surface of the cell membrane. We suggest that this is due to an unmasking of PE and PS molecules which are tightly bound to protein. A protein likely involved in masking these PE and PS molecules is believed to be spectrin. The next experiments suggest that spectrin may be tightly associated with amino-phospholipids on the inner surface of the membrane.

Cross-Linking of Amino-Phospholipids to Membrane Proteins

In order to determine whether membrane proteins, and in particular, spectrin, is closely associated with PE and PS molecules on the inner surface of the membrane, red cells were treated with DFDNB, and the spectrin fraction was isolated and analyzed for convalently bound phosphate and compared to the control spectrin fraction and the spectrin fraction isolated from cells treated with FDNB. First, as seen in Table X, DFDNB treatment led to a loss of total soluble protein obtained from ghosts. This was reflected by a loss in extractable spectrin, which decreased from 20–22% to 8% of the total ghost protein. As seen in Figure 8, the spectrin fraction obtained from control and FDNB-treated cells has less Pi than the spectrin fraction obtained from DFDNB treated cells. DFDNB treatment leads to a cross-linking of approximately a net of 75 nmoles of Pi per milligram protein. This represents about 38 molecules of Pi cross-linked to each molecule

TABLE X. Effect of FDNB and DFDNB on the Extraction of Soluble Proteins and the Spectrin Fraction From the Red Cell Membrane*

	Percentage of ghost protein	
	Total soluble proteins	Spectrin fraction
Control	29 ± 3.6	20 ± 8.9
FDNB treatment	28.2 ± 3.9	22 ± 5.4
DFDNB treatment	10.3 ± 4.7	8 ± 5.5

* Human red cells (10 ml packed cells) were reacted with 0.5 mM FDNB or DFDNB for 30 min at 23°C in 190 ml of 40 mM $NaHCO_3$ – 120 mM NaCl buffer (pH 8.5). Control cells were incubated for 30 min in buffer alone. The preparation of total soluble ghost protein and spectrin fraction is given in the text. Values are the mean ± SD of four experiments.

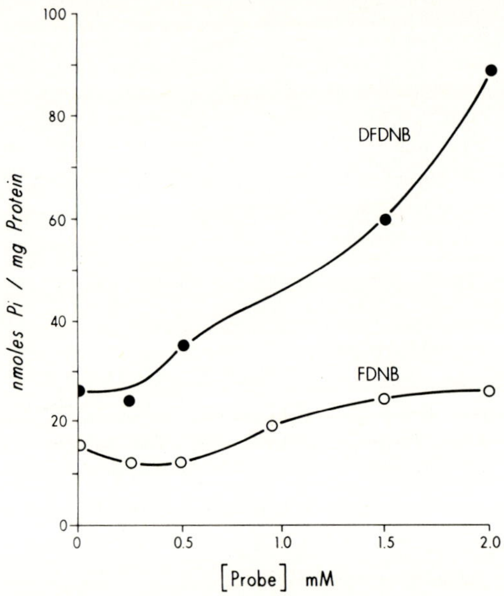

Fig 8. Cross-linking of amino-phospholipids to a spectrin fraction from red cell ghosts. Erythrocytes were reacted with 0.2–2.0 mM FDNB or DFDNB and the spectrin fraction was isolated as explained in Table X. Phosphate determinations were performed as described in text. Each point is the average of duplicate analyses and represents phosphate not extractable with chloroform-methanol.

of spectrin, since 1 mg of spectrin represents about 2 nmoles of spectrin. SDS gel electrophoresis showed that the spectrin from control cells and from FDNB-treated cells gave the identical typical doublet band (bands 1 and 2). The spectrin fraction from DFDNB-treated cells, however, showed most was cross-linked to form high-molecular-weight aggregates which did not enter the gel. It is noteworthy that this cross-linked spectrin was extracted from ghosts and was precipitated at pH 5.1 just like normal spectrin. The spectrin samples from normal and from FDNB- and DFDNB-treated cells did react with purified spectrin antibody. This test showed that the cross-linked proteins, which were obtained by DFDNB treatment and which did not enter the acrylamide gel on electrophoresis, did contain spectrin. However, other proteins may also be present so that we cannot state unequivocally whether the cross-linked phospholipids are wholly or only partly cross-linked to spectrin.

DISCUSSION

It is widely accepted that phosphilipids occur in large part as a bilayer in cell membranes [1, 2]. However, the more detailed structure of the bilayer has been investigated only recently. Bretscher [3, 4] and Gordesky and Marinetti [5] suggested that the aminophospholipids are asymmetrically arranged in the red cell membrane. Bretscher used a short-time pulse-labeling experiment with formylmethionine methylphosphate and compared the labeling of PE in cells to PE in ghosts. Gordesky and Marinetti labeled both cells and ghosts with excess TNBS and FDNB under conditions of saturation of available sites. These studies indicated that at least 70–90% of the PE and nearly 100% of the PS were localized on the inner surface of the membrane. Later, using phospholipases [8] or phospholipid exchange proteins [9, 10, 24] several laboratories confirmed the observations with chemical probes and extended them to include other phospholipids such as phosphatidylcholine and sphingomyelin. These choline phospholipids were presumed to be localized to the extent of 70–80% on the outer surface of the red cell membrane. Soon after these studies, other cell lines and intracellular membranes were studied. The picture which emerged indicated that the asymmetric arrangement of phospholipids was not confined to the red cell membrane but occurred in Golgi membranes [29] and membranes from yeast cells [7], E coli [25], platelets [26, 27], mitochondria [28], microsomes [29], viruses [37], and bacteria [37]. None of these studies gave an unequivocal conclusion, since some of the PE and PS could be localized on either membrane surface and be masked by protein. These findings also raised the question of how the asymmetry is generated in the cell and how it is maintained. Recently the asymmetric arrangement of PE in the microsomal and Golgi membranes has been challenged by Sundler et al [40].

In order to determine whether the phospholipids on each membrane surface occurred in a random array or occurred as clusters, Marinetti studied nearest neighbors of PE and PS in the red cell membrane by cross-linking with DFDNB [11, 12, 30]. These studies indicated that PE and PS occurred in part as nonrandom clusters. Inasmuch as phospholipids have a very rapid lateral mobility in lipid bilayers [31], one has to resolve the difficult question whether the cross-linking pattern observed with DFDNB represents natural partners having a relatively long lifetime or whether the pattern represents cross-linking due to rapid random collision. This is an important problem with cross-linking probes such as DFDNB, which require several minutes to achieve appreciable cross-linking. With artificial bilayers, this time is presumed to be very large relative to the time of lateral mobility of the phospholipids. However, there is uncertainty whether lateral mobility of all phospholipids is rapid, especially in natural membranes where proteins can influence this mobility. Another uncertainty in the problem of nonrandom arrays of lipids in natural membranes is the effect of calcium ions, and the effect of special interactions between the multiple types of phosopholipids. Do studies on phospholipid mobility in artificial bilayers having no proteins and having a simple lipid composition have direct relevance to natural membranes?

In our previous studies on lipid clusters [12] we examined the pattern of cross-linked species of PE-PE, PE-PS, and PS-PS to random and nonrandom arrays based on the lipid composition of the membrane. This approach is a reasonable first approximation but is not definitive. We reasoned that more useful information could be obtained if we were to examine the nature of the molecular species of PE cross-linked to PE. In these studies we found that these cross-linked PE-PE molecules are rich in fatty aldehydes, especially at 37°C. Since the amino group of the diester form of PE should have the same chemical reactivity as the amino group of the plasmalogen form of PE and since these forms of PE occur in about equal amounts and should have the same intrinsic mobility in a bilayer, our observation provides clear evidence of the existence of clusters of plasmalogen PE in the red cell membrane.

The fatty acid and fatty aldehyde analysis of the amino phospholipids cross-linked to membrane protein shows a high concentration of 16:0 and 18:0 fatty acids, suggesting cross-linked PS. Appreciable amounts of fatty aldehydes were also found, indicating cross-linked PE. Therefore both PE and PS are cross-linked to membrane protein. We originally reported that about 33% of the total red cell PS and 3% of the total red cell PE were cross-linked to membrane protein. This was based on phosphate analysis. Our present studies indicate that 30–50% of the amino-phospholipids cross-linked to membrane protein is PE. The amount of PE and PS which becomes cross-linked to membrane protein varies with different samples of red cells, depending in large part on the age of the cell. Which specific proteins become cross-linked to PE and PS remains to be determined definitely. Our preliminary studies suggest that PE and PS become cross-linked to spectrin. This amounts to 38 molecules of amino-phospholipid cross-linked per molecule of spectrin. We suggest that this represents a tight association of spectrin with these PE and PS molecules and that this interaction helps to anchor spectrin to the inner surface of the membrane and may play a role in the spectrin-dependent shape changes of the cell. Our studies on the effect of pH on the labeling of PE and PS by FDNB is consistent with this concept. High pH is reported to release spectrin from the red cell membrane [32].

The molecular species of PE molecules which are localized on the outer surface of the membrane are the same as those on the inner surface. The amount of PE which is localized on the outer surface as determined by labeling with TNBS is about 1.7% at pH 7.4 and 9% at pH 8.5. In both cases, this represents saturation of available PE molecules. Therefore at the higher pH more PE molecules are exposed. Whether this represents unmasking from bound protein or flip-flop of internal PE remains to be determined. At pH 9.0, an additional number of PE and PS molecules on the inner membrane surface become exposed and available to react with FDNB. This effect, we suggest, is due in large part to unmasking of PE by dissociation from bound spectrin. It is noteworthy that the major part of PS and about 15–50% of PE in intact cells are not available to react with certain permeable chemical probes such as MA and FDNB.

The use of probes in sequence has provided new insight into the topology of the phospholipids in the red cell membrane. Reaction of cells to saturation of available sites with MA still allows a certain population of PE molecules to be accessible to TNBS and a different population of PE and PS molecules to be available to FDNB. This indicates heterogeneous domains of PE and PS which differ in hydrophobicity since the hydrophobic neutral probe such as FDNB and to a lesser extent the hydrophobic anionic probe such as TNBS are able to react with these PE molecules whereas the hydrophilic cationic probe MA cannot. Recent work by Bevers et al [33] indicates different pools of phosphatidylglycerol in the plasma membrane of acholeplasma.

Of added interest is our finding that these very small number of PE and PS molecules and/or certain amino groups on specific proteins are involved in the transport of anions (Pi) and cations (K^+). The major evidence for this is that pretreatment of cells to saturation of available sites with MA, which has no effect on Pi and K^+ leak from red cells, does not prevent FDNB or TNBS from exerting their effects on inhibiting Pi leak and enhancing K^+ leak. These results also show that the amino groups regulating Pi leak are localized on the outer surface of the cell membrane, whereas the amino groups regulating K^+ leak are localized primarily on the inner surface of the membrane. Therefore an asymmetric arrangement of anion and cation transport systems occurs in the red cell membrane and it may be related to the asymmetric arrangement of amino phospholipids and proteins. This idea was suggested earlier by Knauf and Rothstein [34], who also provided evidence for SH groups in cation transport.

Valinomycin has been employed to convert the nonpenetrating probe TNBS into a penetrating probe in intact red cells [15]. K^+, Rb^+, or Cs^+ is required for this valinomycin effect. The penetration of TNBS was monitored by the enhanced labeling of PE, PS, and hemoglobin. It is noteworthy that even under these conditions, only 11% of the total membrane PS reacts with TNBS compared to 18% with FDNB. Moreover, the level of labeling of PE by TNBS and FDNB becomes the same (51–52%). These studies are done in intact cells which show very little or no hemolysis and thus the membrane is studied in the native state with minimal perturbation. This is to be contrasted with studies using phospholipases or phospholipid exchange proteins, which must compare cells to ghosts or which can only be done on ghosts.

Alternative Models for Phospholipids in the Red Cell Membrane

The work in this paper suggests that the simple model of a lipid bilayer for cell membranes is not adequate to explain our observations. It is difficult to explain the effects of probes used in sequence on the labeling of PE and PS by the bilayer model. We therefore suggest alternative modifications of the membrane structure to account for our results. These are shown in Figures 9 and 10. In Figure 9, the phospholipids are arranged in a seagull model as suggested earlier by Deamer [42]. Only a relatively small part of the lipid membrane is postulated to have this arrangement, which may be in equilibrium with the major bilayer structure. In the seagull model, some polar head groups of the phospholipids are buried and may be accessible to certain probes and not to others, depending on their charge and hydrophobicity. In the other model, a certain fraction of the phospholipids are shown with polar head groups burried. These phospholipids are considered to be in transit during flip-flop. Again, this would represent a relatively small number of phospholipid molecules whose polar head groups would have access primarily to hydrophobic probes.

In Figure 10 are shown protein arrays in the bilayer which lead to masking of polar head groups of phospholipids or which may mask entire phospholipid molecules. These arrangements could explain why an appreciable fraction of PS molecules are refractory to several chemical probes.

Finally in Figure 11 is shown a model in which a cluster of PE and PS is tightly associated with spectrin. The PS molecules, because of their negative carboxyl groups, can be bound to spectrin via Ca^{++} bridges. This may explain why EDTA is required to

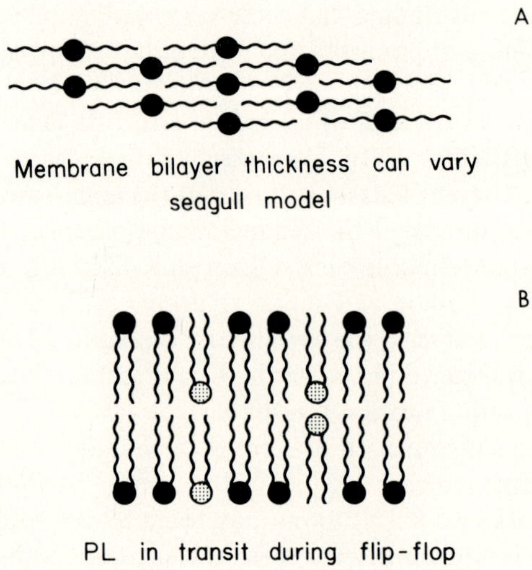

Fig 9. Provisional models of phospholipid arrangements in the red cell membrane. A) Model fashioned after Deamer [42]. We call this the seagull model. The fatty acid chains of the phospholipids run parallel to the plane of the membrane. This model is proposed to account for a small fraction of the phospholipid arrangement in the cell membrane. It may explain the variation in membrane thickness seen on electron micrographs of cell membranes and it shows that certain polar head groups of phospholipids can be buried. B) This model is the typical lipid bilayer and shows certain phospholipid molecules inverted. These represent phospholipid molecules in transit during flip-flop. The symbols or represent phospholipid molecules.

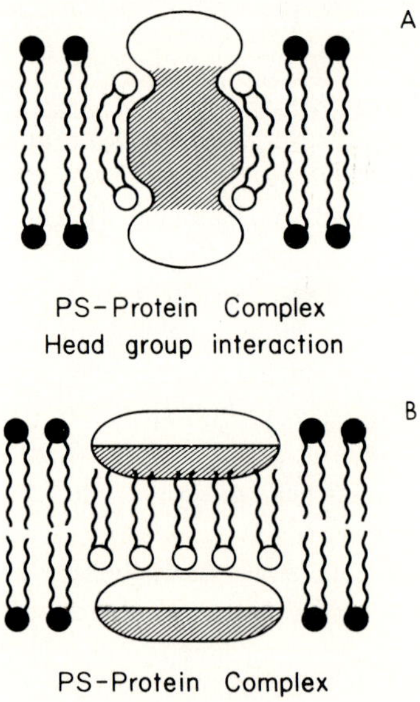

Fig 10. Provisional models of protein-phospholipid interactions in the red cell membrane. A) certain polar head groups of phospholipids (such as PS) interacting with membrane proteins, leading to a masking of these polar head groups. B) Array of amphipathic membrane proteins which are separated by a monolayer of phospholipid. The shaded area represents the hydrophobic part of the protein and the nonshaded area represents the polar portion of the protein which can interact with the polar head group of the phospholipids. Symbols as in Figure 9.

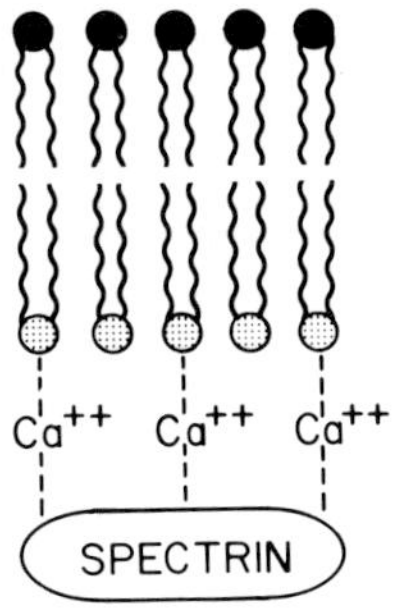

PS-Ca++-Spectrin Complex

Fig 11. Provisional model of the interaction of spectrin with phospholipids of the red cell membrane. This model is suggested to depict how spectrin may interact with clusters of PS and/or PE that are located on the inner surface of the cell membrane. The Ca^{++} bridges are presumed to occur between carboxyl groups of spectrin and carboxyl groups of PS. Symbols as in Figure 9.

release spectrin from the red cell membrane. This model and the one in Figure 10 offer possible roles for phospholipid clusters in cell membranes.

Origin of Phospholipid Asymmetry in Cell Membranes

With very small liposomes made up of two or more phospholipid types, steric and charge factors can lead to asymmetric bilayers. This is not likely to be important with cell membranes except at certain loci where the membrane may have sharp bends and where the radius of curvature can influence packing of specific phospholipids. It is likely that binding to specific membrane proteins may play an important role in maintaining membrane asymmetry. In the case of the red cell we suggest that interaction of PE and PS with spectrin plays a major role in producing and maintaining the asymmetry of PE and PS in the membrane. Base exchange reactions or specific proteins which cause phospholipid translocation may play a role in modifying membrane asymmetry. For example, if the enzyme-catalyzed base exchange of serine and ethanolamine for choline is favored, this can lead to an asymmetry of PE and PS on the surface of cell membranes which face the cytoplasm where these enzymes are located. A balance between phospholipase activity and resynthesis might also lead to an asymmetric membrane. For example, if a phospholipase C specific for lecithin is situated in the cytoplasm and the enzyme which adds phosphorylcholine is located on the opposite side of the membrane, this may lead to an asymmetric arrangement for lecithin, since the diglyceride may readily rotate in the membrane and be converted back to lecithin only on one surface. Lysolecithin is reported to enhance phospholipid flip-flop [35]. Therefore phospholipases which act specifically on certain phospholipids to produce lyso-phospholipids may regulate membrane asymmetry.

Biologic Signficance of Phospholipid Asymmetry and Clusters

The asymmetric arrangement of PE and PS in the red cell membrane and platelet membrane may be important for the control of intravascular clotting. This idea was suggested by several researchers and tested recently by Zwaal, Comfurius, and van Deenen [43]. Their data show that when made available to the exterior surface of inside-out ghosts or disrupted platelets, PE and PS, phospholipids which are important in blood clotting, are able to activate the conversion of prothrombin to thrombin. This is the only case known to the authors where phospholipid asymmetry has a fairly clear biologic role.

Other functions of the phospholipid asymmetry may be related to the maintenance of the membrane potential. PS may play an important role in this regard because of its carboxyl group. This may in part tend to neutralize the carboxyl group of neuraminic acid residues of glycolipids and glycoproteins which are localized on the outer surface of the red cell membrane.

Phospholipid clusters can offer highly charged domains for interaction with specific proteins (eg, anchoring spectrin to the inner surface of the membrane). Phospholipid clusters may also offer channels for transport of ions and small molecules. How this can lead to specific transport is not readily apparent. Acidic clusters of phospholipids may also play a role in binding and sequestering of basic compounds such as histamine, serotonin, or catecholamines. This may be important in the platelet and mast cells which sequester these amines. Clusters of phospholipids may also be involved in the attachment of microfilaments and microtubules to the inner surface of the plasma membrane.

The above ideas are speculative. Similar ideas have been discussed by others [35, 37]. It is hoped that they will generate new concepts of membrane structure and function and lead to new and productive experiments.

Limitations to the Use of Probes for Analysis of Membrane Topology

The following factors should be considered when using either small organic chemical probes or large protein probes.

1. The solubility of the probe in the medium – this is important with chemical probes when attempting to saturate available sites.

2. The stability of the probe in the medium – the probe can undergo hydrolysis or other chemical change which may not allow it to react fully with available sites; the probe may also be modified by enzymes in the membrane preparation.

3. The size and permeability of the probe – this presents different problems for small chemical probes and large protein probes. Small probes may readily penetrate the membrane. It may be difficult to find a chemical probe which does not penetrate the membrane. Large protein probes are likely not to penetrate the membrane; however, their large size may limit their accessibility to all sites on the outer membrane surface. Certain sites may be partially buried and be available to small chemical probes but not to large protein probes.

4. The requirement of other factors for activity of the probe – protein probes such as phospholipases require Ca^{++} ions for activity and are influenced by pH and ionic strength. Chemical probes are less likely to require Ca^{++} ions for activity but may also be influenced by pH and ionic strength. The pH and ionic composition near or on the membrane surface can change markedly from the pH and ionic composition of the bulk phase in the medium.

5. How much the probe perturbs the membrane – all probes will unavoidably perturb the membrane to varying degrees; chemical probes modify functional groups and usually attach other groups of varying size, charge, and hydrophobicity. Phospholipases may induce drastic changes in the phospholipid structure such as removing polar head groups or fatty acids. These changes can lead to rearrangement of membrane components to varying degrees. These changes may induce phospholipid flip-flop, especially when

polar head groups of the phospholipid are removed. Removal of phospholipid polar head groups also will alter the membrane potential and cause rearrangement of membrane components.

6. How stable the membrane components modified by the probes remain – we have found in E coli [25] and with mitochondria mitoplasts [28] that dinitrophenyl and trinitrophenyl derivatives of PE undergo degradation by enzymes and that the fragments such as dinitrophenyl-glycerophosphoryl-ethanolamine and dinitrophenyllysophosphatidylethanolamine can be utilized to resynthesize DNP-PE. Resynthesis may also occur with the degradation products of phospholipids (lysophosphatides, diglycerides, or phosphatidic acid) produced by the action of phospholipases.

7. Specificity of the probe – it would be desirable to have probes which act specifically on certain phospholipids in order to distinguish these from the bulk phospholipids.

8. Time of reaction of the probe – it is desirable to use probes in as short a time as possible to saturate available sites but to minimize membrane alteration; this time factor becomes much more critical in nearest-neighbor analysis in order to distinguish normal partners from random collision of rapidly moving components.

9. The charge and hydrophobicity of the probe – chemical probes can be neutral, cationic, anionic, hydrophobic, or hydrophilic. FDNB and DFDNB are neural and hydrophobic, TNBS is anionic and hydrophobic, MA is cationic and hydrophilic. Differences in charge and hydrophobicity of various regions of the membrane will influence the accessibility and reactivity of each probe to a different extent. These factors can be used to advantage to sense various domains in cell membranes. From the above discussion it is obvious that the judicious use of all the probes will be required to elucidate the fine details of membrane topology.

10. Isolation of cell membranes from disrupted cells – in this case the purity and physical state of the membrane must be determined. Are the membranes isolated entirely as closed vesicles with the same sidedness? Can lipid rearrangement occur independently of protein rearrangement? Are endogenous lipases and proteases present which are activated during cell disruption and these alter the membrane structure?

The advantages and disadvantages of protein and chemical probes has been discussed by Bergelson and Barsukov [35]. Some problems inherent in the use of phospholipases as probes for lipid asymmetry have been pointed out by Martin et al [36]. Carraway [38] and Peters and Richards [39] have discussed the use of chemical probes to study membranes. The combined use of these chemical and protein probes will in the long run provide new insights into membrane structure and function.

ADDENDUM

Combined results of our studies on the human red cell using chemical probes leads us to postulate the following percentage distribution of PE and PS in the membrane:

	Outside surface	Internal membrane matrix	Inside surface
PE	5–10	45–50	40–50
PS	0–2	78–89	11–20

The above distribution of PE and PS is obtained from data on the differential labeling of these amino-phospholipids with FDNB and with TNBS in intact cells. The PE and

PS available on the outer surface are those molecules which react readily with TNBS. The PE and PS which are located on the inner surface are those additional molecules which react with TNBS plus valinomycin or those molecules which react with FDNB minus those molecules which react with TNBS. The molecules of PE and PS which do not react with FDNB or with TNBS + valinomycin are considered primarily to be buried in the membrane matrix and closely associated with protein or possibly to exist to some extent as inverted micelles. The readily reacting molecules of PE and PS are presumed to be in a mobile bilayer. The PE and PS molecules which become cross-linked to protein by DFDNB are considered to be boundary lipids closely associated with membrane protein. Particularly noteworthy is our new finding that clusters of plasmalogen PE occur on the inner surface of the membrane. The above model offers more details than the model proposed by Singer [2].

ACKNOWLEDGMENTS

We acknowledge the work of Dr Stephen A. Kempson (now at the Mayo Foundation, Rochester, Minnesota) on spectrin.

We acknowledge the technical assistance of Ms Kathy Cattieu and Mr Paul Whitman. Dr Richard Mavis, Department of Radiation Biology and Biophysics, University of Rochester, kindly let us use his Hewlett-Packard gas chromatograph.

This work was supported by grant HLB 02063 from the National Institutes of Health.

REFERENCES

1. Stoeckenius W, Engelman DM: J Cell Biol 42:613, 1969.
2. Singer SJ: Ann Rev Biochem 43:805, 1974.
3. Bretscher MS: J Mol Biol 71:523, 1972.
4. Bretscher MS: Nature (New Biol) 236:11, 1972.
5. Gordesky SE, Marinetti GV: Biochem Biophys Res Comm 50:1027, 1973.
6. Gordesky SE, Marinetti GV, Love RJ: Memb Biol 20:111, 1975.
7. Marinetti GV, Love R: Chem Phys Lipids 16:239, 1976.
8. Verklij AJ, Zwaal RFA, Roelofsen B, Comfurius P, Kastelijn D, vanDeenen LLM: Biochim Biophys Acta 323:178, 1973.
9. Bloj B, Zilversmit DB: Biochemistry 15:1277, 1976.
10. Wirtz KWA: Biochim Biophys Acta 334:95, 1974.
11. Marinetti GV, Love R: Biochem Biophys Res Comm 61:30, 1974.
12. Marinetti GV: Biochim Biophys Acta 465:198, 1977.
13. Rey P, McConnell HM: J Am Chem Soc 99:1637, 1977.
14. Lee Y, Chan SI: Biochemistry 16:1303, 1977.
15. Marinetti GV, Skarin A, Whitman P: J Memb Biol 40:143, 1978.
16. Crain R, Marinetti GV: Chem Phys Lipids (In press).
17. Lowry OH, Rosenbrough NJ, Farr AL, Randall RJ: J Biol Chem 193:265, 1951.
18. Dodge JT, Mitchell C, Hanahan OJ: Arch Biochem Biophys 100:119, 1963.
19. Folch J, Lees M, Sloane SGH: J Biol Chem 191:833, 1951.
20. Marchesi VT, Steers E: Science 159:203, 1968.
21. Fairbanks G, Steck TL, Wallach DFH: Biochemistry 10:2606, 1971.
22. Ryan TE, Woods GM, Kirkpatrick FH, Shamoo AE: Anal Biochem 72:359, 1976.
23. Krasne S, Eisenman G, Szabo G: Science 174:412, 1971.
24. Rothman JE, Dawidowicz EA: Biochemistry 14:2810, 1975.
25. Marinetti GV, Love R: Chem Phys Lipids 18:170, 1977.
26. Chap HJ, Zwaal RFA, vanDeenan LLM: Biochim Biophys Acta 467:83, 1975.
27. Shick PK, Kurica KB, Chacko GK: J Clin Invest 57:1221, 1976.

28. Marinetti GV, Senior AE, Love R, Broadhurst CI: Chem Phys Lipid 17:353, 1976.
29. Nilsson OS, Dallner G: Biochim Biophys Acta 464:453, 1977.
30. Marinetti GV, Love R: J Memb Biol 30:213, 1976.
31. Scandella CJ, Devaux P, McConnell HM: Proc Nat Acad Sci USA 69:2056, 1976.
32. Elgsaeter A, Branton D: J Cell Biol 63:1018, 1974.
33. Bevers EM, Singal SA, OpdenKamp JAF, vanDeenen LLM: Biochemistry 16:1290, 1977.
34. Knauf PA, Rothstein A: J Gen Physiol 58:190, 1971.
35. Bergelson LD, Barsukov LI: Science 197:224, 1977.
36. Martin JK, Luthra MG, Wells MA, Watts RP, Hanahan D: J Biochem 14:5400, 1975.
37. Rothman JE, Lenard J: Science 195:743, 1977.
38. Carraway KL: Biochim Biophys Acta 415:379, 1975.
39. Peters K, Richards FM: Ann Rev Biochem 46:523, 1977.
40. Sundler R, Sarcione SL, Alberts AW, Vagelos PR: Proc Nat Acad Sci USA 74:3350, 1977.
41. Rothman JE, Kennedy EP: J Mol Biol 110:603, 1977.
42. Deamer D: Bioenergetics 1:237, 1970.
43. Zwaal RFA, Comfurius P, vanDeenen LLM: Nature 268:358, 1977.

Journal of Supramolecular Structure 8:215–221 (1978)
Normal and Abnormal Red Cell Membranes 25–31

Association of Spectrin With Its Membrane Attachment Site Restricts Lateral Mobility of Human Erythrocyte Integral Membrane Proteins

Velia Fowler and Vann Bennett

The Biological Laboratories, Harvard University, Cambridge, Massachusetts 02138 (V.F.); and Department of Molecular Biology, Wellcome Research Laboratories, Research Triangle Park, North Carolina 27709 (V.B.)

Interactions between spectrin and the inner surface of the human erythrocyte membrane have been implicated in the control of lateral mobility of the integral membrane proteins. We report here that incubation of "leaky" erythrocytes with a water-soluble proteolytic fragment containing the membrane attachment site for spectrin achieves a selective and controlled dissociation of spectrin from the membrane, and increases the rate of lateral mobility of fluorescein isothiocyanate-labeled integral membrane proteins ($>$ 70% of label in band 3 and PAS-1). Mobility of membrane proteins is measured as an increase in the percentage of uniformly fluorescent cells with time after fusion of fluorescent with nonfluorescent erythrocytes by Sendai virus. The cells are permeable to macromolecules since virus-fused erythrocytes lose most of their hemoglobin. The membrane attachment site for spectrin has been solubilized by limited proteolysis of inside-out erythrocyte vesicles and has been purified (V. Bennett, J Biol Chem 253:2292 (1978). This 72,000-dalton fragment binds to spectrin in solution, competitively inhibits association of ^{32}P-spectrin with inside-out vesicles with a K_i of 10^{-7}M, and causes rapid dissociation of ^{32}P-spectrin from vesicles. Both acid-treated 72,000-dalton fragment and the 45,000 dalton-cytoplasmic portion of band 3, which also was isolated from the proteolytic digest, have no effect on spectrin binding, release, or membrane protein mobility. The enhancement of membrane protein lateral mobility by the same polypeptide that inhibits binding of spectrin to inverted vesicles and displaces spectrin from these vesicles provides direct evidence that the interaction of spectrin with protein components in the membrane restricts the lateral mobility of integral membrane proteins in the erythrocyte.

Key words: spectrin, erythrocyte membrane, membrane attachment site, membrane protein mobility

Received for publication May 1, 1978; accepted May 15, 1978.

Address reprint requests to Vann Bennett.

0091/7419/78/0802-0215$01.70

Regulation of membrane protein mobility by transmembrane interactions with cytoplasmic structural proteins has been described for many eukaryotic cells [1, 2]. To study these phenomena at the molecular level it is desirable to have a system in which perturbations of membrane protein mobility can be directly correlated with changes in specific protein-protein associations in the membrane. Fused, hemolyzed human erythrocytes provide a convenient model system to measure membrane protein mobility [3], in which the cytoplasmic side of the membrane is readily accessible to molecular manipulation. In addition, the associations between proteins in the red cell membrane have been characterized in some detail [4, 5] (see below).

Lateral diffusion of erythrocyte integral membrane proteins is relatively restricted compared to other types of cells [3, 6]. Diffusion constants estimated for fresh cells at 37°C range from 4×10^{-11} cm^2/sec for the slowest cells to 10^{-10} cm^2/sec for the fastest [3]. The rates are highly temperature-dependent, and significantly faster in fresh than in ATP-depleted cells [3]. These characteristics suggested that various cellular processes, such as cell aging and metabolism, may regulate the lateral mobility of the membrane proteins in the erythrocyte.

Spectrin, the major peripheral membrane protein in erythrocytes, has been demonstrated by elegant morphological experiments to be associated in some manner with intramembrane particles [7–10], and receptors for colloidal iron hydroxide [11], which structures are thought to be composed of the major integral membrane proteins [9, 12–16]. A high-affinity ($K_d = 10^{-7}M$) interaction between spectrin and a protein component localized on the inner surface of the plasma membrane has been measured in studies of reassociation of pure ^{32}P-spectrin with inside-out vesicles depleted of spectrin and actin [17, 18]. A water-soluble 72,000-dalton proteolytic fragment from spectrin-depleted inverted vesicles has been purified which competitively inhibits binding of ^{32}P-spectrin to vesicles with a K_i of about $10^{-7}M$ [19], which is similar to the K_d for association of ^{32}P-spectrin with membranes. Both inhibitory activity of the fragment and spectrin-binding activity of vesicles are destroyed by either dilute acetic acid or N-ethyl maleimide [19]. The 72,000-dalton fragment comigrates with inhibitory activity on gel filtration with an effective Stokes radius of 39Å, and binds to spectrin in solution with a stoichiometry of 1 mole of fragment per mole of spectrin dimer [19]. Isoelectric focusing of the purified 72,000-dalton fragment partially resolves two peaks of protein and closely associated inhibitory activity with apparent isoelectric points of 4 and 4.4 [19]. The fragment constitutes a minimum of 2.4% of the membrane protein, which is close to the value predicted if spectrin binds in a 1:1 ratio to a 72,000-dalton protein.

It was concluded from these properties that the 72,000-dalton proteolytic fragment represents the membrane attachment site for spectrin [19]. Other polypeptides in the digest, including a 45,000-dalton fragment which has been attributed to the cytoplasmic portion of band 3 [20], do not compete for ^{32}P-spectrin binding to membranes [19]. Moreover, this fragment is released in equal amounts from vesicles prepared from untreated and α-chymotrypsin-digested erythrocytes, even though such external cleavage degrades band 3 to a 60,000-dalton fragment [19]. The 72,000-dalton fragment therefore cannot originate from band 3, and is localized exclusively on the inner surface of the membrane. Glycophorin and the other sialoglycoproteins can also be excluded as a source of this polypeptide, since the periodic acid-Schiff staining profile of vesicles is unchanged by digestion which abolishes binding of ^{32}P-spectrin and releases maximal quantities of the fragment [19].

If an interaction between spectrin and its membrane attachment site constrains the lateral distribution and mobility of the erythrocyte integral membrane proteins, then treatments which displace spectrin from the membrane should correspondingly influence membrane protein mobility. Experimental verification of modulation of diffusional rates of membrane proteins by spectrin has not been heretofore possible, because extraction of spectrin by conventional methods elutes other proteins, including actin, and causes erythrocyte ghosts to disintegrate into small vesicles [7, 13]. Furthermore, in addition to simply dissociating spectrin from the membrane, these methods also destroy proposed spectrin-actin interactions in the membrane [21–25]. We report here that incubation with the 72,000-dalton fragment achieves a selective and controlled dissociation of spectrin from membranes of inside-out vesicles and increases the rate of lateral diffusion of fluoroscein isothiocyanate-labeled integral membrane proteins in fused, hemolyzed human erythrocytes.

METHODS

Human blood stored at 4°C in acid-citrate-dextrose was used within 10 days of drawing. Intact cells were labeled with fluorescein isothiocyanate (FITC; Sigma, Lot No. 114C-5018) and fused to unlabeled cells by Sendai virus as described in Fowler and Branton [3], except that 10 mM Tris, 145 mM NaCl, pH 7.5 Tris-buffered saline (TBS) was used as the fusion buffer. The specific experimental conditions for the incubations are given in the figure legend. Aliquots were withdrawn periodically for observation and counting as described previously [3].

^{32}P-spectrin was prepared and purified as previously described [17, 18]. The 72,000-dalton and the 45,000-dalton fragments were solubilized by limited chymotrypsin digestion of spectrin-actin-depleted inside-out erythrocyte vesicles, and purified as described in Bennett [19]. Measurement of ^{32}P-spectrin reassociation with spectrin-depleted inside-out vesicles was performed as previously described [17–19].

RESULTS

Mobility of membrane proteins was measured as an increase with time in the percentage of uniformly fluorescent cells after fusion of FITC-labeled with unlabeled erythrocytes by Sendai virus [3]. The labeling of erythrocytes with FITC has been shown to be restricted to covalent linkage of the dye with integral membrane proteins (> 70% of the total label is in band 3 and PAS-1) [3]. The fused cells lose most of their hemoglobin and are therefore permeable to macromolecules. Fused erythrocytes preincubated for 2 h at 24°C with 4×10^{-6} M of the 72,000-dalton solubilized attachment site exhibit a marked increase in the rate of redistribution of labeled proteins following elevation of the temperature to 30°C as compared to fused cells incubated in buffer alone (Fig 1). Qualitatively similar results were obtained in several other experiments at the same temperature, at 24°C, or at 37°C. The enhancement of membrane protein mobility is selective, since the 45,000-dalton proteolytic fragment which has been attributed previously to the cytoplasmic portion of band 3 [20] has no effect (Fig 1). Furthermore, no change in rates of mobility is observed following exposure of the 72,000-dalton fragment to dilute acid, a treatment which also abolishes the capacity of the fragment to compete for binding of ^{32}P-spectrin [19].

The solubilized attachment site causes a rapid and complete dissociation of ^{32}P-spectrin from inside-out vesicles (Fig 2) under conditions similar to those under which this polypeptide accelerates lateral mobility of membrane proteins in fused, hemolyzed erythrocytes (Fig 1). The 45,000-dalton fragment of band 3 at equivalent concentrations

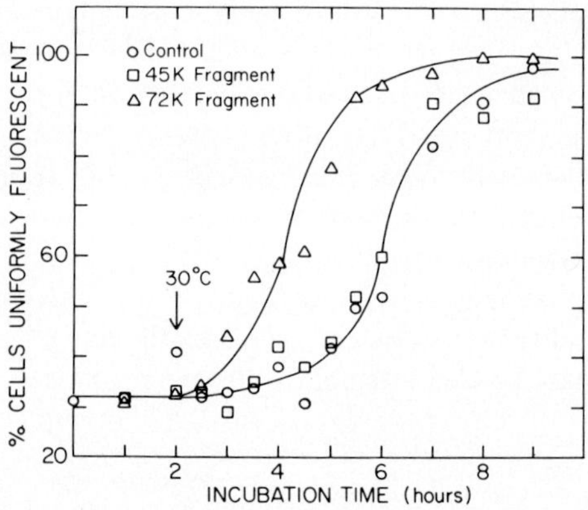

Fig 1. Redistribution of FITC-labeled integral membrane proteins of fused, hemolyzed erythrocytes incubated with 72,000-dalton fragment (△), 45,000-dalton fragment (□), or buffer alone (○), where uniformly fluorescent cells are expressed as a percentage of the total number of fused, hemolyzed cells that are at least partially fluorescent. After fusion, the fused cells were diluted directly into four volumes of TBS, or into TBS containing either the 72,000-dalton (4×10^{-6}M final concentration) or the 45,000-dalton fragment at the same final concentration. After preincubation for 2 h at 24°C, the fused cells were transferred to 30°C as indicated by the arrow.

displaces only a small portion of the reassociated spectrin (Fig 2), and this activity may be due to contamination with the 72,000-dalton fragment [19]. However, incubation of the 72,000-dalton fragment (or the 45,000-dalton fragment) with ghosts or fused cells under conditions similar to those of Figure 1 does not release spectrin or other proteins into the supernatant (as ascertained by polyacrylamide SDS gel electrophoresis; data not shown). This cannot be ascribed simply to trapping of spectrin polypeptides inside the ghosts, since brief sonication does not influence the results. A likely explanation for the difference in displacement of native and reassociated spectrin is that in ghosts additional interactions occur of spectrin with itself or with other proteins (eg, actin; see Refs 21–25) which have not been reconstituted in the binding assay. It is of interest in this regard that the rate of dissociation of spectrin from reconstitued vesicles is greatly reduced if the incubation of spectrin with vesicles is allowed to continue for 90 min before addition of fragment (not shown). It may be implied that spectrin can dissociate from its anchorage site on the membrane, and yet remain bound by secondary interactions. In this event, the initial, rapid rate of dissociation (Fig 2) reflects the true residence time of spectrin with the membrane attachment site.

Incubation of erythrocyte ghosts or fused, hemolyzed cells with the 72,000-dalton fragment under these conditions has no discernable effect on their morphology as determined by phase contrast microscopy. Furthermore, Triton X-100 residues of ghosts [25] are similarly unaffected by incubation with this fragment (not shown). It is therefore reasonable to propose that the 72,000-dalton polypeptide has no major effect on associations of spectrin with other peripheral membrane proteins, and that the increase in lateral motion of membrane proteins is indeed due to perturbation of the association of spectrin with the membrane.

DISCUSSION

The idea that lateral movements of erythrocyte integral membrane proteins are constrained by interactions with spectrin and possibly actin was suggested following

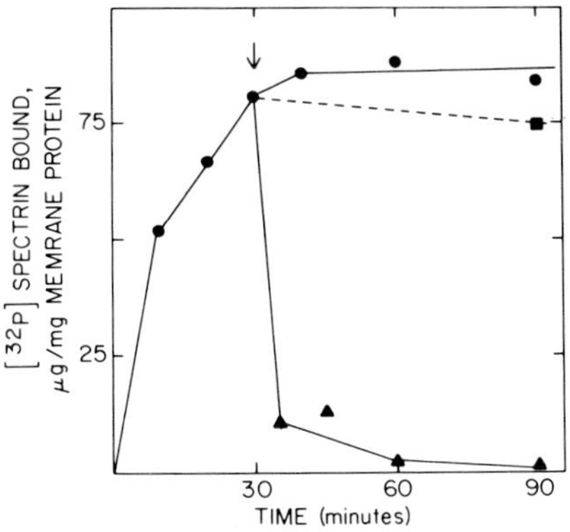

Fig 2. Time course of dissociation of ^{32}P-spectrin from inverted erythrocyte vesicles after addition of 72,000-dalton fragment (▲), 45,000-dalton fragment (■), or no additions (●). ^{32}P-spectrin (40 µg/ml, 1,400 cpm/µg) was incubated at 30°C with inside-out vesicles (100 µg/ml membrane protein) in a buffer containing sodium phosphate (2.5 mM), KCl (30 mM), $MgCl_2$ (0.6 mM), dithiothreitol (0.6 mM), and sucrose (2.4% w/v). At the time indicated by the arrow 72,000-dalton fragment and 45,000 dalton fragment were added at final concentrations of 92 and 99 µg/ml respectively. Aliquots (0.2 ml) were removed from the samples at various times and the membrane-bound ^{32}P-spectrin was determined. The values are corrected for nonspecific binding by subtracting the binding obtained at various times with heat-denatured (5 min, 60°C) ^{32}P-spectrin [17].

observations of factors controlling the aggregatability of intramembrane particles and various surface receptors in the plane of the membrane [7, 8, 10, 11]. Normally, the intramembrane particles are randomly distributed in the plane of the membrane [7, 26]. However, after pretreatment of ghosts under conditions that dissociate spectrin and actin, manipulation of pH or ionic strength induces rearrangement of the particles to form clusters [7, 8]. Also, clustering of colloidal iron hydroxide binding sites (localized primarily on glycophorin) follows the sequestration of antispectrin antibodies inside erythrocyte ghosts [11]. A direct association of spectrin with the intramembrane particles has been proposed on the basis of the results of these antibody experiments [11] and the observation that conditions which promote precipitation of spectrin and actin (low pH, Ca^{2+}, Mg^{2+}, basic proteins) also favor aggregation of particles in membranes partially depleted of spectrin [8]. This hypothesis is supported by the demonstration that the intramembrane particles coaggregate with residual spectrin molecules visualized using ferritin-conjugated antispectrin antibodies [10].

While these sorts of experiments do suggest that under certain conditions close structural associations may occur between spectrin and the integral membrane proteins, studies of protein aggregation are not adequate to analyze the dynamic behavior of membrane proteins, as has been pointed out by Elgsaeter and Branton [7]. In addition, the nonphysiological treatments used to induce particle aggregation may cause nonspecific coprecipitation of proteins in the membrane and may also alter the bulk properties of the membrane lipids. For example, although coaggregation of intramembrane particles with receptors for various lectins [12, 13, 16, 27], influenza virus receptors [12], A antigenic sites [15], anionic sites [28], and surface proteins labeled with a nonspecific hapten, p-diazoniumphenyl-β-D-lactoside [10] invariably occurs in the erythrocyte ghost, anti-concanavalin A antibodies can induce a temperature-dependent redistribution of concanavalin A bound to the cell surface without any effect on the random distribution of the intramembrane particles in intact erythrocytes [29]. An alternative explanation for the restraint of intramembrane particles, which is also consistent with previous data, is that the cytoplasmic portions of these structures are simply trapped within a postulated spectrin-actin meshwork without formation of specific protein-protein associations [5,7,8].

The initial observation that FITC-labeled proteins are mobile in the erythrocyte membrane under conditions where spectrin remains associated with the membrane and particle aggregation does not occur [3] suggested to us that if spectrin controls membrane protein mobility, it must do so by a dynamic and regulatable mechanism. Incubation of ghosts with a water-soluble fragment of the membrane anchorage site for spectrin is a mild and selective method for displacing spectrin from the membrane without perturbing interactions of other proteins with spectrin. The specific enhancement of lateral movement of fluorescent-labeled membrane proteins in fused, hemolyzed erythrocytes by the solubilized attachment site for spectrin, together with the displacement of spectrin from inside-out vesicle membranes, indicates that association of spectrin with its membrane anchorage site does indeed limit the lateral mobility of integral membrane protiens. A minimum diffusion constant for lateral motion (estimated as described in Fowler and Branton [3]) is increased from 10^{-11} cm^2/sec to 2×10^{-11} cm^2/sec in the experiment presented in Figure 1. This value is still low relative to diffusion constants determined for plasma membrane proteins in other cells [30–32], which suggests that erythrocyte integral membrane proteins are only partially freed from constraints by incubation with the solubilized attachment site. This is perhaps not surprising in view of the high local concentration of spectrin in ghost membranes, although the possibility cannot be excluded that other factors (such as possibly a spectrin-actin complex) may regulate membrane protein mobility.

The 72,000-dalton proteolytic fragment does not originate from the major band 3 protein or from PAS-1 [19], whose mobility is monitored in these experiments; moreover, the 45,000-dalton fragment of band 3 is without effect on the lateral movement of these proteins (Fig 1). The anchorage protein for spectrin may itself interact with band 3 and glycophorin and thus could be a heretofore unrecognized component of the intramembrane particles. It is also conceivable, however, that spectrin or the anchorage protein may modify protein mobility through an indirect mechanism, such as altering the physical state of membrane lipids.

ACKNOWLEDGMENTS

The valuable technical assistance of Peter Stenbuck and stimulating discussions with Daniel Branton are gratefully acknowledged.

REFERENCES

1. Edelman GM: Science 192:218, 1976.
2. Nicolson G: Biochim Biophys Acta 457:57, 1976.
3. Fowler V, Branton D: Nature 268:23, 1977.
4. Marchesi VT, Furthmayr H, Tomita M: Ann Rev Biochem 45:667, 1976.
5. Steck TL, J Cell Biol 62:1, 1974.
6. Peters R, Peters J, Tews KH, Bahr W: Biochim Biophys Acta 367:282, 1974.
7. Elgsaeter A, Branton D: J Cell Biol 63:395, 1974.
8. Elgsaeter A, Shotton DM, Branton D: Biochim Biophys Acta 426:101, 1976.
9. Yu J, Branton D: Proc Nat Acad Sci USA 73:3891, 1976.
10. Shotton D, Thompson K, Wofsy L, Branton D: J Cell Biol 76:512, 1978.
11. Nicolson GL, Painter RG: J Cell Biol 59:395, 1973.

12. Tillack TW, Scott RE, Marchesi VT: J Exp Med 135:1209, 1972.
13. Marchesi VT, Tillack TW, Jackson RL, Segrest JP, Scott RE: Proc Nat Acad Sci USA 69:1445, 1972.
14. Grant CWM, McConnell HM: Proc Nat Acad Sci USA 71:4653, 1974.
15. Pinto da Silva P, Douglas SD, Branton D: Nature 232:194, 1971.
16. Pinto da Silva P, Nicolson GL: Biochim Biophys Acta 363:311, 1974.
17. Bennett V, Branton D: J Biol Chem 252:2753, 1977.
18. Bennett V: Life Sci 21:433, 1977.
19. Bennett V: J Biol Chem 253:2292, 1978.
20. Steck TL, Ramos B, Strapazon E: Biochemistry 15:1154, 1976.
21. Tilney LG, Detmers P: J Cell Biol 66:508, 1975.
22. Pinder JD, Bray D, Gratzer WB: Nature 258:765, 1975; 270:752, 1977.
23. Sheetz MP, Painter RG, Singer SJ: Biochemistry 15:4486, 1976.
24. Sheetz, MP, Sawyer D, Jackowski S: In Brewer GJ (ed): "The Red Cell." New York: Alan R. Liss, 1978, pp 431–450.
25. Steck TL, Yu J: J Supramol Struct 1:220, 1973.
26. Pinto da Silva P: J Cell Biol 53:777, 1972.
27. Triche TJ, Tillack TW, Kornfeld S: Biochim Biophys Acta 394:540, 1975.
28. Pinto da Silva P, Moss PS, Fudenberg HH: Exp Cell Res 81:127, 1973.
29. Bächi T, Schnebli HP: Exp Cell Res 91:285, 1975.
30. Edidin M, Zagyansky Y, Lardner TJ: Science 191:466, 1976.
31. Jacobson K, Derzko Z, Wu E-S, Hou Y, Poste G: J Supramol Struct 5:565, 1977.
32. Schlessinger J et al: Proc Nat Acad Sci USA 73:2409, 1976.

Journal of Supramolecular Structure 8:311–324 (1978)
Normal and Abnormal Red Cell Membranes 33–46

The Band 3 Protein of the Human Red Cell Membrane: A Review

Theodore L. Steck

Departments of Biochemistry and Medicine, University of Chicago, Chicago, Illinois 60637

Band 3 is the predominant polypeptide and the purported mediator of anion transport in the human erythrocyte membrane. Against a background of minor and apparently unrelated polypeptides of similar electrophoretic mobility, and despite apparent heterogeneity in its glycosylation, the bulk of band 3 exhibits uniform and characteristic behavior. This integral glycoprotein appears to exist as a noncovalent dimer of two ~ 93,000-dalton chains which span the membrane asymmetrically. The protein is hydrophobic in its composition and in its behavior in aqueous solution and is best solubilized and purified in detergent. It can be cleaved while membrane-bound into large, topographically defined segments. An integral, outer-surface, 38,000-dalton fragment bears most of the band 3 carbohydrate. A 17,000-dalton, hydrophobic glycopeptide fragment spans the membrane. A ~ 40,000-dalton hydrophilic segment represents the cytoplasmic domain. In vitro, glyceraldehyde 3-P dehydrogenase and aldolase bind reversibly, in a metabolite-sensitive fashion, to this cytoplasmic segment. The cytoplasmic domain also bears the amino terminus of this polypeptide, in contrast to other integral membrane proteins. Recent electron microscopic analysis suggests that the poles of the band 3 molecule can be seen by freeze-etching at the two original membrane surfaces, while freeze-fracture reveals the transmembrane disposition of band 3 dimer particles.

There is strong evidence that band 3 mediates 1:1 anion exchange across the membrane through a conformational cycle while remaining fixed and asymmetrical. Its cytoplasmic pole can be variously perturbed and even excised without a significant alteration of transport function. However, digestion of the outer-surface region leads to inhibition of transport, so that both this segment and the membrane-spanning piece (which is selectively labeled by covalent inhibitors of transport) may be presumed to be involved in transport. Genetic polymorphism has been observed in the structure and immunogenicity of the band 3 polypeptide but this feature has not been related to variation in anion transport or other band 3 activities.

Key words: band 3, integral protein, polypeptide, red blood cell, erythrocyte, transport

Received for publication April 25, 1978.

0091-7419/78/0803-0311$02.60

Early high-resolution polyacrylamide gel electrophorograms of human erythrocyte membrane polypeptides in sodium dodecyl sulfate (SDS) revealed a predominant band with a sharp leading edge and diffuse trailing edge, which was variously designated component a, component E, and band 3 [1–8]. Its apparent molecular weight was estimated to be 90,000–100,000, and its prevalence to be $\sim 1 \times 10^6$ copies per ghost membrane [8, 9].

In 1974, Cabantchik and Rothstein [10] demonstrated a close parallel between the inhibition of anion (namely, $^{35}SO_4^{=}$) transport in intact erythrocytes and the rather specific labeling of the band 3 polypeptide. During the ensuing years, numerous structural and functional studies have deepened interest in band 3 and its purported role in anion transport. It is the intent of this review to put this work into perspective.

ISOLATION OF THE BAND 3 POLYPEPTIDE

Band 3 can be assumed to make extensive contact with the apolar core of the membrane lipid bilayer (ie, to be an intrinsic or integral membrane protein) by virtue of the following qualities: 1) It cannot be extracted from the membrane short of dissolving the lipid bilayer itself (eg, with detergents or organic solvents) [5, 24]. 2) Once solubilized, it precipitates in simple aqueous buffers and will eventually aggregate irreversibly in mild detergents such as Triton X-100 [11]; it requires strong detergents such as SDS [1–8] or cetyltrimethylammonium bromide [12] for long-term aqueous solubility. 3) Mild pretreatments of the membrane itself will render band 3 resistant to dissociation in SDS [5]; the molecular basis for this effect is unclear. 4) Band 3 binds considerable Triton X-100 (ie, 0.77 g/g protein), a feature of integral as opposed to nonmembrane proteins, presumably reflecting an extended hydrophobic surface [13]. 5) The amino acid composition of band 3 is distinctly (but not profoundly) enriched in nonpolar residues (Table I; Refs 7, 11, 14). 6) It spans the hydrophobic core of the membrane [15–21] (see also Refs. 9, 22, 23 for review).

Several strategies have been evolved for the purification of this protein.

1. Band 3, and the other integral proteins, can be enriched up to twofold by stripping the membrane of peripheral polypeptides, using denaturing or protein-modifying reagents (eg, mild or strong alkali, lithium diiodosalicylate, or organic mercurials [24]). Some of these treatments appear mild, in that purported transport and liganding activities of the band 3 protein are preserved. (The lipid bilayer may help to stabilize the tertiary structure of integral proteins.)

2. Gently stripped membranes have been treated secondarily with low concentrations of the nondenaturing detergent Triton X-100 so as to solubilize some of the integral proteins (notably, the sialoglycoproteins) while leaving band 3 in the membranous residue. While these membranes can be resealed for use in transport studies, they appear to contain more protein than just band 3 and more functions than just anion transport activity [25].

3. Band 3 can be solubilized from ghosts at higher concentrations of Triton X-100 (eg, $\geq 0.5\%$) or other nondenaturing, nonionic detergents. Purification still requires dissociation of liganded cytoplasmic-surface proteins from band 3 [11]. The protein can then be isolated, still in detergent, by concanavalin A or ricinus communis affinity chromatography [26–30], ion exchange chromatography [11, 31], or immobilization by disulfide-sulfhydryl interchange [32]. (Barratt et al [33] have also isolated band 3 glycoprotein by concanavalin A affinity chromatography in dodecyltrimethylammonium bromide.) It has been observed that band 3 aggregation in mild detergents is significant and increases with

time, temperature, ionic strength, protein concentration, and acidity ([11]; J. Yu and T.L. Steck, unpublished observations). Irreversible adsorption to the chromatography bed frequently leads to reduced yields. Mixed aggregation with other integral proteins in the Triton X-100 extract can reduce purity.

4. Stripped membranes can be dissolved in the denaturing and dissociating detergent SDS and purified by gel filtration [7, 34], hydroxyapatite chromatography [52] or preparative polyacrylamide gel electrophoresis in the same detergent [21, 35]. Aggregation and irreversible binding are not usually a problem, but clean separation from the sialoglycoprotein PAS-1 must be assured. While these preparations are presumably inactive, they are convenient for chemical and even immunologic analysis (see Bhakdi et al [21]).

COMPOSITIONAL ANALYSIS OF THE BAND 3 POLYPEPTIDE

The molecular weight of band 3 has been variously estimated by gel electrophoresis in SDS to be 88,000–105,000 [9]; most recent estimates are compatible with the molecular weight of the polypeptide portion of this glycoprotein being 93,000 ± 3,000 [36]. Electrophoretically, band 3 is characteristically broad and asymmetrical, with a sharp leading edge and a diffuse trailing edge. This dispersion is stable and is not the result of interpeptide associations during electrophoresis [11]. It may be ascribed, at least in part, to variable glycosylation of the polypeptide backbone [11, 26, 28].

There is evidence for multiple minor components, or at least heterogeneous behavior of the polypeptides, in the 90,000- to 100,000-dalton region. There are, for example, three or four minor peripheral polypeptides on the cytoplasmic surface of rabbit erythrocyte membranes which migrate on gel electrophoresis with the bulk of band 3 [37]. A minor trypsin-resistant component in the band 3 region has been observed under some conditions of ghost digestion [21, 38]. Isoelectric focusing has also revealed multiple components in the band 3 region of gels [21, 39]; however, these could as well arise from variations in sialylation or amidation as from heterogeneity in the primary structure of the polypeptides present.

On the other hand, it has been repeatedly observed that the bulk of the band 3 population – perhaps 90% – behaves homogeneously with respect to disulfide cross-linking [36, 40, 41], the binding of glycolytic enzymes [42, 43], selective solubilization [24], and titration with 4,4′-diisothiocyanostilbene-2,2′ disulfonate (DIDS) [44–47]. Those laboratories studying the structure of the band 3 polypeptide by proteolytic dissection, covalent labeling, and partial amino acid sequence analysis thus far have failed to detect significant heterogeneity in individual preparations representing the bulk of the band 3 material [36, 38, 48–51]. For the present discussion, therefore, we shall consider the polypeptide portion of band 3 to be nearly homogeneous.

Our amino acid composition of band 3 is tabulated in column 1 of Table I [35]; similar analyses have been published [11, 14, 21, 34, 48, 51]. It is important that band 3 isolated by a variety of techniques shows uniformity in composition. This may be a reflection of its relative homogeneity. Like many other integral membrane polypeptides, the composition of band 3 is only moderately enriched in hydrophobic and uncharged residues, making its extreme insolubility even more striking.

The carbohydrate content of band 3 has been determined by several groups. As can be seen in Table II, there is considerable variation among these reports in both total carbohydrate content and the relative preponderance of the various sugars. These discrepancies could signify that different laboratories have isolated and analyzed subfractions of the

TABLE I. Amino Acid Composition of Band 3 and Five of its Major Fragments (mole percent)

Residue	Band 3	CH-38	CH-55	CH-17	TR-41	CN-23
Lys	3.4	4.2	2.6	3.5	4.3	2.8
His	2.2	2.1	1.8	1.4	3.1	3.8
Arg	5.2	4.8	5.0	4.2	5.2	4.7
	10.8	11.1	9.4	9.1	12.6	11.3
Asx	6.5	6.1	6.4	6.1	8.1	8.0
Glx	11.9	8.9	12.9	9.6	15.3	18.6
	18.4	15.0	19.3	15.7	23.4	26.6
Thr	5.0	5.5	5.5	5.5	5.5	6.4
Ser	6.8	6.9	7.0	7.1	6.0	5.9
Pro	5.7	6.7	5.9	4.9	5.6	5.0
Gly	7.7	7.7	7.8	9.0	6.4	5.6
Ala	7.4	7.5	7.2	7.1	7.6	6.7
½ Cys	0.7	0.7	0.6	0.9	1.2	0.6
	33.3	35.0	34.0	34.5	32.3	30.2
Val	7.6	8.6	6.4	7.3	6.4	5.5
Met	2.2	3.1	2.1	1.3	1.8	2.6
Ile	4.7	6.0	4.5	6.8	3.8	3.0
Leu	13.4	13.4	14.0	12.6	12.4	12.8
Tyr	3.1	1.9	3.0	3.6	2.4	3.1
Phe	5.5	5.4	6.5	7.5	3.8	3.3
Trp	1.2	0.4	0.8	1.8	1.2	1.8
	37.7	38.8	37.3	40.9	31.8	32.1

The identities of the chymotryptic (CH), tryptic (TR), and S-cyanylation (CN) fragments are given in Figure 1 and in the text. Data are recalculated from Steck et al [35].

TABLE II. Carbohydrate Composition of Band 3 (moles/mole band 3)

Residue	A	B	C	D	E	F
Fucose	8.3	2.5	0.75	1.4	4	7
Mannose	8.3	7.2	3.4	4.3	7	5
Galactose	8.3	12	5.2	4.8	24	16
N-acetylglucosamine	7.6	20	5.5	10.0	25	17
N-acetylgalactosamine	0	0	0.87	3.2	4	2
Sialic acids	1.8	–	0.87	0	5	5
Total	34.3	41.7	16.6	23.7	69	52

Data for columns A–F are taken from References 14, 21, 34, 52, 53, and 65, respectively. Values were normalized to moles/mole band 3, assuming that band 3 has a molecular weight of 93,000 and contains 833 amino acid residues [35]. Values for glucose are considered unreliable and have been omitted.

broad band 3 dispersion relatively enriched or deficient in carbohydrate. Generally, galactose and N-acetylglucosamine were found to be most abundant while N-acetylgalactosamine and sialic acids were present in small amounts.

Gahmberg et al [52] have provided evidence that there are two types of oligosaccharide chains, one unusually large and the other of only a few residues. One of each chain per band 3 polypeptide could account for the entire band 3 carbohydrate content. Their analysis also suggests that the major oligosaccharide may be heterogeneous in composition, which might further broaden the band 3 electrophoretic profile.

Individuals possessing the rare blood type En(a–) appear to lack glycophorin (PAS-1 and -2), yet are clinically normal [52, 53]. Band 3 isolated from these variants exhibited a considerable increase in glycosylation, attributable to a longer major oligosaccharide chain [52]. Its composition resembled that of the wild-type band 3, rather than bearing increased sialic acid in compensation for the loss of the major sialoglycoprotein.

Polypeptides in the band 3 region can be phosphorylated by adding $^{32}PO_4$ to intact cells or by incubating unsealed ghosts with γ-^{32}P-ATP (adenosine triphosphate) [9, 23]. The chemical analysis of phosphate in band 3 isolates, however, amounts to no more than 0.2–0.3 mole/mole [43, 54]. Furthermore, the ^{32}P acceptors in the band 3 region are not identical with the bulk of band 3 and some could be minor and unrelated comigrating polypeptides [28, 55, 56]. All of the ^{32}P incorporated in vitro into the band 3 region appears to be associated with a population of integral molecules [56] which are not bound by concanavalin A affinity columns [28]. Minor fractions of band 3 highly enriched in the ^{32}P incorporated in vitro can be isolated by fractional elution from affinity columns of ricinus communis 1 lectin [30].

The absorption spectrum of band 3 in the nonionic and nonaromatic detergent Ammonyx LO is typical of simple proteins lacking bound chromophores [11].

BAND 3 STRUCTURE

Band 3 spans the erythrocyte membrane asymmetrically [9, 15–23, 35, 50, 51, 58, 59], with its carbohydrate groups confined to the extracellular space [60]. The polypeptides appear to be associated as dimers [40, 41, 61], which correspond in size (~180,000 daltons), prevalence (~6×10^5 per ghost), and disposition (integral and transmembrane) to the ~ 70-Å intramembrane particles visualized in the particle-rich faces of freeze-fracture electron micrographs [62]. Band 3 has also been reported to contain 43% α-helix, as judged from its circular dicroism in a nondenaturing detergent [11].

We have cleaved band 3 in situ into large segments representing outer-surface, transmembrane, and cytoplasmic-surface regions (35, 36; Fig 1). Digestion of intact cells with chymotrypsin cleaves band 3 into 38,000- and 55,000-dalton glycopeptide fragments, whose apparent molecular weights and amino acid compositions sum to that of band 3 (Table I). The former would appear to bear the major oligosaccharide unit and the latter, the smaller [52, 65]. Both fragments are firmly integrated into the membrane and are water-insoluble upon isolation [35, 36]. The hydrophobicity index of both of these pieces is approximately that of band 3 itself (Table I), apparently reflecting a balance between those portions in contact with the aqueous compartment and those buried in the bilayer. The 38,000-dalton segment, unlike the complementary 55,000-dalton piece, does not seem to traverse the membrane. It may contribute to the surface projections seen following the freeze-etching of intact red cells previously digested with proteases [63, 64].

Vigorous chymotryptic digestion at both membrane surfaces leaves a 17,000-dalton subfragment of the 55,000-dalton segment spanning the membrane [35, 36]. The 17,000-dalton fragment is the most hydrophobic of the major proteolytic pieces (Table I); it is also irreversibly integrated into the membrane and is highly water-insoluble upon isolation

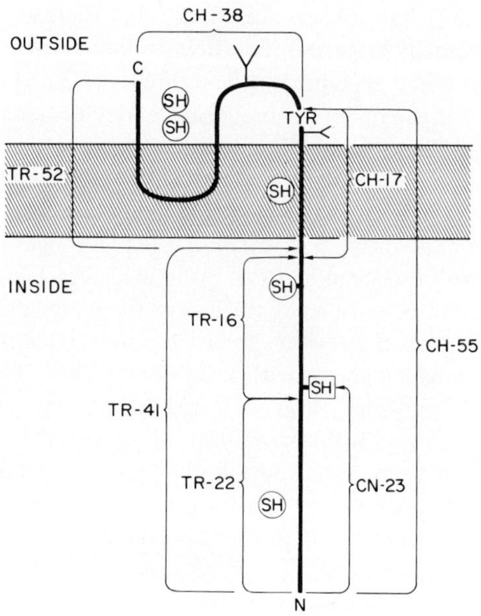

Fig 1. Schematic summary of the disposition of some proteolytic fragments of band 3 in the red cell membrane. Three major, integral fragments are generated by digestion with chymotrypsin (CH). Trypsin (TR) cleaves the polypeptide into a 52,000-dalton integral segment and three major cytoplasmic-surface fragments not anchored in the bilayer. S-cyanylation (CN) of a cysteine residue (SH) cleaves a 23,000-dalton piece from the cytoplasmic-surface, amino-terminal region of band 3. See text for details. Figure adapted from Steck et al [35], with permission.

[35, 65]. These properties render its primary sequence analysis particularly challenging [65]. Since hydrophobic stretches of approximately 20 residues are sufficient to span a lipid bilayer (see, for example, glycophorin [66] or the phage M13 coat protein [67]), this ~ 154-residue segment probably has a complex folding pattern – ie, a globular structure – in the membrane. This would be compatible with the aforementioned freeze-fracture image and with a transport function. Clearly, the position of the several basic residues in the primary structure of this peptide (as well as the other polar residues) will be of great interest.

The cytoplasmic aspect of band 3 is several orders of magnitude more sensitive to proteolysis by trypsin, chymotrypsin, papain, and other proteases than is the extracellular pole [16, 36]. The various fragments so generated are readily released from the membrane in a water-soluble form, still associated with one another in a dimeric ensemble [36]. This domain has a composition distinctly more polar than the remainder of band 3, as illustrated in Table I for the largest of the fragments, a 41,000-dalton tryptic peptide. This piece is seen to roughly complement the 17,000-dalton transmembrane segment when they are compared in size and composition to the presumed parent, the 55,000-dalton chymotryptic polypeptide (Fig 1; Table I; Ref 35).

Major fragments of band 3 have also been generated by chemical cleavage at cysteine residues following their S-cyanylation by 2-nitro-5-thiocyanobenzoate (NTCB) [35, 36, 49–51]. In particular, a 23,000-dalton fragment is released from the cytoplasmic terminus of the band 3 chain, adjacent to which is a 12,000-dalton cyanylation fragment. A ~ 35,000-

dalton segment, apparently the sum of the 23,000 + 12,000 pieces, has also been recovered [49–51]. The composition of the 23,000-dalton fragment is given in Table I.

Drickamer [50, 51] has generated, mapped, and analyzed additional fragments, using S-cyanylation, hydroxylamine, cyanogen bromide, and N-bromosuccinimide to effect chemical cleavage of band 3 molecules previously covalently labeled in various ways from each membrane surface. The outer-surface 38,000-dalton chymotryptic fragment was strikingly unreactive to a variety of probes. In addition, an 11,000-dalton segment of the transmembrane region of band 3 was apparently labeled from both sides of the membrane in a fashion suggesting that this segment looped from the outer surface to the inner and back again.

Tanner and his associates have proposed a somewhat different disposition for the band 3 polypeptide than that shown in Figure 1 [17, 38, 48, 59]. Most notably, an S-shaped structure was suggested, which crosses the bilayer twice and has a large segment of polypeptide duplicated at the two ends of the molecule. My interpretation of these data is that T1 and T2, the two major tryptic fragments which Tanner assumes to be complementary (ie, from different ends of the molecule), are in fact overlapping segments from the same region. I suspect that T2 contains the counterpart of our 17,000-dalton membrane-spanning fragment and is hence a portion of T1 which can be generated in low yield by tryptic digestion of ghosts (see Ref 48 and Fig 4 in Ref 36). Since the readily eluted tryptic fragments we isolate from the cytoplasmic-surface domain of band 3 might have been lost from Tanner's digests during a washing step, and because Tanner's approach was based on autoradiographic analysis of radioiodinated membranes, it is difficult to make a closer comparison of our results at present.

FEATURES OF THE CYTOPLASMIC DOMAIN OF BAND 3

Cross-Linking

Oxidation of ghosts with a variety of reagents, particularly the o-phenanthroline-Cu^{++} chelate complex, converts band 3 into a disulfide-linked dimer [40, 41]. Band 3 probably exists as a stable, noncovalent dimer for these reasons: 1) Dissolution of the membrane in nondenaturing detergents such as Triton X-100 does not reduce the efficiency of the cross-linking reaction despite the profound dilution in local protein concentration attending solubilization [11, 40]. 2) The non-cross-linked and cross-linked forms of Triton X-100-solubilized band 3 have identical sedimentation rates upon sucrose gradient centrifugation [11, 13]. 3) Millisecond flash photochemical cross-linking joins band 3 polypeptides into covalent dimers at a more rapid rate than transient interprotein collisions should allow [61].

The disulfide cross-link has been shown to be confined to the cytoplasmic pole of the polypeptide [36]. Disulfide-cross-linked band 3 can be cleaved by 1 mM CN^- via S-cyanylation to release the same N-terminal 23,000-dalton fragment generated by NTCB [36] (see above). Recently Miyakawa, Takemoto, and Fox [68], using a completely different membrane-impermeable reagent, tartryl-di(glycylazide) (TDGA), also found that band 3 was cross-linked only from the cytoplasmic surface.

At present, there is no evidence as to whether the membrane-integrated portions of the band 3 dimer are intimately apposed.

The Amino Terminus of the Band 3 Polypeptide Is Confined to Its Cytoplasmic Pole

A current concept of the integration of membrane-spanning proteins [69] is an adaptation of the model proposed by Blobel and his colleagues for secreted proteins [70]. The amino terminus of the nascent polypeptide, led by an excisable "signal peptide," is threaded directly from a membrane-bound ribosome through the bilayer into the cisternal space of the endoplasmic reticulum. In this way, the N terminus comes to reside on the outer surface of the plasma membrane. Glycosylation of such proteins would be confined to their amino terminal segment, the carboxyl terminus of the molecule never leaving the cytoplasmic space. This paradigm clearly applies to glycophorin A [66], histocompatibility antigens [71], and perhaps the envelope glycoprotein of vesicular stomatitis virus [72].

In contrast, band 3 exhibits a different pattern. Drickamer [50] has shown that the 23,000-dalton fragment generated from band 3 by S-cyanylation with ^{14}C-NTCB is not radioactively labeled, as is the complementary 71,000-dalton polypeptide. Since every newly generated N terminus should be labeled by this cleavage reaction, the original amino terminus of band 3 would appear to reside in the cytoplasmic, 23,000-dalton piece. Fukuda et al [49] have confirmed this result.

Jenkins and Tanner [48] have adduced complementary evidence favoring the same conclusion. They found that their fragment, 3f (which appears to be very similar to the 55,000-dalton chymotryptic fragment discussed above), shares a blocked amino terminus with band 3. In our view (Fig 1), but not Tanner's, the shared N terminus would be at the cytoplasmic end of band 3. More recently, Steck et al [35] reported that the 23,000-dalton cyanylation fragment and the 22,000-dalton tryptic fragment, both of which map at the cytoplasmic pole of band 3, also have unreactive amino termini, as does the parent band 3 molecule. Thus, four laboratories are in agreement concerning this unexpected orientation of band 3. Furthermore, it seems that the glycosylation of band 3 is confined to its C-terminal section, despite one argument to the contrary [48]. It is interesting that integral intestinal brush border membrane hydrolases may share this "reversed polarity" with band 3 [73]. The mechanism of insertion of these proteins into membranes will obviously be of great interest.

Immunogenicity

Two laboratories have recently reported that rabbit antibodies prepared against band 3 react only with immunodeterminants within the cytoplasmic domain of the molecule [31, 49]. Since immunization was carried out with whole ghosts and with band 3 dissolved in either Triton X-100 (a nondenaturing detergent) or SDS (a denaturing detergent), this specificity cannot be ascribed to the mode of polypeptide preparation. However, evidence for antigenic determinants in the extracellular portion of band 3 has also been reported [21].

Genetic Polymorphism

Mueller and Morrison [74] have observed altered gel electrophoresis patterns in band 3 and certain of its fragments obtained from a small fraction of normal individuals. They ascribe this feature to a ~ 3,000-dalton increase in the size of the cytoplasmic domain of this polypeptide, presumably of genetic origin.

Köhler and associates have recently reported that the 23,000-dalton cytoplasmic-terminal segment of band 3 is both structurally and immunologically heterogeneous among normal human donors [75, 76]. The composition of this fragment showed unexpected variation, particularly in glutamate (or glutamine) content. Furthermore, the amino acid sequence of a specific pentapeptide from this region varied among normal donors [76]. Finally, mutual inhibition among various 23K preparations in a radioimmunoassay with rabbit anti-23K antisera showed antigenic variation within the donor population [75].

Phosphorylation

Phosphorylation of polypeptides in the band 3 region has been repeatedly observed in intact cell and isolated membranes [9, 23, 54–57]. The phosphate bond is stable – apparently of the ester type. Labeling is not stimulated by cyclic AMP (adenosine monophosphate) in vitro. The phosphate appears to be introduced only from the cytoplasmic surface [77]. Drickamer [50, 51] has found that phosphorylation occurs primarily within 10,000 daltons of the cytoplasmic N terminus of band 3, but that some $^{32}P_i$ can also be detected in fragments ascribed to the center of the polypeptide chain.

Associations

The cytoplasmic pole of band 3 appears to provide binding sites for several other proteins. The most tenaciously bound is the membrane polypeptide termed band 4.2 [42]. This peripheral protein [24], which behaves as a homotetramer in cross-linking studies [40], is of unknown function; unlike the other band 3 ligands discussed below, its binding has not been shown to be reversed by electrolytes or metabolites. Its binding stoichiometry might be as low as one tetramer per 20 band 3 polypeptides [9].

Band 3 provides the membrane binding site for both glyceraldehyde 3-P dehydrogenase (G3PD) [42] and aldolase [43] in vitro; the extent to which these associations occur in the intact cell has yet to be established. The binding reactions are reversible and sensitive to both the elevation of ionic strength and to specific metabolites. The patterns of elution suggest that the associations of these enzymes with band 3 utilize known binding sites for substrates or allosteric effectors. Binding is confined to the cytoplasmic pole of band 3 and has a stoichiometry of one enzyme tetramer per band 3 protomer. There are more than enough copies of band 3 to bind all of the G3PD plus aldolase in the cell. Interestingly, the catalytic activity of aldolase is inhibited reversibly upon binding to ghosts, isolated band 3, or cytoplasmic surface fragments of band 3 [43].

Recently hemoglobin was shown to bind to ghosts with a stoichiometry of 1.2–1.3 $\times 10^6$/membrane [78], suggesting that band 3 provides the liganding site. Since this association was only observable in the acidic pH range at low ionic strength, its physiologic significance is unclear.

Branton and his colleagues have presented freeze-fracture evidence that the lateral distribution of the A (PF) face intramembrane particle population (believed to contain principally band 3) is influenced by spectrin [79, 80]. However, a study by Cherry et al [81] on the rotational freedom of band 3 in the intact cell suggested that it is not immobilized, as would be expected if it were bound to an extended spectrin network. Furthermore, Bennett and Branton [82, 83] have reported that the membrane binding site for spectrin is not associated with the bulk of band 3 molecules. The importance of transient interactions between the spectrin-actin system and integral proteins such as band 3 is obviously an important topic for future research.

Ultrastructure

As discussed, a ~40,000-dalton cytoplasmic-surface segment of the band 3 polypeptide can be readily released from the membrane by mild proteolysis [36]. This domain would amount to 80,000-daltons per band 3 dimer, and should thus be visible in situ in the electron microscope. Recent freeze-etch studies of the true cytoplasmic face of human red cell ghosts and inside-out vesicles have indeed revealed such projections [63, 64]. Their prevalence was compatible with the predicted ~ 600,000-dalton band 3 dimers present per ghost. Furthermore, these projections could be decorated with G3PD, which forms specific associations with band 3 [42]. The projections (and the G3PD decoration) were abolished by mild proteolysis sufficient to cleave away the cytoplasmic aspect of band 3. It is interesting that similar cytoplasmic-surface projections have also been visualized in preparations of Na^+, K^+-ATPase [84], and Ca^{++}-ATPase [85]. This finding can be added to other similarities among these molecules; ie, they are all membrane-spanning oligomeric transport proteins containing disulfide-linkable polypeptides of ~ 10^5 molecular weight [86, 87].

BAND 3 FUNCTION

Several functions have been attributed to the band 3 region of the electrophoretic profile. Bellhorn, Blumenfeld, and Gallop [88] found the erythrocyte acetylcholinesterase (radiolabeled with diisopropylfluorophosphate) in this gel region; however, more recent work has shown that this enzyme, while an integral membrane glycoprotein, is clearly distinguishable from band 3 in its electrophoretic and chromatographic behavior both in Triton X-100 and in SDS [11, 89].

A rather indirect line of evidence, based primarily on the binding of cytochalasin B to the integral proteins of stripped ghost membranes, suggested that glucose transport activity was an attribute of band 3 [90–92]. However, recent studies have clearly identified an integral glycoprotein of 45,000–55,000 daltons as the likely glucose transporter [93–95] (see also the reports of D.C. Sogin and P.C. Hinkle [95a], and of M.A. Zoccoli et al [95b] in this Symposium).

The ~ 10^5-dalton polypeptide of the Na^+,K^+-ATPase has been identified in the band 3 electrophoretic region as the acyl-^{32}P covalent intermediate [96]; however, this polypeptide contributes roughly 10^2 of 10^6 polypeptides to the band 3 zone [97].

Elsewhere in this symposium, both Branton and Sheetz have argued that a minor fraction of the band 3 region which remains associated with spectrin-actin residues following Triton X-100 solubilization of the bulk of band 3 could be the membrane binding site for spectrin. The relationship of this material to the bulk of band 3 therefore warrants careful evaluation.

Osmotic water flow in intact red cells can be inhibited by the sulfhydryl reagent 5,5′-dithio-bis-(2-nitrobenzoate) with a concomitant and highly selective labeling of band 3 [98]. The relationship of water transport to band 3 is thus an intriguing question.

The relationship of band 3 to anion transport is discussed extensively by Rothstein [110] elsewhere in this symposium and in other recent reviews [44, 99–101]. Briefly, the major evidence linking band 3 to anion transport is twofold. First, covalent inhibitors of anion exchange, notably stilbene disulfonates such as DIDS, label band 3 rather selectively [10, 14]. Ignoring early discrepancies, complete inhibition occurs when roughly 1.2×10^6 DIDS molecules are bound per cell – ie, one DIDS molecule per band 3 [44–47]. Secondly, partially purified preparations of band 3 confer anion transport activity on lipid vesicles [25, 27]. While neither line of evidence rigorously excludes a minor protein as the anion transporter, no such alternate candidate has been implicated. That band 3 is the anion transporter is thus a strong working hypothesis, consistent with what is known about the structure of this molecule.

The behavior of the anion transporter is that expected of a fixed and asymmetrical membrane-spanning protein like band 3. The kinetic constants for anion transport appear to be different at the two membrane surfaces [102, 103; Gunn RB, Froehlich O, Steck TL: Manuscript in preparation]. Furthermore, mild oxidation, which cross-links band 3, leads to differential changes in the apparent kinetic constants at the two sides of the membrane [102, 103]. Finally, various inhibitors have been shown to act differentially at one membrane surface or the other [101, 103–105].

Papain and pronase digestion at the outer surface of intact red cells inhibits anion transport profoundly [44]. Since the 55,000-dalton membrane-spanning segment of band 3 remains intact following such treatment, it seems reasonable to conclude that some aspect of the degraded 38,000-dalton region is necessary for transport activity. Chymotrypsin digestion of intact cells does not inhibit transport although it cleaves band 3 into 38,000-dalton and 55,000-dalton segments (Fig 1). We may infer that native tertiary structure is retained in the protein mildly cleaved with chymotrypsin but not following the more extensive papain or pronase digestion. Freeze-etch electron micrographs suggest that the outer-surface projections attributable to band 3 dimers survive even vigorous proteolysis of intact cells [63, 64], so that this aspect of the molecule apparently does not fall to pieces upon cleavage.

Recent studies have indicated that two covalent inhibitors of anion flux selectively bind to the 17,000-dalton, membrane-spanning portion of band 3 [50, 106], making this domain a prime target for studies on the structural basis for anion transport.

While the integral outer and membrane-spanning segments of band 3 appear to be involved in anion exchange activity, the 40,000-dalton cytoplasmic-surface domain can be excised without significant effects on transport [103, 106]. The binding of G3PD and aldolase to this portion of the molecule also does not alter transport kinetics significantly [103]. Furthermore, antibodies directed against the 23,000-dalton cytoplasmic terminus of band 3 fail to inhibit anion transport [31].

It is commonly held that the interface between the protomers in oligomeric transport proteins might provide a polar pathway through which solutes traverse the membrane (eg, Singer [107]). This implies that the functional unit of band 3 is the dimer rather than the individual protomers. However, the correlation of the fractional labeling of band 3 polypeptides by DIDS with the fractional inhibition of anion transport is quite linear and has a slope of unity [44–47]. This finding suggests that either 1) each protomer contributes equally and independently to transport activity, 2) there is a very high degree of positive cooperativity in the binding of DIDS to band 3 such that the ligand is essentially added pairwise to dimers, or 3) that DIDS modification of the first protomer of a functional dimer happens to lower the activity of the unit to one-half and that the second bound DIDS molecule completes the inactivation. In the absence of discriminating data, the first alternative seems the most likely. This is not an unreasonable inference, since many soluble oligomeric enzymes are composed of identical, nonintereacting subunits.

How does the anion transporter function? Kinetic evidence suggests a double displacement (ping-pong) mechanism [108]. Presumably, single anions are alternately transported from one compartment to the other in a reciprocating cycle, probably conformational in nature. This hypothesis is consistent with studies of differential inhibitor binding at the two membrane surfaces [101, 110]. For Cl^- and HCO_3^-, the rate constant for such a conformational change would be vastly greater for the substrate-loaded as opposed to the unloaded form of the transporter [101, 109]. Consequently, Cl^- transport and HCO_3^- transport are almost entirely one-for-one; the net movement of these anions, arising from cycles with an empty return step, would occur about once in 10^5 exchange cycles under conditions where membrane potential gradients are dissipated by a diffusable cation system. This behavior is quite compatible with the purported physiological functions of the red cell anion transport system: 1) the exceedingly rapid 1:1 exchange of Cl^- and HCO_3^- required for efficient CO_2 disposal; 2) the slow net anion movements accompanying rate-limiting cation movements in cell volume adjustment; 3) the slow transport of metabolically important anions, such as phosphate and lactate.

An integrated understanding of band 3 structure and function seems at present to be a distant but increasingly realizable goal.

ACKNOWLEDGMENTS

Original studies presented here were supported by American Cancer Society grant BC-95E and F and USPHS grant GM 22722. The author is a Faculty Research Awardee of the American Cancer Society.

REFERENCES

1. Berg HC: Biochim Biophys Acta 183:65, 1969.
2. Lenard J: Biochemistry 9:1129, 1970.
3. Furthmayr H, Timpl R: Eur J Biochem 15:301, 1970.
4. Bretscher MS: J Mol Biol 58:775, 1971.
5. Fairbanks G, Steck TL, Wallach DFH: Biochemistry 10:2606, 1971.
6. Trayer HR, Nozaki Y, Reynolds JA, Tanford C: J Biol Chem 246:4485, 1971.
7. Tanner MJA, Boxer DH: Biochem J 129:333, 1972.
8. Guidotti G: Ann Rev Biochem 41:731, 1972.
9. Steck TL: J Cell Biol 62:1, 1974.
10. Cabantchik ZI, Rothstein A: J Memb Biol 15:207, 1974.
11. Yu J, Steck TL: J Biol Chem 250:9170, 1975.
12. Fairbanks G, Avruch J: J Supramol Struct 1:66, 1972.
13. Clarke S: J Biol Chem 250:5459, 1975.
14. Ho MK, Guidotti G: J Biol Chem 250:675, 1975.
15. Bretscher M: J Mol Biol 59:351, 1971.
16. Steck TL: In Fox CF (ed): "Membrane Research." New York: Academic, 1972, p 71.
17. Boxer DH, Jenkins RE, Tanner MJA: Biochem J 137:531, 1974.
18. Shin B, Carraway KL: Biochim Biophys Acta 345:141, 1974.
19. Mueller TJ, Morrison M: J Biol Chem 249:7568, 1974.
20. Reichstein E, Blostein R: J Biol Chem 250:6256, 1975.
21. Bhakdi S, Bjerrum OJ, Knüfermann H: Biochim Biophys Acta 446:419, 1976.
22. Carraway KL: Biochim Biophys Acta 415:379, 1975.
23. Marchesi VT, Furthmayr H, Tomita M: Ann Rev Biochem 45:667, 1976.
24. Steck TL, Yu J: J Supramol Struct 1:220, 1973.
25. Wolosin JM, Ginsburg H, Cabantchik ZI: J Biol Chem 252:2419, 1977.
26. Findlay JBC: J Biol Chem 249:4398, 1974.
27. Ross AH, McConnell HM: Biochem Biophys Res Commun 74:1318, 1977.
28. Roses AD: J Supramol Struct 4:481, 1976.
29. Adair WL, Kornfeld S: J Biol Chem 294:4696, 1974.
30. Wong P, Roses AD: Brewer GJ (ed): "The Red Cell." New York: Alan R Liss, 1978; p 479.
31. England B, Steck TL: J Supramol Struct (Suppl)2:212, 1978.
32. Kahlenberg A: Anal Biochem 74:337, 1976.
33. Barratt DG, Sharom FJ, Thede A, Grant CWM: Biochim Biophys Acta 465:191, 1977.
34. Furthmayr H, Kahane I, Marchesi VT: J Memb Biol 26:173, 1976.
35. Steck TL, Koziarz JJ, Singh MK, Reddy G, Köhler H: Biochemistry 17:1216, 1978.

36. Steck TL, Ramos B, Strapazon E: Biochemistry 15:1154, 1976.
37. Vimr ER, Carter JR Jr: Biochem Biophys Res Commun 73:779, 1976.
38. Jenkins RE, Tanner MJA: Biochem J 161:131, 1977.
39. Conrad MJ, Penniston JT: J Biol Chem 251:253, 1976.
40. Steck TL: J Mol Biol 66:295, 1972.
41. Wang K, Richards FM: J Biol Chem 249:8005, 1974.
42. Yu J, Steck TL: J Biol Chem 250:9176, 1975.
43. Strapazon E, Steck TL: Biochemistry 16:2966, 1977.
44. Passow H, Fasold H, Lepke S, Pring M, Schuhmann B: In Miller MW, Shamoo AE (eds): "Membrane Toxicity." New York: Plenum, 1977, p 353.
45. Halestrap AP: Biochem J 156:193, 1976.
46. Ship S, Shami Y, Breuer W, Rothstein A: J Memb Biol 33:311, 1977.
47. Lepke S, Fasold H, Pring M, Passow H: J Memb Biol 29:147, 1976.
48. Jenkins RE, Tanner MJA: Biochem J 161:139, 1977.
49. Fukuda M, Eshdat Y, Tarone G, Marchesi VT: J Biol Chem 253:2419, 1978.
50. Drickamer LK: J Biol Chem 251:5115, 1976.
51. Drickamer LK: J Biol Chem 252:6909, 1977.
52. Gahmberg CG, Myllyla G, Leikola J, Pirkola A, Nordling S: J Biol Chem 251:6108, 1976.
53. Tanner MJA, Jenkins RE, Anstee DJ, Clamp JR: Biochem J 155:701, 1976.
54. Wolfe LC, Lux S: J Biol Chem 253:3336, 1978.
55. Hosey MM, Tao M: J Supramol Struct 6:61, 1977.
56. Roses AD, Appel SH: J Memb Biol 20:51, 1975.
57. Avruch J, Fairbanks G: Biochemistry 13:5507, 1974.
58. Whiteley NM, Berg HC: J Mol Biol 87:541, 1974.
59. Jenkins RE, Tanner MJA: Biochem J 147:393, 1975.
60. Steck TL, Dawson G: J Biol Chem 249:2135, 1974.
61. Kiehm DJ, Ji TH: J Biol Chem 252:8524, 1977.
62. Weinstein RS: In Surgenor DM (ed): "The Red Blood Cell." New York: Academic, 1974, vol 1, p 213.
63. Weinstein RS, Khodadad JK, Steck TL: In Brewer GJ (ed): "The Red Cell." New York: Alan R Liss, 1978. p 413.
64. Weinstein RS, Khodadad JK, Steck TL: J Supramol Struct (Suppl) 2:211, 1978.
65. Koziarz JJ, Köhler H, Steck TL: J Supramol Struct (Suppl) 2:215, 1978.
66. Tomita M, Marchesi VT: Proc Nat Acad Sci USA 72:2964, 1975.
67. Wickner W: Proc Nat Acad Sci USA 73:1159, 1976.
68. Miyakawa T, Takemoto LJ, Fox CF: J Supramol Struct 8:303–310, 1978.
69. Rothman JE, Lenard J: Science 195:743, 1977.
70. Blobel G, Dobberstein B: J Cell Biol 67:835, 1975.
71. Springer TA, Strominger JL: Proc Nat Acad Sci USA 73:2481, 1976.
72. Katz FN, Rothman JE, Lingappa VR, Blobel G, Lodish HF: Proc Nat Acad Sci USA 74:3278, 1977.
73. Maroux S, Louvard D: Biochim Biophys Acta 419:189, 1976.
74. Mueller TJ, Morrison M: J Biol Chem 252:6573, 1977.
75. Köhler H, Singh M, Steck TL, Murashige J: J Supramol Struct (Suppl) 2:211, 1978.
76. Singh MK, Köhler H, Steck TL: Fed Proc 37:1507, 1978.
77. Rubin CS, Rosenfeld RD, Rosen OM: Proc Nat Acad Sci USA 70:3735, 1973.
78. Shaklai N, Yguerabide J, Ranney HM: Biochemistry 16:5585, 5593, 1977.
79. Yu J, Branton D: Proc Nat Acad Sci USA 73:3891, 1976.
80. Shotten D, Thompson K, Wofsy L, Branton D: J Cell Biol 76:512, 1978.
81. Cherry RJ, Bürkli A, Busslinger M, Schneider G: Nature 263:389, 1976.
82. Bennett V, Branton D: J Biol Chem 252:2753, 1977.
83. Bennett V: J Biol Chem 253:2292, 1978.
84. Vogel F, Meyer HW, Grosse R, Repke KRH: Biochim Biophys Acta 470–497, 1977.
85. Stewart PS, MacLennan DH: J Biol Chem 249:985, 1974.
86. Liang S-M, Winter CG: J Biol Chem 252:8278, 1977.
87. Murphy AJ: Biochem Biophys Res Commun 70:160, 1976.
88. Bellhorn MB, Blumenfeld OO, Gallop PM: Biochem Biophys Res Commun 39:267, 1970.
89. Niday E, Wang C-S, Alaupovic P: Biochim Biophys Acta 469:180, 1977.

90. Lin S, Spudich JA: Biochem Biophys Res Commun 61:1471, 1974.
91. Kahlenberg A: J Biol Chem 251:1582, 1976.
92. Zala CA, Kahlenberg A: Biochem Biophys Res Commun 72:866, 1976.
93. Kasahara M, Hinkle PC: J Biol Chem 252:7384, 1977.
94. Batt ER, Abbott RE, Schachter D: J Biol Chem 251:7184, 1976.
95. Lienhard GE, Gorga FR, Orasky JE Jr, Zocolli MA: Biochemistry 16:4921, 1977.
95a. Sogin DC, Hinkle PC: J Supramol Struct (In press).
95b. Zoccoli MA, Baldwin SA, Lienhard GE: J Supramol Struct, (Suppl) 2:216, 1978.
96. Avruch J, Fairbanks G: Proc Nat Acad Sci USA 69:1216, 1972.
97. Hoffman JF: J Gen Physiol 54:343, 1969.
98. Brown AP, Feinstein AB, Sha'afi RI: Nature 254:523, 1975.
99. Gunn RB: In Hoffman JF (ed): "Membrane Transport Processes." New York: Raven Press, 1978, vol 1, p 61.
100. Rothstein A, Cabantchik ZI, Knauf P: Fed Proc 35:3, 1976.
101. Cabantchik ZI, Knauf PA, Rothstein A: Biochim Biophys Acta (In press).
102. Rice WR, Steck TL: Biochim Biophys Acta 433:39, 1976.
103. Rice WR, Steck TL: Biochim Biophys Acta 468:305, 1977.
104. Kaplan JH, Scorah K, Fasold H, Passow H: FEBS Lett 62:182, 1976.
105. Zaki L, Fasold H, Schuhmann B, Passow H: J Cell Physiol 86:471, 1975.
106. Grinstein S, Ship S, Rothstein A: Biochim Biophys Acta 507:294, 1978.
107. Singer SJ: J Supramol Struct 6:313, 1977.
108. Gunn RB, Froehlich O: J Supramol Struct (Suppl)2:213, 1978.
109. Knauf PA, Fuhrmann GF, Rothstein S, Rothstein A: J Gen Physiol 69:363, 1977.
110. Rothstein A, Knauf PA, Grinstein S, Shami Y: In Lux S, Marchesi VT, Fox CF (eds): "Normal and Abnormal Red Cell Membranes." New York: Alan R Liss (In press).

Journal of Supramolecular Structure 8:325–335 (1978)
Normal and Abnormal Red Cell Membranes 47–57

Fine Structure of the Band 3 Protein in Human Red Cell Membranes: Freeze-Fracture Studies

Ronald S. Weinstein, Jena K. Khodadad, and Theodore L. Steck

Department of Pathology, Rush Medical College and Rush-Presbyterian-St Luke's Medical Center, Chicago, Illinois 60612 (R.S.W., J.K.K.); and Departments of Biochemistry and Medicine, The University of Chicago, Chicago, Illinois 60637 (T.L.S.)

The major red cell membrane protein, band 3, is a glycoprotein which extends across the membrane from the extracellular space into the cytoplasmic compartment. It is widely held that band 3 is a component of the intramembrane particles (IMP) which can be demonstrated by freeze-fracture electron microscopy. In this study, we find that the outer surface poles of the IMP can be seen by freeze-etching after they are unmasked by proteolysis under conditions which excise the surrounding sialopeptides from the membrane. The poles appear as distinctive projections, 30–50 Å in diameter, the "ES particles." The ES particles remain associated with the outer surface of the membrane following cleavage of the band 3 polypeptide by chymotrypsin or pronase. This is consistent with previous biochemical studies which have shown that the 38,000-dalton outer surface segment of band 3 is intercalated in the lipid bilayer. A granulofibrillar component at the inner surface of the membrane is provisionally identified as the 40,000-dalton inner-surface domain of band 3.

Key words: **band 3 protein; freeze-fracture electron microscopy; glyceraldehyde-3 phosphate dehydrogenase; integral membrane protein; intramembrane particle; membrane proteins, unmasking; spectrin**

The band 3 polypeptide demonstrated on polyacrylamide gels represents the major protein constituent of the red cell membrane. It comprises approximately one-quarter of the total membrane protein [1] and exists in the membrane as a noncovalent dimer [2–4]. The 93,000-dalton band 3 polypeptide can be proteolytically dissected into three large subfragments. These have been partially characterized and consist of outer-surface, transmembrane, and cytoplasmic surface domains with apparent molecular weights of approximately 38,000, 17,000, and 40,000 daltons respectively (Fig 1) [5, 6]. The fragment generated at the outer surface is a glycopeptide which intercalates into the bilayer, where it is anchored by hydrophobic associations. It remains firmly embedded within the lipid bilayer after proteolysis; however, the association of this segment with the remainder of the molecule is unknown. The transmembrane segment extends through the

Received for publication April 20, 1978; accepted April 28, 1978.

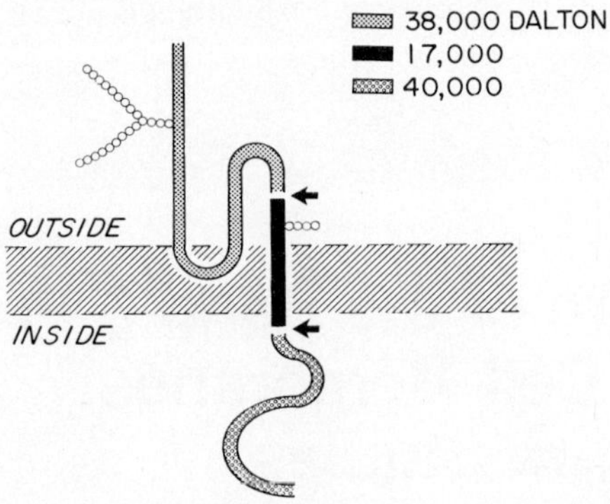

Fig 1. Highly schematic representation of the red cell protein band 3 showing the disposition of three large subfragments which are generated by proteolysis with chymotrypsin. Arrows indicate the sites of proteolysis. This is based on biochemical data reviewed by Steck [22] and ultrastructural data described in this paper.

hydrophobic core of membrane and can only be liberated from the bilayer with detergents. In contrast, the inner cytoplasmic domain is readily released from the membrane by proteolysis [5, 6].

Although the three-dimensional configuration of the band 3 protein within the membrane is unknown at the present time, it is established that this polypeptide spans the membrane asymmetrically and that it extends into the aqueous compartments at both membrane surfaces [1]. The studies described below represent an effort to visualize the morphologic counterparts of the band 3 polypeptide at the outer and inner membrane surfaces by freeze-fracture deep-etch electron microscopy.

MATERIALS AND METHODS

Red Blood Cells

Blood was obtained by venipuncture from a single human donor (TLS), washed three times with 150 mM NaC1–5 mM sodium phosphate buffer, and processed immediately for ultrastructural and biochemical analyses. The results of some experiments were confirmed on outdated blood from the blood bank. Unless otherwise stated, experimental procedures were performed at 0–5°C, and centrifugations were performed in a Sorvall SS-34 rotor.

Ghosts and Vesicles

Sealed ghosts were prepared by lysing red cells in 40 volumes of 5 mM sodium phosphate buffer (pH 8). After centrifugation, the pellet was incubated in an equal volume of 0.3 M NaC1–10 mM Na phosphate buffer (pH 8) at 37°C for 1 h and washed twice in 150 mM NaC1–5 mM sodium phosphate buffer. Unsealed ghosts were prepared by lysing cells in 40 volumes of 5 mM sodium phosphate buffer (pH 8) and washing twice in the same buffer [7, 8]. To prepare inside-out (IO) vesicles, open ghost pellets were mixed with 39 volumes of 0.5 mM sodium phosphate buffer (pH 8.3). After 30 min on ice, the suspension was centrifuged at 15,000 rpm for 30 min. The supernatant was removed and the pellets were incubated overnight at 5°. Pellets were homogenized by five passes through a 27-gauge hypodermic needle [7, 9]. Aliquots (1.2 ml) of homogenate were layered over a 2-ml barrier of Dextran 110 (Pharmacia) in 0.5 mM sodium phosphate buffer (pH 8) (density 1.01 g/ml). The samples were centrifuged at 15,000 rpm for 1 h at 5°. The band at the top of the dextran barrier was taken to be the IO vesicle fraction. The membranes were washed in 0.5 mM sodium phosphate buffer (pH 8.0) by centrifugation at 18,000 rpm for 30 min. The pellet was resuspended in a small volume of 0.5 mM sodium phosphate buffer (pH 8.0). Acetylcholinesterase and glyceraldehyde-3-phosphate dehydrogenase (G3PD) accessibility in the input homogenate as well as in the gradient-purified IO vesicle fraction were quantified to estimate the percentage of vesicles of inside-out orientation [7, 9].

Proteolysis of Intact Cells, Ghosts, and Vesicles

Packed suspensions of intact red cells, ghosts, or vesicles were digested for 1 h with an equal volume of fresh chymotrypsin (Sigma) or trypsin (Worthington) at a final concentration of 0.1 or 1.0 mg/ml. Diisopropylfluorophosphate (DFP: Sigma) was added (to a final concentration of 1 mM for red cells and ghosts and 0.5 mM for IO vesicles) to terminate enzyme activity. Other experiments were performed with pronase (Sigma) at a final concentration of 1 mg/ml. Following proteolysis, membrane preparations were incubated at 0°, 23°, or 37°C for 1–4 hours to enhance IMP clustering. Aliquots of each sample were taken for SDS-polyacrylamide gel electrophoresis, performed according to Fairbanks, Steck, and Wallach [8], as modified by Steck and Yu [10].

Freeze-Fracture Electron Microscopy

Samples were fixed in PBS-buffered 1% glutaraldehyde (pH 8.0) at 0°C for 30 min, and then washed three times in distilled water. Specimens were placed either in 20% glycerol or water and rapidly quenched in Freon 22 to –150°C [11]. Freeze fracturing and freeze etching were done in a Balzer Model BAF 301 freeze-etch unit. The stage temperature was maintained at –100° for 60–90 sec for deep etching. Replication was with platinum-carbon for 1 sec at a 45° angle, followed by carbon coating for 10–12 sec. Some specimens were rotary-shadowed at a 25° angle, with a Balzers rotary shadowing unit [12]. Replicas were floated on saline, cleaned with Chlorox, rinsed in water, and collected on 100-mesh copper grids. Replicas were photographed in either a Philips EM-300 or 301 electron microscope. For measurements of intramembrane particle diameters, electron micrographs of unidirectionally shadowed membranes were printed at a final magnification of 150,000 ×. Measurements were made perpendicular to the direction of platinum shadowing for 200–300 consecutive particles.

RESULTS

Effects of Proteolysis on Electrophorograms

Gel electrophoresis of red cell ghosts and IO vesicles dissolved in SDS showed that band 3 is not diminished by the vesiculation procedure, although the amount of spectrin (bands 1 and 2) is markedly reduced. Proteolysis of unsealed ghosts and IO vesicles with chymotrypsin or trypsin (0.1 or 1.0 mg/ml) at 0° for 1 h produced extensive digestion of the major membrane proteins (Fig 2).

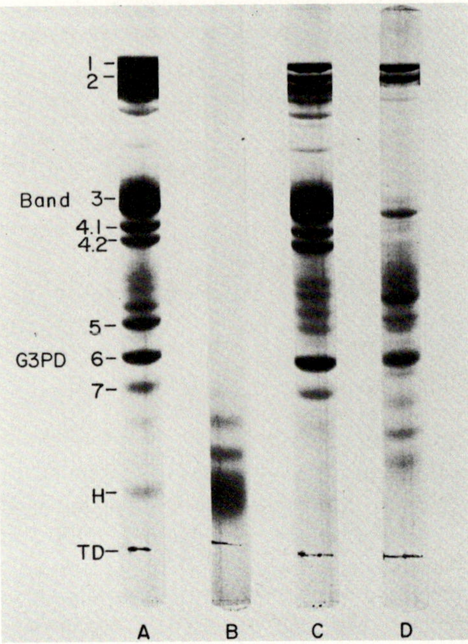

Fig 2. SDS-polyacrylamide gels of membrane preparations. H) residual hemoglobin; TD) tracking dye. Gel A, fresh ghosts. Gel B, unsealed ghosts digested with chymotrypsin (1 mg/ml) for 1 h at 0°C; there is extensive digestion of all major membrane proteins. Gel C, sealed inside-out vesicle fraction. Acetylcholinesterase [7] and G3PD accessibility assays [9] demonstrated that 88% of the vesicles had an inside-out orientation. The remainder were right-side-out vesicles. Most of the spectrin (bands 1 and 2) and actin (band 5) have been eluted. Gel D, sealed inside-out vesicle fraction digested with trypsin (5 μg/ml) for 1 h at 0°. Band 3 is markedly reduced. The residual band 3 protein may be in right-side-out vesicles which contaminate the fraction.

Freeze-Fractured Red Cell Membranes

Four membrane surfaces are revealed by freeze-fracture electron microscopy. According to recently standardized nomenclature, the natural surfaces of the membrane are designated ES for the extracellular or outer surface, and PS for the protoplasmic or inner surface [13]. The fracturing process generates two novel surfaces: PF, the fracture face of the protoplasmic leaflet of the membrane; and EF, the fracture face of the extracellular leaflet of the membrane. The two fracture faces bear populations of intramembrane particles (IMP), designated IMP_P on PF and IMP_E on EF surfaces [14, 15]. An asymmetrical distribution of the IMP persists when membranes are fragmented into right-side-out and inside-out vesicles and thus serves as a useful marker of membrane orientation [16].

Ultrastructure of Intramembrane Particles

In high-quality replicas of intact red cell membranes, the IMP_P and IMP_E appeared somewhat pleomorphic. In unidirectionally shadowed replicas, there was variability in the apparent diameters of the IMP_P (Fig 3), although this could occur if the IMP are asymmetrical. However, this variability of diameters was also observed in rotary-shadowed preparations in which the majority of IMP_P appeared symmetrical in the plane of the membrane (Fig 4). Therefore, the variability cannot be ascribed to IMP asymmetry alone.

Measurements of IMP diameters confirmed the impression that the IMP are somewhat variable in size as is reflected in the standard deviations of the measurements. In 1% glutaraldehyde-fixed, glycerinated intact red cells, the mean IMP_P diameter was 66 ± 12 Å (±SD). The mean diameter of IMP_E was 74 ± 13 Å. Although the large majority of IMP on a given fracture face fall within a relatively narrow size range, there may be subpopulations which have a different morphology. This was supported by the demonstration of previously undescribed short rods at fracture faces by rotary shadowing (Fig 4).

The ultrastructure of the IMP in isolated red cell membranes was examined before and after protease digestion. Proteolysis with chymotrypsin, trypsin, and pronase cleaved the membrane polypeptides into small segments and released 50–80% of the protein from the membrane. However, the IMP remained morphologically intact (Figs 5–8).

IMP clustering was not observed in intact red cells, although there was occasionally mild clustering in undigested isolated ghost membranes. Proteolysis of isolated membranes at 0° produced significant clustering, which was enhanced by incubation of isolated membranes at 23° or 37° either during or subsequent to proteolysis. Proteolysis of intact human cells did not induce a redistribution of IMP_P.

Unmasking of the Outer Surface Pole of the IMP

The extracellular surface (E surface) of deep-etched intact red cells, isolated membranes, and IO vesicles appeared smooth or finely granular (Fig 5). There was a suggestion

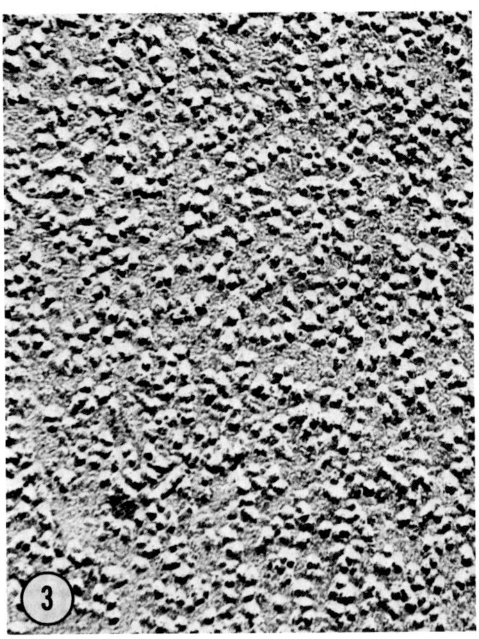

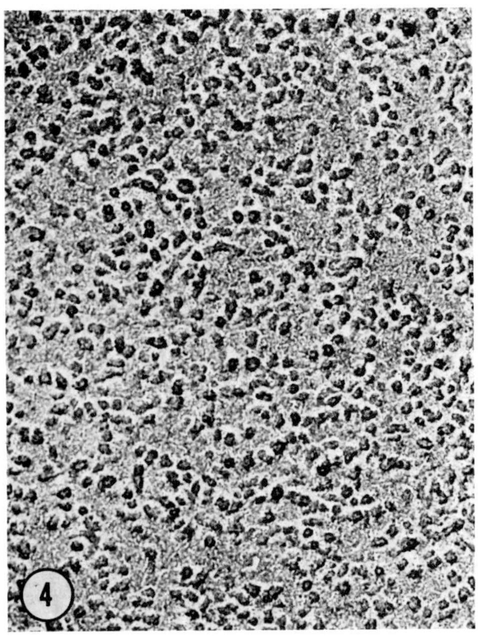

Fig 3. Electron micrograph of the PF surface of a human red cell fixed in 1% glutaraldehyde and glycerinated prior to freeze-fracturing. The surface was unidirectionally shadowed with platinum-carbon at a 45° angle. The IMP_P vary in diameter and cast shadows of different lenghts (× 150,000).

Fig 4. PF surface of a human red cell prepared as in Figure 3 but rotary-shadowed at a 25° angle. The variability in IMP_P sizes is confirmed. In addition to the round particles, many short rods are demonstrated at the PF surface by rotary shadowing (× 150,000).

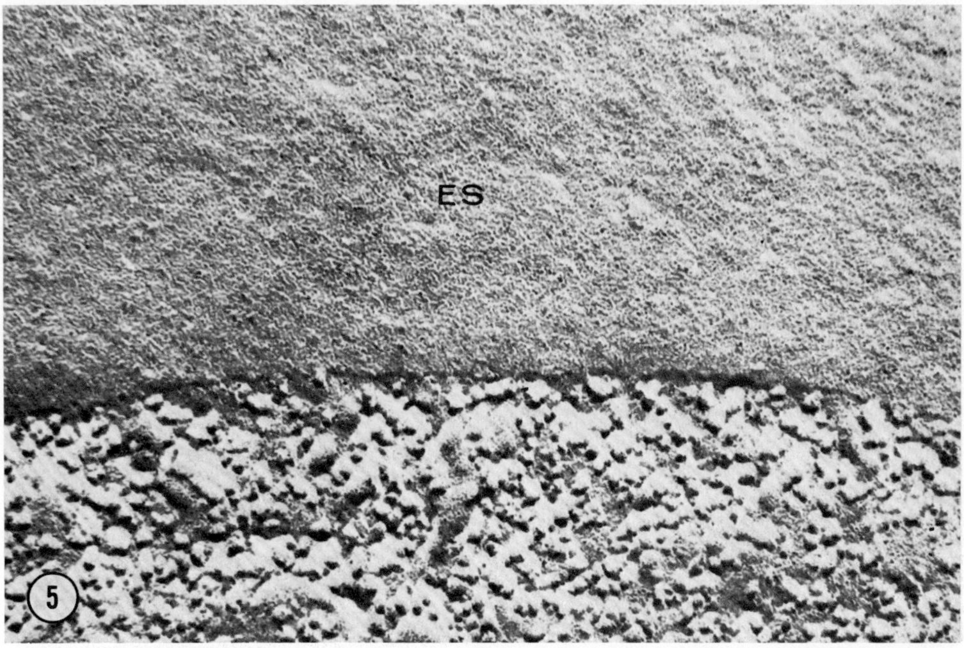

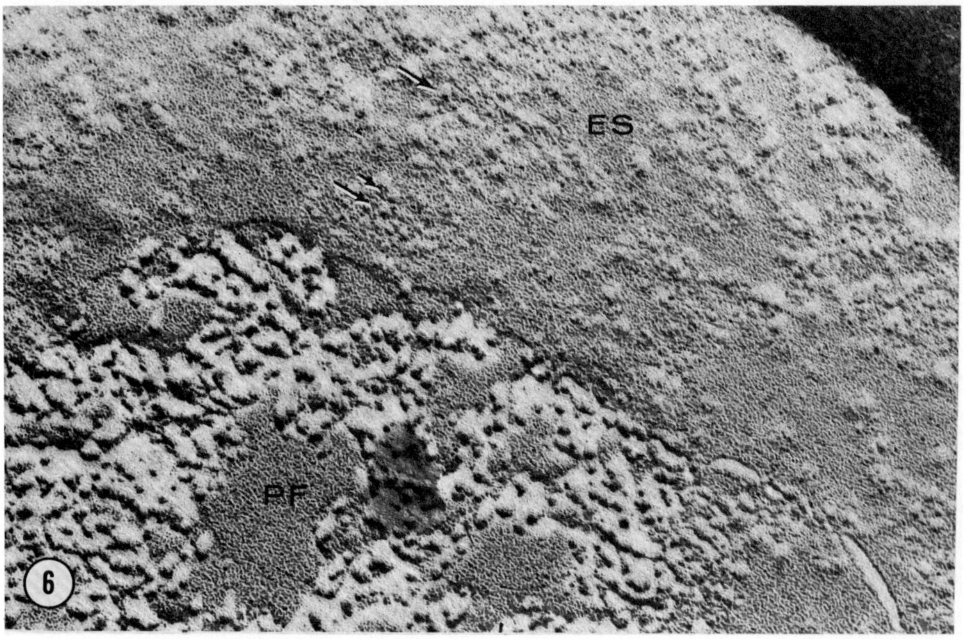

Fig 5. Freeze-fractured, deep-etched open ghost without proteolysis. The outer or extracellular surface (ES) of the membrane is nearly devoid of substructure. IMP_P (bottom) are non-clustered (× 156,000).

Fig 6. Open ghost following digestion with chymotrypsin (1 mg/ml) for 1 h at 0°C. Many 30- to 50-Å particles (arrows) are present at the E surface (ES). The ES particles are mildly clustered, as are the IMP_P at the P face (PF), following proteolysis at 0° (× 156,000).

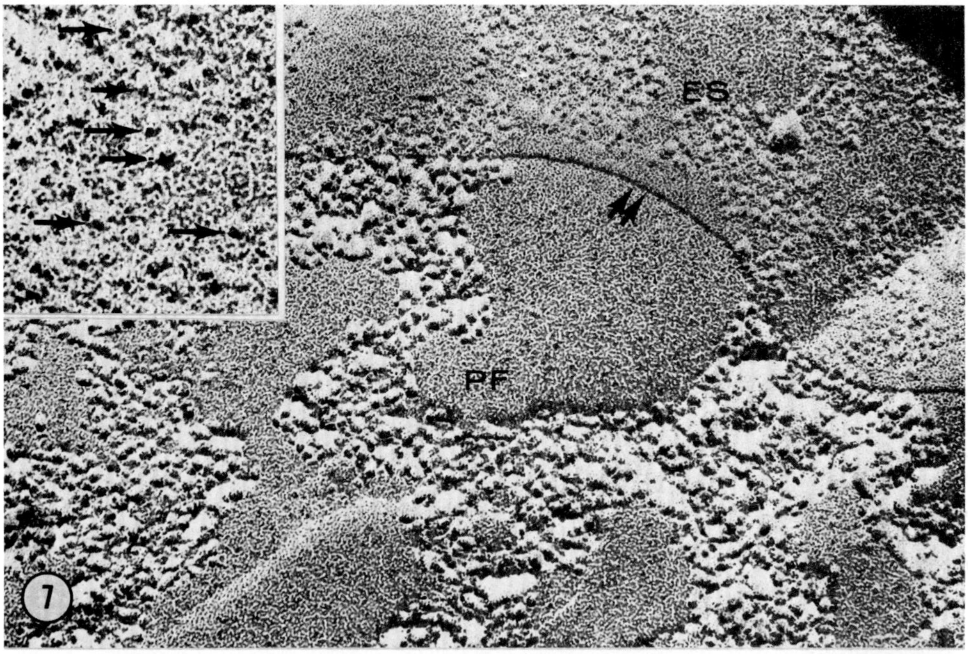

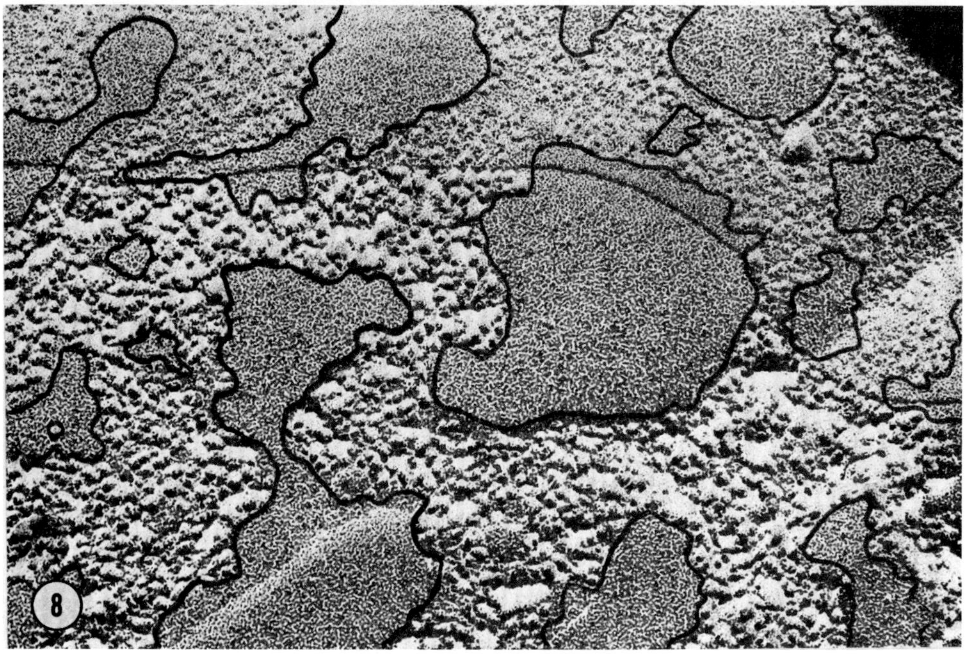

Fig 7. Top: Open ghost following digestion with pronase (1 mg/ml) at 0° for 4 h. Double arrows show where the fracture passes from the interior of the membrane (PF) to the extracellular surface (ES). The IMPp and the ES particles are clustered (× 156,000). Insert: High magnification of ES particles (arrows). The particles are small and cast long shadows (× 310,000).

Fig 8. Duplicate print of the electron micrograph in Figure 7 (× 156,000). Boundaries have been drawn with a pen between ES-particle-containing areas and smooth areas on the extracellular surface (ES), and between IMPp-rich areas and smooth areas on the protoplasmic face (PF). Particle-containing areas have the same topographical distribution at the PF and ES surfaces.

of discrete particles at the E surface, but particles casting long shadows were not observed. Amorphous mounds were present overlying the IMPp aggregates at the E surface of isolated membranes in which mild IMPp clustering was induced by incubation at 37°C in the absence of protease [15].

A discrete population of 30- to 50-Å particles, designated ES particles, was observed at the outer surface of the membranes following proteolysis (Figs 6, 7). These ES particles cast long shadows, indicating that the structures they represent project well above the adjacent membrane. The ES particles were somewhat difficult to quantitate in freeze-fracture replicas because of their small size, but they appear to be represented in numbers similar to the IMPp (Weinstein, Khodadad, and Steck, manuscript in preparation). Their topography also closely resembled that of the IMPp (Figs 7, 8). Based upon these observations, we can hypothesize that the ES particles are the outer surface poles of the IMPp, revealed by proteolysis.

Since the IMPp have been ascribed to band 3, it follows that the ES particles may contain the outer surface domain of the molecule. It is conceivable that following proteolysis, the constituent polypeptides of the IMPp and ES particles might be dissociated by lateral diffusion in the membrane if they are merely linked covalently (Fig 9). Therefore, we subjected isolated red cell membranes to proteolytic digestion with pronase or chymotrypsin at 0° under conditions which cleave every copy of band 3. Following proteolysis, we encouraged the differential redistribution of the IMPp and ES particles by incubating the digested membranes at 23° or 37° for up to 4 h. The two populations of particles consistently cosegregated, implying that there are stable noncovalent associations between the IMPp and the ES particles. Furthermore, that segment of the band 3 polypeptide represented in the ES particles may contribute to the image of the IMPp. The emergence of ES particles following proteolysis is consistent with the observation that IMPp morphology is unaffected by such treatment.

Band 3 at the Protoplasmic Surface

In an attempt to visualize band 3 protein at the protoplasmic surface (P surface) of the membrane, we examined deep-etched inside-out vesicles which were depleted of nearly all of their spectrin and actin. The P surface of the vesicles contained two prominent components: a granulofibrillar component; and a population of discrete particles (PS particles) having an average diameter of approximately 90 Å (Fig 10). Digestion with trypsin, chymotrypsin, or pronase under conditions which result in the release of the 40,000-dalton segment of band 3 from the cytoplasmic surface, without producing a further reduction in residual spectrin and actin, also caused the removal of the granulofibrillar component leaving intact the 90-Å PS particles (Fig 11).

DISCUSSION

These freeze-fracture studies support the view that the red cell membrane protein band 3 is a component of the IMPp as postulated previously by many other investigators [1, 17–19]. In the past, it has been difficult to reconcile the relatively flat, structureless appearance of the outer surface of the red cell membrane with the concept of glycopeptides extending into the extracellular compartment [14]. A number of explanations which might account for the lack of detailed structure at the outer surface of the mem-

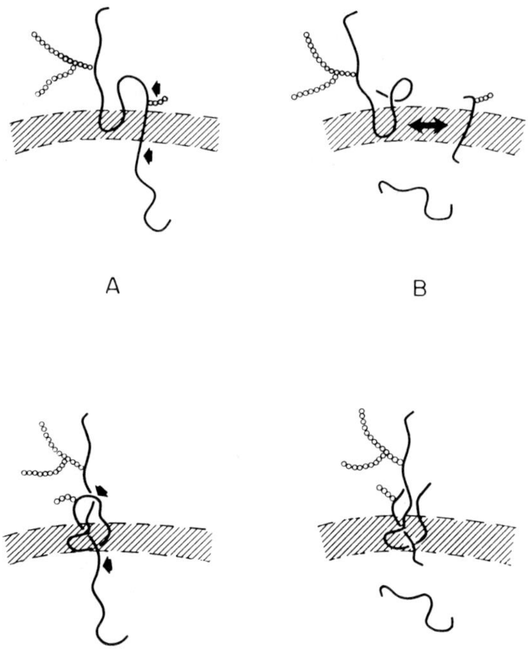

A B C D

Fig 9. Scheme depicting two possible fates of a proteolytically cleaved glycoprotein, corresponding to the IMP and the ES particles which are visualized by freeze-fracture and deep-etch electron microscopy. A) Glycoprotein *without* noncovalent associations between the extracellular and transmembrane domains of the polypeptide. Arrows show the locations of extracellular and intracellular protease-sensitive sites. B) Molecule corresponding to "A" following proteolysis. The extracellular domain has dissociated from the membrane-spanning segment, but remains intercalated in the lipid bilayer. The inner surface segment, which does not intercalate into the bilayer, is shed. C) Glycoprotein *with* noncovalent associations between the extracellular and transmembrane domains of the polypeptide. Arrows show the locations of protease-sensitive sites. D) Molecule corresponding to "C" following proteolysis. The extracellular domain remains noncovalently associated with the transmembrane domain. The inner surface segment is shed.

brane have been considered on theoretical grounds, but none have been fully substantiated experimentally [20].

We have now demonstrated that a distinctive particulate component, the ES particle, can be "unmasked" at the outer surface of the red cell membrane by proteolysis. There are several observations which indicate that these outer surface particles and the IMP_P are structurally related. First, the ES particles appear to overlie the IMP_P and coaggregate with them when IMP_P clustering is produced experimentally. Secondly, these two populations of particles seem to be present in approximately equivalent numbers, although precise quantitation of the ES particles is difficult because of their small size. These observations suggest that the ES particles may be the outer surface poles of the IMP_P. If the band 3 polypeptide is represented in the IMP_P (an idea which is consistent with available evidence), then the band 3 molecule is likely to be a component of the ES particles as well.

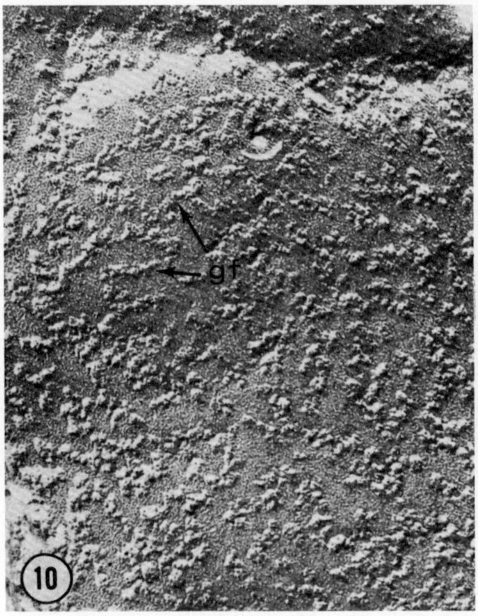

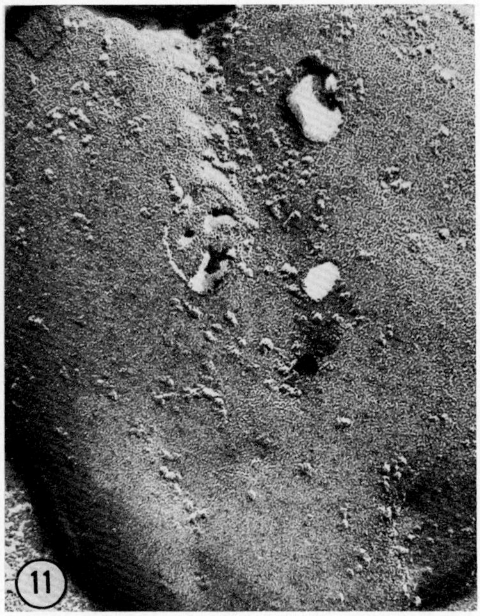

Fig 10. P surface of an inside-out vesicle. A granulofibrillar component (gf) is prominent on this deep-etched surface. PS particles are present, but are relatively inconspicuous prior to proteolysis (× 110,000).

Fig 11. Inside-out vesicle after digestion with trypsin (5 μg/ml). The granulofibrillar component of the P surface (inner surface) of the membrane has been cleaved away. Protease-resistant 90-Å particles are prominent after trypsinization has removed the granulofibrillar component (× 110,000).

The mechanism by which partial proteolysis reveals the ES particles is uncertain. However, there are several possibilities that merit discussion. The first possibility is that the ES particles represent residual proteolytic enzymes; this possibility was eliminated by polyacrylamide gel electrophoresis of SDS-solubilized membranes. Bands corresponding to the molecular weights of trypsin, chymotrypsin, and pronase were not represented on these gels. A second possibility is that the emergence of ES particles is due to an intramolecular rearrangement of partially digested band 3 molecules. This is unlikely because the ES particles are made visible by proteolysis of resealed ghosts by trypsin under conditions which do not permit cleavage of the band 3 polypeptide [5, 6, 21]. A third possibility is that proteolytically sensitive sialoglycoproteins are released from the membrane, unmasking the stable outer surface domains of band 3. This explanation is the most plausible in view of the differential sensitivity of band 3 and sialoglycoproteins to proteolysis at the extracellular surface of the cell [21].

Several lines of evidence support the hypothesis that the granulofibrillar component at the inner surface of the membrane contains the 40,000-dalton intracytoplasmic extension of the band 3 polypeptide.

1. The granulofibrillar component persists after all peripheral membrane proteins, including spectrin and actin, are removed from vesicle membranes with either dimethylmaleicanhydride or para-chloromercuribenzene sulfonate [15].

2. The granulofibrillar component can be selectively decorated with glyceraldehyde-3-phosphate dehydrogenase (G3PD) [15], which binds exclusively to the cytoplasmic

domain of band 3 [3]; with proteolysis, binding as well as decoration with G3PD is abolished concomitantly with the release of the 40,000-dalton fragment.

3. The band 3 polypeptide and the granulofibrillar component are both exquisitely sensitive to proteolysis.

4. The topographical distribution of the granulofibrillar component of the PS array at the inner surface of the membrane and the IMP_P within the membrane are similar.

In summary, proteolytic digestion has different effects on the ultrastructure of the outer surface, the inner surface, and the interior of the red cell membrane. The images of individual IMP_P are unaffected by proteolysis at 0°. Structures which we have tentatively identified as the outer surface projections of the IMP_P, the ES particles, become apparent after proteolysis, whereas the corresponding PS projections, the granulofibrillar component, disappears. This behavior can be accounted for by current knowledge of the disposition of the band 3 polypeptide in the membrane (see Steck [22]).

ACKNOWLEDGMENTS

This study was supported by funds from the Otho S.A. Sprague Memorial Institute, contract No. N00014-C-0596 from the Office of Naval Research, and grant No. BC-95 E and F from the American Cancer Society.

The excellent technical assistance of Ms Elaine Sundin, Mrs Benita Ramos, and Mr William Leonard is gratefully acknowledged. We also wish to thank Ms Jayne Adams for the photography.

REFERENCES

1. Steck TL: J Cell Biol 62:1, 1974.
2. Steck TL: J Mol Biol 66:295, 1972.
3. Yu J, Steck TL: J Biol Chem 250:9176, 1975.
4. Peters K, Richards FM: Ann Rev Biochem 46:5232, 1977.
5. Steck TL, Ramos B, Strapazon E: Biochemistry 15:1154, 1976.
6. Steck TL, Koziarz JJ, Singh MK, Reddy G, Köhler H: Biochemistry 17:216, 1978.
7. Steck TL: Methods Memb Biol 2:245, 1974.
8. Fairbanks G, Steck TL, Wallach DFH: Biochemistry 10:2606, 1971.
9. Steck TL, Kant JA: Meth Enzymol 31:172, 1974.
10. Steck TL, Yu J: J Supramol Struct 1:220, 1973.
11. Moor H: Int Rev Exp Pathol 5:179, 1966.
12. Margaritis LH, Elgsaeter A, Branton D: J Cell Biol 72:47, 1977.
13. Branton D, Bullivant S, Gilula NB, Karnovsky MJ, Moor H, Mühlethaler K, Northcote DH, Packer L, Satir B, Satir P, Speth V,Staehelin LA, Steere RL, Weinstein RS: Science 190:54, 1975.
14. Weinstein RS: Cancer Res 36:2518, 1976.
15. Weinstein RS, Khodadad JK, Steck TL: In Brewer G (ed): "The Red Cell." New York: Alan R. Liss, 1978, pp 413–427.
16. Steck TL, Weinstein RS, Straus JH, Wallach DFH: Science 168:255, 1970.
17. Guidotti G: Ann Rev Biochem 41:731, 1972.
18. Yu J, Branton D: Proc Nat Acad Sci USA 73:3891, 1976.
19. Cherry RJ, Burkli A, Busslinger M, Schneider G, Parish GR: Nature (London) 263:389, 1976.
20. Weinstein RS: In Surgenor D MacN (ed): "The Red Blood Cell." New York: Academic, 1974, pp 213–268.
21. Steck TL: In Fox CF (ed): "Membrane Research." New York: Academic, 1972, p 71.
22. Steck TL: J Supramol Struct 8:311, 1978.

Journal of Supramolecular Structure 8:337–347 (1978)
Normal and Abnormal Red Cell Membranes 59–69

Distribution of Glycophorin on the Surface of Human Erythrocyte Membranes and Its Association With Intramembrane Particles: An Immunochemical and Freeze-Fracture Study of Normal and En(a–) Erythrocytes

Carl G. Gahmberg, Georg Tauren, Ismo Virtanen, and Jorma Wartiovaara

Department of Bacteriology and Immunology (C.G.G., G.T.), and Department of Pathology (I.V., J.W.), University of Helsinki, Haartmaninkatu 3, 00290 Helsinki 29; and Department of Electron Microscopy, University of Helsinki, Malminkatu 20, 00100 Helsinki 10, Finalnd (I.V., J.W.)

Human erythrocyte membranes of the En(a–) blood group lack the major sialoglycoprotein (glycophorin). By absorption of a crude antiglycophorin antiserum with En(a–) membranes a specific antiglycophorin antiserum was obtained. By immune electron microscopy we showed that glycophorin is randomly distributed on the surface of normal erythrocytes. When polycationized ferritin, which mainly binds to glycophorin, was used as a marker a similar even labeling of normal erythrocyte membranes was seen. En(a–) membranes bound much less of this marker. In freeze-fracturing the intramembrane particles of both membrane types had a similar distribution and appeared in equal amounts. However, partial removal of spectrin from these membranes, followed by incubation at pH 6 resulted in more extensive aggregation of the particles in En(a–) membranes than in normal membranes. The results may be interpreted as glycophorin contributing by electrostatic repulsion to the random distribution of the intramembrane particles in normal cells. This repulsion is weakened in En(a–) cells by the lack of glycophorin.

Key words: **erythrocyte membranes, glycophorin, intramembrane particles**

The human erythrocyte membrane has been extensively studied and serves as a model for plasma membranes in general [1–3]. It contains four major integral glycoproteins and many minor glycoproteins [4, 5], which have their carbohydrate located only on the outside [6–8] and many if not all of the glycoproteins penetrate the membrane [9, 10]. The major sialoglycoprotein, PAS 1 [4] or glycophorin [11], contains 60%

Received for publication March 5, 1978; accepted April 4, 1978.

0091-7419/78/0803-0337$02.30

carbohydrate, including a large proportion of the sialic acid of the cell. Though its primary structure has been determined [12] its physiologic function remains unclear.

The exact arrangement of glycophorin in the membrane is unknown. Attempts to localize glycophorin have been made using polycationized ferritin [13], influenza virus [14], and phytohemagglutinin [11, 14], but the results were complicated by the possible binding of these reagents to surface molecules other than glycophorin.

The major integral glycoprotein, band 3 [4], contains a few percent carbohydrate with little or no sialic acid [15–17]. It probably exists as a dimer in the membrane [18] and constitutes 20–25% of the membrane protein. It is probably involved in transport of anions [16, 19] and possibly in glucose transport through the membrane [20].

When membranes are freeze-fractured along their hydrophobic interior, characteristic intramembrane particles (IMP) are seen [21]. These are probably formed by integral glycoproteins and in the erythrocyte membrane mainly band 3 and glycophorin have been claimed to constitute the particles [22, 23].

We and others recently found that the membrane of the rare human blood group En(a–) [24, 25] lacks glycophorin [17, 26, 27]. We have taken advantage of this fact to obtain a specific antiglycophorin antiserum by absorption of a crude antiserum with En(a–) membranes. We here report that glycophorin is randomly distributed on the cell surface both when studied by an immunoferritin technique and with polycationized ferritin. In addition we have found that the distribution of the IMPs of En(a–) cells and normal cells is identical in isolated ghosts, but when spectrin [28] is partially removed, the IMPs more easily form aggregates in En(a–) membranes than in normal membranes.

METHODS

Cells

Normal human erythrocytes (AB Rh+) and En(a–) erythrocytes (AB Rh+) were obtained through the Finnish Red Cross Blood Transfusion Service, Helsinki. The cells were processed within two weeks of blood donation.

Surface Labeling of Cells and Isolation of Membranes

Normal and En(a–) erythrocytes were labeled by the neuraminidase-galactose oxidase/NaB^3H_4 technique [7, 17]. Membranes were isolated and aliquots counted for radioactivity as described previously [7].

Production of Antiglycophorin Antiserum

A glycophorin preparation was isolated from normal erythrocytes by chloroform-methanol extraction [29]. One major band was present on gel electrophoresis in the presence of sodium dodecyl sulfate (SDS) with an apparent molecular weight of 85,000. Rabbits were immunized three times at two-week intervals subcutaneously with 0.5 mg of this preparation in 0.5 ml of PBS (0.15 M NaCl–0.01 M sodium phosphate, pH 7.4) emulsified in 1 ml of Freund's adjuvant (Difco). Ten days after the last injection the rabbits were bled. One milliliter of the serum was absorbed two times with 1 ml of packed En(a–) membranes at 4°C for 24 h. After absorption the serum was centrifuged at 100,000g for 1 h and stored at 4°C with 0.02% sodium azide.

Immunoprecipitations With Protein A-Containing Staphylococcus aureus Strain Cowan I

Normal and En(a–) erythrocyte membranes, labeled by the neuraminidase-galactose oxidase/NaB^3H_4 technique, were solubilized in PBS containing 1% Triton X-100, 2 mM phenylmethylsulfonyl fluoride (Sigma), and 1% ethanol. The samples were centrifuged at 10,000g for 30 min and the supernatants recovered. To 0.2 ml of these were added 5 μg mouse IgG and 5 μl of rabbit anti-mouse IgG antiserum, prepared by standard techniques. All subsequent incubations were done at 0°C. After 1 h, 100 μl of a 10% suspension of Staphylococcus aureus Cowan I strain (obtained from Dr P. Landwall, Stockholm) [30] was added and the tubes incubated for 30 min. The samples were then centrifuged at 3,000 rpm for 10 min and the supernatants recovered. Five μl of the antiglycophorin antiserum or preimmunization serum was added and the tubes incubated for 2 h. Then 0.2 ml of the staphylococcal suspension was added and the incubation continued for 1 h. The bacteria were then washed three times in the Triton X-100-containing buffer, and the proteins eluted from the staphylococci by boiling in 1% SDS for 1 min.

Polyacrylamide Gel Electrophoresis

Membrane or protein samples were dissolved in electrophoresis sample buffer, boiled for 2 min, and electrophoresed on 8% cylindrical acrylamide gels according to Laemmli [31] The cylindrical gels were sliced and counted after NCS solubilization [7] or stained according to Weber and Osborn [32].

Immunoelectron Microscopy

Sheep anti-rabbit IgG, purified by affinity chromatography on Sepharose 4 B-coupled rabbit IgG [33], was conjugated to ferritin (Sigma) using the two-step method of Otto, Takamiya, and Vogt [34] as described earlier [35]. For immunoelectron microscopy the erythrocytes and the membranes were first reacted with the antiglycophorin antiserum (10 μl/0.1 ml packed cells or membranes) for 60 min at 0°C. The specimens were then washed three times in PBS and incubated with ferritin-conjugated anti-rabbit IgG for 60 min at 0°C. After washing three times in PBS, the samples were fixed at 0°C for 60 min in 2.5% glutaraldehyde buffered with 0.1 M sodium cacodylate at pH 7.2. After dehydration in ethanol the samples were embedded in Epon 812, thin-sectioned, poststained with uranyl acetate and lead citrate, and examined in a Jeol 100 B electron microscope.

Labeling of Cells With Polycationized Ferritin

The cells were labeled with polycationized ferritin (Miles-Yeda, Rehovoth, Israel) at a ferritin concentration of 0.1 mg/ml in PBS at 22°C for 60 min. Thereafter the cells were fixed in 2.5% glutaraldehyde buffered with 0.1 M sodium cacodylate (pH 7.2) for 60 min and processed for thin sectioning as described above.

Freeze-Fracturing Studies

The following samples of membranes were studied by freeze-fracturing: a) isolated membranes of normal and En(a–) cells left after isolation at 0°C; and b) membranes which were depleted of spectrin. Two different methods were used to achieve spectrin removal: 1) Normal and En(a–) membranes were incubated in a 50-fold volume of 0.1 mM ethylenediaminetetraacetate (EDTA), pH 8.0, at 4°C for 16 h [28]. After incubation the membranes were pelleted by centrifugation in a Sorvall centrifuge at 12,500 rpm for 30 min. The membranes were then incubated in PBS at 37°C for 30 min to achieve possible redistribution of the IMPs. 2) Membranes of both cell types were incubated for 16 h at 37°C in 20 mM sodium phosphate (pH 8.5) containing 0.02% sodium azide [36]. Thereafter the membranes were pelleted by centrifugation. The samples were pretreated for electron microscopy by incubation in 0.05 M sodium phosphate (pH 6.0) for 30 min. The membranes were fixed in 2.5% glutaraldehyde as above, washed twice with PBS, and impregnated with 30% glycerol in PBS at 4°C for 16 h. The samples of membrane suspensions were rapidly frozen in liquid Freon 22 cooled to its freezing point by liquid nitrogen. The freeze-fracture replicas were prepared in a Balzers 360 M apparatus by electron gun evaporation of Pt-C and C.

Protein Determinations

Protein was determined according to Lowry et al [37] with bovine serum albumin as a standard.

RESULTS

Surface Labeling of Normal and En(a–) Erythrocytes

Normal and En(a–) erythrocytes were surface-labeled and the membranes isolated and studied on cylindrical polyacrylamide gels. In normal cells PAS 1 (glycophorin dimer [38]) and PAS 2 (mainly glycophorin monomer) were strongly labeled (Fig 1 A), whereas these peaks were absent from En(a–) membranes (Fig 1 B). The mobility of band 3 from En(a–) membranes was slower and it was more strongly labeled than in normal membranes.

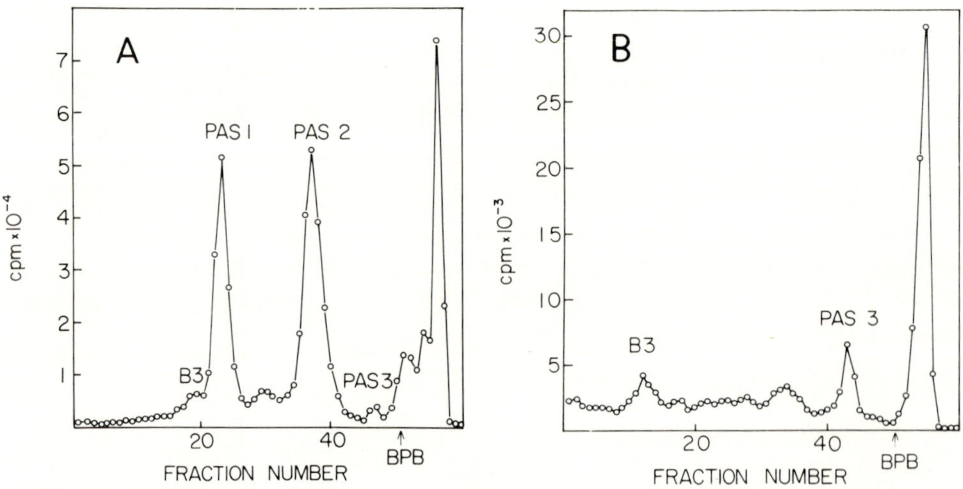

Fig 1. Polyacrylamide gel patterns of surface-labeled normal and En(a–) erythrocyte membranes. A) Pattern of normal membranes; B) pattern of En(a–) membranes. B3) band 3; PAS 1–3) the periodic acid-Schiff-positive sialoglycoproteins (PAS 1 = glycophorin dimer, PAS2 = glycophorin monomer (predominantly). BPB) position of bromophenol blue marker dye.

Distribution of Glycophorin in Normal Erythrocytes as Revealed by Immunoferritin Technique

Glycophorin was visualized by an indirect immunoferritin method using specific antiglycophorin antiserum. The specificity of the antiserum was shown as follows: When normal erythrocyte membranes were solubilized and treated with the antiglycophorin antiserum and were immune-precipitated with protein A-containing staphylococci and studied by polyacrylamide gel electrophoresis, the only peak observed corresponded to the monomer of glycophorin, or PAS 2 (Fig 2 A). No peak was obtained from labeled En(a–) membranes (Fig 2 B) nor did rabbit preimmunization serum precipitate any antigen from normal membranes (not shown). When normal erythrocytes were stained by the immunoferritin technique, ferritin particles were seen along the entire cell surface (Fig 3 A). Notably, when isolated membranes from normal erythrocytes were similarly labeled, a distinct asymmetric labeling of the membranes was observed on the external surface (Fig 3 B), judged from the fibrillar material marking the cytoplasmic face of the membranes.

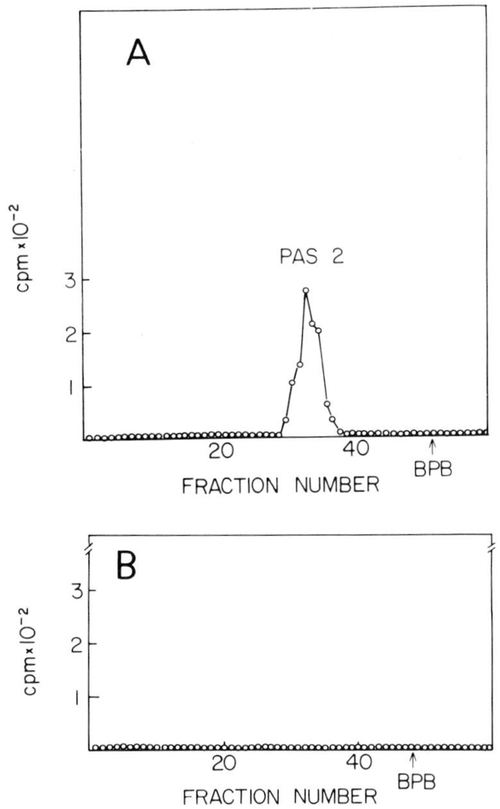

Fig 2. Polyacrylamide gel patterns of surface-labeled normal erythrocyte membranes precipitated with antiglycophorin antiserum and preimmunization serum. A) Pattern obtained from normal membranes after treatment with antiglycophorin antiserum and protein A-containing staphylococci; B) pattern obtained from normal membranes after treatment with preimmunization serum and staphylococci.

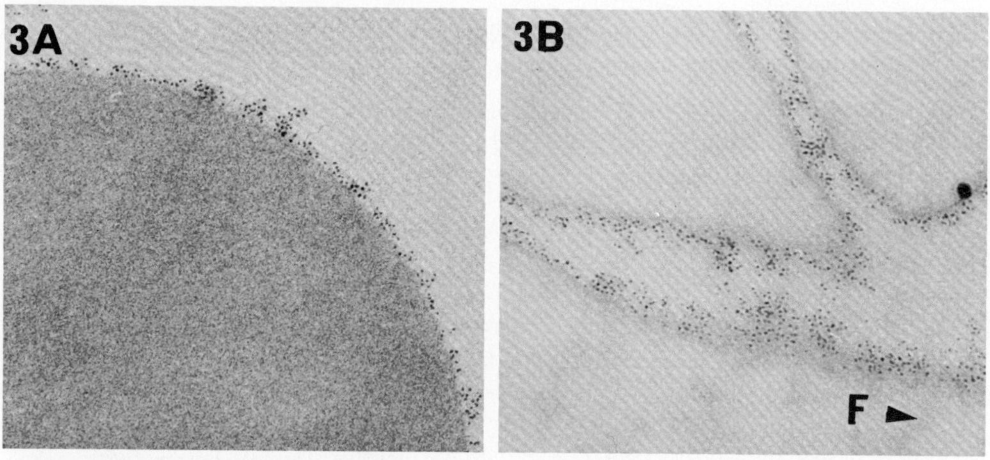

Fig 3. Visualization of glycophorin distribution by indirect immunoferritin technique. A) Normal erythrocyte surfaces are densely labeled with ferritin; B) isolated membranes of normal erythrocytes show label on the external membrane surface. Note the fibrillar material (F) indicating the cytoplasmic surface of the membranes. (Magnification 70,000 ×).

Distribution of Anionic Sites on Normal and En(a–) Membranes as Seen With Polycationized Ferritin

When normal erythrocytes were incubated with polycationized ferritin, a dense, uniform distribution of ferritin particles was seen on the cell surface (Fig 4). In contrast to this, En(a–) cells showed less binding and more uneven binding of the marker (Fig 5). The difference in the labeling of the two cell types was consistent and evident both in tangential (Fig 4 A, 5 A) and transverse (Fig 4 B, 5 B) sections of the membranes.

Distribution of Intramembrane Particles in Freeze-Fractured Membranes of Normal and En(a–) Erythrocytes

When erythrocyte membranes were freeze-fractured, a random distribution of intramembrane particles was seen both in normal (Fig 6A) and in En(a–) (Fig 6B) membranes. When spectrin was partially removed by incubation of the isolated membranes at 37°C in 20 mM sodium phosphate (pH 8.5) and the membranes were then transferred to pH 6.0 before freeze-fracturing, normal membranes showed a slight and variable aggregation of the intramembrane particles (Fig 6C), whereas the particles on En(a–) membranes were clearly and consistently more aggregated (Fig 6D). When membranes were depleted of spectrin by incubation with EDTA, they formed small vesicles. With this treatment there was an extensive aggregation of intramembrane particles in both normal (Fig 6E) and in En(a–) (Fig 6F) membranes.

DISCUSSION

The structure of glycophorin is remarkably well known. The primary structure of the polypeptide has been determined [12]. It contains three major regions, including a hydrophobic amino acid stretch, which probably is located within the lipid bilayer. The NH_2-terminal portion shows amino acid acid substitutions which depend on the MN antigen activity [39], and it carries the carbohydrate of the protein.

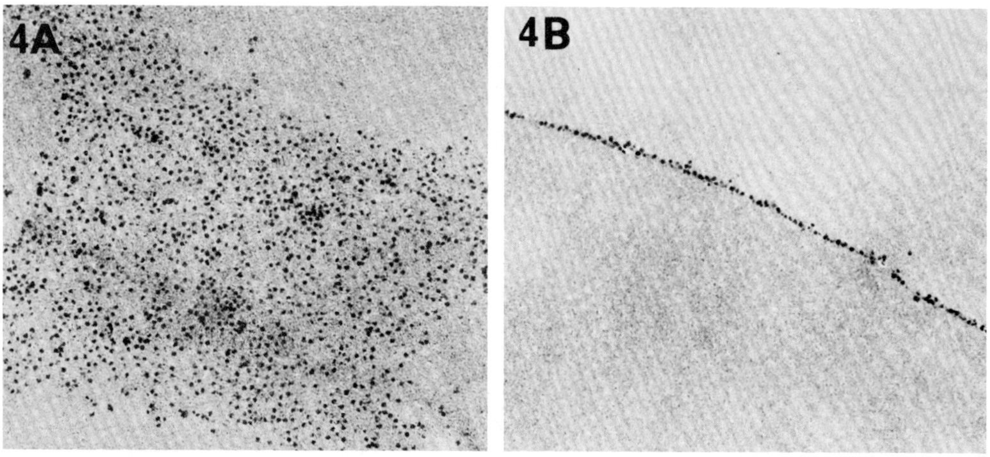

Fig 4. Normal erythrocyte membranes labeled with polycationized ferritin. A) In tangential section a dense and uniform labeling is seen; B) in transverse section a continuous labeling of the cell surface is evident. (Magnification 70,000 ×.)

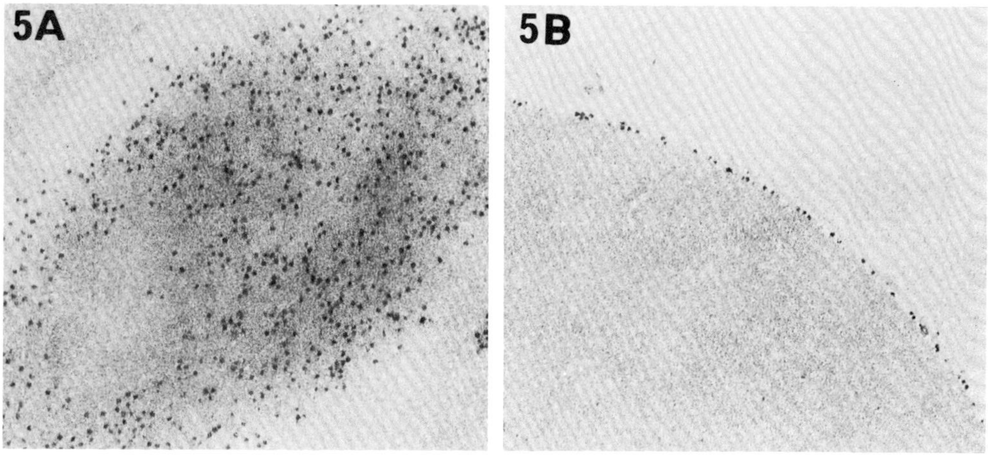

Fig 5. En(a–) erythrocytes labeled with polycationized ferritin. A) In tangential section a relatively sparse and more uneven labeling than in Figure 4A is evident; B) in transverse section a clearly discontinuous staining of the cell surface is seen. (Magnification 70,000 ×.)

The precise location of glycophorin in the membrane has been difficult to determine. We have approached this problem by the use of erythrocytes of the rare blood group En(a–). Erythrocyte membranes of this blood group lack glycophorin. This was first shown by protein staining and radioactive labeling techniques [17, 26, 27] and recently Furthmayr arrived at the same conclusion by use of a radioimmunologic method [39].

In the present experiments the polycationized ferritin marker was more sparsely distributed on the surface of En(a–) membranes than on normal membranes. The difference in the patterns of normal and En(a–) membranes should be due to glycophorin and it can be concluded that its surface distribution seems to be random. A similar result was obtained with the indirect immunoferritin technique using antiglycophorin antiserum and ferritin-conjugated sheep anti-rabbit IgG antiserum. It should be noted that the antibodies reacted exclusively with the outer surface of the membranes and thus with the NH_2-

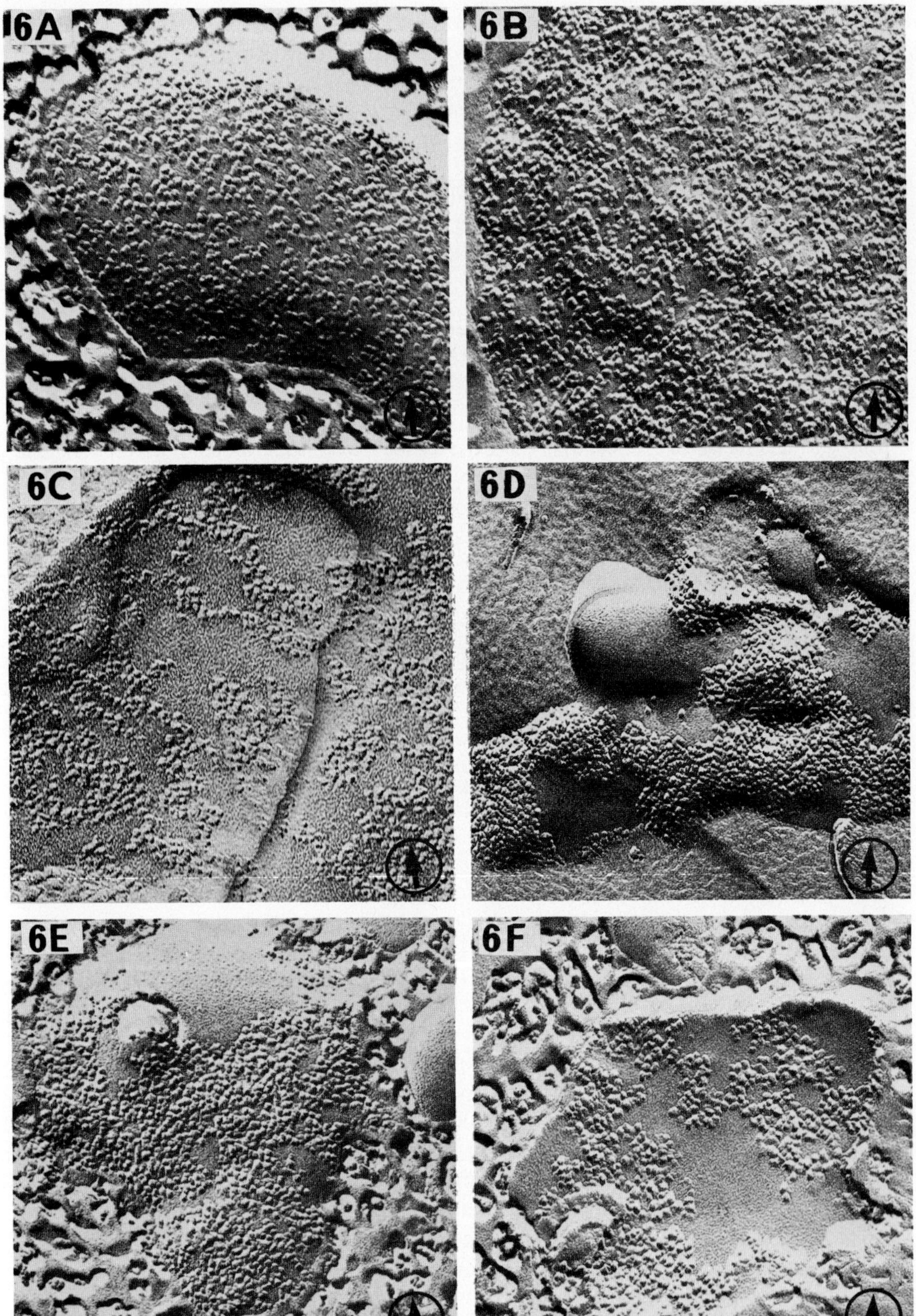
6A
6B
6C
6D
6E
6F

terminal portion. This is in contrast to the antibodies produced by Cotmore, Furthmayr, and Marchesi [40], which were raised against the COOH-terminal fragment of glycophorin and actually only reacted with the cytoplasmic surface of the membrane.

By use of En(a–) membranes we have approached the problem whether glycophorin is a component of the IMPs seen in freeze-fracturing of the membranes. We have been able to confirm the results of Bächi et al [41] that untreated En(a–) membranes contain IMPs evidently of normal size, distribution, and number. Therefore glycophorin is not an essential or a major component of these particles. Both band 3 and glycophorin preparations have been reconstituted into lipid vesicles, and particles resembling IMPs have been observed [22, 42, 43], but the significance of these results is still unclear.

It is obvious that the IMPs somehow are associated with spectrin. After removal of spectrin the IMPs can be aggregated [36], and we have recently shown with selective cross-linking of spectrin by periodate, that the IMPs are aggregated [44]. It is also known that antibodies against spectrin redistribute surface anionic sites which mainly are due to glycophorin [45], and recently Shotton et al [46] showed that antispectrin antibodies aggregate the IMPs. It is evident, however, that the attachment of IMPs to spectrin cannot be mediated solely by glycophorin, because then one would expect a nonrandom distribution of IMPs in En(a–) cells even under conditions when spectrin is not removed. We favor the hypothesis that this connection is mainly formed by band 3.

After treatment with 20 mM phosphate followed by incubation at pH 6 there was a more extensive aggregation of IMPs in En(a–) membranes than in normal membranes. This further indicates that glycophorin normally is a constituent of the particles and is involved in part in keeping the particles dispersed. This assumption is supported by the fact that neuraminidase treatment enhances the aggregation of the IMPs in normal cells [36], and Shotton et al [46] recently published evidence that most major surface proteins are involved in the formation of the IMPs.

A schematic model of the structure of IMPs and their relation to band 3, glycophorin, and spectrin is shown in Figure 7. The major part of the particles is formed by band 3 proteins. Both band 3 and glycophorin exist as dimers and penetrate the membrane, but only band 3 is more closely associated with spectrin, perhaps by intercalation between spectrin fibers [47]. Our results are only suggestive, and only when IMPs are isolated in pure form can definite knowledge of their composition be obtained.

ACKNOWLEDGMENTS

This study was supported by the Academy of Finland, the Finnish Cancer Society, and the Sigrid Jusélius Foundation. The skilful technical assistance of Anneli Asikainen and Elina Waris is acknowledged.

Fig 6. Cleaved fracture faces of normal and En(a–) erythrocytes. Both in membranes from normal (A) and En(a–) (B) erythrocytes a similar even distribution of the intramembrane particles is seen. When membranes of normal cells were depleted of spectrin by incubation in 20 mM sodium phosphate (pH 8.5) at 37°C for 16h and then transferred to 0.05 M sodium phosphate (pH 6.0) and incubated at 37°C for 30 min, a slight aggregation of IMPs is seen (C). After a similar treatment of En(a–) membranes a clear aggregation is seen (D). When membranes were depleted of spectrin by incubation in 0.1 mM EDTA (pH 8.0) at 4°C for 16 h and then incubated in PBS at 37°C for 30 min, an extensive aggregation of the IMPs occurred both in normal (E) and En(a–) (F) membranes. Shadowing direction is indicated by circled arrow. (Magnification 75,000 ×.)

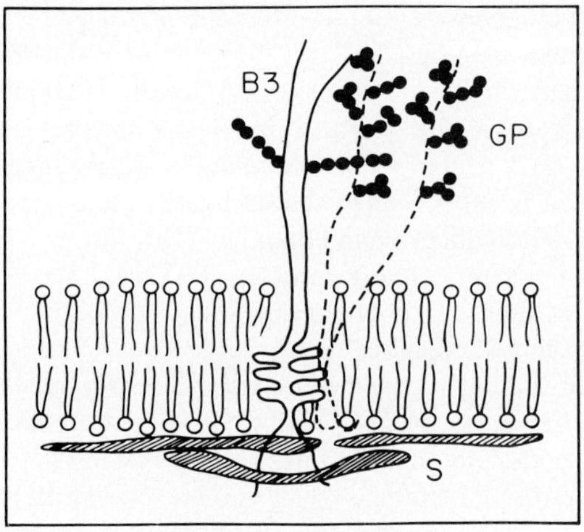

Fig 7. Schematic drawing of the normal erythrocyte membrane showing the band 3 (B3) and glycophorin (GP) dimers forming the intramembrane particles, and the intercalation of band 3 between the spectrin fibers (S).

REFERENCES

1. Steck TL: J Cell Biol 62:1, 1974.
2. Marchesi VT, Furthmayr H, and Tomita M: Ann Rev Biochem 45:667, 1976.
3. Gahmberg CG: In Poste G, Nicolson GL (eds): "Dynamic Aspects of Cell Surface Organization." Amsterdam: North-Holland, 1977, p 371.
4. Fairbanks G, Steck TL, Wallach DFH: Biochemistry 10:2606, 1971.
5. Gahmberg CG: J Biol Chem 251:510, 1976.
6. Nicolson GL, Singer SJ: J Cell Biol 60:236, 1974.
7. Gahmberg CG, Hakomori S: J Biol Chem 248:4311, 1973.
8. Steck TL, Dawson G: J Biol Chem 249:2135, 1974.
9. Bretscher MS: Nature New Biol 231:229, 1971.
10. Mueller TJ, Morrison M: J Biol Chem 249:7568, 1974.
11. Marchesi VT, Tillack TW, Jackson RL, Segrest JP, Scott RE: Proc Nat Acad Sci USA 69:1445, 1972.
12. Tomita M, Marchesi VT: Proc Nat Acad Sci USA 72:2964, 1975.
13. Nicolson GL: J Cell Biol 57:373, 1973.
14. Tillack TW, Scott RE, Marchesi VT: J Exp Med 135:1209, 1972.
15. Tanner MJA, Boxer DH: Biochem J 129:333, 1972.
16. Ho MK, Guidotti G: J Biol Chem 250:675, 1975.
17. Gahmberg CG, Myllylä G, Leikola J, Pirkola A, Nordling S: J Biol Chem 251:6108, 1976.
18. Steck TL: J Mol Biol 66:295, 1972.
19. Cabantchik ZI, Rothstein A: J Membrane Biol 15:207, 1974.
20. Kahlenberg A: J Biol Chem 251:1582, 1976.
21. Branton D: Proc Nat Acad Sci USA 55:1048, 1966.
22. Yu J, Branton D: Proc Nat Acad Sci USA 73:3891, 1976.
23. Pinto da Silva P, Moss PS, Fudenberg HH: Exp Cell Res 81:127, 1973.
24. Darnborough J, Dunsford I, Wallace JA: Vox Sang 17:241, 1969.
25. Furuhjelm U, Myllylä G, Nevanlinna HR, Nordling S, Pirkola A, Gavin J, Gooch A, Sanger R, Tippett P: Vox Sang 17:256, 1969.
26. Tanner MJA, Anstee DJ: Biochem J 155:701, 1976.
27. Dahr W, Uhlenbruck G, Leikola J, Wagstaff W, Landfried K: J Immunogen 3:329, 1976.
28. Marchesi VT, Steers E Jr, Science 159:203, 1968.

29. Hamaguchi H, Cleve H: Biochem Biophys Res Commun 47:459, 1972.
30. Landwall P: "Dialysis Cultivation of Bacteria. Optimization of Yields of Bacteria and Their Products." Doctoral thesis, Karolinska Institute, Stockholm, 1977.
31. Laemmli UK: Nature 227:680, 1970.
32. Weber K, Osborn M: J Biol Chem 244:4406, 1969.
33. March SC, Parikh I, Cuatrecasas P: Anal Biochem 60:149, 1974.
34. Otto H, Takamiya H, Vogt A: J Immun Meth 3:137, 1973.
35. Virtanen I, Miettinen A, Wartiovaara J: J Cell Sci 29:287, 1978.
36. Elgsaeter A, Branton D: J Cell Biol 63:1018, 1974.
37. Lowry OH, Rosebrough NJ, Farr AL, Randall RJ: J Biol Chem 193:265, 1951.
38. Marton LSG, Garvin JS: Biochem Biophys Res Commun 52:1457, 1973.
39. Furthmayr H: Nature 271:519, 1978.
40. Cotmore SF, Furthmayr H, Marchesi VT: J Mol Biol 113:539, 1977.
41. Bächi T, Whiting K, Tanner MJA, Metaxas MN, Anstee DJ: Biochim Biophys Acta 464:635, 1977.
42. Sharom FJ, Barratt DG, Grant CWM: Proc Nat Acad Sci USA 74:2751, 1977.
43. Segrest JP, Gulik-Krzywicki T, Sardet C: Proc Nat Acad Sci USA 71:3294, 1974.
44. Gahmberg CG, Virtanen I, Wartiovaara J: Biochem J 171:683, 1978.
45. Nicolson GL, Painter RG: J Cell Biol 59:395, 1973.
46. Shotton D, Thompson K, Wofsy L, Branton D: J Cell Biol 76:512, 1978.
47. Cherry RJ, Bürkli A, Busslinger M, Schneider G, Parish GR: Nature 263:389, 1976.

Journal of Supramolecular Structure 8:349–360 (1978)
Normal and Abnormal Red Cell Membranes 71–82

Molecular Characteristics of the Transferrin-Receptor Complex of the Rabbit Reticulocyte

Hsiang-Yun Yang Hu and Philip Aisen

Departments of Biophysics and Medicine, Albert Einstein College of Medicine, Bronx, New York 10461

A macromolecular complex of transferrin and a membrane component was isolated by gel filtration chromatography from Triton X-100-solubilized ghosts of reticulocytes previously incubated with ^{125}I-labeled transferrin. This complex is believed to be transferrin specifically associated with its primary receptor. Following the procedures of Clark [14], the complex in Triton X-100 was found to behave as an asymmetric molecule with a molecular weight of approximately 250,000 and an axial ratio of 9:1. On SDS-polyacrylamide gel electrophoresis the complex displays, in addition to transferrin, components of molecular weights 176,000 and 95,000, respectively. The larger component may be a dimer of the smaller. Each appears to cross-link, with dimethyl suberimidate, to transferrin. These results are compatible with the hypothesis that the transferrin receptor itself has a molecular weight near 175,000 and may be a dimer of two smaller components each of molecular weight near 95,000.

Key words: transferrin, receptor, reticulocytes, cross-link, membrane, detergent

Probably the most important, and certainly the best known, function of transferrin is to provide iron for the biosynthesis of hemoglobin. Indeed, transferrin is the only known effective source of iron for hemoglobin synthesis by reticulocytes [1], and presumably for other immature erythroid cells as well. The initial event in the interaction of transferrin with reticulocytes is the binding of the protein to specific receptors on the cell surface. These transferrin-binding receptors are lost, along with the capacity to synthesize hemoglobin, as the reticulocyte matures into a circulating erythrocyte [2]. They are vulnerable to proteolytic attack, so that cells treated with trypsin or Pronase lose the ability to bind transferrin and remove its iron [3, 4]. Until recently, little more was known about the chemistry of transferrin receptors and the nature of their interaction with the iron-binding protein.

The development of detergent-based methods for solubilizing membrane proteins with preservation of function has led to a resurgence of interest in the transferrin receptors of erythroid cells. A number of groups have reported studies of transferrin-binding

Received for publication March 5, 1978; accepted April 19, 1978.

components of red cell membranes [5–13]. As yet, however, an agreed-upon model of the transferrin receptor, and the chemical nature of the transferrin-receptor interaction, has not emerged. Our own work has been prompted by the recent studies of Clarke in which methods are developed for characterizing the molecular properties of impure membrane proteins in detergent solution [14]. In presenting our data, we will also try to point out explicitly areas of agreement and discord with the work of others.

EXPERIMENTAL PROCEDURES

Materials

Deuterium oxide (99.8%) was obtained from Stohler Isotope Chemicals. Triton X-100 was purchased from New England Nuclear, while dimethyl suberimidate and sodium dodecyl sulfate (Sequanal grade) were products of the Pierce Chemical Co. Carrier-free ^{125}I was supplied by Amersham/Searle. Ultrapure sucrose was from Schwarz/Mann, and Ultrogel AcA22 from LKB Instruments. Pig heart fumarase, porcine thyroglobulin, yeast alcohol dehydrogenase, bovine liver catalase, lactoperoxidase, o-nitrophenyl-β-D-galactopyranoside, L-malic acid, and β-nicotinamide adenine dinucleotide were supplied by the Sigma Chemical Co. Rabbit muscle phosphorylase a and E coli β-galactosidase were from the Worthington Biochemical Corp. Other chemicals were analytical grade, or the highest-quality commercially obtainable. Doubly distilled water was used for all experiments and preparations.

Preparation of ^{125}I-labeled Transferrin and the Putative Transferrin-Receptor Complex

Transferrin was isolated from rabbit serum by the method of Baker, Shaw, and Morgan [15] and radioiodinated to high specific activity using sepharose-bound lactoperoxidase as described by David and Reisfeld [16]. Reticulocytosis of 15–25% was induced in rabbits by repeated bleeding. Ghosts from reticulocytes previously incubated with ^{125}I-labeled transferrin were prepared by the method of Dodge, Mitchell, and Hanahan [17] and extracted with Triton X-100 according to the procedure of Leibman and Aisen [13]. A complex of transferrin and a membrane constituent, thought to be the primary transferrin receptor of the reticulocyte, was purified from such extracts by gel filtration chromatography on a 1.6 × 81 cm column of Ultrogel AcA22. The column was equilibrated with 0.2% Triton X-100 in pH 7.4, 5 imosm phosphate buffer [17] containing 0.02% sodium azide and eluted with the same buffer. Two peaks of radioactivity were observed in the chromatograms. The slower-moving peak eluted at the position of free transferrin, and it presumably represents uncomplexed protein released from its association with the cell membranes. The faster peak, accounting for about 60% of the radioactivity supplied to the column, moved with ferritin (MW ∿440,000; Stokes radius, 61 Å) and is considered to represent the complex of transferrin and its receptor. This peak was proportionately greater in columns run at 4°C than in columns at 18°, in keeping with the tendency of transferrin to remain associated with its receptor at low temperature [10]. For subsequent studies, fractions totaling about 6 ml in volume were taken from the crest of the faster-moving peak.

Sucrose Gradient Ultracentrifugation

The procedures of Clarke [14] were followed to obtain molecular parameters of the transferrin-receptor complex in detergent. Sucrose gradients 5–20% (w/v) in 5 imosm sodium phosphate and 0.1% Triton X-100, were prepared in H_2O and D_2O in cellulose nitrate tubes (0.5 X 2 inches, Beckman) and stored over night at 5°. Samples (100 μl) of the purified, concentrated transferrin-receptor were carefully layered on top of each gradient and centrifuged in the SW65 rotor of a Beckman L5-65 preparative ultracentrifuge at a speed of 34,000 rpm at 5°. A running time of 17 h was used for gradients in H_2O, and 26 h for gradients in D_2O. After the run, five-drop fractions were collected from the bottom of each tube for radioactivity counting, with aliquots taken for enzymatic assay of the marker proteins in 0.1 M sodium phosphate buffer, pH 7.6, at room temperature (following the Worthington Enzyme Manual) and for determination of density from refractive index measurements in a Zeiss Abbe refractometer.

Partial Specific Volume and Sedimentation Coefficient of the Transferrin-Receptor Complex

Again, the experimental and computational procedures developed by Clarke provided the model for our studies [14]. Assuming that the ^{125}I-transferrin-receptor complex binds the same amount of Triton X-100 in H_2O and in D_2O, its partial specific volume can be obtained from the measured sedimentation coefficients (s), densities (ρ), and viscosities (η) of the complex in the sucrose gradient at the position of half-distance of travel (r_{avg}), Equation 1:

$$\bar{v}_H = \frac{\dfrac{S_H \eta_H}{S_D \eta_D} - 1}{\rho_D \dfrac{S_H \eta_H}{S_D \eta_D} - \rho_H} \qquad (1)$$

Here, subscripts H and D refer to quantities measured in H_2O and D_2O respectively. Sedimentation coefficients at the position r_{avg} were calculated from Equation 2:

$$S_{r_{avg}} = [(r - r_0)/t]/\omega^2 r_{avg} \qquad (2)$$

where r_0 is the distance of the applied sample from the center of rotation, r is the distance of the peak of interest at time t, and ω is the angular velocity of the rotor. Since the density of the medium is a linear function of sucrose concentration, $\rho_{r_{avg}}$ may be determined from the measured refractive index of the fractions collected after ultracentrifugation and a reference plot of the densitites of standard solutions versus their refractive indices. The viscosity of the medium at the position r_{avg} of the transferrin-receptor complex was obtained from interpolation of the values for the marker protein calculated from Equation 3:

$$\frac{\eta_{r_{avg}}}{\eta_{20,w}} = \frac{s_{20,w}(1 - \bar{v}\rho_{r_{avg}})}{s_{r_{avg}}(1 - \bar{v}\rho_{20,w})} \qquad (3)$$

Values of $s_{20,w}$ (Svedberg units) and $\bar{v}$ (cm^3/gm), respectively, for the marker proteins used in these calculations are: β galactosidase, 16.0 and 0.73 [18]; catalase, 11.4 and 0.73 [19]; fumarase, 9.09 and 0.738 [20]; alcohol dehydrogenase, 7.40 and 0.73 [21]; and transferrin, 4.97 and 0.725 [22, 23].

Once $\bar{v}$ is calculated from Eq (1), $s_{20,w}$ of the transferrin-receptor complex can be obtained from Equation 4:

$$s_{20,w} = s_H(\eta_H/\eta_{20,w})(1-\bar{v}_H\,\rho_{20,w})/(1-\bar{v}_H\,\rho_H) \quad (4)$$

The peak of interest in these studies is taken to be the faster-moving, ^{125}I-bearing peak of Figure 1.

The Stokes Radius of the Transferrin-Receptor Complex

The Stokes radius of the transferrin-receptor complex in Triton X-100 was determined by gel filtration on a column of Ultragel AcA22 equilibrated with 5 imosm sodium phosphate buffer (pH 7.4) containing 0.1% of the detergent, 10% sucrose (the concentration at the position of the transferrin-receptor complex in the sucrose gradient centrifugation study), and 0.02% sodium azide. The column was run and calibrated with standard proteins at 18° (Fig 2). The buffer used for equilibration was also used for elution. For better accuracy, elution positions were measured by weight rather than volume [24]. Void weight was estimated with blue dextran, and included weight with DNP-alanine. Results were expressed as $\mathrm{erf}^{-1}(1-K_d)$, of which the Stokes radius is generally a linear function:

$$R_s = A + B\,\mathrm{erf}^{-1}(1-K_d) \quad (5)$$

where A and B are empirical constants for a given chromatographic system [24].

Cross-Linking of the Transferrin-Receptor Complex

Reaction conditions were similar to those of Wang and Richards [25]. The purified complex of ^{125}I-labeled transferrin and its receptor was concentrated about five times by ultrafiltration with the Schleicher and Schuell ultrafiltration apparatus, and made 25 mM in sodium phosphate buffer (pH 8.0). Dimethyl suberimidate was added to a concentration of 3 mg/ml. The reaction mixture was kept at 0° for 20 min, and at room temperature for 30 min. The cross-linking reaction was then stopped by addition of ammonium acetate to a final concentration of 0.2 M, with stirring for 10 min. After removing Triton X-100 with Bio-Beads SM-2 [13], the preparation was taken for electrophoresis in SDS polyacrylamide gel.

SDS Polyacrylamide Gel Electrophoresis

The methods of Fairbanks, Steck, and Wallach [26] were followed, with minor modifications. Gels measured 0.5 × 11 cm, and contained 4% polyacrylamide. Samples were in electrophoresis sample buffer containing 2% SDS, with or without 3% β-mercaptoethanol, and were incubated at 37°C for 2 h before electrophoresis. Gels were calibrated for estimations of molecular weight with thyroglobulin (subunit MW 335,000), β-galactosidase (130,000), phosphorylase a (92,000), transferrin (77,000), catalase (57,000), and ovalbumin (43,000). Gels containing ^{125}I-labeled transferrin, or its complex with the transferrin receptor, were cut into 3.0-mm slices and counted for ^{125}I activity in a Searle model 1195 automatic gamma counter.

RESULTS

Molecular Size and Shape of the Transferrin-Receptor Complex

Results of sucrose gradient ultracentrifugation studies are shown in Figure 1 and Table I. Water-soluble proteins, which in general do not bind Triton X-100 [14], were used as markers to calibrate the gradients. The peaks of greater density are taken to represent the transferrin-receptor complex, while the peaks of lower density correspond to free transferrin, presumably dissociated from the receptor during the course of experimental manipulation.

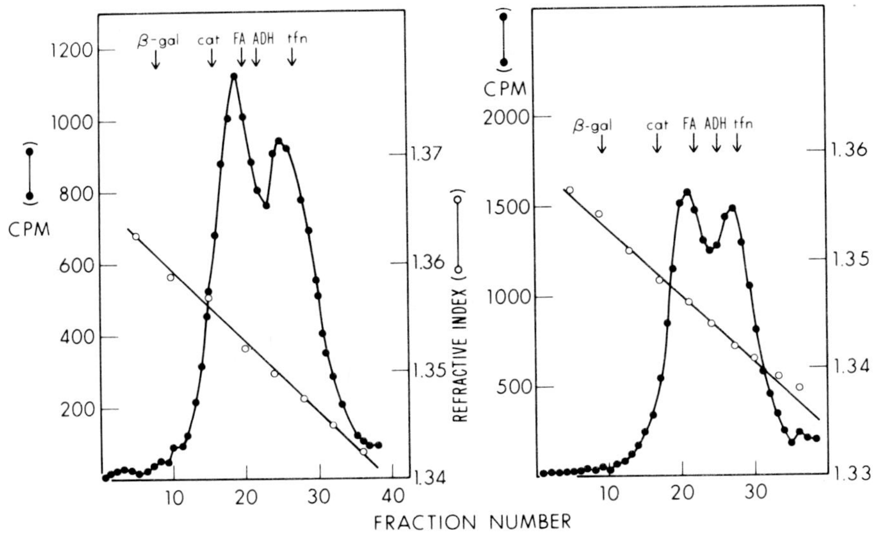

Fig 1. Ultracentrifugation profile of transferrin-receptor complex of rabbit reticulocytes in 5–20% (w/v) sucrose gradient containing 5 imosm sodium phosphate and 0.1% Triton X-100 (pH 7.4) in H_2O (left) and D_2O (right) at 5°. β-gal) β-galactosidase, cat) catalase, FA) fumarase, ADH) alcohol dehydrogenase, tfn) transferrin.

TABLE I. Parameters Obtained for Calculation of the Partial Specific Volume of the Transferrin-Receptor Complex by Sucrose Gradient Ultracentrifugation in 0.1% Triton X-100

Parameter	H_2O	D_2O
Sedimentation coefficient, s (S)	5.062	3.037
Density, ρ (g/cm^3)	1.035	1.135
Viscosity, η (cP)	1.692	1.953

The transferrin-receptor complex migrated to a position between catalase and fumarase, the relative position of the complex with respect to these markers being virtually the same in H_2O as in D_2O. Thus, the partial specific volume of the complex must be similar to those of the marker enzymes. The sedimentation coefficients, densities, and viscosities for the transferrin-receptor complex at the half-distance of travel in H_2O and D_2O, calculated from the ultracentrifugation data as indicated under Methods, are shown in Table I. The partial specific volume, $\overline{v}$, was then obtained from these calculated values according to Equation 1, assuming that the complex binds Triton X-100 equally in H_2O and D_2O. With $\overline{v}$ known, the sedimentation coefficient $s_{20,w}$, shown in Table II, is obtained.

In order to estimate the molecular weight of the transferrin-receptor complex from the Svedberg equation

$$M = \frac{6\pi\eta_{20,w} R_s N S_{20,w}}{1-\overline{v}\,\rho_{20,w}} \qquad (6)$$

the Stokes radius of the complex must be known. This was obtained (Table II) by gel filtration using an Ultrogel AcA22 column calibrated with soluble protein standards. Since high concentrations of sucrose may change the amount of Triton X-100 bound to proteins or their state of aggregation [27], these gel filtration studies were carried out in the same buffer used for ultracentrifugation, made 10% (w/v) in sucrose, the approximate concentration at the position of the transferrin-receptor peak after ultracentrifugation. The elution profile of the column is shown in Figure 2, and its calibration plot in Figure 3. The elution weight of the transferrin receptor complex remains very close to that of apoferritin, the same result obtained in earlier studies when the column buffer contained no sucrose [13]. It seems likely, therefore, that the perturbing effects of sucrose on the complex, if any, are minimal, and its Stokes radius is therefore taken as that of apoferritin – 61 Å as calculated from the hydrodynamic data in Crichton [28]. The molecular weight of the complex, as given in Table II, may then be calculated from Equation 2. Two other physical parameters of interest, the frictional ratio f/f_0. and the diffusion coefficient $D_{20,w}$, are also shown in Table II. These were obtained from knowledge of its Strokes radius, partial specific volume and molecular weight by the following relationships:

$$D_{20,w} = \frac{kT}{6\pi\eta_{20,w} R_s} \qquad (7)$$

$$f/f_0 = \frac{R_s}{(3\overline{v}M/4\pi N)^{1/3}} \qquad (8)$$

where k is the Boltzmann constant and T the absolute temperature. The high frictional ratio of the transferrin-receptor complex, 1.46, suggests that it is an asymmetric molecule

TABLE II. Molecular Characteristics of Putative Transferrin-Receptor Complex of Rabbit Reticulocyte in Triton X-100

Physical parameter	Transferrin-receptor complex	Receptor
Partial specific volume, $\bar{v}$ (cm^3/g)	0.735	0.739
Sedimentation coefficient, $s_{20,w}$ (S)	9.49	
Stokes radius, R_S (Å)	61	
Molecular weight, M	250,000	175,000
Frictional ratio, f/f_0	1.46	
Diffusion coefficient, $D_{20,w}$ (cm^2/s)	3.50×10^{-7}	

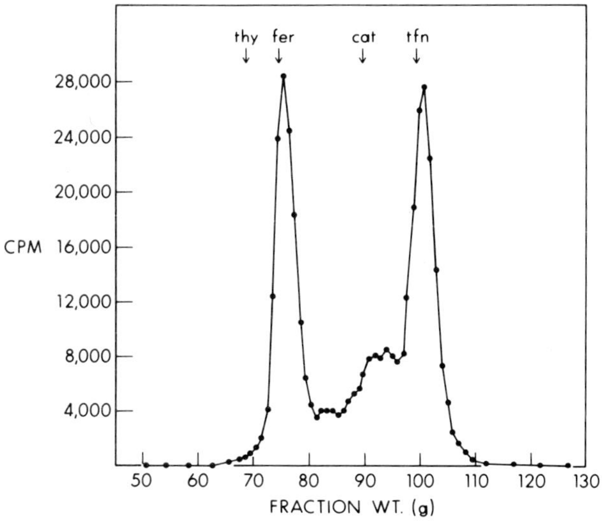

Fig 2. Gel filtration chromatogram of Triton X-100-solubilized rabbit reticulocyte membranes prepared from cells incubated with ^{125}I-labeled rabbit transferrin on Ultrogel AcA22 (1.6 × 81 cm) column. The column was equilibrated and eluted with 5 imosm sodium phosphate buffer (pH 7.4) containing 0.1% (v/v) Triton X-100 and 10% (w/v) sucrose at 18°; thy) thyroglobin, fer) apoferritin, cat) catalase, tfn) transferrin.

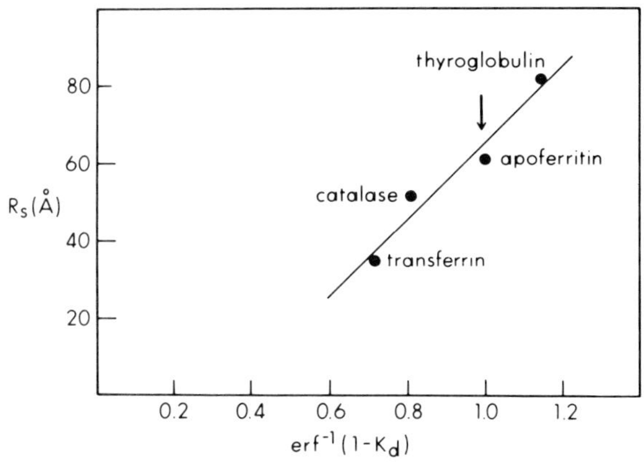

Fig 3. Calibration plot for determination of the Stokes radius of the transferrin receptor complex by gel filtration on Ultrogel AcA22. The arrow indicates the position of the transferrin-receptor complex.

deviating substantially from globular shape. Assuming no solvation by H_2O, the axial ratio of an ellipsoid of revolution approximating the shape of the complex is about 9, as obtained from Perrin plots [29]. If one molecule of receptor is taken to bind one molecule of transferrin, the partial specific volume and molecular weight of the receptor itself in Triton X-100 can be deduced, and these too are shown in Table II.

Cross-Linking of the ^{125}I-Transferrin-Receptor Complex With Dimethyl Suberimidate

In previous work, three prominent components were identified by SDS-gel electrophoresis in dithiothreitol of the transferrin-receptor complex: a band of molecular weight 77,000, corresponding to free transferrin; another at molecular weight 95,000; and a third at molecular weight 176,000 [13]. To determine which, if any, of these are directly complexed to transferrin, ^{125}I-transferrin-receptor complexes, purified by gel filtration, were treated with the cross-linking reagent dimethyl suberimidate and then subjected to SDS-gel electrophoresis. Three radioactive components were found (Fig 4). In the absence of the disulfide-disrupting reagent β-mercaptoethanol, the apparent molecular weight of these were 60,000, 128,000, and 260,000. Incubation with β-mercaptoethanol before electrophoresis shifted the apparent molecular weight of these components to 76,000, 180,000, and 280,000 respectively. In a control study, free transferrin at concentrations of 0.2–0.5 mg/ml (much greater than that in transferrin-receptor complex) was treated with dimethyl suberimidate and in each case gave only one radioactive band on SDS gel. This had an apparent molecular weight of 60,000 in the absence of β-mercaptoethanol, and 77,000 when preincubated with the sulfhydryl reagent. We believe, therefore, that the three radioactive bands observed in dimethyl suberimidate-treated transferrin-receptor complexes correspond to free transferrin, transferrin linked to the 95,000 mol wt component, and possibly transferrin linked to the 176,000 mol wt component. In one experiment, the relative amount of the 176,000 mol wt component in the

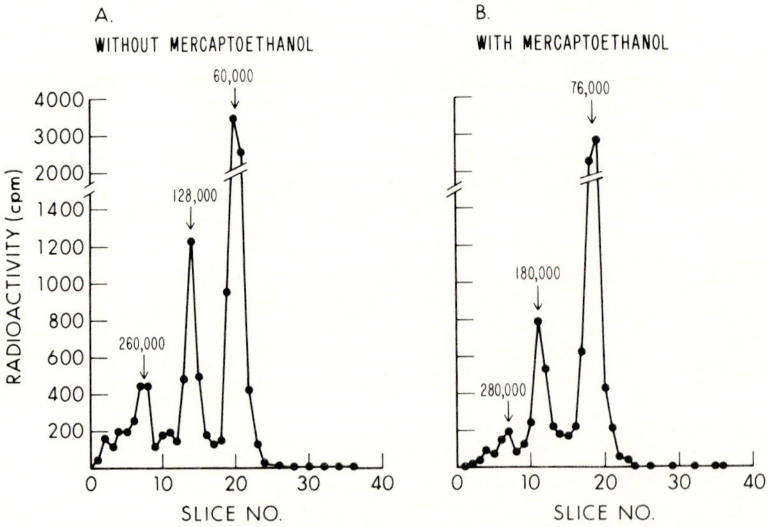

Fig 4. Radioactivity patterns of sodium dodecyl sulfate gel electrophoresis of transferrin-receptor complex purified by gel filtration and treated with dimethyl suberimidate. A) Without β-mercaptoethanol; B) with β-mercaptoethanol in sample buffer.

transferrin-receptor complex increased on prolonged preincubation without β-mercapto-ethanol, while the 95,000 mol wt component became hardly detectable, perhaps suggesting that the smaller component may dimerize to form the larger.

DISCUSSION

The Existence of Surface Receptors for Transferrin on Erythroid Cells

By now, the existence of specific transferrin-binding receptors on the membranes of developing, hemoglobin-synthesizing erythroid cells is beyond question. These receptors are specific for transferrin [10]; they are vulnerable to attack with proteases [3], and hence a) they are located at the external surface of the cell membrane and b) they have protein moieties as essential components, and they have been identified on circulating reticulocytes, on erythroid cells of bone marrow, and on Friend erythroleukemic cells [2, 30, 31]. Evidence has also been obtained for similar transferrin-receptors on the surface of placental cells [32]. Since the first stage in the interaction of transferrin with erythroid cells to provide iron for the biosynthesis of hemoglobin entails specific binding of the protein to its receptor, the fundamental importance of the transferrin receptor in the physiology of iron metabolism is clear.

Because of its accessibility in the peripheral circulation the reticulocyte, induced by bleeding or by injection of acetyl phenylhydrazine, is often taken as a model of the hemoglobin-synthesizing, iron-requiring cell. Transferrin-specific receptors of the reticulocyte are saturable so that their behavior can be described by the Michaelis-Menten formalism commonly applied to enzymic reactions. By such analyses, the number of binding sites for homologous transferrin on the reticulocyte membrane has been variously estimated as 50,000 for the human cell, and from 26,000 to 560,000 for the rabbit cell [2, 33, 34]. The reasons for this variability are not clear, although recently it has been suggested that artifactual binding of transferrin to plastic ware may be at fault [35]. The avidity of red cell precursors for transferrin also varies with their stage of maturation, earlier cells binding more protein [36]. The means by which reticulocytosis is brought about is another factor affecting transferrin binding [37]. In our laboratory we generally find that reticulocytes induced by bleeding bind, at saturation, about 125,000 transferrin molecules per cell, and we take this to be the number of available receptor sites.

As the reticulocyte develops into a mature erythrocyte, functioning surface receptors for transferrin disappear [2] and transferrin-binding activity is no longer demonstrable in detergent-solubilized membranes [13]. The fate of the receptor during maturation is unknown, although it has been suggested that an alteration in its carbohydrate content may be associated with its loss of function [13].

Transferrin-Binding Components of Erythroid Cell Membranes

Probably the first to utilize detergents to solubilize membranes of reticulocytes incubated with labeled transferrin in a search for the transferrin receptor were Garrett, Garrett, and Archdeacon [5]. Using Triton X-100, deoxycholate, and SDS, these investigators found by gel filtratron chromatography a macromolecular complex of transferrin and a membrane component(s) which may have included the primary transferrin receptor. Pursuing this approach with Triton X-100, the gentlest and most effective detergent used by Garrett and associates for solubilizing transferrin-bearing complexes, Speyer and Fielding identified a transferrin-bearing component from membranes of human reticulocyte incubated with labeled transferrin [6]. This fraction had an apparent molecular sizeof 230,000 by gel chromatography and was thought to represent the transferrin-receptor complex. An obligatory step in the Speyer-Fielding isolation entailed passage of the detergent-solubilized reticulocyte membranes through a column of Sepharose 2B, a procedure not found necessary by most other investigators [10]. However, the findings of Speyer and Fielding were substantially confirmed by van der Heul, Kroos, and van Eijk [38], using rat reticulocytes.

In general, remarkably little agreement has prevailed among the several groups attempting to characterize the transferrin receptor of erythroid cells. Sly, Grohlich, and Bezkorovainy found a 200,000 mol wt complex of transferrin and a membrane component from rabbit reticulocytes induced by injection of acetyl phenylhydrazine [8]. On SDS-urea gel electrophoresis this complex yielded bands of molecular weight 120,000, 77,000 (free transferrin), and 60,000, and showed the presence of carbohydrate not accounted for by the transferrin. Witt and Woodworth [7], in contrast, found a 35,000 mol wt protein in chick embryo red cells, capable of binding to photoaffinity-labeled ovotransferrin. Using affinity chromatography, Light [12] identified, in Triton X-100 solubilized rabbit reticulocyte ghosts, a 35,000 mol wt protein which formed a dimer capable of associating with transferrin, and argued that this represented the basic unit of the transferrin receptor [12]. Ecarot-Charrier et al, taking a different tack, used antibodies to rabbit transferrin to precepitate the apparent transferrin-receptor complex from solubilized rabbit reticulocyte membranes [39]. The nontransferrin component of this complex migrated electrophoretically as a single peak, but no estimate of its molecular weight was published. Finally, Morgan's group identified a macromolecular complex of transferrin and a component of the rabbit reticulocyte membrane by gel chromatography using the detergent Teric 12A9 (polyethoxylated lauryl alcohol) [10]. This component was shown to be present in reticulocytes and not in mature erythrocytes, and it bound transferrin in reversible and saturable manner. The complex migrated on column chromatography with an apparent molecular weight of 350,000, so that the receptor itself appeared to be a protein of molecular weight near 275,000.

Some Molecular Characteristics of the Putative Transferrin-Receptor Complex

Because of these inconsistencies in the reported properties of these transferrin-associating membrane components we have undertaken to characterize the transferrin-receptor complex by the more rigorous approaches of Clarke [14]. Our starting material was a complex of transferrin and a component of the rabbit reticulocyte membrane, isolated by Ultrogel AcA22 chromatography in Triton X-100 [13]. Over 60% of the radioactivity of ^{125}I-labeled transferrin bound to reticulocyte ghosts is recoverable in this complex, in which transferrin is associated in a reversible and saturable manner. We believe it likely, therefore, that we are dealing with the specific complex of transferrin and its membrane receptor.

The molecular parameters of this complex, in Triton X-100, are presented in Table II. Perhaps of greatest interest, its molecular weight is 250,000, or, subtracting the contribution of transferrin and assuming a 1:1 stoichiometry of receptor binding to transferrin, 175,000 for the receptor itself. The hydrodynamic or Stokes radius of the complex, has a value measured by gel filtration chromatography (Fig 2) close to that of ferritin, a hollow spherical molecule 61 Å in radius and of about 440,000 mol wt. Since this is probably a lower limit of the true Stokes radius [40], it is evident that the transferrin-receptor complex departs greatly from spherical symmetry. Assuming that water of hydration makes a negligible contribution to hydrodynamic behavior, which seems probable for a complex largely composed of a membrane protein, the axial ratio for a hydrodynamically equivalent prolate ellipsoid of revolution is about 9:1 [29]. Such an ellipsoid would be 40 Å × 360 Å, so that it could readily span the cell membrane. The asymmetric nature of the transferrin-receptor complex may also help account for the apparent discrepancies in its molecular size reported by various groups, since small variations in methods used for solubilization might induce appreciable changes in hydrodynamic properties.

As much as 6% of the total membrane protein of a reticulocyte bearing 125,000 transferrin receptors of 175,000 mol wt could, from the estimate of total membrane protein in the erythrocyte ghost given by Fairbanks, Steck, and Wallach [26], consist of the specific transferrin receptor.

The partial specific volume of the transferrin-receptor complex, 0.735 cm^3/g, falls in the range of most proteins. Since the partial specific volume of Triton X-100 is 0.91 cm^3/g, it appears that, once solubilized, the complex binds very little detergent. Attempts to verify this experimentally were unsuccessful, as it was not possible to attain concentrations of the complex sufficiently high to measure reliably its ability to bind detergent. It seems likely, however, that the transferrin receptor falls into the class of peripheral or extrinsic membrane proteins [41] which bind only small amounts of detergent, and in monomeric rather than micellar form [42].

Subunit Structure of the Transferrin Receptor

In earlier SDS gel electrophoresis studies of the transferrin-receptor complex, three major protein components were identified: a band of 176,000 mol wt, another of 95,000 mol wt, and a band corresponding to free transferrin. The experiments with dimethyl suberimidate reported in this paper provide evidence that the 95,000 mol wt component is in sufficiently close proximity to transferrin to be cross-linked to it. Our results are not sufficiently compelling, however, to indicate whether the same is true of the 176,000 mol wt component. Since the molecular weight of the transferrin receptor itself is about 175,000, it is unlikely that the receptor is composed of two different subunits of 95,000 and 176,000 mol wt respectively. A more attractive possibility is that the heavier component is a dimer of the smaller, incompletely dissociated by the procedure for SDS-gel electrophoresis, and that the functional receptor consists of this dimer. It should again be noted that both the 95,000 and 176,000 mol wt components can be identified in membrane fractions of mature erythrocytes which no longer bind transferrin, and no longer cross-link to it [11]. We have previously suggested that the loss of transferrin-binding activity may be due to alteration in the carbohydrate content of these components [13], but definitive evidence for this is still not available.

Our results are not in complete accord with those reported by Nunez et al in studies of transferrin cross-linked to intact reticulocytes [11]. These investigators found a 125,000 mol wt complex of transferrin and a membrane component in the absence of mercaptoethanol, migrating with an apparent molecular weight of 140,000 in its presence. In our studies, in which the apparent molecular weight of a cross-linked product increased from 128,000 to 180,000 after reduction, the treatment with sulfhydryl reagent was carried out for 2 h rather than 20 min, perhaps accounting for some of the discrepancy. We have also chosen to work with purified transferrin-receptor complexes rather than whole cells in the belief that nonspecific cross-linking would be minimized. It is possible, however, that a cross-linking component is present in intact membranes which we fail to detect in purified complexes.

REFERENCES

1. Hemmaplardh D, Morgan EH: Biochim Biophys Acta 373:84, 1974.
2. Jandl JH, Katz JH: J Clin Invest 42:314, 1963.
3. Jandl JH, Inman JK, Simmons RL, Allen DW: J Clin Invest 38:161, 1959.
4. Hemmaplardh D, Morgan EH: Biochim Biophys Acta 426:385, 1976.
5. Garrett NE, Garrett RJB, Archdeacon JW: Biochem Biophys Res Comm 52:466, 1973.
6. Speyer BE, Fielding J: Biochim Biophys Acta 332:192, 1974.
7. Witt DP, Woodworth RC: In Crichton RR (ed): "Proteins of Iron Storage and Transport in Biochemistry and Medicine." Amsterdam: North Holland, 1975, pp 133–140.
8. Sly DA, Grohlich D, Bezkorovainy A: In Crichton RR (ed): "Proteins of Iron Storage and Transport in Biochemistry and Medicine." Amsterdam: North Holland, 1975, pp 141–146.
9. van Bockxmeer FM, Hemmaplardh D, Morgan EH: In Crichton RR (ed): "Proteins of Iron Storage and Transport in Biochemistry and Medicine." Amsterdam: North Holland, 1975, pp 111–119.
10. van Bockxmeer FM, Morgan EH: Biochim Biophys Acta 468:437, 1977.
11. Nunez MT, Fischer S, Glass J, Lavidor L: Biochim Biophys Acta 490:87, 1977.
12. Light ND: Biochim Biophys Acta 495:46, 1977.
13. Leibman A, Aisen P: Biochemistry 16:1268, 1977.
14. Clarke S: J Biol Chem 250:5459, 1975.
15. Baker E, Shaw DC, Morgan EH: Biochemistry 7:1371, 1968.
16. David GS, Reisfeld RA: Biochemistry 13:1014, 1974.
17. Dodge JT, Mitchell C, Hanahan DJ: Arch Biochem Biophys 110:119, 1963.
18. Craven GR, Steers E Jr, Anfinsen CB: J Biol Chem 240:2468, 1965.
19. Martin RG, Ames BN: J Biol Chem 236:1372, 1961.
20. Hill RL, Taipel JW: In Boyer P (ed): "The Enzymes." 3rd Ed. New York: Academic, 1971, vol 5, pp 539–571.
21. Kuff EL, Hogeboom GH, Steubich MJ: J Biol Chem 212:439, 1955.
22. Roberts RC, Makey DK, Seal US: J Biol Chem 241:4907, 1966.
23. Oncley JL, Scatchard G, Brown A: J Phys Colloid Chem 51:184, 1947.
24. Fish WW: Meth Membrane Biol 4:189, 1975.
25. Wang K, Richards FM: J Biol Chem 249:8005, 1974.
26. Fairbanks G, Steck TL, Wallach DFH: Biochemistry 10:2606, 1971.
27. Simons K, Helenius A, Garoff H: J Mol Biol 80:119, 1973.
28. Crichton RR: Struct Bond 17:67, 1973.
29. Tanford C: "Physical Chemistry of Macromolecules." New York: Wiley, 1961, p 326.
30. Kailis SG, Morgan EH: Br J Haemat 28:37, 1974.
31. Hu H-YY, Gardner J, Aisen P, Skoultchi AI: Science 197:559, 1977.
32. King BF: Anat Rec 186:151, 1976.
33. Kornfeld S: Biochim Biophys Acta 194:25, 1969.
34. Baker E, Morgan EH: Biochemistry 8:2954, 1969.
35. Phillips JL: Biochim Biophys Res Comm 71:726, 1976.
36. Nunez MT, Glass J, Fischer S, Lavidor LM, Lenk EM, Robinson SH: Br J Haemat 36:519, 1977.
37. Workman EF Jr, Graham G, Bates GW: Biochim Biophys Acta 399:254, 1975.
38. van der Heul C, Kroos MJ, van Eijk HG: In Brown E, Aisen P, Crichton RR, Fielding J (eds): "Proteins of Iron Metabolism." New York: Grune & Stratton, 1977, pp 299–304.
39. Ecarot-Charrier B, Grey V, Wilczynska A, Shulman HM: In Brown E, Aisen P, Crichton RR, Fielding J (eds): "Proteins of Iron Metabolism." New York: Grune & Stratton, 1977, pp 291–298.
40. Nozaki Y, Schecter NM, Reynolds JA, Tanford C: Biochemistry 15:3884, 1976.
41. Helenius A, Simons K: Biochim Biophys Acta 415:29, 1975.
42. Clarke S: Biochem Biophys Res Comm 79:46, 1977.

Journal of Supramolecular Structure 8:361–373 (1978)
Normal and Abnormal Red Cell Membranes 83–95

Physical-Chemical Studies of Spectrin

G.B. Ralston

Department of Biochemistry, University of Sydney, Sydney, NSW, 2006, Australia

In recent years considerable progress has been made in the understanding of the structure and function of the red blood cell membrane. The protein spectrin, of high molecular weight and propensity for self-association, appears to play a major role, in concert with actin, in maintaining the shape and integrity of the membrane. A study of the physical-chemical properties of spectrin, and its size, shape, self-association pattern, and its interaction with other components, leads to a plausible model for the way this protein performs its biological role. The evidence from the structure and interactions of spectrin suggests a structure which is relatively symmetrical yet highly expanded, and which allows extensive, two-dimensional network formation with actin. In these respects, the structure of spectrin is quite different from that of myosin, to which it has often been likened.

Key words: spectrin, actin, hydrodynamic properties, structure of spectrin

When Marchesi and his colleagues first isolated spectrin back in 1969 [1, 2], they recognised from the way the red cells fragmented after extraction of the protein that spectrin probably plays an important role in maintaining the integrity and shape of the cell. Sedimentation velocity studies on the isolated spectrin showed the presence of multiple boundaries [2, 3] and suggested that spectrin was capable of self-association. A study of the physical-chemical properties of spectrin, and its size, shape, self-association behaviour, and its interaction with other components of the membrane, is a prerequisite for an understanding of the functional role of spectrin.

Before an unambiguous analysis of the properties of spectrin could be undertaken, the isolation of a pure preparation was essential. In early studies with this protein, spectrin was isolated from other components in the water-soluble extract by the use of gel filtration on Sephadex G-200. Although this allows the removal of many of the contaminating proteins, chiefly hemoglobin, it is now clear that not all other proteins are removed by this means. Traces (up to 5%) of other components, chiefly component 5, are eluted with the spectrin in the void volume fraction from the Sephadex G-200 columns [4–6]. Furthermore, the spectrin prepared this way is itself heterogeneous, as was indicated in Marchesi's sedimentation analysis [2].

Received for publication March 5, 1978; accepted April 24, 1978.

Rechromatography of the void volume fraction from the G-200 columns on 4% agarose gels, a medium capable of resolving globular proteins up to 15×10^6 daltons, revealed a series of components occupying elution positions from the void volume through almost the entire fractionation range of the column [4]. Figure 1 shows the elution profile for a sample of the water-soluble proteins prepared at low temperature. The peaks labelled "tet" and "di" correspond to a tetramer of 960,000 daltons and a dimer of 480,000 daltons, respectively [4]. These oligomers do not appear to interconvert on prolonged storage in moderate salt concentrations and at temperatures below 30°C. In other words, the elution profile represents discrete, nonequilibrating species, rather than a reversible interaction pattern.

The void volume peak, V_0 (Fig 1), has been shown to contain small amounts of components 4.5 and 5, in addition to spectrin [7]. We observe a constant stoichiometry for the components of this fraction, one molecule of component 4.5 and two molecules of component 5 for each spectrin tetramer, over a large number of different preparations. This ratio is the same as that for the whole membrane, or for the pellet after Triton X-100 extraction. The constant stoichiometry, and our inability to separate the spectrin from the other components by physical means, leads us to believe that the void volume fraction is a well-defined complex, rather than a series of separate, large homotropic polymers of the individual components. Since this material also elutes in the void volume from 2% agarose columns (G.B. Ralston and J.C. Dunbar, unpublished results), it would appear to be of very large size and very highly agregated.

A small peak near 190 ml (Fig 1) comprises a number of nonspectrin proteins, chiefly components from the 3 region, and components 5 and 7. The elution position of these proteins suggests that they all exist in oligomeric forms, with molecular weights near one million.

The presence of these multiple components in the void volume fraction from Sephadex G-200 columns, and thus in the preparations of "spectrin," may in large part explain the variability in the physical properties of the protein isolated in this way

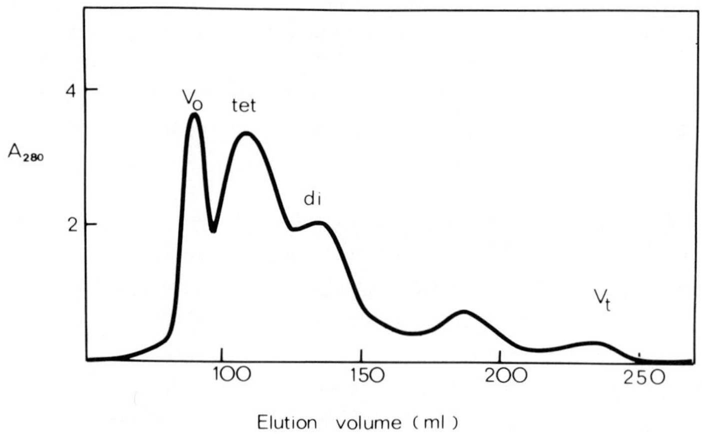

Fig 1. Elution of a crude spectrin preparation from a column (2.5 × 60 cm) of 4% agarose gel beads. The water-soluble proteins, prepared from human erythrocyte ghosts at 4°C, were eluted from the column with 0.1 M NaC1, 0.01 M sodium phosphate, 5 mM EDTA, and 5 mM mercaptoethanol (pH 7.5). V_0) the void volume peak; tet) the spectrin tetramer; di) the spectrin dimer; V_t) the total volume peak.

(compare Refs 2 and 3). In particular, the size of the very highly aggregated complex, and its variable proportion in different preparations [4] would be expected to influence markedly the properties of the preparation. In addition, further complications can arise from a temperature-dependent dissociation of the tetramer to the dimer and monomer [8], so that preparations made at 37°C will not be directly comparable with those made at low temperature.

In spite of the probable variation in the composition of the spectrin preparations from different laboratories, a number of consistent points emerge. Major components of low-temperature preparations are of approximately 9 S and 12 S [2, 4, 6, 8], corresponding to the dimer and tetramer, respectively [4], while 37°C preparations seem to comprise mainly the 9 S component, together with another of from 4 to 7 S, presumably the monomer [4, 6, 8].

THE EFFECTS OF SALT

A number of early reports claimed that spectrin is aggregated in moderate concentrations of salt: Clarke [3] reported that sodium chloride concentrations above 10 mM caused aggregation. These conclusions have generally been based on the increase in sedimentation coefficient that is seen when the salt concentration is raised from very low levels, and they are questionable on two counts. First, the primary charge effect would be expected to operate at very low salt concentrations, and this effect may be large. Second, the preparations used in some of the earlier studies were almost certainly heterogeneous, such that a single peak in the sedimentation pattern at low salt concentrations may not represent only a single component. The appearance of several, faster boundaries on addition of salt may thus arise from both the swamping of the charge effect and the improved resolution of the several species already present.

The above interpretation has been confirmed in studies with isolated oligomers of spectrin. The change in sedimentation coefficient of both the tetramer and the dimer, on increasing the salt concentration, follows very closely the relationship derived by Pedersen [9] for the primary charge effect: The sedimentation coefficient decreases linearly with the inverse of the solution conductance. In addition, the effect is linearly dependent on the protein concentration, again as required by the primary charge effect. The dependence of sedimentation coefficient on the protein concentration, in both low and high salt concentrations (Fig 2), is quite different from that to be expected from aggregation.

Support for this interpretation has come from gel filtration experiments, which have shown that as the salt concentration is raised from very low values up towards 0.1 M, both the tetramer and dimer elute at increasingly greater elution volumes. This behaviour is quite the reverse of aggregation, and again is better explained in terms of the operation of charge exclusion phenomena in the gel matrix [10]. The tetramer and dimer components in total water-soluble protein extracts behave identically with the isolated oligomers, eliminating the possibility of changes having taken place in the proteins during isolation [10].

Although salt does not appear to induce the aggregation of spectrin, there is increasing evidence for salt-dependent conformation changes in spectrin. The limiting sedimentation coefficient for spectrin in low-ionic-strength solution is not identical with that in the presence of 0.1 M NaCl (G.B. Ralston, unpublished results). This effect is

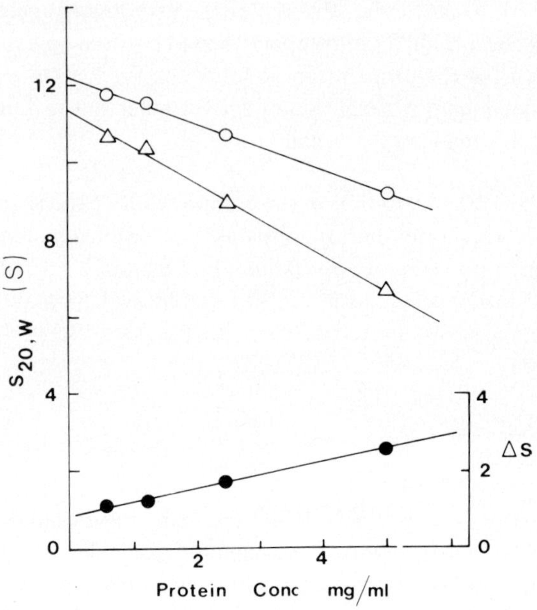

Fig 2. Effect of salt and protein concentration on the sedimentation coefficient of the spectrin tetramer. ○—○) 0.1 M NaC1, 0.01 M sodium phosphate, pH 7.5; △—△) 5 mM sodium phosphate, pH 7.5; ●—●) the difference in sedimentation coefficient, Δs, (right-hand ordinate) as a function of protein concentration.

demonstrated for the tetramer in Figure 2. Similar effects have been seen with the isolated dimer (J.C. Dunbar and G.B. Ralston, unpublished results). Bennett and Branton [11], in density gradient sedimentation velocity studies, find a lower sedimentation coefficient for the spectrin dimer in 0.3 mM phosphate buffer (7S) than after the addition of 20 mM KC1 (8 S). These data are supported by the results of analytical ultracentrifugation studies by Shotton and Branton (quoted in Ref 11).

THE TETRAMER OF SPECTRIN

The tetramer appears to be the largest homopolymeric aggregate of spectrin to be isolated from the red cell membrane. The tetramer, purified by gel filtration on 4% agarose gels, appears to be homogeneous by the criteria of gel filtration, sedimentation velocity, acrylamide gradient electrophoresis, and sedimentation equilibrium [12]. Electrophoresis in dodecyl sulphate yields only the two spectrin components of 220,000 and 250,000 daltons, respectively, in equal amounts (Fig 3).

This purified tetramer has a molecular weight of 960,000 determined both by sedimentation equilibrium and sedimentation/diffusion [4, 12].

The sedimentation coefficient of 12.2 S for this material (Table I) is a great deal lower than the value of approximately 35 S expected for a compact globular protein of this molecular weight, and it corresponds to a frictional ratio of 2.8. Similarly, the elution of the tetramer from agarose columns is considerably earlier than expected.

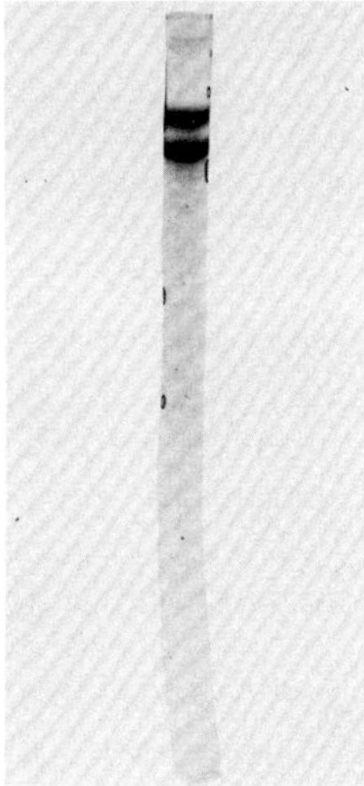

Fig 3. Electrophoresis of the purified tetramer of spectrin. Electrophoresis was performed in 5.6% acrylamide gels containing 1% SDS, essentially by the method of Fairbanks, Steck, and Wallach [23].

TABLE I. Hydrodynamic Properties of Spectrin*

Property	Tetramer (a)	Dimer (b)	Monomer (c)
MW	960,000 [4, 12]	480,000 [4] 430,000 [6]	225,000 [6]
$s^{\circ}_{20,w}$	12.2 S [12] 12.6 S [6]	9.7 S [6] 9.3 S	4.4 S [6] ~ 7 S [4]
$D^{\circ}_{20,w}$ ($cm^2 sec^{-1}$)	1.1×10^{-7} [12]	1.75×10^{-7}	–
f/f_0	2.8	2.1 [6] 2.3	2.9 [6]
$K_S/[\eta]$	1.33 [12]	1.15	–
a/b (0.5 g/g hydration)	–	5 [6]	13 [6]
a/b (from $K_S/[\eta]$)	4	7	–

*Values not referenced are unpublished results of J.C. Dunbar and G.B. Ralston

The anomalous hydrodynamic properties have traditionally been explained by proposing a long rod shape for spectrin [3]. A model of this nature has also appeared attractive in the light of supposed similarities between myosin and spectrin [13] and of possible contractile roles for spectrin [14].

However, because asymmetry and expansion can both give rise to an increase in the frictional ratio, it is notoriously difficult to determine both the size and shape of a molecule from hydrodynamic properties alone. If a shape is known, the dimensions of this shape can be determined from the frictional coefficient. Usually, a compact ellipsoid of rotation is chosen to represent the shape of the molecule, partly because of the daunting complexity of the calculation for other shapes. Moderate values of the frictional ratio are taken to indicate a globular particle with a degree of "hydration" or departure from truly spherical. Very large values of the axial ratio in this treatment generally are taken to indicate a long, rod-like molecule. However, if the molecule is not compact but is highly expanded, this treatment is not satisfactory, resulting in an anomalous, high value of the axial ratio. By these criteria, for example, a spherically symmetrical random coil appears to have a high axial ratio.

There is some theoretical basis for use of the ratio $K_s/[\eta]$, the ratio of the concentration-dependence of the sedimentation coefficient to the intrinsic viscosity, as a measure of symmetry of the molecule. Creeth and Knight [15] have tested this relationship empirically and found that for the spherical particles, ranging from denatured proteins in guanidine hydrochloride to latex spheres, $K_s/[\eta]$ was close to 1.6, while for rod-like particles the value of $K_s/[\eta]$ decreased with increasing axial ratio, approaching zero for very long rods. For a number of proteins of known shape, $K_s/[\eta]$ appeared to be a function of axial ratio [15].

When this treatment is applied to spectrin, a value of 1.33 (Table I) was found for the tetramer [12], a value very different from that of 0.2 for myosin; it indicates a shape no more asymmetric than serum albumin or glutamate dehydrogenase, with a probable axial ratio no more than about 4, estimated by use of the empirical relationship quoted by Creeth and Knight.

It is therefore unlikely that the spectrin tetramer can be represented adequately by the model of a long rod. The unusual hydrodynamic properties may then be due more to a highly expanded but basically symmetrical structure than a grossly elongated one [12]. On the basis of a symmetrical model, hydrodynamic data from viscosity, diffusion, and gel filtration all suggest a particle radius of about 200 Å [12].

THE DIMER

A number of laboratories have used the more rapid method of preparing spectrin by means of extraction at low ionic strength at 37°C. Although this method removes most of the spectrin within 15 min rather than many hours, the spectrin so isolated is in a dimer form, of molecular weight about 480,000 [6, 8].

The dimer produced in this way appears to be very similar to that isolated from low-temperature preparations, but sufficient study has not yet been made to determine whether the two forms are identical. Gratzer and Beaven [6] measured the sedimentation coefficient of the dimer of human spectrin as 9.7 S, and in our laboratory (J.C. Dunbar, unpublished results) a value of 9.3 S has been obtained, both for low-temperature and 37°C preparations. Clarke [3] reported a limiting sedimentation coefficient for her spectrin preparations in the range of 8–10 S, and although this preparation may have been contaminated with higher aggregates of spectrin, it would appear that the dimer was a prominent component.

Gratzer and Beaven [6] also reported the presence of monomeric spectrin in their 37° preparations. This species appeared to have a sedimentation coefficient of 4.4 S, and its proportion increased with time of storage and on freezing and thawing the ghosts. The monomer and dimer were stable aggregates, and like the tetramer and dimer system from low temperature preparations they did not appear to be in rapid equilibrium [6].

The sedimentation coefficient of the dimer corresponds to a frictional ratio of 2.1 [6]. Allowing for 0.5 g/g hydration Gratzer and Beaven [6] calculate an axial ratio of about 5 for the dimer, and about 13 for the monomer (Table I). However, they admit that the prolate ellipsoid is not a very realistic model and suggest that a flexible coil may be a better approximation. Certainly, the physical properties of the dimer are again quite different from those of myosin.

Recently we have subjected the dimer of spectrin to the Creeth-Knight analysis for symmetry [15]. With the dimer from 37°C preparations, the value of 1.15 for $K_s/[\eta]$ indicates a more asymmetric structure for the dimer than was seen for the tetramer, but still not a grossly asymmetric one. A value of 7.2 can be estimated for an axial ratio of the dimer, if a prolate ellipsoid is a valid model, using the empirical equation given by Creeth and Knight [15]. This value is in reasonable agreement with that of 5 estimated by Gratzer and Beaven [6] (Table I).

Results somewhat different from these have been obtained by Schechter et al [16] with spectrin in the detergent, deoxycholate. These workers have found that in this solvent, the dimer and monomer of spectrin have very similar sedimentation coefficients: between 5.5 and 6 S. These data are consistent with dimerisation as an end-to-end association of monomers, since the frictional coefficients of rod-like molecules of constant diameter increase almost linearly with the length of the rod. Although this interpretation is not in dispute, it is very unlikely that the protein in deoxycholate is similar in overall conformation to that of the protein in the absence of detergents. In fact, Schechter et al [16] report that the aqueous extract was heterogeneous, but with an average sedimentation coefficient near 8 S. Addition of deoxycholate resulted in dissociation and a decrease in sedimentation coefficient to about 6 S. Furthermore, addition of deoxycholate caused a decrease in the mean residue ellipticity of about 15%. Although Schechter et al [16] suggest that this is not a major conformational change, it is nevertheless a significant one that may be expected to alter the hydrodynamic properties of the protein. The changes, both in optical properties and in the sedimentation coefficient, indicate that the conformation of spectrin in the presence of deoxycholate is not the same as that in its absence.

SECONDARY STRUCTURE

The chiroptical properties of spectrin have been examined in a number of different studies, but again there has been a marked variation in the results from different laboratories, as indicated by the data of Table II. Most experiments have been done with the void volume peak from Sephadex G-200 chromatography, a preparation already shown to be heterogeneous. The results reported by Brandts et al [17] were made on the unfractionated water-soluble extract. It is not possible unequivocally to determine which of the oligomers predominated in the preparations used for the data of Table II.

Although methods such as sedimentation velocity, in which a partial separation of components occurs, can still give reasonable estimates of the properties of noninteracting components in a mixture, the optical properties of components in such a mixture can not easily be extracted. It is likely that the data of Table II underestimate the helical content of spectrin. Schechter et al [16] report that a crude extract of spectrin in deoxycholate had a mean residue ellipticity of $-19{,}000\ \mathrm{deg \cdot cm^2 \cdot dmole^{-1}}$, while after purification the same sample in the same solvent showed an increase in the magnitude of the trough to about $-23{,}000\ \mathrm{deg \cdot cm^2 \cdot dmole^{-1}}$, a change of approximately 20%. Since the presence of deoxycholate appeared to reduce the magnitude of the circular dichroism (CD) trough [16], it is likely that the magnitude of this trough is even greater for aqueous solutions.

Measurements on the purified tetramer in our laboratory [12] were originally made on rather dilute solutions in the visible region, where the optical rotation is very small. These studies indicated about 45% α-helix. We have since repeated these measurements on very carefully prepared samples, over a range of protein concentrations. These results (Table III) indicate an α-helix content close to 60% for both the tetramer and the dimer, based on the Moffitt-Yang b_0 parameter. The fit of the data to the Moffitt-Yang plots is very good, with correlation coefficients in the region of 0.9995. The specific rotation at the mercury 578 line is very low, about −6°. Within the limits of accuracy of these measurements, we are unable to detect a difference in the optical rotatory dispersion of the tetramer and dimer.

However, studies on the purified proteins in the far UV circular dichroism spectrum indicate an even greater apparent helix content, and significant differences between the tetramer and dimer (Fig 4). The molar ellipticity of the tetramer (−28,600 deg · cm^2 · $dmole^{-1}$) is quite a bit greater in magnitude than any of the values listed in Table II.

To some extent, this difference presumably reflects the greater purity of the sample in the latter case, but there may well be other factors involved, such as differences between the tetramer and dimer, temperature and solvent effects on the proteins, and perhaps conformational changes.

TABLE II. Chiroptical Properties of Spectrin

a. Circular dichroism	$-[\Theta]_{222} \times 10^{-4}$ deg · cm^2 · $dmole^{-1}$	% helix[a]
Pinder et al [5]	1.9	54
Gratzer and Beaven [6]	1.6–1.8	45–50
Schechter et al [16]	2.2	60
Vincentelli et al [18]	–	61
Brandts et al [17]	2.1	63
b. Optical rotatory dispersion	$-[m']_{233} \times 10^{-3}$ deg · cm^2 · $dmole^{-1}$	% helix[b]
Reynolds and Trayer [27]	3	25
Brandon [19]	5.95	48

[a]Based on $[\Theta]^H_{222} = -39{,}000$ [21].
[b]Based on $[m']^H_{233} = -14{,}600$ for polylysine [21].

TABLE III. Chiroptical Properties of Spectrin Oligomers*

	Dimer (a)	Tetramer (b)
$[\alpha]_{578}$	−6 ± 2°	−6 ± 2°
b_0	−382°	−385°
% helix (b_0)	60 ± 5	60 ± 5
$[m']_{233} \times 10^{-3}$	−9.62°	–
% helix (ORD)	66	–
$[\Theta]_{222} \times 10^{-3}$	−26.7°	−28.6°
% helix (CD)	68	73

*All measurements made in 0.1 M NaCl, 0.01 M sodium phosphate (pH 7.5), 25–27°C.

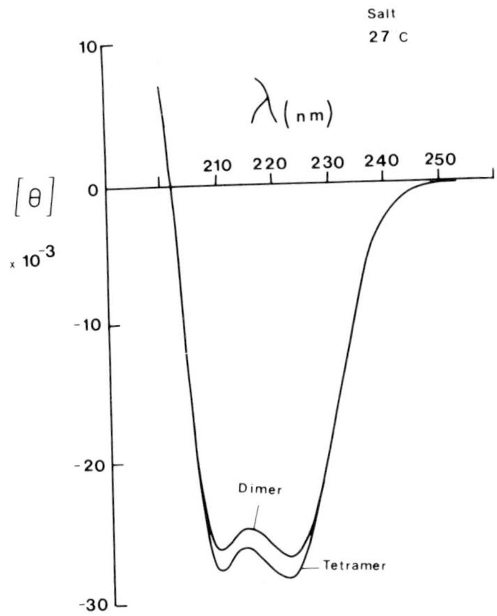

Fig 4. Circular dichroic spectra for the tetramer and dimer of spectrin in 0.1 M NaC1, 0.01 M sodium phosphate, pH 7.5. Spectra were recorded in a Cary 60.01 polarimeter, with cells of 1 mm pathlength. Protein concentrations: tetramer, 0.42 mg/ml; dimer, 0.37 mg/ml.

Chen, Yang, and Martinez [20] have developed a method for the calculation of helical and β-structure content in proteins from the circular dichroism spectrum. This method is based on the average properties of structured regions in a number of different proteins, whose structures are known from crystallographic studies. Structure distributions determined in this way are thought to be more meaningful for globular proteins than those determined from the use of long helical models such as polyamino acids. However, when the apparent helical content is as high as it appears to be in spectrin, there are good grounds for retaining the use of polyamino acids as models. This procedure has been adopted in the present case, with the use of the summarized values for polyamino acids listed by Jirgensons [21], and yields an α-helical content of 73% for the tetramer and 68% for the dimer, both in 0.1 M NaCl at 27°C.

The CD spectrum of spectrin, in an undefined oligomeric state, has been analysed in detail by Vincentelli, Devogel, and Leonis [18] with the use of the method of Chen, Yang, and Martinez [20]. Their analyses suggest 61% helix and 20% β-structure. The helical content is lost rapidly and almost completely on heating to 100°C, but the β-structure appears to be surprisingly stable. Brandts et al [17] also find a residual structure, resistant to heating. However, both of these studies were performed on unfractionated mixtures, so the conclusions must be tempered with caution.

CONFORMATION CHANGES

The chiroptical properties of spectrin are markedly dependent on salt concentration and temperature. In the presence of 0.1 M NaC1 and at temperatures between 15° and 40°C, the optical rotating dispersion (ORD) and CD spectra of spectrin are relatively constant, the magnitude of the rotation or ellipticity decreasing by only a small amount with increasing temperature, as shown for the specific rotation in Figure 5. At higher temperatures, thermal denaturation appears to occur with a midpoint near 50°C. This transition has been observed calorimetrically and by circular dichroism by Brandts et al [17] using unfractionated spectrin. At even higher temperatures, there appears to be a further structure change, centered near 60°C (Fig 5), but this change does not appear to correspond to changes in enthalpy. Aggregation phenomena, as well as further unfolding, may contribute to this high temperature transition.

In very low salt concentration, the temperature-dependent changes are more interesting. At 20°C, the lower salt concentration seems to result in a small conformational change, reflected in about a 5% decrease in the magnitude of the ellipticity. This optical change seems to correspond to the change in sedimentation coefficient as the salt concentration is lowered, and may reflect a slight expansion of the molecule, promoted by the increased electrostatic free energy. As the temperature is raised, however, further, more substantial changes take place. Instead of the slight decrease in laevorotation with increasing temperature seen in 0.1 M NaCl, laevorotation in low salt concentrations steadily increases (Fig 5). By 37°C, the optical rotation has already undergone a substantial change.

These temperature-dependent changes in low salt concentrations parallel the dissociation from the tetramer to the dimer. Possibly, the change in optical rotation reflects a change in conformation that is required to enable the dissociation step. The presence of salt prevents this change, stabilizing the tetramer conformation, and thus inhibiting dissociation.

What is not clear at present is why the dissociation is apparently irreversible. Gratzer and Beaven [6] have also noted that dissociation of the dimer to monomers is not a reversible process: Reversible unfolding in guanidine hydrochloride regenerates only dimers

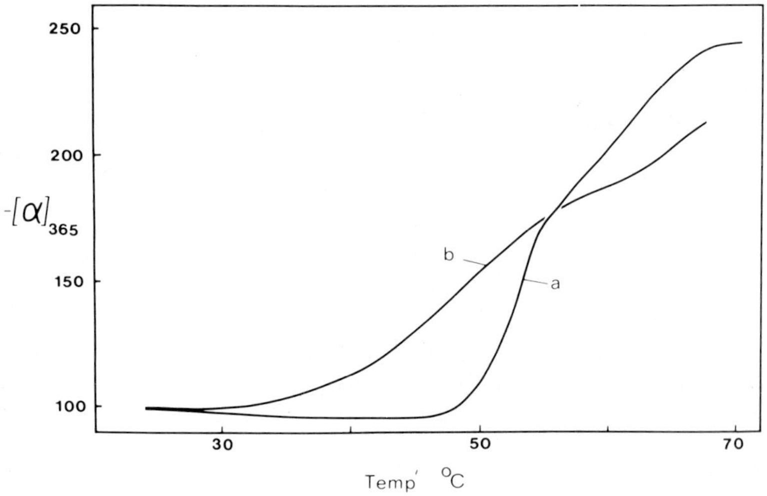

Fig 5. Temperature dependence of specific rotation for the spectrin tetramer. Measurements were made on a Perkin-Elmer polarimeter, model 241, with cells of pathlength of 10 cm. a) Tetramer in 0.1 M NaCl, 0.01 M sodium phosphate, pH 7.5; b) Tetramer in 5 mM sodium phosphate, pH 7.5. The temperature plotted is that of the circulating water bath and has not been corrected for the temperature differential between the interior of the cell and the bath.

from dimers, and only monomers from the monomers. It is possible that irreversible changes in covalent bonds, either peptide bonds, or phosphoryl groups, may accompany the dissociation process, but evidence is lacking at present.

A MODEL FOR SPECTRIN

On the basis of the hydrodynamic properties, a number of models for the structure of spectrin can be eliminated. The compact globular structure is eliminated by the high frictional ratio, and the long-rod model is inconsistent with the value of $K_S/[\eta]$. Any model that is proposed must also be consistent with increasing symmetry as the monomer units associate to form dimers and tetramers. A side-by-side association of rods with axial ratios of about 13 may satisfy the data, but a structure like this is not consistent with other requirements.

The tetramer is the largest known homotropic association state of spectrin. Higher association states seem to comprise actin in the ratio of one actin molecule for each two chains of spectrin. This stoichiometry suggests a continuous two-dimensional network of spectrin and actin, in which each actin molecule links two adjacent spectrin monomers. The spectrin monomers are envisaged as being organized into tetramer units. In order to satisfy the spectrin-actin stoichiometry, and to allow two-dimensional continuity, a cross structure is proposed, as shown in Figure 6. A structure like this has two-dimensional symmetry and would be expected to behave quite differently than a rod. The dimer and monomer dissociation states, however, would show increasing asymmetry. The radius of the cross would be expected to be near 200 Å, the Stokes radius of the tetramer. Given, then, the area of a single tetramer "cell" as 1.6×10^5 Å^2 and the number of copies of the

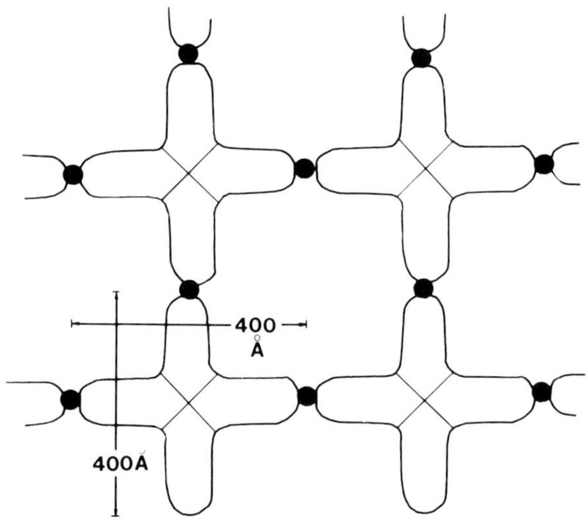

Fig 6. A model for the spectrin-actin network. The spectrin tetramer is envisaged as being composed of monomers arranged such that one actin molecule can bridge two adjacent monomer "arms." The "unit cell" of the repeating network is approximately 400 Å × 400 Å, based on the Stokes radius of the tetramer.

tetramer per erthyrocyte as approximately 8.5×10^4 [23], the total area that the spectrin network can cover is 1.36×10^{10} Å^2, in excellent agreement with estimates of the surface area of the ghost [24].

This model has certain points of similarity with that proposed by Kirkpatrick [28], but differs in the important respects of the shape of spectrin (allowing better membrane coverage), and the interaction with actin (allowing two-dimensional network formation).

As a further check on the validity of the model, it is possible to calculate the sedimentation coefficient of a structure that can be approximated by an assemblage of spherical subunits [25]. The cross structure can be approximated by an arrangement of nine spherical subunits, each of mass 100,000 daltons, and of radius 60 Å. The diameter of this cross will be 600 Å, and the total mass 900,000 daltons. The dimer can be approximated by two adjacent arms, and the monomer by a single linear arm. For these structures, the sedimentation coefficents are shown in Figure 7, together with the experimental values. Although the dimensions and arrangements of this structure are rather arbitrary and crude, nevertheless such a structure is reasonably consistent with the experimental data.

The proposed structure for the dimer is also consistent with the "C" structures seen in negative contrast preparations in the electron microscope [22] and with the three-domain structures, approximately 500 Å long, seen in high-resolution low-angle shadowing experiments (D. Branton and D. Shotton, personal communication).

Very recently, Hainfeld and Steck [26] have shown scanning electron micrographs of a "sub-membrane reticulum," appearing as a continuous web over the cytoplasmic face of the membrane. The size and arrangement of the components of this reticulum bear a surprising and gratifying resemblance to the sort of structure just proposed for spectrin. This is a very welcome convergence from two completely different experimental approaches.

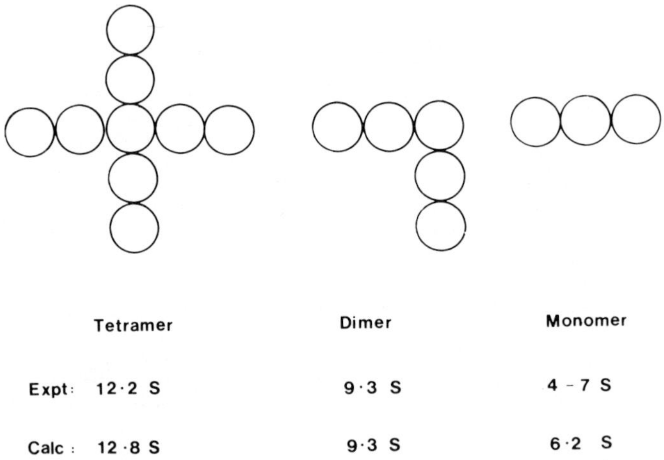

Fig 7. Model representations of the spectrin oligomers. The tetramer, dimer, and monomer were represented by arrangements of spherical subunits, for the purposes of calculation of approximate sedimentation coefficients. Each spherical subunit has a radius of 60 Å and a mass of 100,000 daltons. For each oligomer, the experimental and calculated sedimentation coefficients are compared.

ACKNOWLEDGMENTS

The original research described in this review was supported by grants from the Australian Research Grants Committee and the University of Sydney Consolidated Medical Research Fund.

REFERENCES

1. Marchesi VT, Steers E Jr: Science 159:203, 1968.
2. Marchesi SL, Steers E, Marchesi VT, Tillack TW: Biochemistry 9:50, 1970.
3. Clarke M: Biochem Biophys Res Commun 45:1063, 1971.
4. Ralston GB: Aust J Biol Sci 28:259, 1975.
5. Pinder J, Tidmarsh S, Gratzer WB: Arch Biochem Biophys 172:654, 1976.
6. Gratzer WB, Beaven GH: Eur J Biochem 58:403, 1975.
7. Dunbar JC, Ralston GB: Biochim Biophys Acta (In press).
8. Ralston G, Dunbar J, White M: Biochim Biophys Acta 491:345, 1977.
9. Pedersen KO: In Svedberg T, Pederson KO: "The Ultracentrifuge." Oxford: Clarendon Press, 1940, pp 23–29.
10. Ralston GB: Biochim Biophys Acta 443:387, 1976.
11. Bennett V, Branton D: J Biol Chem 252:2753, 1977.
12. Ralston GB: Biochim Biophys Acta 455:163, 1976.
13. Sheetz MP, Painter RG, Singer SJ: Biochemistry 15:4486, 1976.
14. Guidotti G, Ann Rev Biochem 41:731, 1972.
15. Creeth JM, Knight CG: Biochim Biophys Acta 102:549, 1965.
16. Schechter NM, Sharp M, Reynolds JA, Tanford C: Biochemistry 15:1897, 1976.
17. Brandts JF, Erickson L, Lysko K, Schwartz AT, Taverna RD: Biochemistry 16:3450, 1977.
18. Vincentelli J, Devogel M, Leonis J: Arch Int Physiol Biochim 84:682, 1976.
19. Brandon DL: FEBS Lett 58:349, 1975.
20. Chen YH, Yang JT, Martinez HM: Biochemistry 11:4120, 1972.
21. Jirgensons B: "Optical Activity of Proteins and Other Macromolecules." Berlin: Springer-Verlag, 1973.
22. Tilney LG, Detmers PJ: Cell Biol 66:508, 1975.
23. Fairbanks G, Steck TL, Wallach DFH: Biochemistry 10:2606, 1971.
24. Weinstein RS: In Surgenor DM (ed): "The Red Blood Cell." New York: Academic, 1974, pp 324–368.
25. Bloomfield V, Van Holde KE, Dalton WO: Biopolymers 5:149, 1967.
26. Hainfeld JF, Steck TL: J Supramol Struct 6:301, 1977.
27. Reynolds JA, Trayer H: J Biol Chem 246:7337, 1971.
28. Kirkpatrick FH: Life Sci 19:1, 1976.

Journal of Supramolecular Structure 8:375–389 (1978)
Normal and Abnormal Red Cell Membranes 97–111

Vesicles Isolated From ATP-Depleted Erythrocytes and out of Thrombocyte-Rich Plasma

Hans U. Lutz

Laboratory for Biochemistry, Federal Institute of Technology, ETH, Universitätstrasse 16, CH 8092 Zürich, Switzerland

When human erythrocytes are depleted of endogenous ATP they release spectrin-free vesicles as a light vesicle fraction [Lutz et al: J Cell Biol 73: 548, 1977] and chains of rounded vesicles as well as flattened myelin forms in a heavy vesicle fraction. The heavy fraction retains some spectrin, and glycophorin is partially degraded. The release of both types of fragments is not dependent upon added Ca^{+2}, and 50 μM EGTA does not prevent the vesicle release. Concomitant with vesicle release, a large fraction of the major protein components of the cell is found in disulfide-bonded aggregates.

A protocol is outlined to recover erythrocyte-specific fragments from thrombocyte-rich plasma. It allows detection of spectrin-free vesicles in whole blood stored under blood bank conditions for 12 days. In freshly drawn blood no such vesicles are observed, but particles are obtained that are different from thrombocyte fragments and that show a prominent glycoprotein running slightly faster than glycophorin.

Key words: **thrombocyte-rich plasma, disulfide-bonded protein aggregates, erythrocyte fragmentation, human erythrocytes, in vitro aging, ATP-depletion, spectrin-free vesicles, fragments of erythrocytes.**

ATP-depleted human erythrocytes display a series of structural [1–3] and functional [3–6] alterations that are likely to help us understand the requirements to be fulfilled by a structurally intact, deformable, and functionally active erythrocyte membrane. If erythrocytes are depleted of ATP for more than 20 hours erythrocytes have become echinocytes [1–3], and some of these blebs are lost as spectrin-free vesicles [7]. Evidence has been presented which suggests that echinocytic blebs represent a membrane in which the lateral mobility of antigens is not restricted as in the rest of the membrane [8]. A similar behavior is expected for antigens in spectrin-free vesicles. Therefore echinocytes may contain part of their membrane in a state similar to that found in spectrin-free

Abbreviations: EGTA – ethyleneglycol bis (β-aminoethylether)-N,N′-tetraacetic acid; ATP – adenosine triphosphate; CPD – citrate-phosphate dextrose solution used to preserve whole blood; SDS – sodium dodecylsulphate; DDT – dithiothreitol.

0091-7419/78/0803-0375$02.90

vesicles, and thus their functional properties could well be an average of those found in vesicles and in ATP-loaded erythrocyte. However, the spectrin-free vesicles, named "microspheres" by morphologists [9], are not the only membrane fragment being released from ATP-depleted cells [9]. Thus a detailed study of functional properties of released fragments requires the myelin forms to be characterized as well. In this presentation some insight on both release of spectrin-free vesicles and myelin forms is given. The requirements for their release are analyzed and compared with those known to induce a release of spectrin-free vesicles when erythrocytes are incubated with Ca^{+2} and ionophore A23187 [10].

Spectrin-free vesicles are such a defined and easily derived structural entity from human erythrocytes that it would be interesting to know whether such vesicles have physiological significance. Some evidence along this line has been given for spectrin-free vesicles being released from erythrocytes stored under blood bank conditions [11]. In this study a protocol is worked out to search for erythrocyte-specific fragments in thrombocyte-rich plasma.

MATERIALS AND METHODS

Human blood collected in CPD was obtained from the Red Cross. If not otherwise indicated the donors had the following blood group: O, Rh^+, M/M.

ATP-Depletion Experiments

Whole blood was centrifuged for 7 min at 2,000 rpm in a Sorvall-SS34 rotor. The supernate was withdrawn as thrombocyte-rich plasma for the experiments described later. The buffy coat was removed and the cells made up to 50% hematocrit in 5 mM phosphate 150 mM NaCl (pH 7.4). This suspension was passed through a cottom column to remove most of the white cells and residual thrombocytes. The eluate was washed three times in the same buffer and was incubated at 20% hematocrit in a medium containing 60 mM glycylglycine (or 50 mM glycylglycine when 5 mM phosphate was added), 110 mM NaCl, 5 mM Kcl, 250 mg/liter penicillin G, and 300 mg/liter streptomycin. The pH was adjusted with 1 N NaOH to pH 7.5. The cell suspensions were placed in dialysis bags and these were immersed in 10 volumes of the same medium. The Erlenmeyer flasks containing the dialysis bags were incubated in a shaking water bath at 37° C. After 6, 12–15, and 18–24 hours, the pH was readjusted to 7.4 in the surrounding medium. At the given times the content of the dialysis bags was centrifuged for 7 min at 2,000 rpm in a Sorvall-SS34 rotor. The supernates collected were diluted up to 10-fold with isotonic buffered saline and centrifuged for 1–2 hours at 45,000g. The vesicle pellets were resuspended in the same buffer and analyzed; samples of these suspensions were layed on isotonic dextran step gradients consisting of two solutions with the densities $\rho = 1.05$ and $\rho = 1.085$ (not corrected for added salt). These gradients were centrifuged overnight in swing-out buckets at 100,000g. The following day the light fraction at the interface and the heavy one as the trailing fraction above the pellet were withdrawn from the top and washed once in a large volume of buffered saline. In some experiments the erythrocytes have been surface-labeled with ^{125}I using lactoperoxidase and glucose oxidase [12]. Under these conditions only the integral membrane proteins, glycophorin and protein component 3, are labeled.

Gel Electrophoresis

SDS-polyacrylamide slab gels (8 × 2.7%) were performed in a system similar to that described by Neville [13], with a running gel in 0.38 M Tris and 0.1% SDS at pH 8.8. The stacking gel had a pH of 6.8, and the electrode buffer was 0.025 M Tris 0.3 M glycine and 0.1% SDS. The samples were incubated prior to electrophoresis for 30 min at 37° C in a medium containing 1% SDS, 40 mM DTT (if not otherwise indicated) 25% glycerol, 0.06 M Tris (pH 6.8) (final concentration).

Gels were stained for glycoproteins according to Eckhardt et al [14], and for proteins with Coomassie blue in 50% methanol, 10% acetic acid. Quantitation of protein components was carried out with a gel scanner Integraph (Bender and Hobein, Zürich) on Coomassie blue stained and dried gels. Quantitation of glycoproteins was performed on photographic negatives taken from gels stained with the fluorescent dansylhydrazine [14].

Isolation of Vesicles From Whole Blood

The protocol used is described in Figure 5. The filtration of thrombocyte-rich plasma was performed on a laminar flow Sartorius ultrafiltration system by using 3 filter units with a pore size of 0.8 μm. The filters were washed prior to use with water and isotonic saline. The completely liquid-filled system was connected to the flask containing the plasma to be filtered, and care was taken to avoid air from being trapped. The plasma was passed through the filter without artificially increasing the pressure.

The filtrate was centrifuged for 2 h at 45,000g. The pellet was resuspended in a small volume of buffered saline and 1 mg/ml aprotinin (a plasmin inhibitor, Novo, Copenhagen) was added. This suspension was layered on top of a dextran step gradient as outlined above.

A light and heavy fraction were collected from the gradient and washed once. The material thus obtained was resuspended in a small volume divided in three equal fractions and antisera added along with 1–2 mg aprotinin per ml. Commercially available anti-M and anti-N (Merz and Dade, Bern) have been used in a 1/1 dilution having agglutination titers of 1/8–1/12. Following the addition of sera, the samples were incubated for 30 min at 37° C and then pelleted in an Eppendorf centrifuge. These pellets were kept for several hours at 4° C and then they were resuspended and pelleted for 30 sec in a table centrifuge, the supernatant removed and the remaining pellets 3 times washed with buffered saline. The final pellets were made 1% in SDS and stored frozen.

Thrombocyte membranes were a gift from Dr Clemetson, Bern [15].

RESULTS

Light and Heavy Fractions of Vesicles Released From ATP-Depleted Human Erythrocytes

When human erythrocytes are depleted of endogenous ATP they release vesicular material that does not pellet upon centrifugation of the cell suspension for 7 min at 2,000 rpm in a Sorvall-SS34 rotor. The supernate thus obtained can be separated into a light and heavy fraction by a dextran step gradient (see Methods). With this step gradient the light fraction is found at the interface, and the heavy fraction is found as a trailing fraction above a tiny pellet containing some residual erythrocytes. The light fraction has the properties of the previously described spectrin-free vesicles, with an average density of ρ = 1.062 [7] with no obvious signs of proteolytic damage (Fig 1B, compare background in the lower half of the gel with Fig 1A). However, the heavy fraction, which appears to have a similar protein composition, shows extended proteolysis evident from the high background in the trace of bound Coomassie blue in the lower half of the gel (Fig 1C). In addition, glycophorin from these vesicles is partially degraded (see arrows for glycophorin and its major breakdown product in Fig 1C). The number of vesicles found in the heavy fraction can be diminished by including phosphate in the incubation mixture, but their properties remain unchanged (Table I). Thus the diffuse Coomassie blue staining bands

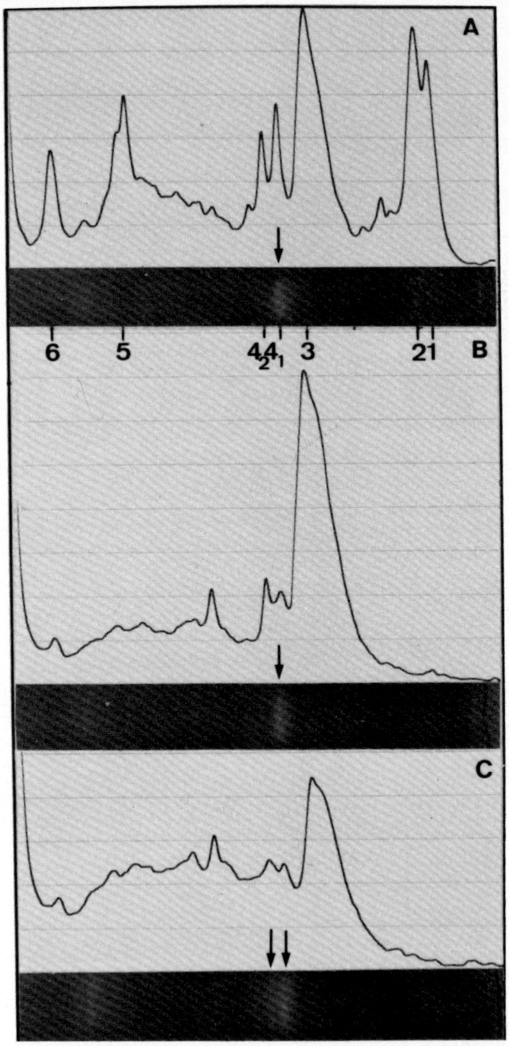

Fig 1. Protein compositions of light and heavy fractions of vesicles released from ATP-depleted human erythrocytes. Experimental details are given in Table I for assays with phosphate. Each graph consists of a scan from the dried Coomassie blue stained gel and of a photograph from the same gel previously stained for glycoproteins. A) fresh ghosts; B) light vesicle fraction; C) heavy vesicle fraction. The numbers listed below gel A refer to the major protein components of human erythrocytes. The arrows indicate the position of glycophorin and its major breakdown product where present.

TABLE I. Properties of Light and Heavy Vesicle Fractions From ATP-Depleted Human Erythrocytes

Addition to incubation mixture	Type of fraction	Membrane protein (μgm/10 ml supernate)	Content of protein component 3 (%)	Extent of proteolytic damage to glycophorin (%)	Predominant structures observed on electron micrographs
None	Light	68	47	0	Rounded vesicles
	Heavy	152	21	10	Myelin forms and rounded vesicles in chains
5 mM phosphate	Light	80	49	2	Rounded vesicles
	Heavy	78	26	16	Myelin forms and rounded vesicles in chains

Erythrocytes were ATP-depleted for 45 hours as outlined in Methods, except that the cells were not passed through a cotton column but were washed 5 times in isotonic saline supplemented with phosphate only for those cells incubated in phosphate thereafter. Membrane protein was determined from Coomassie blue stained gels as outlined in ref 7. The content of protein component 3 was determined by scanning Coomassie blue stained and dried gels (see Methods). The extent of proteolytic damage to glycophorin was quantified by calculating the relative amount of stain found in the lower molecular weight form (see arrows in Fig 1) as a percentage of the total stain detected in both glycophorin and breakdown product for ghosts and vesicles. The observed percentage for ghosts was set at zero, and the difference between numbers determined for vesicles and for ghosts was listed.

in the lower half of the gel may originate from high-molecular-weight proteins that cause the high buoyant density of these vesicles.

On the other hand, when erythrocytes are washed thoroughly free of white cells and plasma (see Methods), the heavy vesicle fraction retains a small amount of spectrin (6% of the total membrane protein including bands 7 and 8) and does not show a diffuse Coomassie blue stained zone (gel 2b, Fig 2). Although no signs of extended proteolysis are seen on Coomassie blue stained gels, glycophorin is still partially degraded (data not shown). Addition of phenyl methane sulfonyl fluoride (10–20 mg/liter) does not prevent glycophorin from being degraded in the heavy vesicle fraction under optimum conditions (not shown). Further evidence for some proteolysis to persist even under optimum conditions for ATP-depletion is clearly obtained from cells that have been surface-labeled with

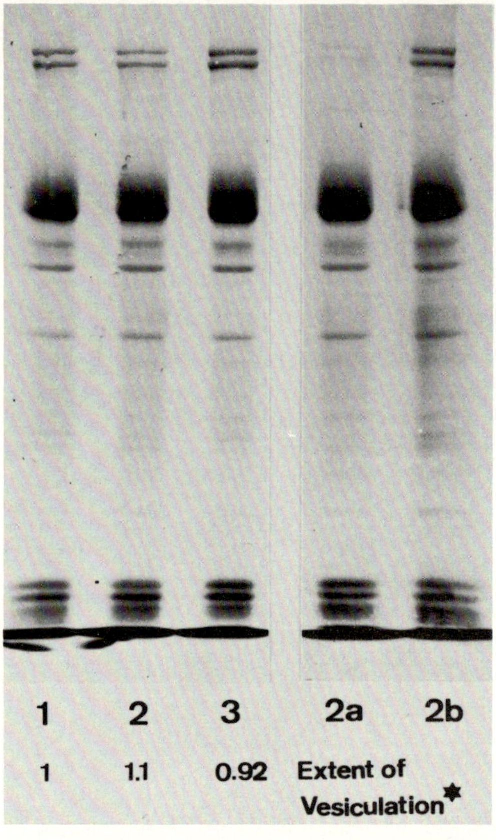

Fig 2. Extent of vesiculation and protein composition of vesicles released from ATP-depleted human erythrocytes in the presence of Ca^{+2} or EGTA. Erythrocytes were washed as outlined in Methods and surface-labeled with ^{125}I [12] prior to incubation. ATP-depletions were carried out for 38 hours in the medium given in Methods supplemented with 5 mM phosphate and with no further addition in experiment 1, with 50 μM $CaCl_2$ in experiment 2, and with 50 μM EGTA in experiment 3. 2a refers to the light vesicle fraction; 2b, to the heavy vesicle fractions.

*Extents of vesiculation are listed as relative numbers based on the number of cpm from ^{125}I recovered in the vesicle pellet originating from 10 ml of supernate from ATP-depleted cells. Extent 1, listed for the control (experiment 1), corresponds to 16,712 cpm recovered in the vesicle pellet. Extent data shown for experiments 1 and 2 are averages from two separate experiments. Radioactivity and protein were determined in triplicate.

^{125}I. Whereas ghosts from fresh cells contained 91,396 cpm per mg protein, those of ATP-depleted cells retained only 59,670 cpm per mg protein. The vesicles recovered from ATP-depleted cells account for an estimated fraction of 12% of the loss.

Most interesting is the morphology of the two fractions. The light one displays rounded vesicles, as previously described, and the heavy one shows rounded vesicles mostly in chains, and some vesicles appear to carry with them fragments of erythrocytes (Fig 3A). Among these structures elongated strands or flattened myelin forms are detected (Fig 3B) that are abundant in preparations revealing extended proteolysis (not shown).

Effect of Calcium on the Release of Spectrin-Free Vesicles

In view of the finding [10] that spectrin-depleted vesicles are released from human erythrocytes within 90 min following the addition of calcium and ionophore A23187, the question arose whether calcium that is known slowly to enter ATP-depleted cells [16] is necessary for the release of spectrin-free vesicles during ATP-depletion. Thus erythrocytes were depleted of ATP with varying concentration of calcium chloride in media not containing phosphate. All Ca^{+2} concentrations exceeding 50 μM resulted in enhanced hemolysis and proteolytic damage to vesicles and cells, but up to this concentration the activity of acetylcholinesterase found in the supernates after pelleting the cells was comparable to that found in the absence of Ca^{+2}, reaching 32% higher levels at 50 μM Ca^{+2}. Since the addition of 50 μM Ca^{+2} did not significantly enhance the release of vesicles, only traces of Ca^{+2} might be needed to induce the release. Such low concentrations of Ca^{+2} could have been introduced as Ca^{+2} adsorbed to washed cells or as contaminant in sodium chloride. Therefore the release of spectrin-free vesicles was studied in the presence of EGTA as well. In these experiments cells were surface labeled with ^{125}I (see Methods) to quantify integral membrane proteins. The extent of vesiculation was almost identical

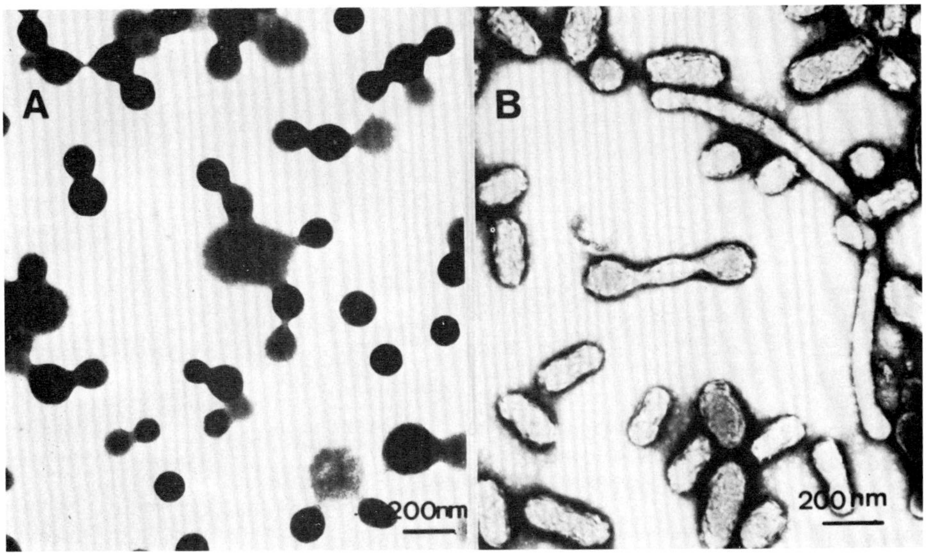

Fig 3. Electron micrographs from heavy fractions obtained following staining with uranylacetate. A) 15-sec staining revealing the electron-dense material trapped within vesicles; magnification ×33,000. B) 60-sec staining, focused on the surface of these structures; magnification ×40,000.

in preparations with or without Ca^{+2}, as well as with 50 μM EGTA when the amount of ^{125}I was measured in washed vesicle pellets from supernates of ATP-depleted cells (including both light and heavy fractions) (Fig 2, gels 1–3). The protein compositions of all three vesicle pellets are identical as are the compositions of all light and heavy fractions respectively demonstrated in Figure 2 for the assay with Ca^{+2} (gel 2a and 2b). Consequently the release of spectrin-free vesicles is not dependent upon added calcium and thus occurs by a different series of phenomena than that observed with calcium and ionophore.

Formation of Disulfide-Bonded Protein Aggregates in ATP-Depleted Erythrocytes That Have Released Spectrin-Free Vesicles

Introduction of calcium with ionophores causes the endogenous transglutaminase to be activated [17, 18] and ATP to be rapidly depleted [19]. Thus ATP-depletion and transglutaminase-dependent protein cross-linking precede the release of spectrin-free vesicles when calicum is introduced with ionophore. A similar pair of events occurs during in vitro aging: ATP is depleted [7] and disulfide-bonded protein aggregates are formed, irrespective of added Ca^{+2} or EGTA. This is shown in Figure 4 in erythrocytes that have released spectrin-free vesicles. (A thorough analysis of these aggregates has been published by Liu and Palek [20]). Since disulfide formation is dependent on oxidative conditions, the release of spectrin-free vesicles, as found in the light fraction, is partially inhibited by

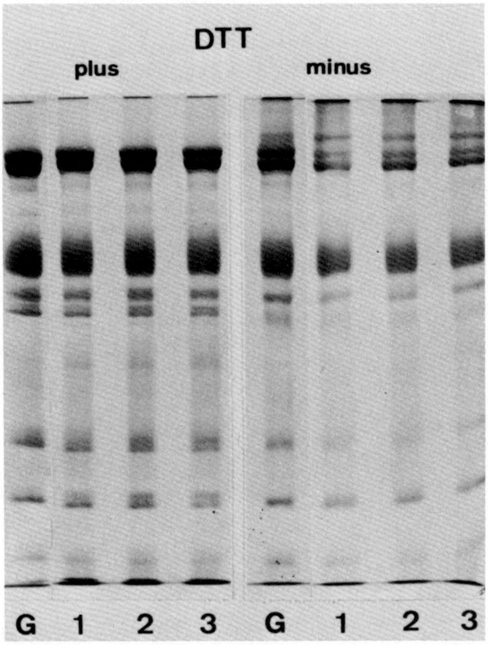

Fig 4. Formation of disulfide-bonded protein aggregates in ATP-depleted erythrocytes that have released vesicles. The conditions were as outlined in Figure 2. After having removed the vesicles from ATP-depleted cells, the cells were washed once and ghosts were isolated and frozen in 1% SDS without addition of NEM, which would have eliminated the slight formation of aggregates seen in ghost proteins electrophoresed without prior reduction. Each sample applied to the gel contained 15 μg of protein and was electrophoresed with or without prior reduction with DTT. 1) ghosts from ATP-depleted cells; 2) ghosts from ATP-depleted cells with 50 μM $CaCl_2$; 3) ghosts from ATP-depleted cells with 50 μM EGTA. G, fresh ghosts.

nitrogen, but the release of vesicles found in the heavy fraction is not affected (Lutz and Müller, unpublished results, December 1977).

Isolation of Vesicles From Whole Blood

Whole blood stored for more than 12 days in CPD contains spectrin-free vesicles that can be isolated from thrombocyte-rich plasma following the protocol outlined in Figure 5. The light and heavy fractions (Fig 6) retain proteins reminiscent of thrombocyte membranes (compare with gel T Fig 7A) and of spectrin-free vesicles. After agglutination of the particles from these fractions with rabbit anti-M and anti-N sera and repeated washing of the agglutinated and pelleted material, the protein composition of these pellets is similar to that of spectrin-free vesicles isolated from in vitro aged human erythrocytes (Fig 6), except that they retain actin (component 5) but very little spectrin. In spite of using blood from a donor with a homozygous genotype M/M, anti-N agglutinates these vesicles to some degree and anti-M reacts weakly with vesicles. These data suggest the vesicles to have lost some of the antigens, although they contain glycophorin (evident from gels stained for glycoproteins, not shown). When thrombocyte-rich plasma from whole blood stored under blood bank conditions for 4 weeks is processed the same way, light and heavy fractions following the step gradient reveal a protein composition

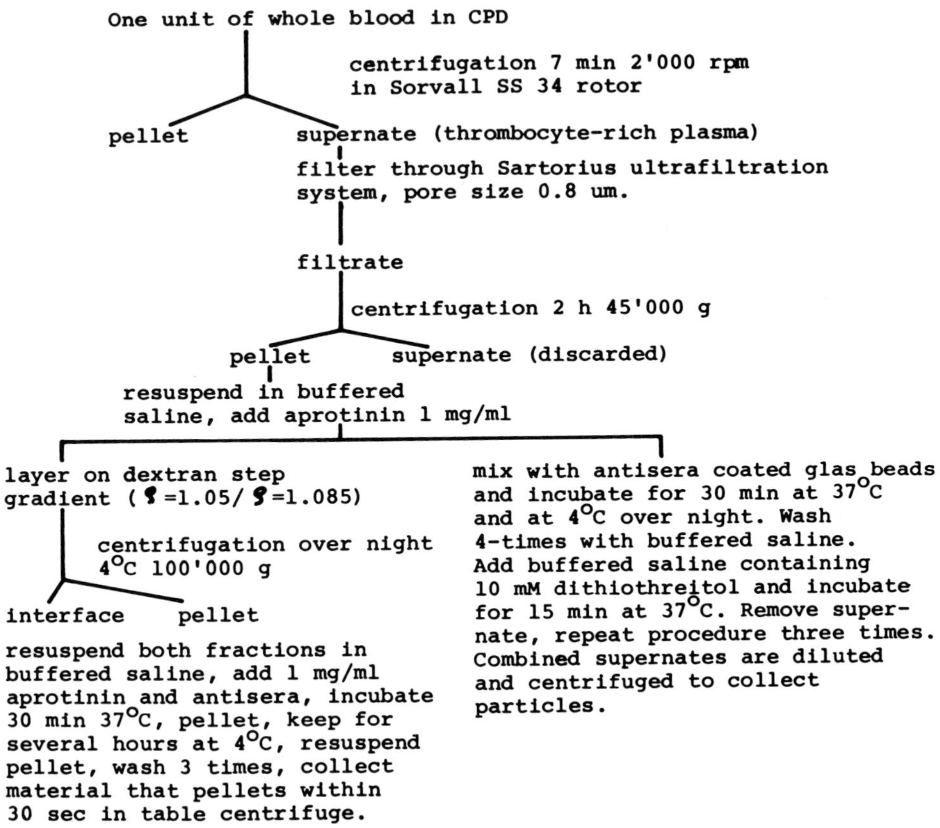

Fig 5. Isolation of erythrocyte-specific fragments.

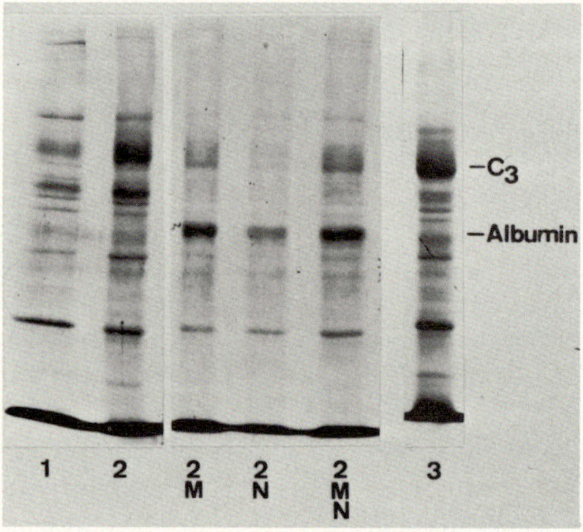

Fig 6. Spectrin-free vesicles from whole blood stored under blood bank conditions. Whole blood stored for 13 days was treated as outlined in Figure 5. Protein compositions are shown in gel 1 for the light vesicle fraction; in 2, for the heavy vesicle fraction of the dextran step gradient. Equal amounts of the heavy fractions were agglutinated with M/N blood group antisera and the protein composition of the agglutinated and pelleted material shown in 2_M, 2_N, 2_{MN}. M refers to added anti-M;N, to anti-N. C_3 denotes protein component 3.

similar to spectrin-free vesicles without further purification by agglutination (shown for heavy fraction in Fig 6).

Thrombocyte-rich plasma from fresh blood collected in CPD and processed in the same day according to the protocol in Figure 5 does not contain spectrin-free vesicles, but both light and heavy fractions show many protein bands originated from thrombocytes. However, when the heavy fraction from the dextran step gradient is agglutinated with antisera M or N, a prominent protein band (see arrow in Fig 7A) is enriched in the pellet that has no counterpart in thrombocyte membrane proteins. Both M and N antisera seem to have the same effect. The prominent band appears to be a glycoprotein running slightly faster than glycophorin (Fig 7B). The prominent band does not originate from added sera, nor is it a degradation product of thrombocyte glycoprotein because the thrombocyte protein pattern remains unchanged when thrombocyte membranes are incubated with antisera (T_M Fig 7A and B). Identical results are obtained when thrombocyte-rich plasma from an N/N homozygous donor is used (data not shown).

In order to avoid agglutination and copelleting of thrombocyte fragments, preliminary experiments have been performed using immunadsorption to antisera-coated glass beads. Anti-M and anti-N sera from MRC Blood Group Reference Lab in London (titer 1/124 and 1/64, respectively) were covalently coupled by dithiobis succinimidyl propionate (Pierce) to aminoalkyl glass beads (Pierce) following the protocol from Lomant and Fairbanks [21]. Since the antibodies were reversibly coupled, the washed beads could be treated with reducing agent to release antisera and bound material. The supernate after this reduction was diluted and centrifuged to collect particles. In two preliminary experiments the pellets thus obtained reveal the prominent glycoprotein and serum albumin but decreased amounts of protein bands originating from thrombocytes (Fig 8). However, the binding capacity of the glass beads was low, such that the supernate still contained a large fraction of this protein. The amount of protein that can be agglutinated or adsorbed to immobilized antisera is very low and does not exceed 30 μgm per unit of blood. Although this material behaves like a vesicle, it may be of other origin than erythrocytes. Experiments are in progress to check whether this glycoprotein is partially identical to glycophorin.

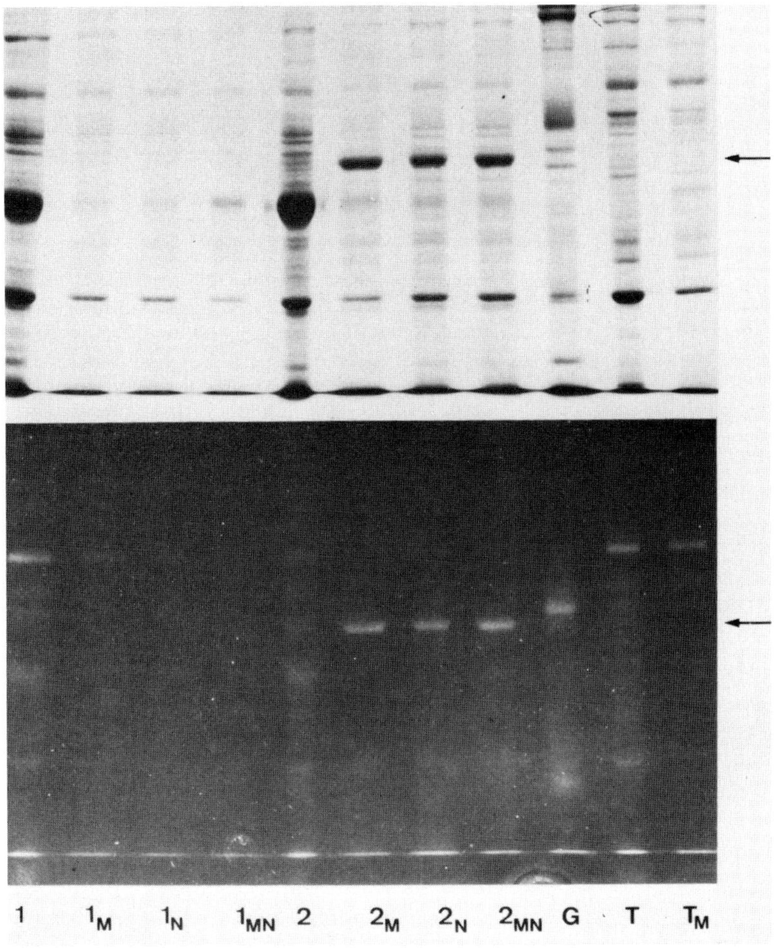

Fig 7. A) Protein composition of light and heavy particle fractions isolated from fresh thrombocyte-rich plasma. Plasma was processed as outlined in Figure 5 except that 20 mg/liter PMSF was added to the plasma prior to filtration. The light and heavy fractions following the dextran step gradient were divided in three equal parts, and anti-sera were added as indicated by subscript M or N (anti-M or anti-N). 1, supernate collected from all three agglutination assays from the light fraction; 2, supernate collected from all three agglutination assays from heavy fraction; 1_M, 1_N, 1_{MN}, agglutinated and pelleted material from the light fraction; 2_M, 2_N, 2_{MN}, agglutinated and pelleted material from the heavy fraction; G, 15 μgm protein of fresh human erythrocyte membranes; T, 15 μgm protein of thrombocyte membranes; T_M, thrombocyte membranes incubated with anti-M and pelleted.

B) Glycoprotein composition of light and heavy particle fraction isolated from the fresh thrombocyte-rich plasma.

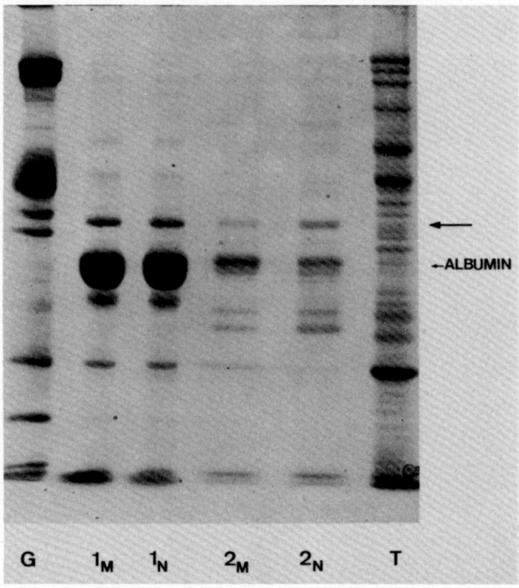

Fig 8. Protein composition of particles derived from fresh thrombocyte-rich plasma adsorbed to anti-M- or anti-N-coated glass beads. Fresh whole blood M/M was processed as outlined in Figure 5 and given in Methods. 1_M shows the protein composition of the material not bound to glass beads coated with anti-M; 2_M shows the protein composition of the particles that were bound and released by adding reducing agent; 1_N and 2_N show the equivalent results obtained with anti-N-coated glass beads (when antisera-coated glass beads were processed without adding the particles obtained after filtration and centrifugation of the filtrate, no protein could be found pelleted after reduction of the glass beads); G, 20 μgm protein of human erythrocyte membranes; T, 20 μgm protein of thrombocyte membranes. The arrow points to the prominent glycoprotein found in these particles (see also Fig 7).

DISCUSSION

Light and Heavy Vesicles

ATP-depleted erythrocytes release two types of fragments, a light fraction containing essentially spectrin-free vesicles, or microspheres, and a heavy fraction that contains chains of rounded vesicles and flattened myelin forms. The heavy fraction retains a small portion of spectrin and shows several indications of proteolytic damage, even under optimum conditions. Since myelin forms are abundant in preparations with extended proteolysis, it is likely that these structures have evolved from chains of rounded vesicles by proteolytic damage. Whereas spectrin-free vesicles from the light fraction do not show obvious signs of proteolysis, the heavy vesicle fraction and the residual cells do. These results are compatible with earlier findings that ATP-depleted cells release low-molecular-weight glycopeptides [22, 23]. However, the question remains unsettled why the light vesicle fraction hardly undergoes proteolysis and the heavy one is extensively proteolyzed. Whether this difference is due to potential proteases being trapped along with spectrin in the heavy vesicle fraction is not known. It is still not even clear whether the residual spectrin found in heavy vesicles is located in the chains of rounded vesicles or in the scarcely seen fragments of erythrocytes.

Requirements For Vesicle Release From ATP-Depleted Human Erythrocytes

During in vitro aging of human erythrocytes 50 μM Ca^{+2} does not enhance vesicle release and 50 μM EGTA has no inhibitory effect. Thus the well-documented endogenous transglutaminase that requires at least 0.5 mM Ca^{+2} to be active [17, 18] remains inactive during in vitro aging. Instead the proteins undergo disulfide-bonded aggregation that prevents spectrin from being trapped in vesicles. Although these changes are occurring concomitantly with vesicle release, they are not absolute requirements for vesicle release; under nitrogen, disulfide formation and release of spectrin-free vesicles are partially inhibited, but heavy vesicles are still formed (Lutz and Müller, unpublished results). We have previously shown that ATP has to be depleted for spectrin-free vesicles to be released. We then hypothesized that during ATP-depletion more and more of the yet unknown connections between integral membrane components and spectrin are destroyed. Such connections could well involve a phosphorylated site of spectrin that has recently been shown to play an important role in maintaining erythrocyte shape [6].

Although a loss of interaction between integral and peripheral membrane proteins is obviously necessary and theoretically conceivable, we lack similarly simple perceptions concerning the other major alteration that seems to be required: the formation of phosphatidate. We found phosphatidate to be enriched in spectrin-free vesicles from in vitro, aged human erythrocytes when its relative content was compared to that found in fresh erythrocytes. Allan et al [10] did not detect phosphatidate in spectrin-depleted vesicles induced by Ca^{+2}-ionophore A23187, but they report a stimulated phosphatidate labeling capacity due to diacylglycerol formed [24]. Phosphatidate found in spectrin-free vesicles from in vitro, aged erythrocytes can hardly be formed from diacylglycerol because ATP is depleted before vesicles are released.

Although the protein composition of the two types of spectrin-free vesicles is very similar, the lipid composition as well as the events favoring release differ. However, ATP-depletion is common to both types.

Isolation of Erythrocyte-Specific Fragment From Whole Blood

Since microspheres have been observed in blood stored under blood bank conditions [25] (and even in situ during erythrocyte phagocytosis [26]) and in fresh blood from certain patients [25], it is obvious to analyze such microspheres for their protein composition. On the other hand, it is unlikely that in vivo aged erythrocytes release spectrin-free vesicles to a large extent in circulation because their cellular ATP is not known to drop sufficiently to induce vesicle release [27]. Nevertheless a sensitive method has been worked out to test this possibility, taking advantage of the M/N bloodgroup antigens that occur only on erythrocytes and involve glycosylated side-chains as well as the N-terminus of glycophorin [28]. Using the protocol outlined in Figure 5, spectrin-free vesicles can be purified to some degree from thrombocyte-rich plasma of blood stored under blood bank conditions. The weak agglutinability observed with anti-M when M/M cells are used and the partial agglutination found with anti-N are not unexpected because it is known that blood stored under these conditions loses antigenic material to the supernate.

The vesicles isolated from stored blood differ from those obtained from washed cells upon ATP-depletion in their retention of protein component 5 and the appearance of a new protein band with an apparent molecular weight of 140,000. Overall their composition appears to be comparable to that reported for microvesicles from stored blood as reported by Rumsby et al [11] in a drawing of a gel. Thus it can be concluded that blood stored in CPD undergoes vesiculation leading to spectrin-free vesicles. This vesiculation may be reduced by supplementing CPD with adenine, which has been shown to maintain high cellular ATP levels and erythrocyte survival rates after transfusion [29, 30]. It may well be that storage of blood under nitrogen further improves the survival, because under these conditions at least the release of spectrin-free vesicles is partially inhibited.

When the protocol outlined in Figure 5 is applied to thrombocyte-rich plasma from freshly drawn blood, particles are agglutinated that differ in protein composition from thrombocyte membranes and spectrin-free vesicles. They contain a prominent glycoprotein that has a slightly lower apparent molecular weight than glycophorin. Although the total amount of protein found in this particle fraction from one unit of blood was very low and thus did not allow chemical characterizations exceeding gel electrophoresis, the same results were obtained repeatedly for both M/M and N/N erythrocytes. Immunoadsorption using antisera-coated glass beads resulted in retention of the prominent glycoprotein, whereas some other proteins seen in agglutinated particles that clearly originated from thrombocytes were reduced. However, the reversible immunoadsorption technique has to be improved, because only a fraction of the prominent protein found in the particle suspension was adsorbed. Thus an erythrocyte-specific antiserum must be used that is not identical to M/N antisera.

In preliminary experiments using immunreplica techniques with antibodies against glycophorin, Claude Bron (Lausanne) and I have obtained some evidence that the particles isolated from thrombocyte-rich plasma contain protein components that form precipitations with anti-glycophorin. These studies will show whether particles containing a glycophorin breakdown product are released from erythrocytes in circulation presumably as a mode to correct for suffered damage.

ACKNOWLEDGMENTS

The author thanks Mrs N. v. Fischer for technical assistance, Dr T. Bächi, Institute for Medical Microbiology, University of Zürich for the electron micrographs, and Drs M. Metaxas and M. N. Metaxas from the Red Cross in Zürich for helpful discussions concerning the use of antibodies and for providing typed blood units. This work has been supported by SNSF grant 3.022-0.76, Berne.

REFERENCES

1. Nakao M, Nakao T, Yamazoe S: Nature 187:945, 1961.
2. Féo CJ, Leblond PF: Blood 44:639, 1974.
3. Weed R, Lacelle P, Merrill E: J Clin Invest 48:795, 1969.
4. Tadano K, Hellums JD, Lynch EC, Peck EJ, Alfrey CP: Blood Cells 3:163, 1977.
5. Sheetz M, Singer SJ: J Cell Biol 73:638, 1977.
6. Birchmeier W, Singer SJ: Cell Biol 73:647, 1977.
7. Lutz HU, Liu SC, Palek J: J Cell Biol 73:548, 1977.
8. Gordon JA, Marquardt MD: Nature 258:346, 1975.
9. Bessis M, Mandon P: N Rev Fr Hematol 12:443, 1972.

10. Allan D, Billah MM, Finean JB, Michell RH: Nature 261:58, 1976.
11. Rumsby RH, Trotter J, Allan D, Michell RH: Biochem Soc Trans 5:126, 1977.
12. Reichstein E, Blostein R: J Biol Chem 250:6256, 1975.
13. Neville D: J Biol Chem 246:6328, 1971.
14. Eckhardt AE, Hayes CE, Goldstein IJ: Anal Biochem 73:192, 1976.
15. Clemetson KJ, Pfueller SL, Luscher EF, Jenkins CSP: Biochim Biophys Acta 464:493, 1977.
16. Palek J, Church A, Fairbanks G: In Bolis L, Hoffmann JF, Leaf A (eds): "Membranes and Disease." New York: Raven Press, 1976, pp 41.
17. Lorand L, Weissmann LB, Epel DL, Brunner-Lorand J: Proc Natl Acad Sci USA 73:4479, 1976.
18. Anderson DR, Davis JL, Carraway KL: J Biol Chem 252:6617, 1977.
19. Taylor D, Baker R, Hochstein P: Biochem Biophys Res Commun 76:205, 1977.
20. Palek J, Liu SC, Snyder LM: Blood 51:385, 1978.
21. Lomant AJ, Fairbanks G: J Mol Biol 104:243, 1976.
22. Brovelli A, Suhail M, Pallavicini G, Sinigaglia F, Balduini C: Biochem J 164:469, 1977.
23. Brovelli A, Pallavicini G, Sinigaglia F, Balduini CL, Balduini C: Biochem J 158:497, 1976.
24. Allan D, Michell RH: Biochem J 166:495, 1977.
25. Weed RI, Reed CF: Am J Med 41:681, 1966.
26. Essner E: J Biophys Biochem Cytol 7:329, 1960.
27. Boron ER: J Lab Clin Med 62:263, 1963.
28. Wasniowska K, Drzeniek Z, Lisowska E: Biochem Biophys Res Commun 76:385, 1977.
29. Dawson RB: Transfusion 17:242, 1977.
30. Zuck TF, Bensinger TA, Peck CC, Chillar RK, Beutler E, Button LN, McCurdy PR, Josephson AM, Greenwalt TJ: Transfusion 17:374, 1977.

Journal of Supramolecular Structure 8:391–397 (1978)
Normal and Abnormal Red Cell Membranes 113–119

The Exchangeability of Human Erythrocyte Membrane Cholesterol

Yvonne Lange and Josephine S. D'Alessandro

Biophysics Division, Boston University School of Medicine, Boston, Massachusetts 02118

A new method has been used to determine what fraction of human erythrocyte cholesterol is available for exchange with plasma unesterified cholesterol. Erythrocytes labeled with ^{3}H-cholesterol by this exchange process were incubated with sonicated phosphatidylcholine vesicles, giving rise to a net movement of cholesterol out of the cells. The specific activity of cholesterol taken up by the vesicles depended on the length of time of incubation. Initially the specific activity in the vesicles was greater than that in the cells, but after approximately 10% of cell cholesterol had been removed, the specific activity of subsequently removed cholesterol was equal to that of the remaining erythrocyte cholesterol. We conclude from these data that a) all of the cholesterol in the erythrocyte is exchangeable with plasma, and b) approximately 10% of erythrocyte cholesterol is in a more rapidly exchangeable pool than the remainder.

Key words: **cholesterol exchange, erythrocyte membrane, cholesterol pools**

Since the original studies which showed that unesterified cholesterol readily exchanges between erythrocytes and plasma [1, 2], numerous authors have attempted to determine what proportion of membrane cholesterol participates in this exchange process [3–6]. These measurements all were based on a study of the equilibration of radiolabeled cholesterol between erythrocytes and plasma lipoproteins, all the label being in one or the other component at the outset of the experiment. The results of these studies are divided between those that observed complete exchange of erythrocyte cholesterol [3, 4] and those that found that a portion of erythrocyte cholesterol does not participate in the exchange process [5, 6]. A resolution of these contradictory findings would be of value, as the extent to which erythrocyte cholesterol is available for exchange has important implications with regard to membrane structure.

In a recent paper [7] we showed that the transfer of labeled cholesterol between human erythrocytes and plasma occurred by the same mechanism and involved the same pool of molecules whether the transfer involved no net movement of cholesterol (exchange)

Received for publication March 30, 1978; accepted May 15, 1978.

or whether a net movement of cholesterol out of the cells took place. In spite of the fact that this study did not reveal some of the details of exchange reported here, it provided the basis for a new, extremely simple technique for the determination of the amount of exchangeable erythrocyte cholesterol. In the experiments described in this paper, erythrocytes labeled with ^{3}H-cholesterol by exchange were incubated with sonicated phosphatidylcholine vesicles so as to deplete the cells of cholesterol. Because exchange and depletion are manifestations of the same process, the cholesterol molecules removed from the membrane in this way came from the pool which was labeled by the exchange process and the fraction of total membrane cholesterol which was labeled by exchange could be determined by measuring the specific activity of the cholesterol taken up by the vesicles. This study demonstrates that cholesterol in human erythrocytes is in two distinct kinetic pools, one of which contains approximately 10% of the cell cholesterol and exchanges rapidly with plasma, while the other contains the bulk of cell cholesterol and exchanges with plasma at a slower rate. Furthermore, the results demonstrate that all of human erythrocyte cholesterol is exchangeable with plasma.

METHODS

Blood from healthy human donors was collected in heparin (4,000 USP units/liter blood). Plasma and the "buffy coat" were separated from the cells after 15 min centrifugation at 1,500g. The red cells were washed three times in 10 volumes of the following buffer, which was used in all experiments: 150 mM NaCl, 5 mM KCl, 5.5 mM Na_2HPO_4, 0.8 mM NaH_2PO_4, 0.5 mM $CaCl_2$, 5 mM glucose, pH 7.4. Plasma was preheated for 50 min at 56°C to destroy lecithin:cholesterol acyltransferase activity [8] and then labeled with ^{3}H-cholesterol as described by Murphy [9]. Labeling of erythrocytes with ^{3}H-cholesterol by exchange from plasma was performed as follows. Erythrocytes were incubated at 37°C at a hematocrit of 30% in buffer containing approximately 4% labeled plasma. In some experiments plasma was labeled with ^{3}H-cholesterol "indirectly," as follows. Erythrocytes labeled by exchange from autologous ^{3}H-cholesterol plasma were washed extensively in autologous unlabeled plasma and then incubated with a fresh aliquot of the same plasma for 16 h. This plasma then was used to label erythrocytes to be used in the experiment. Low density lipoproteins (LDL) were isolated from the plasma of fasting human donors using established procedures [10]. LDL was labeled by incubation with ^{3}H-cholesterol-labeled erythrocytes for 16–18 h.

Egg phosphatidylcholine (grade I) was purchased from Lipid Products (Redhill, Surrey, UK) and gave a single spot after thin-layer chromatography on silica gel. Vesicles were prepared by lyophilization of the lipid from benzene, dispersion in buffer, and sonication for 20 min with a Branson sonifier under N_2 in a water-jacketed cell at 4°C. The sonicate was centrifuged at 15,000g for 20 min to remove titanium particles shed from the probe.

"Inside out" membrane vesicles (IOVs) were prepared and assayed for sidedness as described by Steck [11]. Sidedness and sealing of IOV preparations were assessed before and after incubation with phosphatidylcholine vesicles using acetylcholinesterase as a membrane marker. Purity was between 80 and 90%. Incubations of erythrocytes or IOVs labeled with ^{3}H-cholesterol with sonicated vesicles were carried out at a hematocrit of approximately 20% in a shaking water bath at 37°C. Streptomycin sulfate was added as an antibacterial agent. Approximately 15 μM vesicle phospholipid was added to 5 μM membrane phospholipid. After 1–3 h the vesicles were removed for the assay of the specific activity of the cholesterol they had taken up and replaced with a fresh aliquot of the same vesicle preparation. By incorporation of ^{14}C-labeled phosphatidylcholine into the vesicles during their preparation, it was shown that no significant loss of vesicles from the supernatant occurred under the conditions of these experiments. Incubations were terminated by centrifugation for 10 min at 1,500g or for 15 min at 17,000g to pellet the erythrocytes and IOVs respectively. The supernatant containing the vesicles then was centrifuged for 20 min at 27,000g to remove any membrane fragments resulting from the small amount of hemolysis which occurred in some experiments. This supernatant then was concentrated under N_2 in a magnetically stirred cell using an Amicon Diaflo ultrafilter and the lipids were extracted [12]. Erythrocyte lipid extraction and cholesterol assays were performed as described [7]. Due to the large amount of phospholipid present in the supernatant lipid extracts, it was found necessary to carry out a saponification step followed by hexane extraction prior to cholesterol assay of these samples. Radioactive PC, the generous gift of Dr Trevor Redgrave, was synthesized from enzymatically prepared phosphatidic acid and choline chloride (methyl-^{14}C) [13]. ^{3}H-cholesterol and ^{14}C-choline chloride were purchased from New England Nuclear, Boston, Massachusetts.

RESULTS

When erythrocytes labeled with ^{3}H-cholesterol by exchange from plasma were incubated with egg lecithin vesicles, cholesterol was taken up by the vesicles, in consonance with the findings of others [14]. The specific activity of the cholesterol removed from the erythrocytes was found to depend on the time of incubation, that is, on the extent of cholesterol depletion. To obtain precise data on the specific activity changes, vesicles were incubated with erythrocytes until they had taken up sufficient cholesterol to permit the assay of specific activity and then were replaced with fresh vesicles to remove more erythrocyte cholesterol. It was found that the cholesterol initially removed from the cells had specific activity higher than that of the cholesterol in the erythrocytes. As more cholesterol was removed from the cells, the specific activity of this cholesterol decreased until it was equal to that of the remaining erythrocyte cholesterol (see experiment 1, Table I and Fig 1a). The equality of specific activity of removed cholesterol and remaining cholesterol was reached after the removal of approximately 10% erythrocyte cholesterol.

Several control experiments were carried out to rule out the possibility that the high-specific-activity cholesterol removed initially from the erythrocytes represented a highly labeled plasma component that had remained stuck to the cell surface in spite of the washes carried out after the incubation to exchange ^{3}H-cholesterol into the cells from plasma. Cells that had been labeled by incubation with ^{3}H-cholesterol labeled plasma were washed thoroughly with unlabeled plasma, and these cells – putatively freed of any adsorbed labeled plasma – were used to label a further aliquot of plasma. In turn this plasma was used to label erythrocytes, which then were incubated with vesicles to remove cholesterol. The high specific activity of initially removed cholesterol still was observed (experiment 2, Table I and Fig 1a). A similar method was used to label purified human plasma low-density lipoprotein, which then was used to label erythrocytes. This method of labeling erythrocytes prior to cholesterol depletion also gave the same result (experiment 3, Table I and Fig 1a).

We conclude that the high-specific-activity cholesterol initially removed from erythrocytes in the depletion experiments is a manifestation of a true membrane phenomenon.

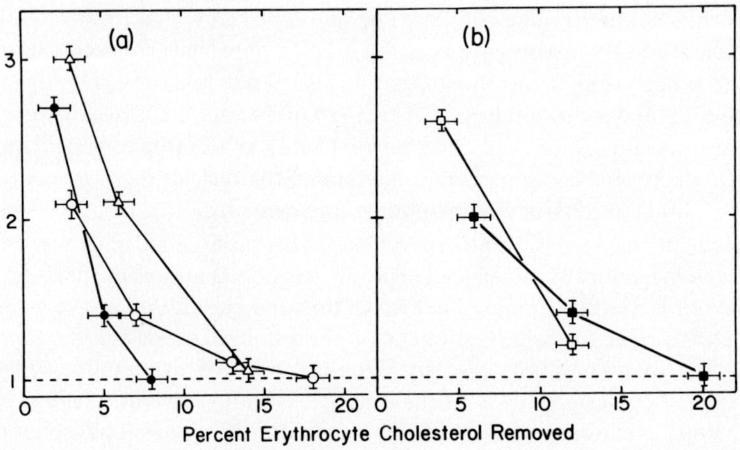

Fig 1. Results of cholesterol depletion experiments using a) intact erythrocytes (RBC) labeled directly from plasma (○); indirectly from plasma (●); from LDL (△); b) IOVs prepared from labeled RBC (■) or labeled after preparation (□). r is the cholesterol specific activity in vesicles at the end of an incubation, expressed relatively to the final specific activity in RBCs after an experiment consisting of 2–4 sequential incubations of vesicles with membranes. For each incubation the value of r is plotted versus the percentage of membrane cholesterol which had been removed by the end of that incubation.

TABLE I. Specific Activity of Cholesterol Removed From Erythrocytes (RBC) and Inside-Out Membrane Vesicles (IOV) by Incubation With Vesicles*

Experiment no.	Membrane system	Labeling method	Incubation no.	% RBC cholesterol removed	Specific activity (10^5 dpm/mg cholesterol) Vesicles	Initial RBC	Final RBC	r
1	Intact RBC	Direct plasma	1	3	16.9	9.1	8.2	2.1
			2	7	11.6			1.4
			3	13	9.0			1.1
			4	18	8.1			1.0
2	Intact RBC	"Indirect" plasma	1	2	12.4	5.1	4.6	2.7
			2	5	6.3			1.4
			3	8	4.6			1.0
3	Intact RBC	LDL	1	3	5.7	2.1	1.9	3.0
			2	6	4.1			2.1
			3	14	2.2			1.1
4	IOV	Labeled after preparation	1	4	56.2	25.4	21.7	2.6
			2	12	25.2			1.2
5	IOV	Prepared from labeled RBC	1	6	15.3	8.6	7.5	2.0
			2	12	10.3			1.4
			3	20	7.6			1.0

*Vesicles were incubated with membranes for 1–3 h, removed, and replaced with fresh vesicles. Column 5 shows the amount of cholesterol removed from RBC by the end of a given incubation with vesicles. The specific activity of the cholesterol taken up by the vesicles during each incubation is given in column 6 and the ratio (r) of this specific activity to the final RBC specific activity is given in column 9.

The experimental findings can be described by the following model. Erythrocyte cholesterol exists in two kinetically distinct pools, one of which contains approximately 10% of the total cholesterol and exchanges more rapidly with plasma cholesterol than does the other pool, which constitutes approximately 90% of erythrocyte cholesterol. During the initial incubation, in which ^{3}H-cholesterol was exchanged into the cells for a period of 16–19 h, the small, more rapidly exchangeable pool was closer to equilibrium with plasma cholesterol than was the larger pool, and the former therefore had reached higher specific activity at the end of the incubation. The cholesterol initially removed from the cells by incubation with vesicles came from the more rapidly exchangeable pool and therefore had high specific activity. After the pool was emptied out, cholesterol removed subsequently had lower specific activity, reflecting the presence of the larger, more slowly exchangeable pool.

We investigated the effect of the duration of the incubation to label the erythrocytes on the specific activity of cholesterol in the two pools. It was found that doubling the labeling period from 10 to 22 h did not alter the specific activity of the cholesterol initially taken up by the vesicles, that is, the cholesterol in the smaller pool (see experiment 6, Table II). However, the specific activity of cholesterol in the larger pool increased somewhat. These results are consistent with the model, since the small pool already had equilibrated with plasma during the 10-h incubation, whereas the specific activity of the large pool continued to increase between 10 and 20 h.

The following experiment was carried out to determine whether any exchange occurred between the two cholesterol pools. Erythrocytes were labeled by incubation with ^{3}H-cholesterol-labeled plasma for 6 h. An aliquot of these cells was incubated immediately with lecithin vesicles to sample the specific activity of the cholesterol in the small pool. Another aliquot of the same labeled cells was kept in buffer at 37°C for 18 h. After this delay the cells were incubated with lecithin vesicles to sample the specific activity of the cholesterol in the small pool. The results of this experiment are shown in Table II (experiment 7). It can be seen that the specific activity of the cholesterol in the

TABLE II. Time Dependence Studies of Specific Activity of Cholesterol Removed From Erythrocytes by Incubation With Sonicated Vesicles*

Experiment no.	Time of labeling incubation (h)	Incubation no.	% RBC cholesterol removed	Specific activity (10^5 dpm/mg cholesterol): Vesicles	Initial RBC	Final RBC	r
6	10	1	3	28.6	16.3	14.6	2.0
		2	8	17.0			1.2
		3	14	14.3			1.0
	22	1	5	29.2	24.1	20.9	1.4
		2	10	20.3			1.0
7	6 No delay	1	4	41.3	20.6	ND	
	18-h delay	1	6	35.2			

*See text and caption of Table I for explanation. In experiment 6 the durations of the incubations with sonicated vesicles were the same in both samples.
ND: Not determined.

small pool had decreased by approximately 15% as a result of the 18 h delay period. Even in the absence of any mechanism within the erythrocyte for exchange between the two pools, one would expect some decrease in the specific activity of the small pool due to exchange between erythrocytes. It follows that cholesterol exchange between the two pools occurs extremely slowly, if at all.

To determine whether the small cholesterol pool is accessible from both sides of the membrane, cholesterol depletion experiments were carried out with the inside-out membrane vesicle preparation described by Steck [11]. It was found that whether the membrane vesicles were prepared from ^{3}H-cholesterol labeled erythrocytes or labeled after their preparation from unlabeled erythrocytes, the specific activity of the cholesterol removed from the membrane depended on the amount of cholesterol removed in a manner qualitatively similar to that observed in intact erythrocytes (see experiments 4 and 5, Table I and Fig 1b).

It is possible that rather than reflecting two cholesterol pools in each erythrocyte, these experiments indicate two types of cells – 10% of the cells having very fast exchange characteristics compared to the rest. Differences in cholesterol exchange due to the age distribution in the erythrocyte population were investigated as follows. Erythrocytes were incubated in ^{3}H-cholesterol-labeled plasma for a period of 1 h – a time chosen so as to label predominantly the rapidly exchangeable pool. The cells then were centrifuged at 37,000g for 1 h in a tube 7 × 700 mm – a procedure which leads to the separation of erythrocytes according to age, the youngest cells having the lowest density [15]. Erythrocytes in the top 10% and the bottom 10% fractions of the tube were extracted and the specific activity of their cholesterol was determined. No difference between the fractions was observed.

DISCUSSION

Previously reported measurements of erythrocyte exchangeable cholesterol were based on experiments in which erythrocytes and plasma lipoproteins were incubated together until equilibration of labeled cholesterol, initially present in one or the other component, had occurred [3–6]. Such experiments necessitate lengthy incubations (up to 24 h) and suffer from the further disadvantage that knowledge is required of how much of the unesterified cholesterol in plasma is exchangeable. In contrast, the experiments described in this paper involve only relatively short incubations of erythrocytes and provide a precise and sensitive measure of the size of the exchangeable cholesterol pool.

In principle, a careful study of the kinetics of ^{3}H-cholesterol exchange between erythrocytes and lipoproteins would reveal the presence of the rapidly exchangeable pool we report here. However, the fact that this pool constitutes only about 10% of total cell cholesterol would make it difficult to observe in such a study, and it is therefore not surprising that it has not been reported hitherto.

There are two possible explanations for our findings. First, it is possible that the cell population is not homogeneous with respect to the characteristics of cholesterol exchange. We have shown that the rapidly exchangeable pool cannot be accounted for in terms of an inhomogeneity in cholesterol exchange characteristics due to cell age. Further study is needed to determine whether some other cell population variable could be involved.

The alternative possibility is that erythrocyte membrane cholesterol exists in two pools within the cell membrane. The finding that the small pool is still present in IOVs suggests that it is associated with the membrane bilayer. It seems unlikely that the small pool is cholesterol bound to intrinsic membrane protein, although this possibility cannot be ruled out at present. It has been reported recently that band 3 protein from human erythrocytes interacts strongly with cholesterol [16]. However, all evidence to date suggests that lipid associated with intrinsic membrane proteins, although in a different state from bulk membrane lipid, is readily exchangeable with other membrane lipid [17, 18]. Further study is required to determine if the more rapidly exchangeable molecules differ from the rest of the cell cholesterol in their interaction with some other membrane constituent or if they form an isolated cholesterol pool within the membrane.

Our studies of cholesterol depletion of ^{3}H-cholesterol-labeled erythrocytes have shown that after the removal of the small amount of high-specific-activity cholesterol, subsequently removed cholesterol has the same specific activity as that of the erythrocytes. This demonstrates that all of the erythrocyte cholesterol must have been labeled and therefore that it all is exchangeable with plasma. Previous studies [19, 20] have shown that transbilayer movement of cholesterol occurs in the human erythrocyte membrane with a half-time of less than 50 min at 37°C. Since cholesterol exchange occurs at the outer half of the membrane bilayer and it is extremely unlikely that all membrane cholesterol is located in this half of the membrane, the finding of the present paper indicates that cholesterol in both halves of the membrane is exchangeable with plasma. This provides further demonstration, based on an entirely different experimental approach, that cholesterol can move between the two halves of the bilayer in the erythrocyte membrane.

ACKNOWLEDGMENTS

This work was supported by grants from the National Institutes of Health, HL20303 and HL 18623.

REFERENCES

1. Hagerman JS, Gould RG: Proc Soc Exp Biol Med 78:329, 1951.
2. London JM, Schwartz H: J Clin Invest 32:1248, 1953.
3. Basford JM, Glover J, Green C: Biochim Biophys Acta 84:764, 1964.
4. Quarfordt SH, Hilderman H: J Lipid Res 11:528, 1970.
5. Bell FP, Schwartz CJ: Biochim Biophys Acta 231:553, 1971.
6. D'Hollander F, Chevallier F: J Lipid Res 13:733, 1972.
7. Lange Y, D'Alessandro JS: Biochemistry 16:4339, 1977.
8. Lichtman MA, Marinetti GV, Gordseky SE: Nouv Rev Fr Hematol 14:5, 1974.
9. Murphy J: J Lab Clin Med 60:571, 1962.
10. Deckelbaum RJ, Shipley GG, Small DM: J Biol Chem 252:744, 1976.
11. Steck TL: In Korn E (ed): "Methods in Membrane Biology." New York: Plenum, 1974, vol 2, p 245.
12. Folch J, Lees M, Stanley GHS: J Biol Chem 226:497, 1957.
13. Sears B, Hutton WC, Thompson TE: Biochemistry 15:1635, 1976.
14. Bruckdorfer KR, Edwards PA, Green C: Eur J Biochem 4:506, 1968.
15. Borun ER, Figueroa WG, Perry SM: J Clin Invest 36:676, 1957.
16. Klappauf E, Schubert D: FEBS Lett 80:423, 1977.
17. Warren GB, Toon PA, Birdsall NJM, Lee AG, Metcalfe JC: Proc Nat Acad Sci USA 71:622, 1974.
18. Hesketh TR, Smith GA, Houslay MD, McGill KA, Birdsall NJM, Metcalfe JC, Warren GB: Biochemistry 15:4145, 1976.
19. Lange Y, Cohen CM, Poznansky MJ: Proc Nat Acad Sci USA 74:1538, 1977.
20. Kirby CJ, Green C: Biochem J 168:575, 1977.

Journal of Supramolecular Structure 8:399–412 (1978)
Normal and Abnormal Red Cell Membranes 121–134

Triton Shells of Intact Erythrocytes

Michael P. Sheetz and David Sawyer

Physiology Department, University of Connecticut Health Center, Farmington, Connecticut 06032

About 40% of human erythrocyte membrane protein is resistant to solubilization in 0.5% Triton X-114. These components comprise a structure called a Triton shell roughly similar in size and shape to the original erythrocyte and thus constitute a cytoskeleton. With increasing concentrations of Triton the lipid content of the Triton shell decreases dramatically, whereas the majority of the protein components remain constant. Exceptions to this rule include proteins contained in band 3, the presumed anion channel, and in band 4 which decrease with increasing Triton concentration. The Triton-insoluble complex includes spectrin (bands 1 and 2), actin (band 5), and bands 3′ and 7. Component 3′ has an apparent molecular weight of 88,000 daltons as does 3; but unlike 3, it is insensitive to protease treatment of the intact cell, has a low extinction coefficient at 280 nm, and is solubilized from the shells in alkaline water solutions. Component 7 also has a low extinction coefficient at 280 nm. Spectrin alone is solubilized from the Triton shells in isotonic media. The solubilized spectrin contains no bound Triton and coelectrophoreses with spectrin eluted in hypotonic solutions from ghosts. Electron micrographs of fixed Triton shells stained with uranyl acetate show the presence of numerous filaments which appear beaded and are 80–120 Å in diameter. The filaments cannot be composed mainly of actin, but enough spectrin is present to form the filaments. Triton shells may provide an excellent source of material useful in the investigation of the erythrocyte cytoskeleton.

Key words: **Triton, cytoskeleton, spectrin, actin, erythrocyte membrane**

Two independent reports have shown that nonionic detergents solubilized the majority of integral membrane proteins from erythrocyte ghosts, leaving an insoluble fraction which contained the major portion of the peripheral proteins, spectrin and actin, and several other components [1–3]. Yu, Fischman, and Steck [2] showed that these proteins were organized in a shell which had a form similar to that of the original ghosts. Lux, John, and Karnovski [4] have further shown that the shape of irreversibly sickled cell ghosts is preserved in the shells obtained after Triton extraction. Therefore, the shell left after Triton extraction of the membrane may be regarded as part of the cytoskeleton of the ghosts.

Received for publication April 21, 1978; accepted June 1, 1978.

0091-7419/78/0804-0399$02.60

The shape and deformability of the erythrocyte are thought to depend upon the properties of this cytoskeleton adherent to the undersurface of the cell. For example, in the mouse model of hereditary spherocytosis the red cells are deficient in spectrin, and those cells lose membrane and lyse readily [5]. We have found that bivalent antibodies to spectrin will prevent certain shape changes from occurring in membranes isolated from normal human red cells when added at a concentration equivalent to that of spectrin [6]. At a much lower concentration of bivalent antibody the shape change of erythrocyte membranes induced by adenosine triphosphate (ATP) is accelerated. Since monovalent antibody fragments and control antisera have no effect, the cross-linking of the spectrin network underlying the membrane appears to aid the ATP-dependent shape change. A variety of other experiments also suggest that spectrin and actin have important functions in controlling membrane shape and deformability [7–9]. No doubt other proteins associated with the membrane are also important in the structure and function of the erythrocyte cytoskeleton. For example, the membrane binding site for spectrin [10] may be an oligomer ie, a protein which aids in the creation of a cohesive cytoskeleton.

We have developed a method for preparing cytoskeletons from intact erythrocytes and find that these Triton shells of whole cells are similar to the ghost shells but have several unexpected properties [11]. By working with the intact cells it is possible to maintain constant ionic conditions and to shorten the time required in preparing the shells. In this report we describe further the unusual properties of certain components of Triton shells of intact cells and show that filamentous structures are present in the shells.

MATERIALS AND METHODS

Human erythrocytes were obtained from healthy donors and used within two days. Citrate (10 mM final concentration) was used as an anticoagulant. Cells were washed three times with 146 mM NaCl, 20 mM Tris, pH 7.4 (Iso Tris) and the buffy coat was removed each time. Triton X-114 was obtained from Rohm and Haas and [^{3}H] Triton X-100 was a gift of Dr Phillip Strittmatter. All other compounds were reagent grade or better.

Detergent Extraction Procedure

Washed red cells were suspended in Iso Tris at a 20% hematocrit. In a typical experiment 6 ml of the cells were mixed on ice with 6 ml of a detergent solution containing 5 mM reduced glutathione, 1.0 mM ethylene glycoltetraectic acid (EGTA), 5 mM $MgCl_2$, 140 mM KC1, and 20 mM N-2-hydroxyethyl-piperazine-N′-2-ethane-sulfonic acid (HEPES) (pH 7.0). The mixture was layered on a 25-ml linear sucrose gradient (usually 10–60% sucrose) containing 0.2 mM dithiothreitol (DTT), 140 mM KC1, 5 mM $MgC1_2$, 20 mM HEPES (pH 7.0), and 0.5 mM EGTA. The gradients were normally centrifuged for 1 h at 120,000g max. Fractions (~1ml) were collected dropwise from the bottom of the gradient tube. The sucrose concentration of various fractions was determined from the refractive index. The protein concentration of the fractions was determined by diluting a 100- to 500-λ aliquot to 2.8 ml and precipitating the protein with 0.7 ml of 50% trichloroacetic acid (TCA). The pelleted precipitate (3,000g for 20 min) was solubilized in 200 λ of 1% sodium dodecyl sulfate (SDS) and 10 mM Na_2HPO_4 by incubation at 37°C for 30 min. Protein was then measured by the Lowry assay [12]. In cases where [^{3}H] Triton X-100 was added to the extraction mixture, an aliquot (< 100 λ) of each fraction was added directly to 5 ml of Aqueous Counting Scintillant (ACS) (Amersham Searle) scintillation fluid and counted.

Protease Treatment of Whole Cells

Washed erythrocytes at a 50% hematocrit were incubated with 1.5 mg/ml of chymotrypsin (Sigma) or Streptomyces griseus protease (Sigma) for 1 h at 37°C. The chymotrypsin reaction was stopped by the addition of 420 μg/ml L-1-tosylamide-2-phenylethylcholomethyl ketone (TPCK). Cells were washed twice with Iso Tris before extraction.

pH 11 Extraction

Erythrocyte ghosts were prepared by lysis in 10 mM Tris pH 7.4 (1:100) and pelleting at 25,000g for 10 min, followed by washing two times with the same buffer. Ghosts were then washed (1:100) with the spectrin extraction buffer, 0.2 mM ATP, 0.2 mM EDTA, and 0.2 mM Tris, 0.2 mM DTT (pH 8.0). After overnight extraction the membranes were pelleted and washed once with 0.6 M KCl, 0.1 mM DTT, 10 mM Tris (pH 7.5) to remove band 6. The pellet was washed one time with, and resuspended in, 10 mM glycine, 0.2 mM ATP, and 0.1 mM DTT (pH 11), incubated 16 h on ice, and centrifuged at 100,000 g max for 1 h. The final extract was concentrated by vacuum dialysis and stored as a precipitate in 50% ammonium sulfate.

SDS Gel Electrophoresis

Samples were solubilized by the addition of 2% SDS and 5% β-mercaptoethanol and incubation at 100°C for 2–3 min. The procedure of Fairbanks, Steck, and Wallach [13] was used for the gel electrophoresis in 5.6% acrylamide gels containing 0.1% SDS.

Electron Microscopy of Shells

As the gradients were being collected, some samples were collected in tubes containing 2% glutaraldehyde in 140 mM KCl, 10 mM PO_4 (pH 7.0). After fixation for 1 h on ice, samples were applied to thin carbon films on standard 300-mesh electron microscope grids for 1 min. The grids were then washed twice with Iso Tris by floating them on drops of the buffer and were finally negatively stained with 2% uranyl acetate (pH 4.5). Samples were viewed on a Phillips 300 electron microscope.

RESULTS

Triton Extraction of Whole Cells

When whole erythrocytes were extracted with 0.5% Triton X-114 and centrifuged (120,000 g for 1 h) into a 10–60% sucrose gradient in the same buffer, two light-scattering layers were found as well as a pellet. The pellet was fibrous and incompletely solubilized by SDS and reducing agents. Electron microscope analysis of this material after fixation and embedding revealed structures resembling nuclei, suggesting that the pellet contained nuclear material from contaminating lymphocytes. SDS polyacrylamide gel analysis of the material showed small amounts of protein in the component 3 and 4 region but no spectrin or actin.

The denser light-scattering layer (layer II) was found at a density of 1.185–1.203 g/ml, regardless of whether the sample was centrifugued for 1 or 18 h. The material was in a diffuse layer after 1 h of centrifugation but condensed into a gelatinous wafer after 18 h of centrifugation. Layer II was always white, with no indication of hemoglobin contamination. Layer I was found at the lower edge of (1 h spin) or within (18 h spin) the hemoglobin band at a density of 1.08–1.11 g/ml and was isolated by dilution of the material in buffer and pelleting at 100,000 g for 30 min. Usually no redness was found with the washed pellet. The amount of material in this layer was 2–3 times greater after 18 h than after 1 h of centrifugation.

In a typical experiment 6.8 mg of membrane protein was applied to the gradient [14], 2.0–2.5 mg of protein was recovered in layer II, 0.15–0.5 mg in layer I, and 0.24 mg in the pellet. SDS polyacrylamide gel analysis of the proteins showed that layer I contained components 3 and 4 in approximately equal amounts. Layer II had these two proteins plus spectrin, actin (component 5), component 7, and several minor proteins. From densitometer analysis of the gels it was estimated that layer II was 50–70% spectrin, 6–10% actin, 7–17% component 3, 6–12% component 4, 4–5% component 7, and minor amounts of other membrane proteins. Gels stained for carbohydrate with periodic acid-Schiff reagent (PAS) [13] revealed that less than 10% of the normal content of sialoglycoproteins was present. The components in layer II were organized into shells resembling the erythrocyte in size and form as shown in Fig 1.

If the samples of layer II material were incubated on ice for 36 h, there was a change in the SDS gel pattern of the shells (see Fig 2). As previously reported, there is movement of staining intensity from higher to lower apparent molecular weight in the component 3 and 4 regions [11]. Because these changes may result from proteolysis, shells are normally solubilized with SDS immediately after preparation.

When the concentration of Triton X-114 in the extraction medium is increased from 0.2 to 5%, there is no qualitative change in the SDS gels of the shells stained with Coomassie

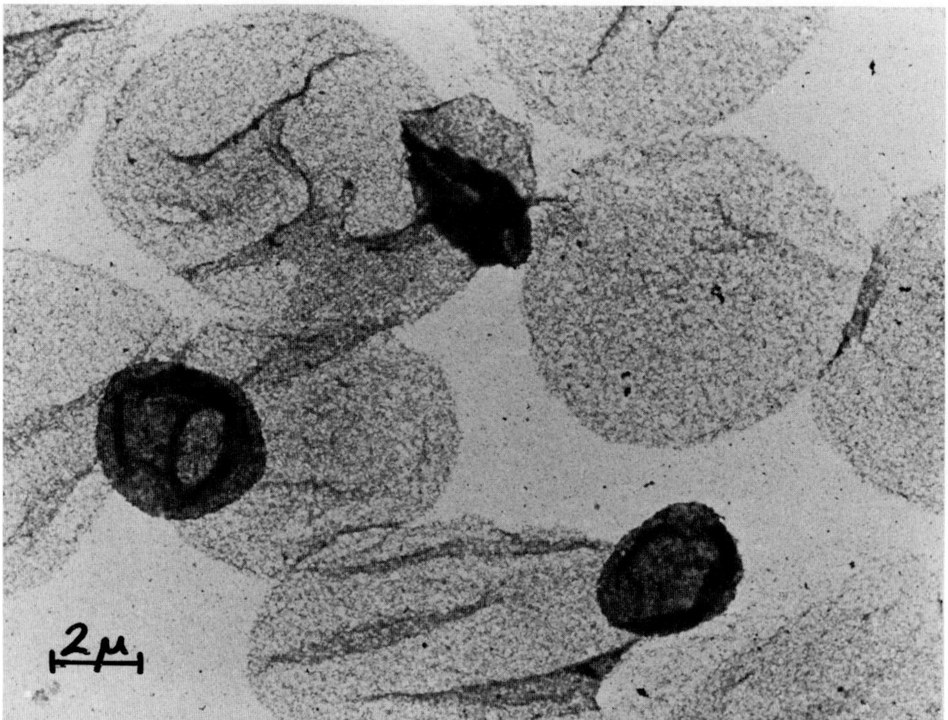

Fig 1. Electron micrograph of Triton shells negatively stained with $UO_2(Ac)_2$ (pH 4.5). magnification 4500 ×.

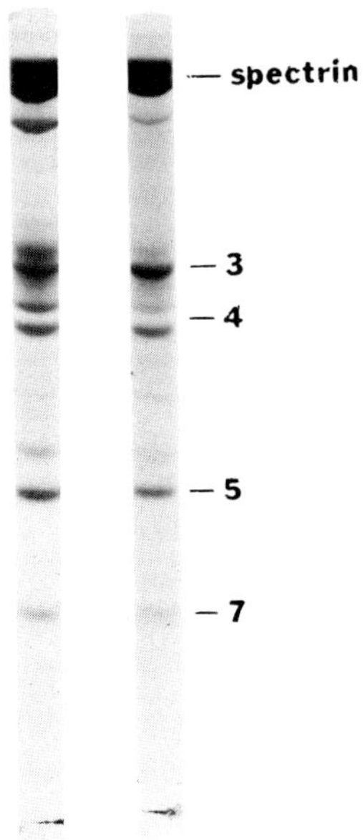

Fig 2. SDS polyacrylamide gels of 0.5% Triton shell material prepared according to the procedure described in Materials and Methods, sec, diluted (1:20) in Iso Tris, 0.5 mM Mg Cl_2, and 0.2 mM DTT, pelleted by centrifugation at 30,000 g for 30 min, and resuspended at a concentration of 1 mg/ml protein in Iso Tris, 0.5 mM $MgCl_2$, and 0.2 mM DTT. Gel a) Material immediately after preparation; gel b) the same material after 36 h on ice (25 μg of protein was applied in each case).

blue [11]. In Figure 3 the densitometer scans, however, show that the intensity of staining in the component 3 and 4 region decreases relative to spectrin and actin when the Triton concentration is increased from 0.5 to 2.0% (Fig 3b and c respectively). By integrating the peak areas through cutting and weighing, the percentages of staining in the component 3 and 4 regions are 17% and 9.5% respectively with 0.5% Triton, whereas with 2% Triton they are 12% and 7.5% respectively. The relative amounts of spectrin, actin, and component 7, however, remain constant within experimental error with a ratio of staining intensities of 1:0. 18:0.065. If we use the published values of the molecular weights of these components to compute their molar ratio [14], then for every mole of spectrin dimer there are 1.7 moles of actin and 1 mole of component 7 in the Triton-insoluble complex.

Component 3′

A component of the shells which electrophoreses in the component 3 region is not proteolyzed when intact cells are treated with trypsin, chymotrypsin, or a nonspecific bacterial protease [11]. Because this protein is distinguishable from the rest of 3 but coelectrophoreses with 3, we have designated it component 3′. Another distinguishing feature of 3′ is that it has a low extinction coefficient at 280 nm which is evident from the densitomer scans in Figure 3d and e. In the scan at 280 nm of an unstained gel of shells from chymotrypsinized cells the absorption in the component 3′ region is much less than that of component 4.2, 5, or the major proteolytic fragment of 3. When the same gel is stained with Coomassie blue and scanned at 550 nm, component 3′ staining is more intense

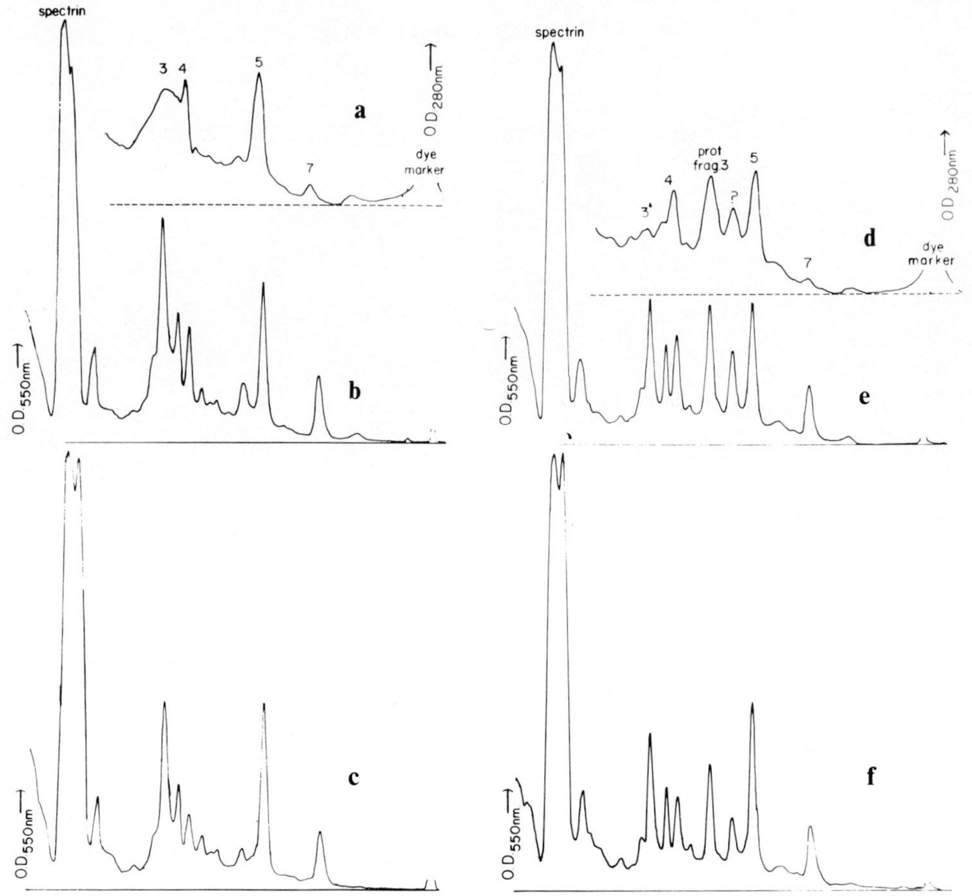

Fig 3. Densitometer scans of SDS polyacrylamide gels of Triton shells SDS-solubilized immediately after isolation and washing (as described in Fig 2). a,b) Gels of 0.5% Triton shells from normal erythrocytes: a) 160 μg of protein was applied and the gel was scanned immediately after electrophoresis at 280 nm; b) 20 μg of protein was applied and the gel was stained with Coomassie blue before scanning at 550 nm. c) Gel of 2% Triton shell material treated analogously to scan b. d, e, f) Shells prepared from chymotrypsinized erythrocytes: d, e) 0.5% Triton shells run as described for the gels a and b; f) 2% Triton shells of chymotrypsinized cells (20 μg of protein applied).

than 4.2, as in Figure 3e, which is a scan of a gel loaded with 20 μg of the same material. If 3′ is a different protein than 3, it may have different solubility properties. Indeed 3′ is released from the shells in 0.5 mM glycine, 0.5 mM EDTA, 0.2 mM DTT (pH 9.0) and is present in the supernatant after centrifugation at 150,000 g for 2 h. Since 3′ may be solubilized from the shells as a complex with Triton, a method was found for isolating 3′ from ghosts. In Figure 4 are densitometer traces at 280 nm and 550 nm before and after Coomassie blue staining, respectively, of the pH 11 extract from membranes which had been preextracted to remove the majority of spectrin and actin. The scan at 280 nm shows absorbing material at the top of the gel which is removed upon fixation with 10% isopropanol and 10% acetic acid. Again the absorbance at 280 nm of the protein which

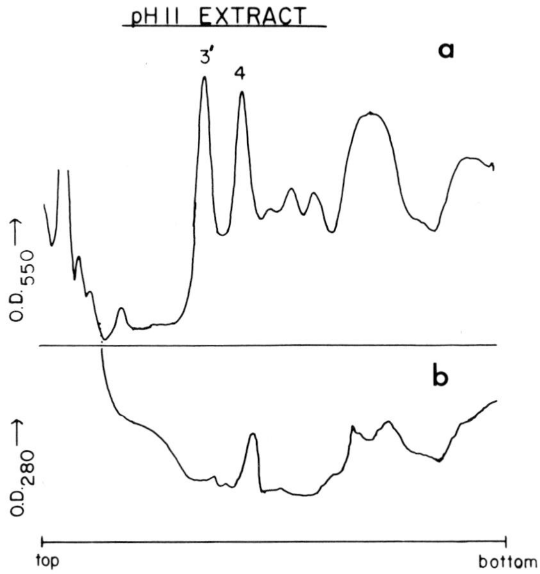

Fig 4. Densitometer scans of the same SDS polyacrylamide gel on which 100 μg of the pH 11 extract (prepared as described in Materials and Methods) was run. Scan b was recorded at 280 nm immediately after electrophoresis and scan a was recorded at 550 nm after staining with Coomassie blue.

electrophoreses in the component 3 region is significantly less than band 4, and this protein has been tentatively called 3′. The lower-molecular-weight components in this extract have not been characterized. Component 3′ is then defined as a protein which coelectrophoreses with band 3 but has a low absorption coefficient at 280 nm and is solubilized in alkaline glycine solutions. Its apparent molecular weight is 88,000 daltons.

Component 3

Since the major chymotryptic fragment of band 3 coisolates with the shells of chymotrypsinized cells, component 3 as well as 3′ may be present in Triton shells normally (Fig 3d). When the concentration of Triton X-114 is increased from 0.5% to 2%, the amount of the chymotryptic fragment of band 3 decreases by 25% in the shells of chymotrypsinized cells whereas the content of 3′ drops only 5% (Fig 3 e,f). As might be expected, higher detergent concentrations removed more of the band 3 fragment than 3′. The decrease in the amount of stain in the 3 region in gels of shells of normal cells prepared by 2% versus 0.5% Triton extraction suggests that band 3 is present (Fig 3b and c). Further indication that 3 is normally in the shells is given by the densitometer scan at 280 nm, which shows that the component in the 3 region absorbs more than 3′ does (Fig 3a).

Band 7

Band 7 is the low-molecular-weight component of the shells, which is present in constant amounts relative to spectrin. The molar ratio of band 7 to spectrin is estimated to be 1:1 from the Coomassie blue staining intensities. But under hypotonic extraction conditions which solubilize spectrin from ghosts, band 7 remains in the ghost. The densitometer tracings at 280 nm reveal that band 7 has a strikingly low absorbance at 280 nm (Fig 3a and b or d and 3).

Spectrin

Washed shells suspended in isotonic media will release a significant but variable fraction of their protein with time. SDS gels of the solubilized protein reveal that it is > 90% spectrin, [11, 15]. As seen in Figure 5 the isotonically solubilized spectrin coelectrophoreses with hypotonic spectrin, and within the precision of the gels (differences of 4,000 daltons could be resolved) the two proteins are identical in molecular weight. The protein may be released as a complex with detergent. To determine if this was the case, spectrin was purified by velocity sedimentation. As seen in Figure 6, the isotonic spectrin sediments as a single species that has the same sedimentation velocity as does hypotonic spectrin in the same ionic conditions. There is no Triton peak associated with the protein peak and from the Triton specific activity there is less than a mole of Triton bound per 2 moles of spectrin dimer. Thus spectrin was released from the shells without detectable proteolysis and free of detergents.

Another parameter of spectrin is its phosphorylation, which occurs in vivo as well as in vitro [16]. We have prelabeled spectrin in intact erythrocytes by incubating with $^{32}P_i$ and have observed that the isotonically solubilized spectrin has a significantly lower specific activity than spectrin in Tris ghosts or hypotonic spectrin [11, 15]. Concomitant with the release of spectrin from shells there is a rise of phosphate label in the non-TCA-precipitable fraction.

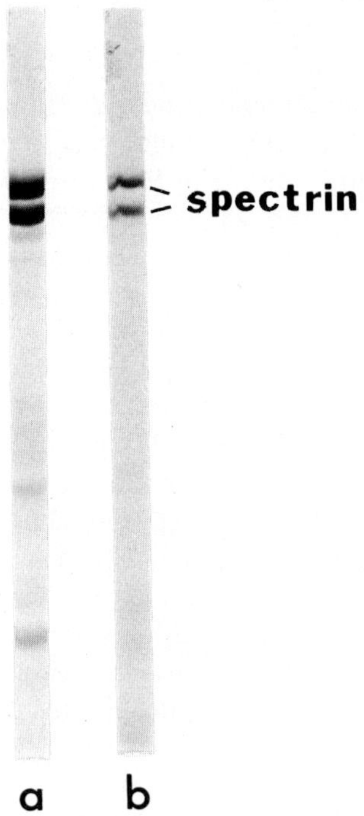

Fig 5. Coomassie blue-stained SDS polyacrylamide gels (3.25% acrylamide) of spectrin prepared a) by hypotonic elution from 10 mM Tris ghosts in 0.1 mM ATP, 0.1 mM EDTA, 0.1 mM DTT, and 0.2 mM Tris (pH 8.0) and b) by isotonic elution from 0.5% Triton shells in Iso Tris, 0.5 mM $MgCl_2$, and 0.2 mM DTT incubated 36 h on ice (20% of the shell spectrin was solubilized in this experiment).

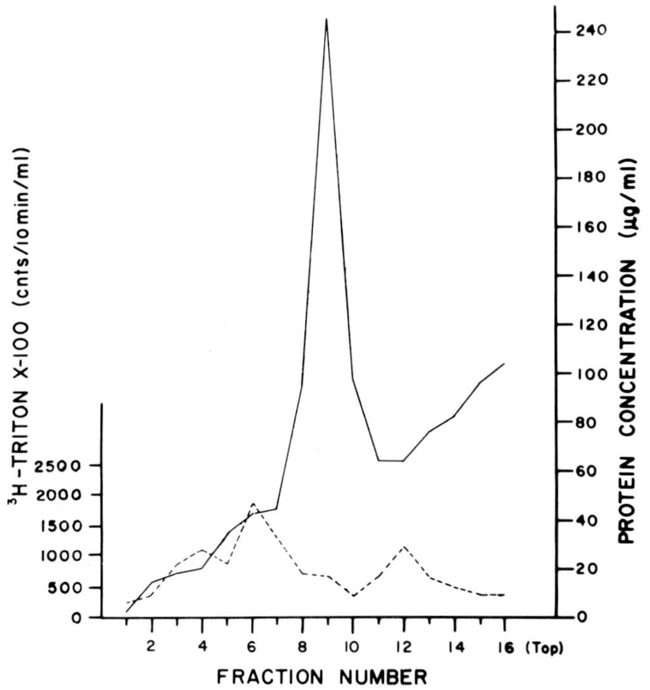

Fig 6. Graph of a velocity sedimentation experiment showing the protein concentration (—) and (^3H) counts (- - -) versus gradient fraction for isotonic spectrin after centrifugation for 16 h at 150,000 g in 10–40% sucrose gradient made with Iso Tris, 0.5 mM $MgCl_2$, and 0.2 mM DTT. The specific activity of the Triton was 461 cpm/μg of Triton, and 0.5 ml of a 500 μg/ml solution of isotonic spectrin was applied to the 4.5-ml gradient.

Electron Microscopy

Earlier electron micrographs of Triton shells of erythrocyte ghosts [8, 10] have not revealed a well-defined reticulum such as has been observed by scanning electron microscopy [17]. A definite reticulum is observed, however, in the shells of whole cells. Special care was taken to shorten the time from lysis until the samples was fixed with glutaraldehyde. After fixation, the samples were negatively stained with uranyl acetate (pH 4.5). As seen in Figure 7a at low magnification the reticulum from a single cell appears unordered over most of its area, particularly where two layers of the network are superimposed. In certain regions, however, where shear has oriented the fibrous elements of the network, a definite order appears in the reticulum. This order is particularly evident where a single layer of the reticulum is viewed, as in Figure 7b. In that figure the shell was torn open and the tearing forces also aligned the fibrous elements of the shells. The fibers are beaded and are 80–120 Å in diameter. Similar structures have been observed in shells stained with phosphotungstic acid (pH 7.4) but the contrast is not as great. From the composition of the shells we can estimate the possible length of actin filaments in the area of the micrograph to be sufficient to go from the top to the bottom of the micrograph four times (Fig 7b); therefore, there is insufficient actin to account for the fibers.

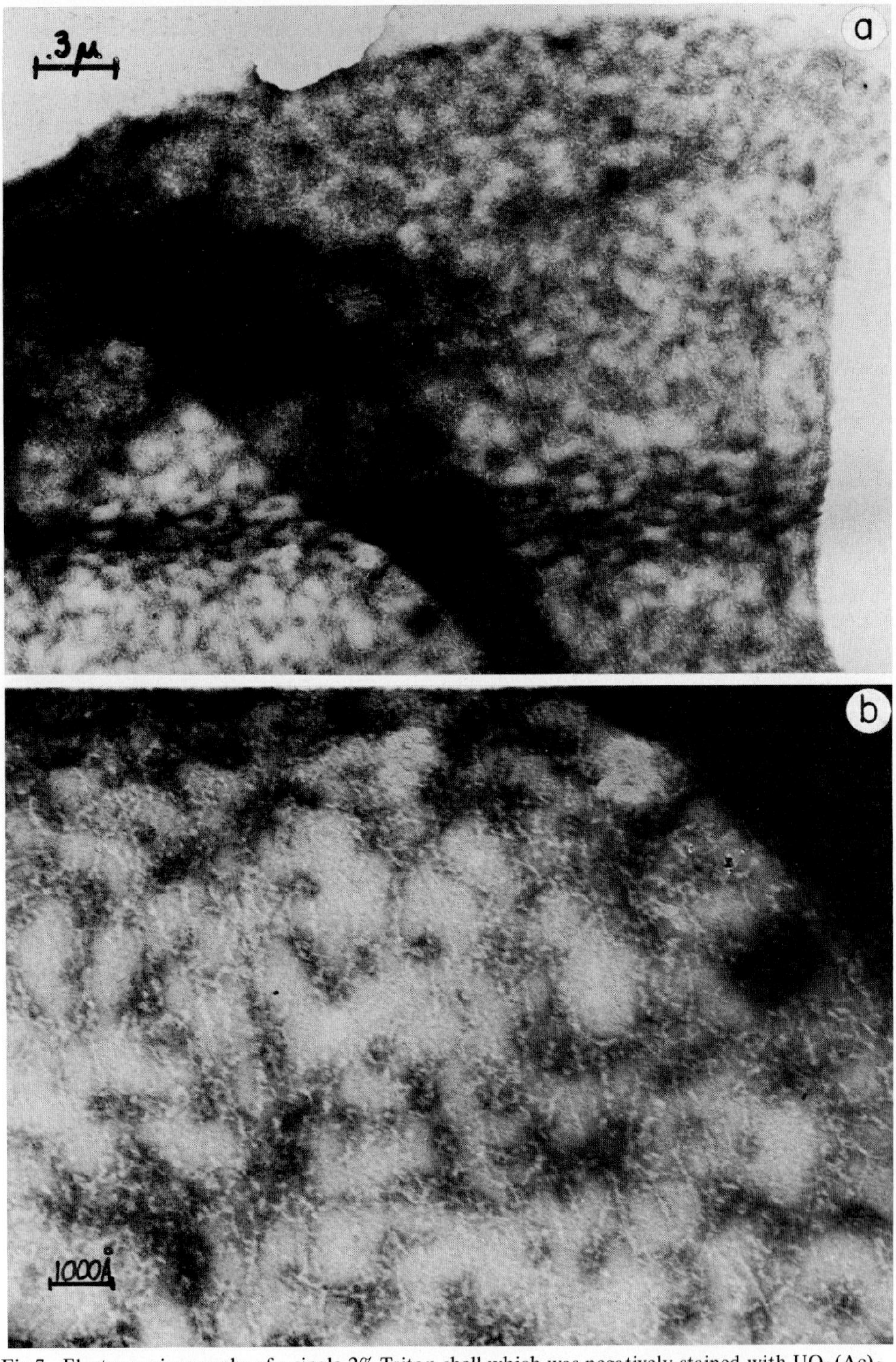

Fig 7. Electron micrographs of a single 2% Triton shell which was negatively stained with $UO_2(Ac)_2$ at pH 4.5 after fixation with glutaraldehyde as described. a) Majority of shell is shown; b) portion of the shell at higher magnification. The second layer of the Triton-insoluble material appears to be torn away in this region, which affords a clearer view of the filamentous structures in the shell.

DISCUSSION

Through the careful dissection of the erythrocyte membrane with nonionic detergents we can understand which complexes exist among the many possible combinations. With this information it will be easier to design reconstitution experiments to understand the bases for the component interactions. In order to isolate complexes which may reflect in vivo structures, we have approximated the ionic environment of the cell cytoplasm during extraction. The nonionic detergent Triton was chosen because it denatures relatively few enzymes [18]. Intact cells rather than ghosts were employed so that the proteins would not be exposed to hypotonic solutions. Because protease contamination was found with whole cell preparations, the proteins of the shells were separated from the detergent, cytoplasm, and solubilized components by sedimentation into a sucrose density gradient of the same ionic composition as the extraction solution. These steps were taken to assure that the shell components would suffer the least possible insult in preparation and to allow for systematic variation of the extraction conditions.

Although the detergent concentration had dramatic effects on the lipid content of the shells, the protein components remained relatively constant. The lipid content was reflected by the shell density and phosphate-to-protein ratio. In shells prepared with 0.5% vs 2.0% Triton X-114 the density was 1.19 vs 1.27 g/ml and the phosphate-to-protein ratio was 0.60 vs 0.04 μmoles P/mg protein [11]. As seen in Figure 3, however, the protein composition of shells extracted with 0.5% vs 2.0% Triton did not change qualitatively. There were significant decreases of staining intensity in the band 3 and 4 region, but those changes can be explained as an increased extraction of the integral membrane protein band 3 and concomitant loss of band 4. In support of this the shells of chymotrypsinized cells extracted with 0.5 vs 2.0% Triton show significant decreases only in the amount of the band 3 proteolytic fragment and band 4. Because we might expect that a complex of peripheral proteins would be relatively insensitive to Triton, it is significant that the amounts of spectrin, actin, band 7, and band 3′ remain roughly proportional in a molar ratio of 1:1.7:1:0.8 in shells prepared with 0.5% or 2% Triton assuming that the staining with Coomassie blue is a true measure of protein concentration. Although the addition of detergent may induce artifactual protein associations, the shell complex is a relatively stable unit and provides a basis to study further the protein components contained in it.

Component 3′ is of particular interest because of its unusual properties. As reported earlier component 3′ is the protein which electrophoreses in the band 3 region, isolates with the shells of intact cells, and is insensitive to chymotrypsin, trypsin, and a nonspecific bacterial protease in the intact erythrocytes [11]. Although a certain portion of the integral protein, band 3, normally appears to coisolate with the shells, band 3′ can be clearly differentiated from that protein. Component 3′ is a water-soluble, ie, peripheral, protein which has a low extinction coefficient at 280 nm. Because 3′ is insensitive to a variety of proteases in the intact cell, it is most likely on the cytoplasmic face of the membrane. In ghosts the amount of 3′ is normally less than the amount predicted from the shells but is variable (Sheetz and Sawyer, unpublished results). The unusual behavior of component(s) 3′ on SDS gels is not understood and raises the possibility that 3′ is several proteins or a major proteolytic fragment of a larger protein. In accord with the latter possibility is the fact that the light meromyosin fragment of myosin has a low absorbance at 280 nm [19]. But the presence of 3′ in ghosts of chymotrypsinized cells does not correlate with the loss of another component nor does 3′ increase appreciably when proteolysis occurs in ghosts or shells. Thus if 3′ is a proteolytic produce of spectrin, then the specific protease must be washed away or inactivated in ghosting and in shell preparation. There is no single high-molecular-weight protein band other than spectrin that is present in enough copies to produce 3′. Again, we assume that Coomassie blue staining gives a true measure of all the proteins present.

Several possible functions for 3′ have been suggested and these functions may be interrelated. Our data suggest that the stimulation of actin polymerization by spectrin is modulated by the erythrocyte casein kinase [20] when 3′ is present (Sheetz and Sawyer, manuscript in preparation). Perhaps related to the actin polymerization activity White and Ralston [21] have solubilized a Mg^{2+} ATPase under conditions which extract 3′ (Sheetz and Sawyer, unpublished results, 1978) and the Mg^{2+} ATPase has an apparent molecular weight similar to 3′. Goodman and Branton [21a] have found that spectrin binds to the vesicles which are left after hypotonic elution of spectrin and actin from the shells; therefore 3′ may form part of the spectrin attachment site in the membrane. Certainly all of these functions are consistent with the present data and indicate that 3′ may have an important role in the functions of the erythrocyte cytoskeleton.

The portion of band 4 associated with the shells immediately after Triton extraction is predominently component 4.1 and with time the staining intensity moves from the 4.1 to the 4.2 region [11]. Since protease will catalyze the same apparent transition in ghosts (Sheetz and Sawyer, unpublished results, 1978), we feel that the conversion is the result of proteolysis. Bennett [22] has observed that proteolysis of inside-out vesicles releases a 72,000-dalton component which coelectrophoreses with 4.2 and competes with the spectrin-binding component on inside-out vesicles. This component may account for the increase in staining in the 4.2 band with time. The amount of band 4, like the amount of band 3, in the shell decreases significantly with higher detergent concentrations in the shells. The content of these two proteins may be coupled since it has been noted previously that they do interact [23, 24].

Another component of the shells which is not well understood is band 7. It is interesting that band 7 is present in stoichiometric amounts with spectrin and that it has a low extinction coefficient at 280 nm. Several calcium-binding proteins – the parvalbumins, troponin C, bovine brain S-100 protein, and bovine intestinal calcium-binding protein – all are low in tyrosine and tryptophan [25]. The calcium-binding proteins are all lower in molecular weight than band 7, but studies are under way to determine if 7 has calcium-binding properties similar to those proteins.

Spectrin is the major component of the shells on the basis of mass, and it is logical to assume that it plays a major role in maintaining the structure of the shell. When spectrin is solubilized either under isotonic conditions or by hypotonic extraction, the shell structure is lost. In isotonic media spectrin alone is solubilized and the reticular structure of the shells disappears [11]. Only vesicles and filaments resembling actin filaments remain after spectrin removal [11]. This suggests that spectrin either constitutes or induces the 80- to 120-Å filaments. Indeed, similar filaments have been observed in spectrin preparations treated with divalent cations [26, 27]. We do not know if shear forces are responsible only for aligning preexisting filaments in the shells or if the filaments are formed as a result of shear stress on the reticulum. The latter possibility raises the point that some bridging structures if not filaments must exist to maintain shell integrity. Numerous attempts have been made to visualize filaments on the cytoplasmic face of the erythrocyte membrane, and only the recent studies of Steck and Hainfeld [17] have revealed an extensive fibrillar network. Again the fibers were visualized best in regions where the network appears to be sheared. The spectrin released from the shells in isotonic media is a dephosphorylated spectrin but does not appear proteolyzed [11, 15]. The phosphorylation of spectrin has been implicated as an important factor in erythrocyte membrane shape changes [28] and in the polymerization of actin stimulated by spectrin [20]. If the dephosphorylation of spectrin causes it to release from the network, then the observed shape changes and loss of actin-polymerizing activity with dephosphorylation could be explained. Rephosphorylation experiments, however, have not resulted in spectrin reaggregation, but certain components necessary for aggregation may be missing.

Although filamentous actin would form a natural bridging structure in the cytoskeleton, several reports suggest that erythrocyte actin may be largely in a globular form [26, 29]. Evidence, however, for the presence of filamentous actin in the erythrocyte is strong. We have repeated the observations of Pinder, Bray, and Gratzer [20], that crude spectrin extracts promote actin polymerization, and Birchmeier and Singer [7] find that actin will polymerize inside the erythrocyte ghosts at concentrations below the critical polymerizing concentration. After spectrin solubilization in isotonic media, actin is always in the pelletable fraction, where numerous 60- to 80 Å-diameter filaments are found. Further we have observed that actin filaments will interact with inside-out but not right-side-out vesicles of erythrocyte membranes (Sheetz and Hom, unpublished results). Figure 7b shows that numerous filaments can be observed in the erythrocyte cytoskeleton which cannot all be accounted for by actin. However, a portion of them which are smaller could be actin filaments. Considerable inferential evidence exists for the presence of globular and filamentous actin in the erythrocyte but neither form has been shown to be involved directly in erythrocyte membrane function.

Since the Triton shells can be simply prepared from intact erythrocytes, they provide a good source of cytoskeletal material which has not been exposed to hypotonic salt solutions. Many of the presumed erythrocyte cytoskeletal components are highly anionic and exposure to hypotonic solutions may alter their native conformation and their subsequent behavior. The Triton-insoluble complex in the shells which is composed of spectrin, actin, and components 3′ and 7 may be a detergent-induced aggregate, but reconstitution studies should test for possible interactions of these components. Whether the presence of component 3 in the shells reflects incomplete extraction or a meaningful interaction with the cytoskeleton is yet to be determined. The isotonic elution of spectrin from the shells provides a means of preparing this protein in physiologic salt conditions, although the protein is in a dephosphorylated form and may have undergone an undetected proteolytic cleavage. Since electron microscopic studies of protein structure are fraught with possible artifacts, we do not assert that the structures in Figure 7b do exist in vivo. The micrograph does depict the cytoskeleton as we imagine it, and it therefore provides a form of model for the cytoskeleton. However, we have refrained from identifying specific proteins with specific structures. The Triton shell of intact erythrocytes provides an excellent starting material for studies of the cytoskeletal structure and components.

ACKNOWLEDGMENTS

We thank Su Ming Hom for his help in the original phases of this work. This project was supported by NIH grant HL-18317.

REFERENCES

1. Steck TL, Yu J: J Supramol Struct 1:232, 1973.
2. Yu J, Fischman D, Steck TL: J Supramol Struct 1:220, 1973.
3. Kirkpatrick FH, Gordesky SE, Marinetti GV: Biochim Biophys Acta 345:154, 1974.
4. Lux SE, John KM, Karnovski MJ: J Clin Invest 58:955, 1976.
5. Lux SE, Pease B, Tomaselli MB, John KM, Bernstein S: J Supramol Struct 6:194a, 1978.
6. Sheetz MP, Singer SJ: J Cell Biol 73:638, 1977.
7. Birchmeier W, Singer SJ: Biochem Biophys Res Commun 77:1354, 1977.
8. Palek J, Liu SC, Snyder LM: Blood 51:385, 1978.
9. Kirkpatrick FH: Life Sci 19:1, 1976.
10. Bennett V, Branton D: J Biol Chem 252:2753, 1977.
11. Sheetz MP, Sawyer D, Jackowski S: In Brewer G (ed): "Erythrocyte Metabolism and Function," 1978, vol 4, p 431.
12. Lowry OH, Rosebrough NJ, Farr AL, Randall RJ: J Biol Chem 193:265, 1951.
13. Fairbanks G, Steck TL, Wallach DFH: Biochemistry 10:2606, 1971.
14. Steck TL: J Cell Biol 62:1, 1974.
15. Sheetz MP, Sawyer D: In Pepe F (ed): "Motility in Cell Function." (In press.)
16. Wolfe LC, Lux SE: Blood 48:963, 1976.
17. Steck TL, Hainfeld JF: In Porter KR (eds): "International Cell Biology, 1976–1977, p6.
17. Steck TL, Hainfeld JF: In Brinkley BR, Porter KR (eds): "International Cell Biology, 1976–1977," 1977, p6.
18. Tanford C, Reynolds JA: Biochim Biophys Acta 457:133, 1976.
19. Lowey S, Slayter HS, Weeds AG, Baker H: J Mol Biol 45:1, 1969.
20. Pinder JC, Bray D, Gratzer WB: Nature 270:752, 1977.
21. White RD, Ralston GB: Biochim Biophys Acta 436:567, 1976.
21a. Goodman SR, Branton D: J Supramol Struct 8:455–463, 1978.
22. Bennett V: J Biol Chem 253:2292, 1978.
23. Yu J, Steck TL: J Biol Chem 250:9176, 1975.
24. Wang K, Richards FM: J Biol Chem 249:8005, 1974.
25. Demaille J, Dutruge E, Caponey JP, Pechere JF: In Drabikowski W et al (eds): "Calcium Binding Proteins," 1974, p 643.
26. Tilney LG, Detmers P: J Cell Biol 66:508, 1975.
27. Kirkpatrick FH, Woods GM, Weed RI, and LaCelle PL: Arch Biochem Biophys 175:367, 1976.
28. Birchmeier W, Singer SJ: J Cell Biol 73:647, 1977.
29. Ralston GB: J Supramol Struct 6:190a, 1978.

Journal of Supramolecular Structure 8:413–430 (1978)
Normal and Abnormal Red Cell Membranes 135–152

Influence of Increased Membrane Cholesterol on Membrane Fluidity and Cell Function in Human Red Blood Cells

Richard A. Cooper

Hematology-Oncology Section, Department of Medicine, Hospital of the University of Pennsylvania, Philadelphia, Pennsylvania 19104

Cholesterol and phospholipid are the two major lipids of the red cell membrane. Cholesterol is insoluble in water but is solubilized by phospholipids both in membranes and in plasma lipoproteins. Morever, cholesterol exchanges between membranes and lipoproteins. An equilibrium partition is established based on the amount of cholesterol relative to phospholipid (C/PL) in these two compartments.

Increases in the C/PL of red cell membranes have been studied under three conditions: First, spontaneous increases in vivo have been observed in the spur red cells of patients with severe liver disease; second , similar red cell changes in vivo have been induced by the administration of cholesterol-enriched diets to rodents and dogs; third, increases in membrane cholesterol have been induced in vitro by enriching the C/PL of the lipoprotein environment with cholesterol-phospholipid dispersions (liposomes) having a C/PL of >1.0. In each case, there is a close relationship between the C/PL of the plasma environment and the C/PL of the red cell membrane. In vivo, the C/PL mole ratio of red cell membranes ranges from a normal value of 0.9–1.0 to values which approach but do not reach 2.0. In vitro, this ratio approaches 3.0.

Cholesterol enrichment of red cell membranes directly influences membrane lipid fluidity, as assessed by the rotational diffusion of hydrophobic fluorescent probes such as diphenyl hexatriene (DPH). A close correlation exists between increases in red cell membrane C/PL and decreases in membrane fluidity over the range of membrane C/PL from 1.0 to 2.0; however, little further change in fluidity occurs when membrane C/PL is increased to 2.0–3.0.

Cholesterol enrichment of red cell membranes is associated with the transformation of cell contour to one which is redundant and folded, and this is associated with a decrease in red cell filterability in vitro. Circulation in vivo in the presence of the spleen further modifies cell shape to a spiny, irregular (spur) form, and the survival of cholesterol-rich red cells is decreased in the presence of the spleen. Although active Na-K transport is not influenced by cholesterol enrichment of human red cells, several carrier-mediated transport pathways are inhibited. We have demonstrated this effect for the cotransport of Na + K

Received for publication April 13, 1978; accepted May 22, 1978.

0091-7419/78/0804-0413$03.20

and similar results have been obtained by others in studies of organic acid transport and the transport of small neutral molecules such as erythritol and glycerol.

Thus, red cell membrane C/PL is sensitive to the C/PL of the plasma environment. Increasing membrane C/PL causes a decrease in membrane fluidity, and these changes are associated with a reduction in membrane permeability, a distortion of cell contour and filterability and a shortening of the survival of red cells in vivo.

Key words: cholesterol, red blood cells, cell membrane, membrane fluidity, fluorescence polarization

Lipids account for approximately 50% of the weight of red cell membranes. Cholesterol and phospholipid are the major lipids (Table I). Small amounts of glycolipids are also present in human red cells, and larger amounts are found in the red cells of other mammalian species. Both glycolipids and phospholipids are polar, whereas cholesterol is a neutral lipid.

A constant feature of mammalian red cell membranes is that the mole ratio of neutral lipid (cholesterol) to polar lipid (phospholipid + glycolipid) is always approximately 0.9–1.0 [1]. However, the relative amounts of glycolipid and phospholipid vary considerably, as do the relative amounts of the various phospholipid classes. Four phospholipids predominate in human red cell membranes: lecithin (phosphatidylcholine), sphingomyelin, phosphatidylserine, and phosphatidylethanolamine. Small amounts of free fatty acids are also present in human red cells, but neither triglycerides nor cholesterol esters are constituents of red cell membranes.

CHOLESTEROL–PHOSPHOLIPID INTERACTIONS

The importance of the association between polar lipids and sterols is emphasized by the fact that the membranes of all higher organisms, including plants and animals, contain both. In those few instances where sterols are known not to occur in prokaryotes and lower eukaryotes, molecules are present which appear to mimic the sterol structure [2]. For example, caratenols are found in certain mycoplasmas and tetrahymanol occurs in tetrahymena piriformis. Cholesterol is the predominant sterol in all cells within the animal kingdom, whereas sterols with an alkylated side chain predominate in plants. The structural requirements for sterols in cell membranes are quite specific. They must possess a β-OH on the third carbon, a $\Delta 5$ double bond, and alternating transantistereochemistry, creating a planar ring structure and an uncyclized side chain at C17 [2, 3].

The molecular interactions which occur between sterols and polar lipids in membranes are not completely understood. Huang has recently proposed that hydrogen bonding occurs between the carbonyl oxygen of the phospholipid acyl side-chains and the 3β-OH of the sterol [4]. This particular model permits an efficient alignment between the acyl chains of phospholipids and the planar sterol nucleus. In most biologic membranes, one of the phospholipid acyl chains is saturated and the other has at least one unsaturated double bond, a cis double bond at C9-10. This asymmetry of acyl chain structure accommodates the asymmetry of the sterol molecule, caused by the protrusion of two angular methyl groups (Cl8 and Cl9) from one face of the sterol nucleus. Models of sterol-phospholipid interaction suggest that phospholipids are capable of accomodating up to 2 moles of cholesterol per mole of phospholipid. For amounts of sterol in excess of a C/P ratio of 2.0, some other molecular configuration is required. This concept is supported by an increasing body of experimental data [5]. It should be noted that, although cholesterol is the usual sterol present in red cell membranes, other sterols which have the structural requirements described above may gain access to the membrane. This has been observed

TABLE I. Lipids of the Normal Human Red Cell Membrane

	μmole/10^{11} cells
Cholesterol	36.1
Phospholipid	38.0
Glycolipid	1.0
Free fatty acid	2.6
	% of total phospholipids
Sphingomyelin	26.0
Lecithin	30.5
Phosphatidylserine (+ phosphatidylinositol)	13.2
Lysolecithin	1.3
Other (polyglycerol phosphatide, phosphatidic acid)	1.7
	Mole/mole
Cholesterol/phospholipid	0.95

in patients who accumulate cholestanol due to an inherited metabolic derangement [6] and in patients who absorb inappropriate quantities of dietary plant sterols, such as β-sitosterol [7].

The interactions between sterols and phospholipids have a number of important consequences for membrane structure. For example, sterols increase the efficiency of packing of phospholipids in artificial membranes [8]. The close interpositioning of sterols with phospholipids causes a degree of immobility to be imposed upon the ten acyl carbon atoms nearest the membrane's surface, while increasing the freedom of motion deep within the hydrophobic core of the membrane [9], thus creating what Chapman has called an "intermediate fluid state" [10]. One manifestation of this effect, which is seen when sterols are added to pure phospholipids, is a dimunition and finally eradication of the endothermic gel to liquid-crystal phase transition which is normally seen upon cooling. Another manifestation is the effect which sterols have on the fluidity of lipid bilayers.

MEMBRANE LIPID FLUIDITY

Under physiologic conditions the lipids of biologic membranes are in a liquid crystalline state. Although the hydrophobic interactions and the hydrogen bonding which occur between lipids maintain the integrity of the lipid bilayer, they also permit appreciable amounts of molecular motion within that bilayer. This motion appears to be greatest within the hydrophobic core of the membrane and least near the hydrocarbon-water interface. It is the process of molecular motion within the membrane that is referred to as "fluidity" and it is this process which imparts viscous properties to the hydrophobic portion of the membrane. This property of membrane lipids is most readily assessed in terms of the motion of small, hydrophobic probes that insert into the membrane and that are detectable by means of nuclear magnetic resonance, electron spin resonance, or fluorescence. The random motion of these probes within the membrane is referred to as rotational diffusion, and this motion is influenced by the viscosity of the microenvironment in which the probe resides. Therefore, measurements of the movement of hydrophobic probes is a means of assessing the viscosity of membrane lipids.

Concepts of membrane fluidity must not be confused with recent studies which have begun to define the membrane's viscoelastic properties. Whereas lipids have viscous properties, they do not have significant elastic properties. The surface viscoelasticity of red cells results from the character of certain membrane proteins, spectrin being the most important, and not from the fluidity of membrane lipids [11].

Membrane fluidity is strongly influenced by the composition of membrane lipids. For example, the number of saturated double bonds within the phospholipid acyl chains in membranes is an important determinant of the membrane's fluid qualities. Indeed, variation in acyl chain saturation is the most common determinant of membrane fluidity in nature. Saturated acyl chains form highly ordered membranes in which fluidity is of low magnitude. Conversely, phospholipids with unsaturated acyl chains form fluid-disordered membranes. Red cell membrane fluidity is also influenced by the amount of cholesterol relative to phospholipid [5, 12, 13] and by the relative amounts of the various phospholipids [14]. Amphiphilic molecules, such as soaps, alcohols, and detergents, partition between aqueous and lipid phases, and have a fluidizing effect on membrane lipids. Lysophosphatides are a naturally occurring amphipathic substance. Local anesthetics, such as procaine, and psychotrophic drugs, such as chlorpromazine, also exert a fluidizing effect under physiologic conditions [15]. Recent studies have suggested that the process of complement lysis is associated with the generation of amphipathic molecules which increase the fluidity of the hydrophobic core of membranes [16].

Because lipid fluidity is very sensitive to temperature, a demand is imposed upon nature to control fluidity under conditions in which temperature changes, for example, in cold-blooded animals exposed to varying ambient temperatures or warm-blooded animals during torpor or hibernation. Similar needs exist in plants which are cold-insensitive. In eukaryotes, sterols buffer the effects of temperature on fluidity by decreasing the activation energy for rotational diffusion, thus permitting less change in fluidity per degree change in temperature than would occur in the absence of sterols. The concept of homeoviscous adaptation is derived from the observation that simple organisms as diverse as bacteria and tetrahymena, are able to maintain membranes having a constant fluidity at a variety of growth temperatures [17–20]. This is achieved by varying the degree of saturation and branching of acyl fatty acids. A similar process of adaptation has been demonstrated in eukaryotic organisms, such as crustacean plankton, which grows in water of widely varying temperatures while maintaining a degree of fatty acid saturation such that the gel-to-liquid crystal phase transition of its membrane lipids is always approximately 2° lower than the ambient temperature [21]. Fish and frogs also vary the saturation/unsaturation ratio of their acyl fatty acids during cold adaptation [22, 23] and this has also been observed in the red cell and mitochondrial membranes of echidna, a primitive mammal, during periods of torpor [24]. Additional mechanisms have been observed in high mammals during hibernation. For example, ground squirrels increase the lysophosphatide content of their cardiac mitochondria [25], and hamsters decrease the cholesterol phospholipid ratio (C/PL) of their brain lipids [26]. All of these changes in membrane lipid composition serve to permit a normal fluidity under conditions of decreased temperature.

SYNTHESIS AND EXCHANGE

Mature red cells lack specific adaptative processes with which to control membrane fluidity. Instead, they depend upon the lipid composition of plasma lipoproteins. Similarities exist between membranes and lipoproteins in the sense that both contain cholesterol and phospholipid in close association with proteins. In addition, plasma lipoproteins contain cholesterol esters and triglycerides. More than two-thirds of the sterol in plasma lipoproteins is in the form of cholesterol esters. From the specific structural requirements for sterols in membranes described above, it is clear that cholesterol esters do not effectively associate with phospholipids in the membrane bilayer.

Two types of exchange diffusion are necessary to describe the movement of cholesterol between plasma lipoproteins and red cell membranes. The first is simple equilibrium exchange in which one molecule of membrane cholesterol exits into plasma in exchange for one molecule of cholesterol in plasma which enters the membrane. This process of equilibrium exchange has a half-time of 2 h, and was first described with isotopically labeled cholesterol by Gould and associates more than 25 years ago [27]. Studies with whole plasma and with isolated plasma lipoproteins in vitro and in vivo have demonstrated that the equilibrium involves the entire free cholesterol pools of both plasma lipoproteins and red cell membranes [28–32].

The second type of exchange diffusion between cholesterol in membranes and plasma lipoproteins concerns the partition of cholesterol within this exchangeable pool; that is, how much cholesterol is in lipoproteins and how much is in membranes.

This partition is best appreciated when it is recognized that cholesterol does not exist as a solute in water, nor does it by itself form micelles or liposomal membranes, as is the case for fatty acids and phospholipids. Sterols are virtually insoluble in water. They are solubilized in lipoproteins and in membranes by amphipathic lipids, such as phospholipids. Therefore, the partition of cholesterol between membranes and lipoproteins is determined by the amount of phospholipid relative to the amount of cholesterol within each compartment, ie, the cholesterol/phospholipid ratio. This has been confirmed by studies in a variety of systems in vivo and in vitro [5, 33, 34]. It is of particular interest because it underlies the pathogenesis of spur cell anemia in man [34] and it may play a role in the development of atherosclerosis in animals fed cholesterol-rich atherogenic diets [35].

SPUR CELL ANEMIA

The syndrome of spur cell anemia represents an abnormality of red cell membrane cholesterol content which results from a primary disorder of plasma lipoprotein metabolism [36]. It occurs in patients with severe liver disease, usually cirrhosis of the alcoholic. Red cells have bizarrely spiculated shapes, and they undergo premature destruction in vivo, primarily in the spleen. Of the two major lipids of the red cell membrane, phospholipids are present in normal amounts but cholesterol is increased by 25–65% [33]. This results in an increase in membrane C/PL from normal values of 0.95 to values as high as 1.60. It is of interest to compare this to values which can be achieved in vitro when cholesterol is mixed with purified phospholipids in water. Under conditions of high lipid concentration and gentle agitation, multilamellar liposomes form in which the maximum C/PL is 1.0 [37]. This value has been considered to be the upper limit of C/PL, and normal membranes have C/PL values which are below 1.0. Values greater than 1.0 can be achieved in vitro when lipids are suspended at a low concentration in water and energy is added, usually in the form of sonication [5, 34, 38, 39]. Thus, although values of less than 1.0 are preferred, values of C/PL greater than 1.0 can be achieved in vitro and are found in disease states in vivo.

Clinical observation has demonstrated that the spur cell membrane phenomonon is acquired, since normal transfused blood develops the abnormality [40]. Similar observations have been made when normal red cells are incubated for 24 h in serum from patients with spur cells [36]. Since cholesterol is transferred from plasma lipoproteins to cell membranes, it was of interest to examine the role of plasma cholesterol concentration in this process. It was observed that the enrichment of red cell membranes with cholesterol did not correlate with the serum cholesterol concentration but correlated strongly with the C/PL of low-density lipoproteins [34] (Fig 1). Thus, by means of equilibrium partition, red cells acquire cholesterol from lipoproteins which have an increased C/PL.

The syndrome of spur cell anemia is not unique to man, but has been described in rodents (guinea pigs and rabbits) [41, 42] and recently in dogs [43] fed cholesterol-rich atherogenic diets. The accumulation of cholesterol is not confined to red cell membranes. In man and in dogs platelet membranes are affected as well [36, 43], and in rodents an increase in C/PL has been observed in the surface membranes of macrophages [44] and liver cells [45]. Moreover, we have recently observed an increase in the C/PL of the surface membrane of lymphoblasts growing as ascites tumors in cholesterol-fed mice. Nor are changes isolated to surface membranes. Cholesterol equilibrates between cell surface membranes and internal membranes [46], causing an increase in the C/PL of microsomal membranes in cholesterol-fed animals [47]. Thus, an increase in the C/PL of plasma lipoproteins leads to an increase in the C/PL of many cell membranes.

CHOLESTEROL ENRICHMENT IN VITRO

Studies have been carried out in vitro to examine the equilibrium partition of cholesterol between human red cells and sonicated lipid dispersions containing various quantities of cholesterol [5, 34]. The C/PL of red cell membranes is directly influenced by the C/PL of lipid dispersions containing cholesterol cosonicated with various lecithins and with sphingomyelin. In each case, red cell cholesterol is unaffected by dispersions with a C/PL of 1.0 and is directly proportional to the C/PL of the dispersions over a range of membrane C/PL from 0.4 to 2.7 (Fig 2). Moreover, the addition of cholesterol esters to these dispersions had no influence on the partition of cholesterol. Thus, studies with pure lipid dispersions confirm the conclusions reached with human and experimental spur cell anemia.

If the equilibrium partition of cholesterol in terms of phospholipid was the sole determinant of the C/PL of membranes and lipoproteins, then all structures involved in this exchange should have identical C/PL values. Yet red cells, which have a C/PL of 0.95, are in equilibrium with various phospholipid dispersions with a C/PL of 1.0, and also with low-density lipoprotein, which has a C/PL of 0.8, and high-density lipoprotein, with a C/PL of 0.2. Platelet membranes have a C/PL of 0.6, and the surface membranes of

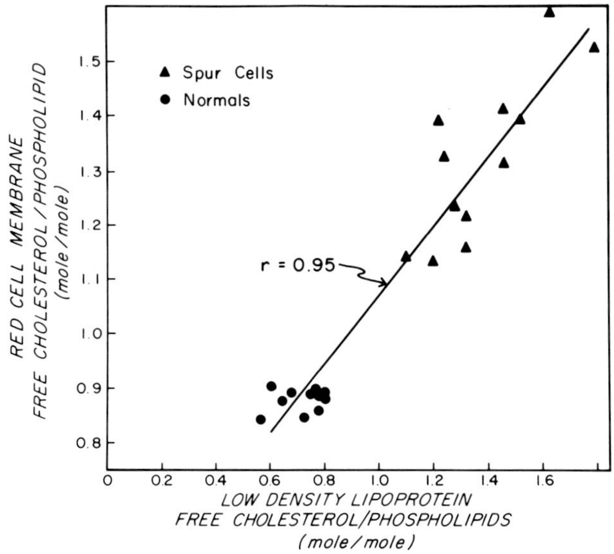

Fig 1. Relationship between the cholesterol/phospholipid (C/PL) mole ratio of red cell membranes of, and serum low-density lipoproteins from, patients with spur cells. A close correlation exists between the C/PL of membranes and lipoproteins [48].

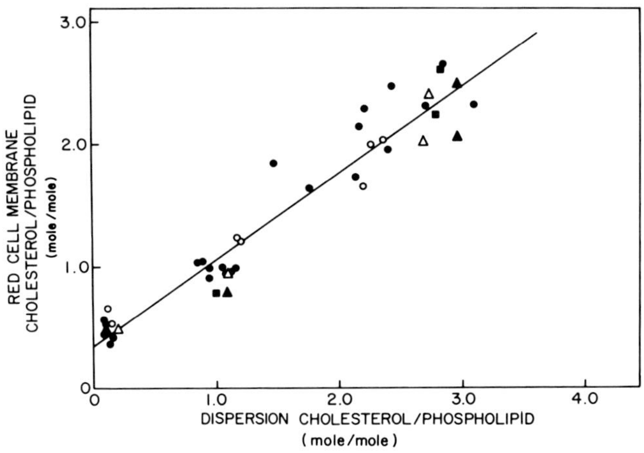

Fig 2. Effect of lipid dispersions on the cholesterol/phospholipid mole ratio of red cell membranes in vitro. Cells were incubated with dispersions for 24 h at 37°C. Phospholipids present in dispersions were •) L-dipalmitoyl lecithin; ○) egg lecithin; ▪) L-dimyristoyl lecithin; ▴) D,L-dipalmitoyl lecithin; △) bovine brain sphingomyelin. The final C/PL of red cell membranes correlated closely with that of lipid dispersions over a broad range of dispersion C/PL, irrespective of the phospholipid present in the dispersion [5].

nucleated cells have C/PL values of 0.4–0.8. Both are in equilibrium with plasma lipoproteins. When high-density lipoprotein is incubated with various phospholipid dispersions, its C/PL remains unchanged in the presence of dispersions with a C/PL of 1.0, and it increases in the presence of dispersions with C/PL values of greater than 1.0 [34]. A part of this seeming disparity results from variable quantities of glycolipids in membranes and lipoproteins. Like phospholipids, these are polar lipids capable of solubilizing cholesterol. In red cells of various mammalian species, glycolipids represent up to 15% of the total membrane lipids. Large amounts are present in the central nervous system. However, glycolipids alone do not account for the wide range of C/PL values observed. It is likely that the association between phospholipids and proteins, which are essential for certain functional and structural properties of both membranes and lipoproteins, occupy some phospholipids in a way which precludes their availability to solubilize cholesterol.

The effect of red cell membrane C/PL on the effective viscosity ($\bar{\eta}$) of red cell membrane ghosts was examined by measuring the rotational diffusion of the fluorescent probe 1,6-diphenyl-1,3,5-hexatriene [5] (Fig 3). A close relation between C/PL and $\bar{\eta}$ was seen through the range of red cell C/PL values extending from 0.5 to 2.0. However, further increases in membrane C/PL to values between 2.0 and 2.7 did not cause a further increase in $\bar{\eta}$. Values for membrane $\bar{\eta}$ ranged from 2.0 P at a membrane C/PL of 0.5 to approximately 6.0 P at C/PL values of 2.0–2.7. No phase transition was apparent over the temperature range 10–40° with red cell membranes at any C/PL studied (Fig 4). The activation energy for rotational diffusion, ΔE, was decreased from 8.3 kcal/mole in normal membranes to 5.8 kcal/mole in cholesterol-rich membranes (C/PL, 2.54), indicative of a high degree of order in the lipid structures of cholesterol-enriched membranes. Conversely, cholesterol depletion increased ΔE to 11.8 kcal/mole at a membrane C/PL of 0.35.

Although a linear relationship exists between the C/PL of dispersions and the C/PL of membranes throughout the broad range of membrane C/PL observed (Fig 2), the influence of C/PL on membrane fluidity was continuous only to a membrane C/PL value of 2.0 (Fig 3). This upper limit of 2.0 in terms of membrane C/PL represents a 1:1 interaction of cholesterol molecules with the acyl chains of phospholipids. It is possible that membranes with C/PL values in excess of 2.0 have domains which include cholesterol in a form that fails to influence membrane fluidity. Alternatively, such domains may exclude DPH, and therefore the dynamics within these domains may not be represented by the rotational diffusion of this probe.

CHOLESTEROL EFFECTS ON CELL CONTOUR

Striking changes in cell contour occur in association with increases in membrane cholesterol. These are characterized by a folding and scalloping of the cell margins (Fig 5). Similar changes occur when normal red cells are enriched with cholesterol by incubation with cholesterol-rich lecithin dispersions or with serum from pateints with spur cells [34, 36]. Moreover, a similar morphology was observed in a patient with spur cells who had undergone splenectomy [48]. The addition of cholesterol to red cells under these circumstances also increases membrane surface area in proportion to the contribution that cholesterol makes to the surface area of normal red cells. The magnitude of this increase in surface area is 0.20–0.25% for each 1.0% increase in membrane cholesterol [32]. Thus, the effect of added cholesterol is to increase surface area and alter cell contour.

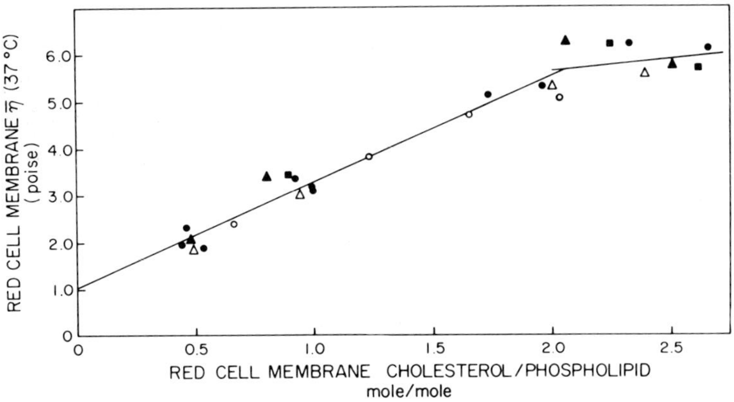

Fig 3. Relationship between the cholesterol/phospholipid mole ratio of red cell membranes and membrane fluidity after incubation of red cells as described in Figure 2. Fluidity was assessed as the rotational diffusion of diphenylhexatriene (DPH) and expressed as the effective microviscosity ($\bar{\eta}$) in poise. A close relationship existed between membrane C/PL and $\bar{\eta}$ to a maximum at a C/PL of 2.0. Thereafter, additional cholesterol did not influence $\bar{\eta}$, as determined with DPH [5].

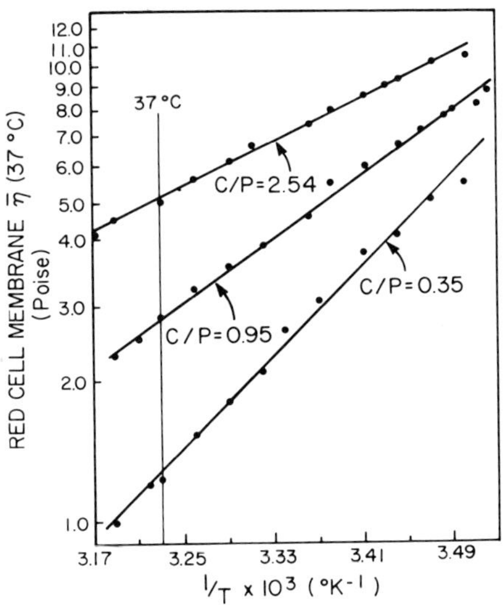

Fig 4. Fluidity of red cell membranes as a function of temperature. Red cells were enriched with or depleted of cholesterol in vitro, as in Figure 3. Effective microviscosity ($\bar{\eta}$) was expressed relative to the reciprocal of the absolute temperature. Cholesterol-enriched membranes had a greater $\bar{\eta}$ at all temperatures. No phase transition was observed [5].

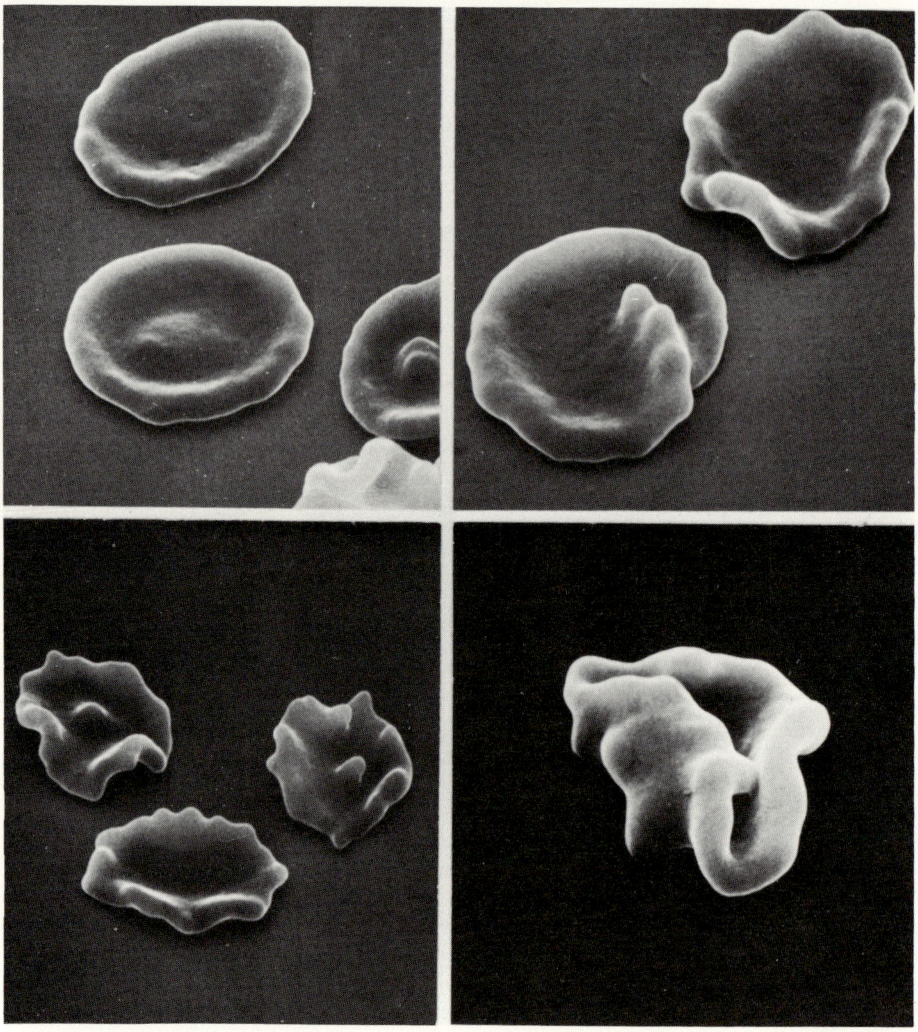

Fig 5. Scanning electron micrographs of red cells enriched with cholesterol in vitro. All photographs are from the same preparation (kindly prepared by Dr R. Weinstein) [34].

Whether due to these gross physical changes in the membrane or whether due to the more subtle changes in fluidity which are also caused by added cholesterol, the flow properties of cholesterol-rich red cells are impaired. This is seen in vitro by a decrease in the red cell's ability to traverse filters of small pore size [34, 36]. In vivo, spur cells are retarded in their circulation through the spleen, where they lose a portion of their surface membrane (Fig 6) and undergo changes in cell contour [36, 48]. This results in a thorny-appearing red cell (the "spur cell"), for which this disorder is named. Membrane remodeling in spur cell anemia is analogous to the loss of membrane that hereditary spherocytes undergo under similar conditions and has been called splenic conditioning [49].

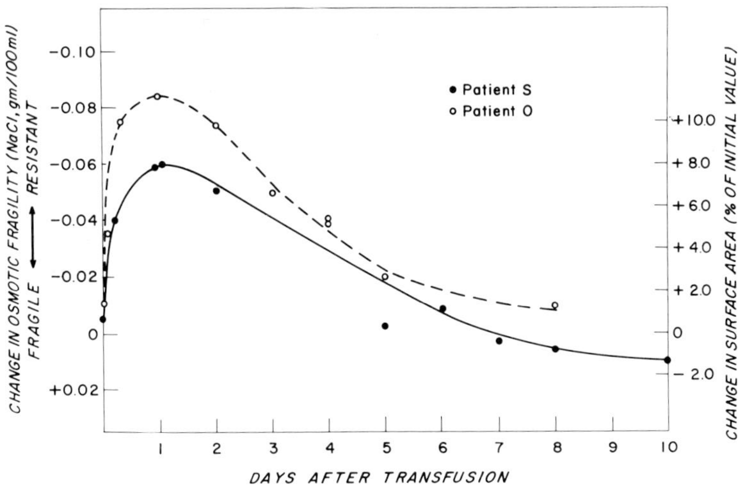

Fig 6. Changes in the surface area of normal ^{51}Cr-labeled red cells after transfusion into two patients with spur cells. Surface area was calculated from a measure of mean osmotic fragility (the concentration of hypotonic NaCl causing lysis of red cells in vitro). An initial increase in surface area resulted from the acquisition of membrane cholesterol by these normal red cells in the circulation of a patient with cholesterol-rich red cells and cholesterol-rich lipoproteins. Subsequent loss of surface area occurred as the spleen eroded the surface of these cholesterol-rich red cells (data reported, in part, in Ref 36).

CHOLESTEROL EFFECTS ON MEMBRANE FUNCTION

The enrichment of membranes with cholesterol has a number of effects on the permeability, transport, and enzymatic activities of the membrane and on the availability of membrane surface receptors. An effect of cholesterol on permeability was first demonstrated using lecithin liposomes containing various sterols, and these studies helped to establish the structural requirements for sterols in membranes [50]. Although not all studies utilizing red cells are in agreement, it appears that increases in membrane cholesterol reduce the passive permeability and facilitated diffusion of a number of electrolytes and nonelectrolytes, whereas cholesterol depletion increases permeability. In contrast, changes in membrane cholesterol do not appear to directly influence the active transport of Na or K. Thus, for example, cholesterol depletion increases the passive permeability of red cells to glycerol, acetate and Na [34, 51]. An apparent increase in active Na flux also accompanies cholesterol depletion. Although this may be explained in terms of a response to the increase in passive Na permeability rather than the primary effect on the transport mechanism [34], an effect of cholesterol on the affinity of the pump for Na has also been demonstrated [52]. In contrast, cholesterol enrichment inhibits the furosemide-sensitive diffusion of Na + K [53], as well as the diffusion of glycerol, erythritol, acetate, and proprionate [54]. Similar decreases in nonelectrolyte permeability have been observed in cholesterol-rich guinea pig red cells [55]. We have not observed any effect of cholesterol enrichment on active Na or K transport [34], although a decrease in active Na flux of very small magnitude was reported in cholesterol-rich guinea pig cells [55]. Thus, modulation of membrane cholesterol has a substantial effect on the cell's permeability to small molecules.

The human platelet has provided additional insight into the relation between membrane cholesterol content and cell function. Shattil and coworkers have shown that human platelets acquire cholesterol when they are incubated with cholesterol-rich lipid dispersions [56]. If the incubation period is short (4–5h) the change in membrane C/PL is confined to the membrane fraction. After 24 h the granule fraction is also cholesterol-enriched. Changes in membrane fluidity parallel changes in C/PL [57]. Associated with this change in membrane lipid composition, platelets become more sensitive to epinephrine and adenosine diphosphate (ADP) such that concentrations of these agents 10–50 times lower than required for inducing normal platelets to aggregate readily induce this aggregation of cholesterol-rich platelets [56] (Fig 7). It is of interest that the C/PL of the membrane (but not granule) fraction of platelets from patients with type II hyperlipoproteinemia is increased [58] and that these platelets are also more sensitive to aggregating agents [59].

The effect of cholesterol on membrane enzymes has been analyzed in rats fed a corn oil diet supplemented with cholesterol [56]. Cholesterol enrichment was found to increase the sensitivity of acetylcholine esterase to fluoride inhibition, decrease the fluoride sensitivity of acetylcholine esterase to fluoride inhibition, decrease the fluoride sensitivity of the Na-K adenosine triphosphatase (ATPase), and cause no change in the fluoride sensitivity of magnesium Mg ATPase. A complex effect of cholesterol on a membrane enzyme, adenylate cyclase, was observed in human platelets [60]. The basal level of this enzyme was increased 2–3 times in cholesterol-rich platelets, and the opposite was seen in platelets with a decreased membrane cholesterol content. Moreover, the stimulation of adenylate cyclase that normally occurs with fluoride or with prostaglandin E_1 was not observed in cholesterol-rich platelets, and prostaglandin E_1 was relatively ineffective in inhibiting platelet aggregation. Effects of membrane cholesterol on membrane enzymes have also been observed in mycoplasma membranes [61, 62].

Three general concepts relate to the mechanism of these cholesterol-induced changes in membrane properties. First is the role of the influence of cholesterol on bulk membrane fluidity. Changes in fluidity may be translated across short distances and influence the range of motion or the potential volume available to a membrane enzyme and its substrate during the enzymatic process. Second is the lipid composition of the immediate environment of the enzyme. Studies with both cytochrome oxidase from mitochondria [63] and Ca-ATPase from sarcoplasmic reticulum [64] have demonstrated a specific boundary layer, or annulus, of phospholipid. Moreover, it appears that cholesterol is specifically excluded from the annulus in sarcoplasmic reticulum. Therefore, in a manner quite distinct from its bulk influence on membrane fludity, cholesterol may influence membrane enzymes by directly interacting with these boundary lipids.

A third general mechanism by which the cholesterol content of membranes may influence membrane enzyme and transport properties relates to the potential effect of membrane lipid composition on the position of proteins, such as enzymes, transport proteins, and receptors, in the plane of the membrane. Shinitzky and co-workers have recently presented evidence which suggests that enrichment of red cell membranes with cholesterol causes an increase in the exposure of membrane proteins to their aqueous environment [65, 66]. If these conclusions can be supported by other techniques, this concept provides a subtle mechanism for the modulation of many membrane events by a primary modulation of membrane lipid composition.

The effects of cholesterol on the permeability and enzymatic properties of membranes cited above emphasize the importance for normal physiology of maintaining

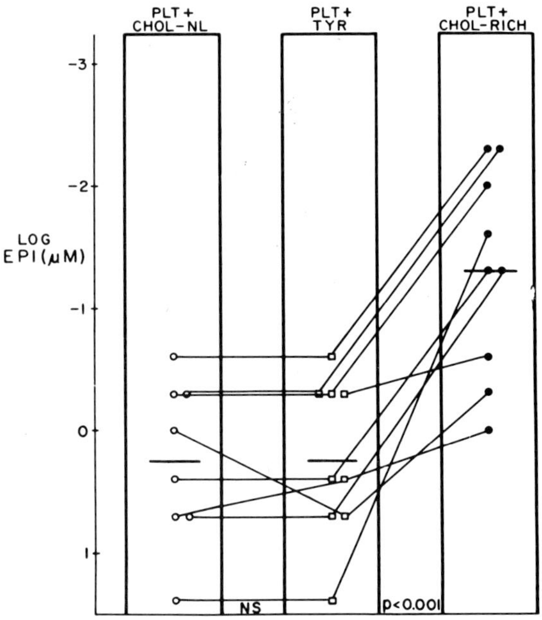

Fig 7. Epinephrine sensitivity of platelets enriched with cholesterol (chol-rich) as compared with platelets incubated with lipid dispersions which induced no change in platelet lipids (chol-nl) and control platelets incubated in tyrodes buffer (tyr). The concentration of epinephrine needed to induce platelet aggregation was decreased 10–100 times in cholesterol-enriched platelets [56].

membrane cholesterol within narrow limits. Mycoplasma membranes which have been adapted to low levels of membrane cholesterol compensate for this by increasing the amount of unsaturated fatty acids associated with their membrane phospholipids [67]. In contrast, it appears that most mammalian cell membranes adapt poorly when exposed to lipoproteins with an increased C/PL. This is evidenced by the accumulation of cholesterol in the membranes of red cells, platelets, liver cells, macrophages, and ascites tumor cells in animals fed a cholesterol-rich diet, as discussed above. These animals also accumulate cholesterol esters in their vessel walls in the form of fatty streaks and atheromatous plaques. The genesis of these lesions is undoubtedly multifactoral, and vessel injury may play an important role. Indeed, it is possible that cholesterol enrichment of endothelial cell membranes may contribute to the process of injury [68]. It is likely that a need exists within cells lining vessel walls to adapt to cholesterol-induced changes in membrane fluidity. Cholesterol esters represent an end product with no functional role. However, esterification of cholesterol does divert cholesterol from a form which is available to enter membranes to a form which is excluded from membrane structure. Cholesterol esterification may represent a form of adaptation to an excess C/PL just as cholesterol synthesis represents an adaptation to a low level of membrane C/PL [69]. In support of this hypothesis we have reported that the rate of cholesterol esterification in the mouse hepatoma cell line Fu5AH bears no relation to the cholesterol concentration of the medium; rather, it is directly related to the C/PL presented to the cells [35] (Fig 8). Thus, it appears that the elevated C/PL of lipoproteins in various animals fed cholesterol-rich atherogenic diets may call forth an adaptative process by some cells whose membranes have become less fluid due to an increase in membrane cholesterol, and that this adaptative process results in the accumulation of cholesterol esters within such cells.

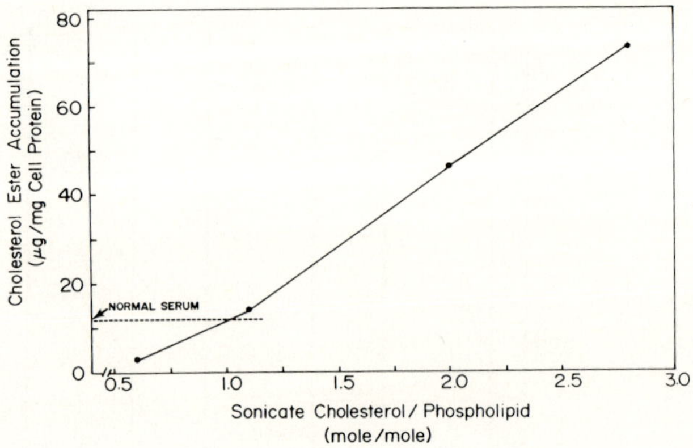

Fig 8. Effect of the cholesterol/phospholipid mole ratio of the medium on cholesterol esterification accumulation in Fu5AH hepatoma cell cultures. The degree of cholesterol ester accumulation correlated directly with the C/PL of lipids in the growth medium. Sonicated lipids with a C/PL of 1.0 caused a degree of cholesterol ester accumulation equivalent to that observed with normal serum [35].

TRANSFER OF CHOLESTEROL PLUS LECITHIN TO RED CELLS

In most patients with liver disease, cholesterol-rich spur cells are not observed. Rather, red cells appear as target cells due to the acquisition of an excess of both cholesterol and phospholipid in proportional amounts [33–70] (Fig 9). Although this has been observed in various forms of liver disease, including hepatitis, cirrhosis, and obstructive jaundice, the changes are most striking in patients with obstructive jaundice or with other forms of liver disease with an obstructive component. The cholesterol increase may be as great as 75% but more commonly ranges between 25 and 50% above normal. Although there is variability from patient to patient, the percentage increase in phospholipid is approximately 60% of the percentage increase in cholesterol, resulting in an increase in the C/PL of approximately 15%. The phospholipid increase is not distributed among the various phospholipids, but rather is confined to lecithin. Thus, cholesterol and lecithin are not only the most exchangeable of the major red cell lipids, but their membrane compartments also undergo the greatest quantitative change in liver disease. In several patients with target cells studied by us thus far, membrane fluidity is normal or actually increased slightly as a result of the acquisition of both cholesterol, which tends to decrease fluidity, and lecithin, which is a very fluid lipid.

It is of interest that a similar abnormality in red cells has been observed in patients with a congenital absence of the serum enzyme lecithin-cholesterol acyltransferase (LCAT) [71]. LCAT deficiency of a variable degree is also quite common in patients with liver disease. However, we have not been able to find any correlation between the serum LCAT activity of patients with liver disease and the abnormalities of lipids within their red cells [33].

Two processes appear to participate in determining the amounts of cholesterol and lecithin in target cells. First is a process analogous to, if not identical with, the isolated transfer of cholesterol from lipoproteins to red cells as dictated by the C/PL of the lipo-

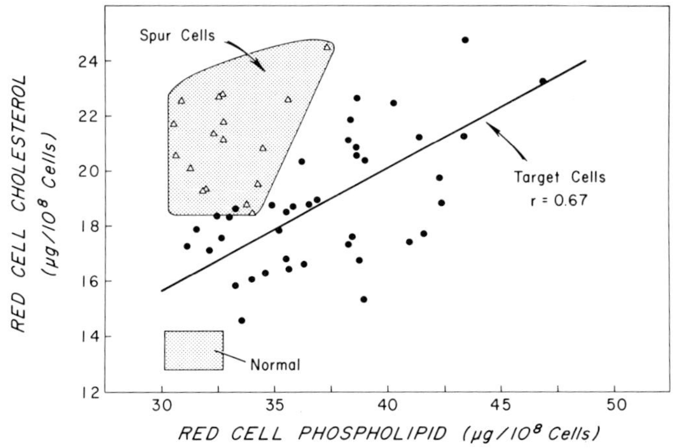

Fig 9. Cholesterol and phospholipid content of red cells from patients with liver disease. Spur cells have a selective increase in cholesterol content, whereas target cells are enriched in both cholesterol and phospholipid [33].

protein. Since the C/PL of low density lipoproteins (LDL) in most patients with liver disease is increased only mildly [33], this accounts for only a small amount of the additional membrane cholesterol. However, this process is readily demonstrable in vitro [33], and it accounts for the increased C/PL of target cells in liver disease [72].

The larger amount of cholesterol and lecithin which is acquired by red cells may involve an independent transfer of lecithin followed by a process of equilibrium during which the C/PL of the red cell (now transiently decreased because of this added lecithin) comes into equilibrium with the increased C/PL of LDL by means of a transfer of cholesterol from LDL to cells. In this regard, it is of interest that the normal phospholipid/protein weight ratio of LDL is approximately 1.0, but it is increased 25% in patients with liver disease [33]. Although an in vitro system has not yet been established to test the importance of phospholipid/protein interactions on the transfer of phospholipid from LDL to cell membranes, it appears likely that the elevated phospholipid/protein of LDL in liver disease underlies the increased lecithin content of target cells. The LDL in patients with spur cells also has a high phospholipid/protein ratio and lecithin also accumulates in spur cells. The fact that the total phospholipid content is not increased in spur cells in vivo appears to result from a loss of membrane phospholipid together with other membrane components as these red cells are conditioned during circulation in vivo [36, 48]. Only the relative increase in lecithin compared with other phospholipids remains in spur cells [33]. Thus, the total content of cholesterol in red cell membranes appears to be a function of 1) the membrane phospholipid content (possibly as influenced by the phospholipid/protein of LDL); 2) the fraction of phospholipid available within each membrane for solubilizing cholesterol (as determined by the amount of membrane phospholipid which is in the form of boundary lipids and other structures strongly related to proteins within the membrane but excluding cholesterol); and 3) by the C/PL of LDL which is in equilibrium with these membranes.

An alternative mechanism for cholesterol and lecithin accumulation in target cells has been suggested by DeGier and his co-workers [70]. This mechanism takes cognizance of the fact that many patients with liver disease, particularly of the obstructive variety, have a discrete lipoprotein (LP-X) which is discoidal in appearance and which is composed primarily of cholesterol and lecithin in equimolar amounts [73, 74]. Similar structures have been observed in LCAT deficiency [75]. DeGier and associates have proposed that these lipoprotein vesicles fuse with the red cell membrane and in this way transfer equivalent quantities of cholesterol and lecithin to the red cell membrane. Moreover, these workers have presented electron micrographs which are interpreted as showing fusion occurring within 2 h in vitro. Although fusion of artificial vesicles with red cells has also been reported, it appears that the presence in the vesicle of a negatively charged phospholipid, such as phosphatidylserine, is an essential requirement for fusion to occur [76]. Lecithin-cholesterol vesicles in liver disease and in LCAT deficiency are neutral. Furthermore, the time course of lipid acquisition by target cells in vivo is slow, with a $T_{1/2}$ of 24 h [33], whereas fusion leading to a 15% increase in surface area was observed with LP-X in vitro in only 2 h [70]. Finally, the process of target cell formation is totally reversible in vivo [33], whereas a fusion process would be irreversible. Thus, it appears unlikely that vesicle fusion with red cells represents a major mechanism whereby a large excess of lecithin is acquired by target cells, and direct transfer of lecithin, followed by equilibration with cholesterol, appears more likely. Further work is needed to resolve this problem.

CONCLUSIONS

The organization of lipids in cell membranes requires specific molecular interactions. Many cell processes occur within the fluid environment created by these membrane lipids. As evolution has proceeded from prokaryotes to eukaryotes and from poikilotherms to homeotherms, cells have developed a decreased tolerance of fluctuations in membrane fluidity. Adaptative mechanisms have developed in order to maintain a normal cell membrane fluidity under conditions which might cause it to change, such as variations in the lipid composition or temperature of the cell's environment. Disease states result when human cells fail to adapt. Red cells are particularly vulnerable to abnormalities in membrane fluidity since they lack specific adaptative mechanisms of their own and must depend for adaptation on the lipid composition of plasma lipoproteins. Exposure of red cells to a lipid environment rich in cholesterol relative to phospholipid leads to an enrichment of red cell membrane cholesterol. This is associated with derangements in membrane fluidity and function and with abnormalities of cell contour and cell survival in vivo.

REFERENCES

1. Rouser G, Nelson GJ, Fleischer S, Simon G: In Chapman D, (ed): "Biological Membranes." New York: Academic, 1968, pp 6–69.
2. Nes WR: Lipids 9:596, 1974.
3. Demel RA, Bruckdorfer KR, Van Deenen LLM: Biochim Biophys Acta 255:311, 1972.
4. Huang C-H: Lipids 12:348, 1977.
5. Cooper RA, Leslie MH, Fischkoff S, Shinitzky M, Shattil SJ: Biochemistry 17:327, 1978.
6. Salen G, Grundy SM: J Clin Invest 52:2822, 1973.
7. Salen G, Ahrens EH Jr, Grundy SM: J Clin Invest 49:952, 1970.
8. Demel RA, DeKruyff B: Biochim Biophys Acta 457:109, 1976.
9. Rothman JE, Engelman DM: Nature New Biology 237:42, 1972.
10. Chapman D (ed): "Biological Membranes: Physical fact and function." New York: Academic, 1968, pp 125–202.
11. Evans EA, Hochmuth RM: J Membrane Biol 30:351, 1977.
12. Shinitzky M, Inbar M: Biochim Biophys Acta 433:133, 1976.

13. Vanderkooi J, Fischkoff S, Chance B, Cooper RA: Biochemistry 13:1589, 1974.
14. Cooper RA, Durocher JR, Leslie MH: J Clin Invest 60:115, 1977.
15. Feinstein MB, Fernandez SM, Sha'afi RI: Biochim Biophys Acta 413:354, 1975.
16. Shattil SJ, Cines DB, Schreiber AD: Clin Res 25:347A, 1977.
17. Sinensky M: Proc Natl Acad Sci 71:522, 1974.
18. Cronan JE Jr, Gelmann EP: Bacteriol Rev 39:232, 1975.
19. McElhaney RN, Souza KA: Biochim Biophys Acta 443:348, 1976.
20. Kitajima Y, Thompson GA Jr: J Cell Biol 72:744, 1977.
21. Farkas T, Herodek S: J Lipid Res 5:369, 1964.
22. Knipprath WG, Mead JF: Lipids 1:113, 1966.
23. Baranska J, Wlodawer P: Comp Biochem Physiol 28:553, 1969.
24. McMurchie EJ, Raison JK: J Thermal Biology 1:113, 1975.
25. Keith AD, Aloia RC, Lyons J, Snipes W, Pengelley ET: Biochim Biophys Acta 394:204, 1975.
26. Goldman SS: Am J Phys 228:834, 1975.
27. Hagerman JS, Gould RG: Proc Soc Exp Biol Med 78:329, 1951.
28. London IM, Schwartz H: J Clin Invest 32:1248, 1953.
29. Gould RG, LeRoy GV, Okita GT, Kabara JJ, Keegan P, Bergenstal DM: J Lab Clin Med 46:372, 1955.
30. Murphy JR: J Lab Clin Med 60:571, 1962.
31. Ashworth LAE, Green C: Biochim Biophys Acta 84:182, 1964.
32. Basford JM, Glover J, Green C: Biochim Biophys Acta 84:764, 1964.
33. Cooper RA, Diloy-Puray M, Lando P, Greenberg MS: J Clin Invest 51:3182, 1972.
34. Cooper RA, Arner EC, Wiley JS, Shattil SJ: J Clin Invest 55:115, 1975.
35. Arbogast LY, Rothblat GH, Leslie MH, Cooper RA: Proc Nat Acad Sci 73:3680, 1976.
36. Cooper RA: J Clin Invest 48:1820, 1969.
37. Bourgès M, Small DM, Dervichian DG: Biochim Biophys Acta 137:157, 1967.
38. Horwitz C, Krut L, Kaminsky L: Biochim Biophys Acta 239:329, 1971.
39. Freeman R, Finean JB: Chem Phys Lipids 14:313, 1975.
40. Silber R, Amorosi E, Lhowe J, Kayden HJ: New Engl J Med 275:639, 1966.
41. Westerman MP, Wiggans RG III, Mao R: J Lab Clin Med 75:893, 1970.
42. Sardet C, Hansma H, Ostwald R: J Lipid Res 13:705, 1972.
43. Cooper RA, Leslie MH, Knight D, Shattil SJ, Detweiler DK: Clin Res 25:454A, 1977.
44. Dianzani MU, Torrielli MV, Canuto RA, Garcea R, Feo F: J Path 118:193, 1976.
45. Grandison AS, Green C: Biochem Soc Trans 4:645, 1976.
46. Bell FP: Biochim Biophys Acta 398:18, 1975.
47. Lang M: Biochim Biophys Acta 455:947, 1976.
48. Cooper RA, Kimball DB, Durocher JR: New Engl J Med 290:1279, 1974.
49. Emerson CP Jr, Shen SC, Ham TH, Fleming EM, Castle WB: Arch Intern Med 97:1, 1956.
50. DeGier J, Mandersloot JG, VanDeenen LLM: Biochim Biophys Acta 150:666, 1968.
51. Grunze M, Deuticke B: Biochim Biophys Acta 356:125, 1974.
52. Giraud F, Claret M, Garay R: Nature 264:646, 1976.
53. Wiley JS, Cooper RA: Biochim Biophys Acta 413:425, 1975.
54. Deuticke B, Ruska C: Biochim Biophys Acta 433:638, 1976.
55. Kroes J, Ostwald R: Biochim Biophys Acta 249:647, 1971.
56. Shattil SJ, Anaya-Galindo R, Bennett J, Colman RW, Cooper RA: J Clin Invest 55:636–643, 1975.
57. Shattil SJ, Cooper RA: Biochemistry 15:4832–4837, 1976.
58. Shattil SJ, Bennett JS, Colman RW, Cooper RA: J Lab Clin Med 89:341–353, 1977.
59. Carvalho ACA, Colman RW, Lees RS: N Engl J Med 290:434–438, 1974.
60. Sinha AK, Shattil SJ, Colman RW: J Biol Chem 252:3310, 1977.
61. Rottem S, Cirillo VP, DeKruyff B, Shinitzky M, Razin S: Biochim Biophys Acta 323:509, 1973.
62. DeKruyff B, VanDijck PWM, Goldbach RW, Demel RA, VanDeenen LLM: Biochem Biophys Acta 330:269, 1973.
63. Jost PC, Griffith OH, Capaldi RA, Vanderkooi G: Proc Nat Acad Sci USA 70:480, 1973.
64. Warren GB, Houslay MD, Metaclfe JC, Birdsall NJM: Nature 255:684, 1975.
65. Borochov H, Shinitzky M: Proc Nat Acad Sci USA 73:4526, 1976.
66. Shinitzky M, Rivnay B: Biochemistry 16:982, 1977.
67. Rottem S, Yashouv J, Ne'eman Z, Razin S: Biochim Biophys Acta 323:495, 1973.

68. Ross R, Harker L: Science 193:1094, 1976.
69. Fogelman AM, Seager J, Edwards PA, Popjak G: J Biol Chem 265:644, 1977.
70. Verkleij AJ, Nauta ILD, Werre JM, Mandersloot JG, Reinders B, Ververgaert PHJ, DeGier J: Biochim Biophys Acta 436:366, 1976.
71. Gjone E, Torsvik H, Norum KR: Scand J Clin Lab Invest 21:327, 1968.
72. Cooper RA, Jandl JH: J Clin Invest 47:809, 1968.
73. Switzer S: J Clin Invest 46:1855, 1967.
74. Hamilton RL, Havel RJ, Kane JP, Blaurock AE, Sata T: Science 172:475, 1971.
75. Glomset JA, Nichols AV, Norum KR, King W, Forte T: J Clin Invest 52:1078, 1973.
76. Papahadjopoulos D, Poste G, Schaeffer BE: Biochim Biophys Acta 323:23, 1973.

Journal of Supramolecular Structure 8:431–438 (1978)
Normal and Abnormal Red Cell Membranes 153–160

The Program of Friend Cell Erythroid Differentiation: Early Changes in Na^+/K^+ ATPase Function

Dixie Mager and Alan Bernstein

Department of Medical Biophysics, University of Toronto, and The Ontario Cancer Institute, 500 Sherbourne Street, Toronto, Ontario, Canada M4X 1K9

Treatment of Friend erythroleukemia cells with several different chemical agents causes an early decrease in the $^{86}Rb^+$ influx mediated by Na^+/K^+ adenosine triphosphatase (ATPase). These agents, which induce Friend cells to differentiate, include dimethylsulfoxide (DMSO), ouabain, hypoxanthine, and actinomycin D. The magnitude of the early decrease in $^{86}Rb^+$ influx correlates with the proportion of cells in cultures of inducible Friend cell clones which later go on to synthesize hemoglobin. Compounds which do not incude differentiation in these cells, such as xanthine, exogenous hematin, and erythropoietin, do not cause a change in $^{86}Rb^+$ influx. A change in the intracellular K^+ ion concentration does not occur during induction by DMSO because, although there is a decrease in K^+ content per cell soon after induction, there is a parallel decrease in cell volume. These results and previous observations from this laboratory are discussed in terms of the posible involvement of the Na^+/K^+ ATPase in Friend cell differentiation.

Key words: **Friend cells, Na^+/K^+ ATPase, K^+ ion levels, transport changes, differentiation**

The study of normal erythropoiesis in vivo is hampered by the inherent cellular heterogeneity of the blood-forming tissues, the difficulty in obtaining large amounts of cells in different stages of development, and the inability to easily maintain long-term cultures of erythroid precursor cells. Thus, many genetic and biochemical studies are very difficult if not impossible to carry out under these conditions. Friend erythroleukemic cells can be stimulated to undergo erythroid differentiation in vitro [15] and therefore provide a useful model system for the genetic and biochemical analysis of the later stages of erythropoiesis.

Friend cells were derived from the spleens of Friend virus-infected mice. They are permanent clonal cell lines which divide every 10–12 h. In 1971, Friend and co-workers

Received for publication April 11, 1978; accepted June 9, 1978.

0091-7419/78/0804-0431$01.70

discovered that these cells could be induced to synthesize hemoglobin by treatment with dimethylsulfoxide (DMSO) [15]. Since that time several other cellular changes that are characteristic of normal erythropoiesis have been found to occur in differentiating Friend cells (Fig 1). As can be seen from this figure, the program of Friend cell differentiation has been extensively characterized. However, knowledge about the initial genetic and molecular mechanisms controlling the induction of this differentiation program is lacking. One major reason for this is the lack of chemical and biologic specificity of the Friend cell-inducing agents.

Besides DMSO and other organic solvents [15, 21–23], certain purines and purine analogs [24], butyric acid [25], and metabolic inhibitors such as actinomycin D [26] also induce Friend cells to differentiate. However, there is no known specific cellular site of action for any of these agents. Thus it has been difficult to ascertain the mechanisms of induction using these compounds. We have observed that ouabain, a specific inhibitor of the plasma membrane-bound enzyme Na^+/K^+ ATPase (adenosine triphosphatase) [27], induces differentiation in Friend cells via direct binding to this enzyme [28]. This is the only case in which interaction of an inducing agent with a specific cellular target, the Na^+/K^+ ATPase, has been shown to be necessary for induction of Friend cell differentiation to occur. Because of this observation, we have been investigating whether an alteration in Na^+/K^+ ATPase activity is a common event during Friend cell differentiation, and if so, whether changes in the function of this enzyme play an important role in the control of differentiation in this system.

MATERIALS AND METHODS

Suspension cell cultures were maintained in α medium [29] supplemented with 10% fetal calf serum (Reheis) as previously described [2]. The $^{86}Rb^+$ uptake experiments were

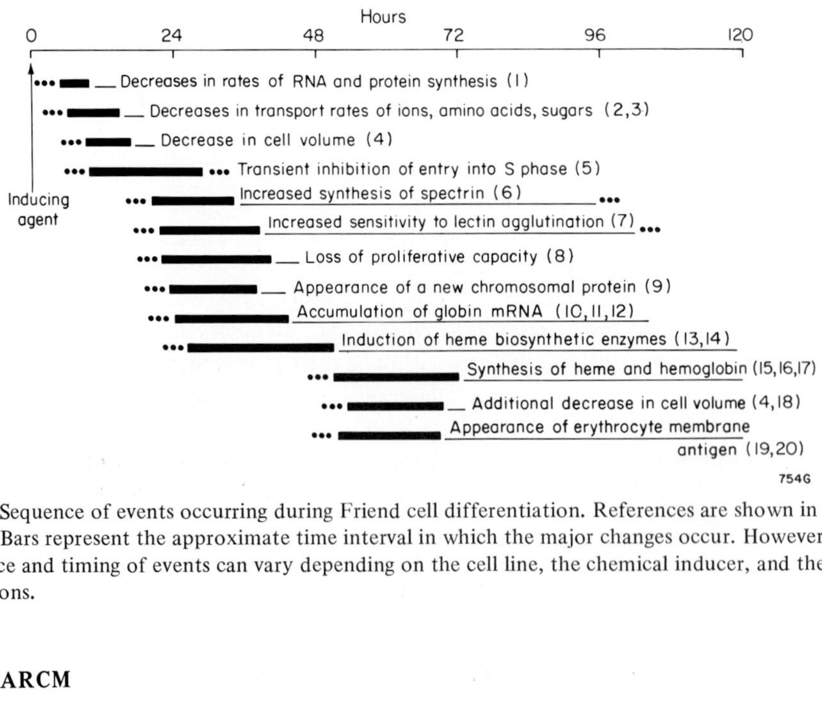

Fig 1. Sequence of events occurring during Friend cell differentiation. References are shown in parentheses. Bars represent the approximate time interval in which the major changes occur. However, the sequence and timing of events can vary depending on the cell line, the chemical inducer, and the culture conditions.

performed using exponentially growing cells as described elsewhere [2]. Cells were stained for hemoglobin by the liquid benzidine staining procedure of Orkin, Harosi, and Leder [30]. Cell volumes were determined with an electronic cell volume spectrometer and pulse-height analyzer as detailed previously [4].

Potassium ion content was measured using a procedure developed by Dr Jim Graves. Duplicate cell samples, containing $(1-2) \times 10^6$ cells, were pelleted and resuspended in 5 ml cold isotonic LiCl. This was quickly layered over 2 ml of a 1:7 mixture of oil (Beckman ultracentrifuge drive oil No. 302411) and dibutylphthalate, and the cells were centrifuged through the oil mixture. The LiCl was aspirated off and the sides of the tube washed several times in distilled water. The oil mixture was aspirated off, the final wash leaving the cell pellet in the bottom of the tube. Then 5 ml of 4 mM CsCl and 0.05% Triton X-100 was added to each tube which was then vortexed, frozen-thawed, and vortexed again. Samples were analyzed using a Perkin-Elmer atomic absorption spectrophotometer (Model 303) with KCl standards between 5 and 40 μM.

RESULTS

Early Changes in $^{86}Rb^+$ Influx During Friend Cell Differentiation

The addition of any one of several chemical inducing agents to cultures of Friend cells results in early decreases in the initial rate of $^{86}Rb^+$ uptake. Figure 2 shows the percentage change in the initial uptake rate of $^{86}Rb^+$ as a function of time after the addition of inducer to the culture medium. As can be seen, such widely different compounds as DMSO, hypoxanthine, and actinomycin D, all of which induce Friend cell differentiation,

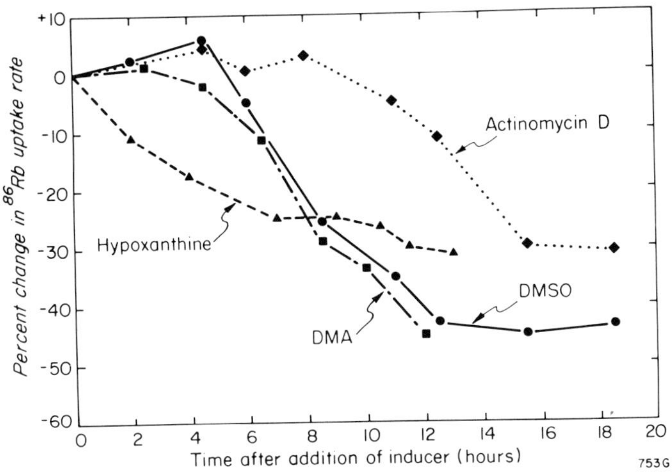

Fig 2. Change in ^{86}Rb uptake rate in response to various chemical inducing agents. At each time point, the initial rate of ^{86}Rb+uptake was determined in both untreated and inducer-treated cells as described previously [2]. The average percentage change in rate in inducer-treated cells relative to the rate in control cells is plotted. The average standard deviation of each percentage point, evaluated at a particular time, varied between 2 and 4%. The inducer concentrations used were 1.5% DMSO (●), 10 mM N,N-dimethylacetamide (DMA) (■), 4 mM hypoxanthine (▲), and 6 ng/ml actinomycin D (♦). The cell line used in all experiments was 745a except for those involving actinomycin D. In these experiments a mutant of 745a, (AIII), resistant to the cytotoxic effect of actinomycin D, was employed.

cause decreases in the initial rate of $^{86}Rb^+$ uptake within 16 h. After this early drop in the influx of $^{86}Rb^+$, which occurs at different times for different inducers, the rate of uptake remains relatively constant for at least 48 h (data not shown). These changes in $^{86}Rb^+$ uptake appear to be due to decreases in the Na^+/K^+ ATPase-mediated influx of $^{86}Rb^+$, since complete inhibition of this enzyme by brief exposure to a high concentration of ouabain reduces the influx of $^{86}Rb^+$ to the same level in both untreated and DMSO-treated cells [2].

Correlation Between the Early Decrease in $^{86}Rb^+$ Influx and the Later Extent of Differentiation in Friend Cells

A number of observations suggest that early changes in transport are an integral part of the program of Friend cell differentiation. First, these transport changes do not occur when cells of other types (chick embryo fibroblasts, human fibroblasts, and mouse L cells) are exposed to the chemical inducers [3]. Second, the time lag between the addition of inducer and the appearance of the early transport changes suggests that these changes in transport in differentiating Friend cells are not the result of a nonspecific effect of the chemical inducers on animal cells in culture. This conclusion is strengthened by the observation that such a widely diverse group of chemical agents all bring about the early changes in transport. Furthermore, the occurrence and magnitude of the early change in $^{86}Rb^+$ influx correlates well with the number of hemoglobin-positive cells observed five days later (Fig 3). For example, xanthine, a compound which is chemically similar to hypoxanthine but does not induce Friend cell differentiation, also does not cause a significant decrease

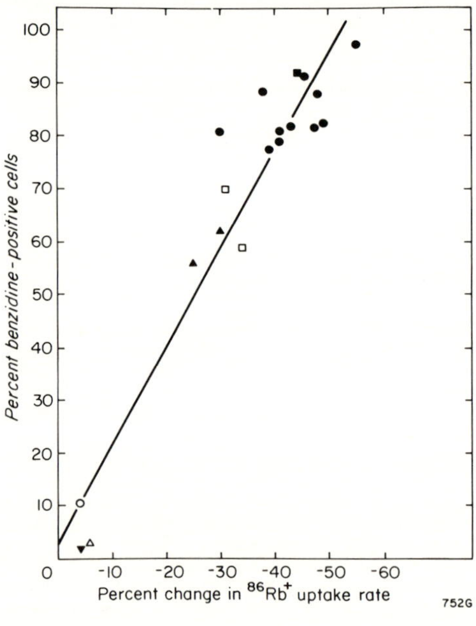

Fig 3. Correlation between the early change in $^{86}Rb^+$ influx, measured 12–16 h after the addition of inducer, and the number of benzidine-positive cells, measured on day 5. The chemicals used were 1.5% DMSO (●), 10 mM DMA (■), 4 mM hypoxanthine (▲), 6 ng/ml actinomycin D (□), 4 mM xanthine (▲), 0.1 mM hematin (△), and 1.0 unit/ml erythropoietin (○). The mutant line AIII was used in experiments involving actinomycin D, whereas 745a was used in all other experiments. The solid line represents the least-squares linear regression line of the data with a correlation coefficient of 0.95.

in $^{86}Rb^+$ uptake [2] (Fig 3). In addition, as can be seen from Figure 3, treatment with erythropoietin, the hormone that controls erythropoiesis in vivo but does not induce Friend cells [31–33], leads to little change in the influx of $^{86}Rb^+$. Treatment of the cells with exogenous hematin, which does not induce hemoglobin synthesis in the Friend cell clones used in this study, also has essentially no effect on $^{86}Rb^+$ influx.

Constancy of Intracellular K^+ Ion Concentration During Friend Cell Differentiation

The Na^+/K^+ ATPase is the enzyme on the cell surface which transports K^+ ions into the cell and Na^+ ions out of the cell against their electrochemical gradients by using ATP as an energy source. Thus, the cell is able to maintain a high (100–200 mM) intracellular K^+ ion concentration and a low (5–20 mM) intracellular Na^+ ion concentration while the reverse situation exists in the outside medium. Inhibition of Na^+/K^+ ATPase activity therefore generally leads to an increase in Na^+ ions and decrease in K^+ ions inside the cell [34–36]. In view of the observations that ouabain induces Friend cells [28], and that several chemical inducers cause early decreases in Na^+/K^+ ATPase function (as measured by decreases in Na^+/K^+ ATPase-mediated $^{86}Rb^+$ influx), the internal K^+ ion content of the cells was measured following induction of differentiation by DMSO. As Figure 4a shows, the intracellular K^+ ion content, expressed on a per cell basis, begins to decrease 8–10 h after the addition of DMSO. However, from Figure 4b, and as shown previously [4], it can also be seen that cell volume is decreasing in parallel. Thus, the intracellular concentration of K^+ ions remains essentially constant for at least the first 24 h of exposure to DMSO (Fig 5). This observation suggests that changes in the internal K^+ ion concentration are not involved in the induction of Friend cell differentiation by DMSO. In addition, these

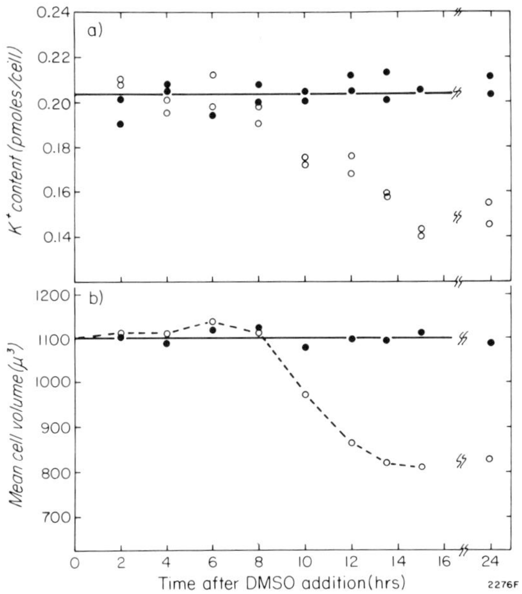

Fig 4. a) Potassium ion content in control (•) and 1.5% DMSO-treated cells (○). At the times indicated, duplicate cell samples were taken from exponentially growing suspension cultures and the K^+ ion content was determined as described in Materials and Methods. The line represents the average K^+ ion content in control cells. b) Mean cell volumes of control (•) and DMSO-treated cells (○). The line represents the average mean volume of control cells.

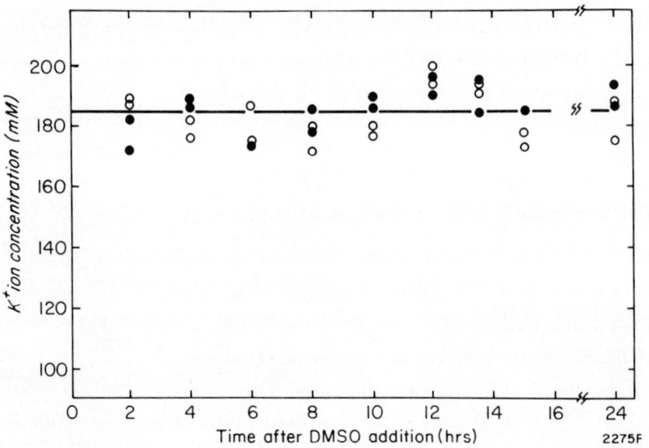

Fig 5. K^+ ion concentration in control (•) and DMSO-treated cells (○). Values were calculated from the data in Figure 4. The solid line represents the average K^+ ion concentration in control cells.

data, together with the observation that the decrease in $^{86}Rb^+$ influx precedes the drop in cell volume by 1–3 h during induction by hypoxanthine and ouabain (unpublished data) as well as DMSO [2], implies that the decrease in cell volume may be a reflection of the the drop in intracellular K^+ ion content.

DISCUSSION

Several observations, presented both here and elsewhere, suggest that a change in the activity of the Na^+/K^+ ATPase may be an important early step in the program of Friend cell differentiation. First, ouabain, a cardiac glycoside that inhibits the activity of the Na^+/K^+ ATPase [27], induces Friend cells to differentiate via direct binding to this enzyme [28]. Other cardiac glycosides, such as K-strophanthin, also induce differentiation in this system (unpublished data). Thus, known inhibitors of Na^+/K^+ ATPase activity can induce Friend cells to differentiate.

Second, as shown here and elsewhere [2], treatment with a wide variety of chemical inducing agents causes an early inhibition of Na^+/K^+ ATPase-mediated $^{86}Rb^+$ influx. Furthermore, a good correlation exists between the magnitude of this early inhibition of transport and the extent of differentiation as measured by the final percentage of hemoglobin-synthesizing cells.

Finally, we have observed that incubation of some Friend cell clones in high (90–100 mM) K^+ ion and low (50–70 mM) Na^+ ion concentrations in the growth medium can induce these cells to differentiate [37, 38]. It has been observed in other systems that monovalent cation concentrations in the same range as those used to induce Friend cells can cause inhibition of Na^+/K^+ ATPase activity [39–41]. Thus it is possible that these inducing conditions also lead to inhibition of the Na^+/K^+ ATPase in Friend cells.

As can be seen from Figure 2, the decreases in $^{86}Rb^+$ influx occur at different times depending on the inducing agent used. Addition of hypoxanthine results in major changes in influx during the first 7 h. However, induction by actinomycin D does not lead to a decrease in transport until 11–15 h after addition of inducer. Thus, the effect on $^{86}Rb^+$ uptake is not immediate as is the case when ouabain is used as an inducing agent. Treatment of the cells with ouabain, at subtoxic doses optimal for induction, results in an immediate inhibition of $^{86}Rb^+$ influx of 30–40% [2, 28]. These results suggest that the inhibition of Na^+/K^+ ATPase function in Friend cells caused by such inducers as hypoxanthine, DMSO, and actinomycin D is probably not due to a direct action of the inducer on the enzyme but rather may be an indirect effect caused by other actions of the inducing agent upon the cell.

Lubin has shown that there is a strict requirement for K^+ ions in the translation of mRNA into protein [42]. Furthermore, it has been suggested that under conditions of decreased protein synthesis mRNAs with a high initiation probability will be preferentially translated [43]. In view of these observations, others have presented evidence which suggests that changes in the intracellular levels of $Na^+$and K^+ ions may be involved in the control of gene expression, possibly by affecting the overall rates of polypeptide chain initiation or elongation and thereby causing preferential translation of certain mRNA, such as immunoglobin [44], viral [45], and δ-crystallin mRNA in embryonic chick lenses [46]. The observation that inhibitors of the Na^+/K^+ ATPase induced differentiation in Friend cells suggested that changes in internal monovalent cation concentrations may play a role in Friend cell differentiation by allowing the preferential translation of certain mRNAs. Since the Na^+/K^+ ATPase transports K^+ into the cell and Na^+ out of the cell, inhibition of this enzyme could lead to a decrease in K^+ ion and/or increase in Na^+ ion content inside the cell. Thus, if such changes in ion content are important events during Friend cell differentiation, incubation in medium in which the relative concentrations of Na^+ and K^+ ions have been reversed ("high K^+, low Na^+" medium) might be expected to interfere with the differentiation process. In fact, however, these ionic conditions actually promote differentiation [37, 38]. Furthermore, as shown here, there is no change in K^+ ion concentration for at least the first 24 h after induction by DMSO (Fig 5). Therefore, changes in monovalent ion content do not appear to be involved in the induction of Friend cell differentiation by the chemical inducers.

The above discussion suggests that if inhibition of Na^+/K^+ ATPase function is a key early step in the induction process, then effects other than changes in the intracellular Na^+ and K^+ ion concentrations may be important. The Na^+/K^+ ATPase utilizes a large proportion of the ATP available in the cell to maintain the asymmetric distributions of Na^+ and K^+ ions across the plasma membrane [47]. Therefore, inhibition of this enzyme could lead to changes in various metabolic processes within the cell. One possibility is that changes in ATP levels may cause changes in the internal levels of cyclic adenosine monophosphate (cAMP), a regulator of several cellular functions in different cell types. The levels of cAMP control the activity of certain protein kinases which regulate the state of phosphorylation of various proteins [48–50]. Thus it is possible to invoke a model for the control of Friend cell differentiation involving early changes in the phosphorylation of certain key proteins. Increased levels of cAMP have been observed early after the induction of Friend cell differentiation (R. Rifkind and P. Marks, personal communication), but no attempt has as yet been made to relate this to the function of the Na^+/K^+ ATPase or to investigate possible changes in the phosphorylation of Friend cell proteins during induction. Studies in this area may gain insight into the molecular mechanisms involved in the control of Friend erythroleukemic cell differentiation.

ACKNOWLEDGMENTS

Dixie Mager is a recipient of a Studentship from the Medical Research Council of Canada. This work was supported by grants from the National Cancer Institute of Canada and the Medical Research Council of Canada.

REFERENCES

1. Sherton CC, Kabat D: Dev Biol 48:118, 1976.
2. Mager D, Bernstein A: J Cell Physiol 94:275, 1978.
3. Germinario RJ, Kleiman L, Peters S, Oliveira M: Exp Cell Res 110:375, 1977.
4. Loritz F, Bernstein A, Miller RG: J Cell Physiol 90:423, 1977.
5. Terada M, Fried J, Nudel U, Rifkind RA, Marks PA: Proc Nat Acad Sci USA 74:248, 1977.
6. Eisen H, Bach R, Emery R: Proc Nat Acad Sci USA 74:3898, 1977.
7. Eisen H, Nasi S, Georgopoulos CP, Arndt-Jovin D, Ostertag W: Cell 10:689, 1977.
8. Gusella J, Geller R, Clarke B, Weeks V, Housman D: Cell 9:221, 1976.
9. Keppel F, Bernard A, Eisen H: Proc Nat Acad Sci USA 74:653, 1977.
10. Ross J, Ikawa Y, Leder P: Proc Nat Acad Sci USA 69:3620, 1972.
11. Ross J, Gielen J, Packman S, Ikawa Y, Leder P: J Mol Biol 87:697, 1974.
12. Gilmour RS, Harrison PR, Windass JD, Affara NA, Paul J: Cell Differ 3:9, 1974.
13. Ebert PS, Ikawa Y: Proc Soc Exp Biol Med 146:601, 1974.
14. Sassa S: J Exp Med 143:305, 1976.
15. Friend C, Scher W, Holland JG, Sato T: Proc Nat Acad Sci USA 68:378, 1971.
16. Ostertag W, Melderis H, Steinheider G, Kluge N, Dube S: Nature New Biol 239:231, 1972.
17. Boyer SH, Wuu KD, Noyes AN, Young R, Scher W, Friend C, Preisler HD, Bank A: Blood 40:823, 1972.
18. Arndt-Jovin DJ, Ostertag W, Eisen H, Klimek F, Jovin TM: J Histochem Cytochem 24:332, 1976.
19. Ikawa Y, Furusawa M, Sugano H: In: Unifying concepts of leukemia. Bibl Haematae 39:955, 1973.
20. MacDonald M, Letarte M, Bernstein A: J Cell Physiol 96:291, 1978.
21. Scher W, Preisler HD, Friend C: J Cell Physiol 81:63, 1973.
22. Tanaka M, Levy J, Terada M, Breslow R, Rifkind RA, Marks PA: Proc Nat Acad Sci USA 72:1003, 1975.
23. Reuben RC, Wife RL, Breslow R, Rifkind RA, Marks PA: Proc Nat Acad Sci USA 73:862, 1976.
24. Gusella JF, Housman D: Cell 8:263, 1976.
25. Leder A, Leder P: Cell 5:319, 1975.
26. Ebert PS, Wars I, Buell DN: Can Res 36:1809, 1976.
27. Glynn IM, Karlish SJD: Ann Rev Physiol 37:13, 1975.
28. Bernstein A, Hunt DM, Crichley V, Mak TW: Cell 9:375, 1976.
29. Stanners CP, Eliceiri GL, Green H: Nature New Biol 230:52, 1971.
30. Orkin SH, Harosi FI, Leder P: Proc Nat Acad Sci USA 72:98, 1975.
31. Goldstein K, Preisler HD, Lutton JD, Zanjani ED: Blood 44:831, 1974.
32. Kluge N, Gaedicke G, Steinheider G, Dube S, Ostertag W: Exp Cell Res 88:257, 1974.
33. Preisler HD, Giladi M: Nature 251:645, 1974.
34. McDonald TF, Sachs HG, Orr CWM, Ebert JD: Exp Cell Res 74:201, 1972.
35. Cuff JM, Lichtman MA: J Cell Physiol 85:209, 1975.
36. Ledbetter MLS, Lubin M: Exp Cell Res 105:223, 1977.
37. Bernstein A, Mager DL, MacDonald M, Letarte M, Loritz F, McCutcheon M, Miller RG, Mak TW: In: "Cold Spring Harbor Conferences on Cell Proliferation," vol 5 (In press).
38. Mager D, MacDonald M, Bernstein A: (Submitted for publication).
39. Skou JC: Biochim Biophys Acta 23:394, 1957.
40. Appel SH, Autilio L, Festoff BW, Escueta AV: J Biol Chem 244:3166, 1969.
41. Brunette DM: Doctoral thesis, University of Toronto, 1972.
42. Lubin M: Nature 213:451, 1967.
43. Lodish HF: Nature 251:385, 1974.
44. Sonenshein GE, Brawerman G: Biochemistry 15:5497, 1976.
45. Carrasco L, Smith AE: Nature 264:807, 1976.
46. Shinohara T, Piatigorsky J: Nature 270:406, 1977.
47. Dahl JL, Hokin LE: Ann Rev Biochem 43:327, 1974.
48. Krebs EG: Curr Top Cell Regul 5:99, 1972.
49. Greengard P: Nature 260:101, 1976.
50. Nimmo HG, Cohen P: Adv Cyclic Nucleotide Res 8:145, 1977.

Journal of Supramolecular Structure 8:439–445 (1978)
Normal and Abnormal Red Cell Membranes 161–167

The Spectrin-Actin Complex and Erythrocyte Shape

Jennifer C. Pinder, E. Ungewickell, D. Bray, and W. B. Gratzer

Medical Research Council Cell Biophysics Unit, 26–29 Drury Lane, London WC2 5RL, England

The effects of phosphorylation of spectrin on the properties of the cytoskeletal network of the human erythrocyte have been studied. A suspension of the cytoskeletal residues obtained after extraction of the ghosts with the nonionic detergent Triton X-100 forms a gel on addition of membrane kinase and ATP. Phosphorylation has no effect on the association state of purified spectrin. No species higher than a tetramer of polypeptide chains is formed in vitro; in the absence of divalent cations, this tetramer is an entity liberated from and evidently present in the membrane. It has not so far proved possible to detect any F-actin in the cytoskeleton before or after phosphorylation. It is suggested that the consequence of phosphorylation is formation of additional interactions between spectrin and monomeric actin molecules. This view is supported by the formation, after phosphorylation of the Triton-extracted cytoskéleton, of an insoluble mass of protein on treatment with a cross-linking reagent. In the absence of divalent cations, a series of oligomeric species is progressively liberated from the cytoskeleton on extraction with solutions of low ionic strength. These oligomers contain actin as well as spectrin, and are thought to result from disruption of the network by random denaturation of the monomeric actin in the absence of divalent metal ions. A schematic view of the effects of phosphorylation on the structure of the cytoskeleton is presented.

Key words: actin, spectrin, spectrin phosphorylation, spectrin-actin association, gelation

It has long been known [1] that the human erythrocyte requires ATP for the maintenance of its discoid shape and that distinct morphologic changes accompany depletion of intracellular adenosine triphosphate (ATP). Recently, Birchmeier and Singer [2] have shown that shape changes in erythrocyte ghosts, which appear to parallel those of intact cells, are related to the phosphorylation of the smaller subunit of spectrin. They postulate that in vivo, spectrin is maintained at an intermediate degree or "steady state" of phosphorylation by the opposing activities of an endogenous kinase and phosphatase, and that this determines the association state of the spectrin network. This raises the possibility that spectrin, alone, is responsible for the maintenance of red blood cell shape.

The identification of the erythrocyte protein band 5 as actin [3], with its familiar role in muscle and nonmuscle contractile systems, indicates that it might be involved in

Received for publication May 1, 1978; accepted May 15, 1978.

0091-7419/78/0804-0439$01.70

erythrocyte shape regulation. The additional observation that erythrocyte actin is extracted and copurifies with spectrin [4] suggests a functional relationship between these two proteins and this led us to search for an interaction in vitro. In our hands [4], spectrin isolated from fresh human red blood cells by conventional methods caused polymerisation of muscle G-actin in solvents which normally depolymerise F-actin, whereas Tilney and Detmers [3] have reported a different manifestation, indicative of an interaction between the same proteins. Subsequently, it became clear that actin-polymerising activity is mediated by phosphorylation of the spectrin [5]. The dramatic nature of the interaction in a model system has been demonstrated [5]: When ghosts are extracted with the nonionic detergent Triton X-100, each leaves behind an insoluble cytoskeletal residue [6, 7], which contains predominantly spectrin and actin, with traces of other proteins and a small amount of phospholipid. These residual shells, when dispersed in buffer by homogenisation, retain their integrity, and on addition of Mg^{2+}, ATP, and a preparation [8] of a cAMP-independent erythrocyte membrane kinase, gelation of the suspension occurs. This suggests that new intermolecular interactions result from the phosphorylation. The inhibition of the gelation process by DNAase I, which is known to sequester G-actin [9], implies that the changes involve an actin response to spectrin phosphorylation. Experiments described here give evidence that in isolation phosphorylation of spectrin does not influence its association state and cannot alone account for the ATP changes in erythrocyte shape.

SPECTRIN PHOSPHORYLATION AND THE CYTOSKELETON

Spectrin with its associated actin may be seen as forming a two-dimensional network, or probably a rather irregular lattice, on the cytoplasmic surface of the membrane [7]. On phosphorylation of the smaller subunit, the pattern of protein-protein contacts is evidently changed [5]. If no minor protein constituents participate in this process, it must involve changes in spectrin-spectrin, actin-actin, or spectrin-actin interactions, or combinations of these.

Direct evidence that neither the conformation nor the association state of spectrin is affected by phosphorylation has been obtained (Ungewickell and Gratzer, Eur J Biochem, in press). In brief, we find that spectrin in solution is an equilibrium mixture of two association states – a (presumed) heterodimer, which is not readily dissociated into single chains, and a tetramer. Interconversion between dimer and tetramer is slow at room temperature and below, and if spectrin is prepared by extraction of ghosts at low ionic strength in the cold, the tetrameric species is predominantly recovered. This, however, represents a metastable state, for at 37°C the equilibrium strongly favours the dimer (Fig 1). It therefore follows that the tetramer must be stable in situ, and thus represents a fundamental unit of the network. Studies on spectrin phosphorylated in solution with membrane kinase, and on preparations dephosphorylated with bacterial alkaline phosphatase, show that the dimer-tetramer equilibrium is unperturbed by changes in the phosphorylation state. Moreover, no higher association states are generated in solution at any accessible protein concentration, except at high concentrations (in the millimolar range) of divalent cations. This effect again is independent of the degree of phosphorylation. We thus arrive at a view of the spectrin in situ, involving the attachment of tetramers to specific sites in the membrane, containing presumably a transmembrane spectrin-binding protein [10]; the tetramers may be in contact with one another (as indicated by cross-linking experiments [11]), and the stability of the system may also depend on the rather high cytoplasmic magnesium concentration.

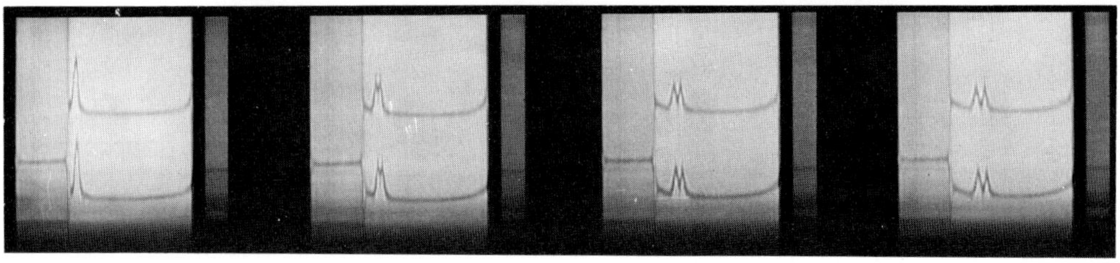

Fig 1. Sedimentation velocity of equilibrium mixture of spectrin dimer and tetramer, phosphorylated (wedge cell) and dephosphorylated (plane cell). The solvent is 0.10 M sodium chloride, 0.05 M Tris, pH 7.6. Velocity, 60,000 rpm.

We cannot entirely rule out the formation of new actin-actin associations, contingent on phosphorylation. Certainly in solutions containing spectrin and muscle actin, phosphorylation of the spectrin provokes polymerisation of the actin [5]. We have been unable so far to establish the mechanism of this process; possibly the spectrin provides a template on which actin monomers can be immobilised, and thus affords an entropically driven stabilisation of the oligomeric nuclei [12] for the polymerisation reaction. In the Triton-extracted ghost, in which the proteins are disposed in a filamentous network, gelation does not appear to be accompanied by polymerisation of the actin. At all events the dispersed gel is not birefringent and does not show actin-like filaments in negative stained preparations examined in the electron microscope (unpublished observations). Any mechanism of cell shape control based on a G→F-actin transformation would place stringent restrictions on the disposition of actin in the membrane. Given the slow diffusion of proteins in the plane of the erythrocyte membrane [13], the formation of nuclei for polymerisation (a reaction of high order) and the propagation of the association reaction would be much too slow to be useful.

The most likely consequence of phosphorylation would seem to be a change in the spectrin-actin interaction, without polymerisation, but with the formation of new intermolecular contacts. We have some evidence in favour of such a view from cross-linking experiments. It is well known that bifunctional reagents bring about extensive cross-linking of proteins in the erythrocyte membrane (see for example, Wang and Richards [14]), with the formation of many complex species. We have worked instead on the simpler system afforded by the Triton-extracted ghosts. After exposure to reagents in the series of bifunctional imidoesters [15] – dimethylsuccinimidate, dimethyladipimidate and dimethylsuberimidate, containing respectively methylene chains of two, four, and six carbon atoms – cross-linked species are recognised on extraction of the network with sodium dodecyl sulphate and gel electrophoresis. These species comprise oligomers of spectrin, as found in whole ghosts [11], and the extent of reaction is independent of phosphorylation state. At a critical chain length, however, viz eight carbons (dimethylsebacimidate), a striking effect of phosphorylation sets in: treatment of cytoskeletons from phosphorylated cells with the reagent leads to the formation of a product, insoluble in boiling sodium dodecyl sulphate, with a white fibrous appearance. No such insoluble material is formed from cytoskeletons of phosphorus-depleted cells. Estimation of the recovery of soluble proteins from the former material by solubilisation in hot sodium dodecyl sulphate shows that some 60% of the total protein is rendered insoluble after exposure to dimethylsebacimidate at 1 mg/ml. There is some uncertainty in estimating the distance spanned in practice by a cross-linking reagent containing a flexible chain of methylene groups. If the chain were fully extended, the distance between the functional groups would be about 11 Å in dimethylsuberimidate and 14 Å in dimethylsebacimidate. However, the mean end-to-end distance is probably a better measure of the effective span, and this can be estimated [16] as 5.4 and 6.2 Å for the two reagents, respectively. These distances are relatively small in comparison with the principal dimensions of the molecules making up the network. It thus appears that phosphorylation establishes a new type of intermolecular contact in the cytoskeleton, which is repeated throughout the network, and allows extensive cross-linking to occur.

ATTEMPTS AT IDENTIFICATION OF THE REPEATING UNIT

As suggested above, the spectrin tetramer is a recognisable entity in the membrane. Attempts were made to solubilise the Triton-extracted cytoskeletal ghost network in aqueous solutions of low ionic strength, such as those used for extraction of spectrin from intact membranes. In the absence of EDTA, no significant quantities of protein are liberated over a period of several days in the cold. When EDTA is added, however, protein progressively appears in the supernatant, and the dissolution of the cytoskeleton is accompanied also by the progressive appearance of a precipitate identified by gel electrophoresis as actin. The solubilised fraction can be analysed by agarose electrophoresis in nondenaturing conditions and by sedimentation velocity. A typical schlieren pattern is shown in Figure 2. A series of boundaries can be seen, which clearly correspond to protein oligomers, consisting predominantly of spectrin. These components are poorly resolved in preparative sucrose gradient sedimentation, but samples taken across the distribution reveal that all

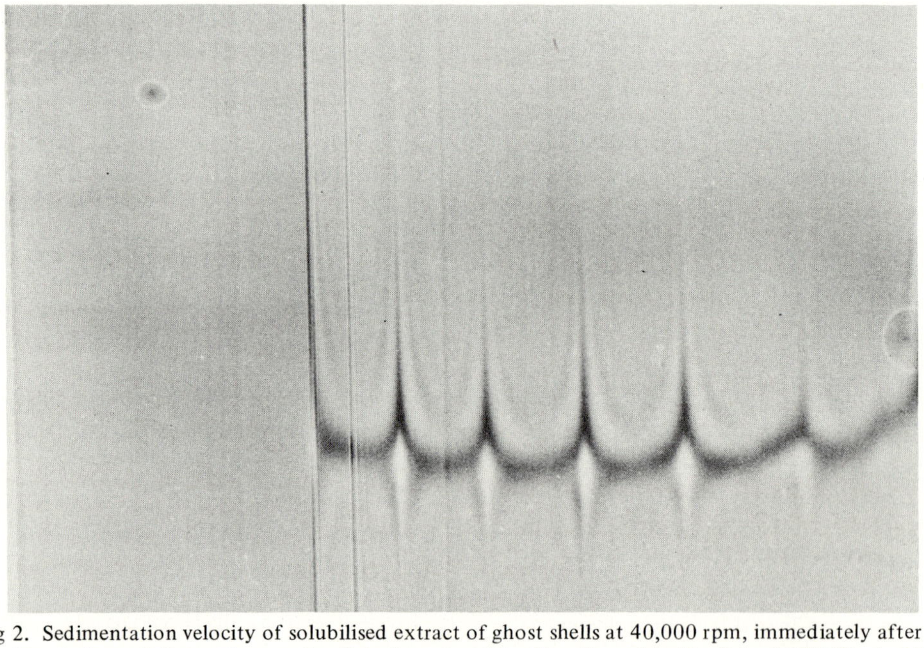

Fig 2. Sedimentation velocity of solubilised extract of ghost shells at 40,000 rpm, immediately after reaching full speed. Extraction was by dialysis against 10 mM sodium chloride, 0.1 mM EDTA, 1mM Tris, pH 7.5, for 12 h, followed by distilled water for 24 h. The salt concentration was brought to 0.1 M before sedimentation analysis.

contain actin. The mole ratio of actin to spectrin (dimer) is in the range 1.1–1.7. Since spectrin itself forms no associated species in solution beyond the tetramer, it would seem to follow that the spectrin tetramers in the oligomeric components are linked by unpolymerised actin. Because G-actin is conformationally unstable in the absence of divalent cations [17], one may infer that the progressive denaturation of actin monomers allows disruption of the network, so that parts of it are progressively liberated.

NATURE OF CYTOSKELETAL PROTEINS

Recently evidence has accrued [18] which indicates that the metabolic exhaustion of the intracellular ATP is followed only after a considerable interval by the progressive loss of the discoid character. This argues against an ATPase-linked mechanism of shape control, such as might be required by an actomyosin-like contractile element in the membrane. Additionally, the view propounded by earlier authors (see, for example, Guidotti [19] and Brandon [20]) that spectrin resembles, and may be regarded as a form of myosin, cannot be sustained in the light of recent studies of its physical properties (see, for example, Kam et al [21]). It is evidently a molecule of relatively low asymmetry, and bears no physical resemblance to myosin. The erythrocyte actin has been found (Fig 3) to be of the β type (in disagreement with another report [22] stating it to be a mixture of the

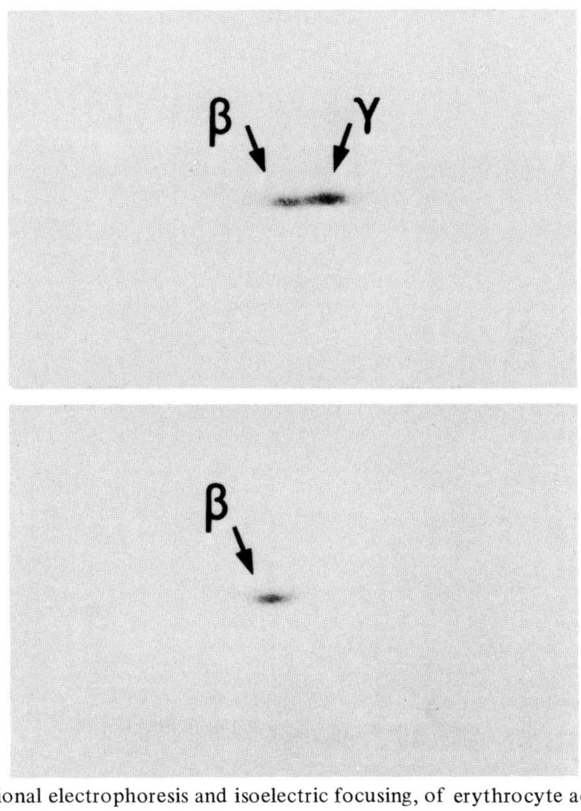

Fig 3. Two-dimensional electrophoresis and isoelectric focusing, of erythrocyte actin (lower panel), stained with Coomassie Brilliant Blue G. The upper panel shows for comparison an autoradiogram of the same gel, which contained ^{35}S-labelled actin from chicken neurones. Both β and γ actin species are present [23] (provided by Q.L. Choo).

β and γ variants); this is not the species present in either striated or smooth muscle, which contain α and γ actin respectively. Other membrane proteins (bands 4.1, 4.2, 4.9, and 3′) are also relatively prominent in gel electrophoresis patterns of the cytoskeletal residue; however, none of these is thought to play any direct role in the in vitro spectrin-actin interaction. A comparison with skeletal myofibril proteins shows that none of the minor proteins can be identified with actinin.

CONCLUSIONS

The arguments we have outlined suggest that the ATP-dependent mechanism of erythrocyte shape control is a function primarily of the cytoskeletal network of spectrin and actin. The balance of the evidence so far indicates that the actin, though capable of polymerising in vitro, is unpolymerised in the membrane, and that it functions by a mechanism quite different from that in known contractile systems. The spectrin is present as a series of tetramers, linked to each other either directly or by way of other cytoskeletal protein constitutents, but also to monomers of actin. On spectrin phosphorylation an additional type of affinity is generated, and a new spectrin-actin bond is formed; in the cytoskeletal extract this is accompanied by gelation. In Figure 4 we give a schematic and tentative representation of the structure of the cytoskeleton as a function of spectrin phosphorylation.

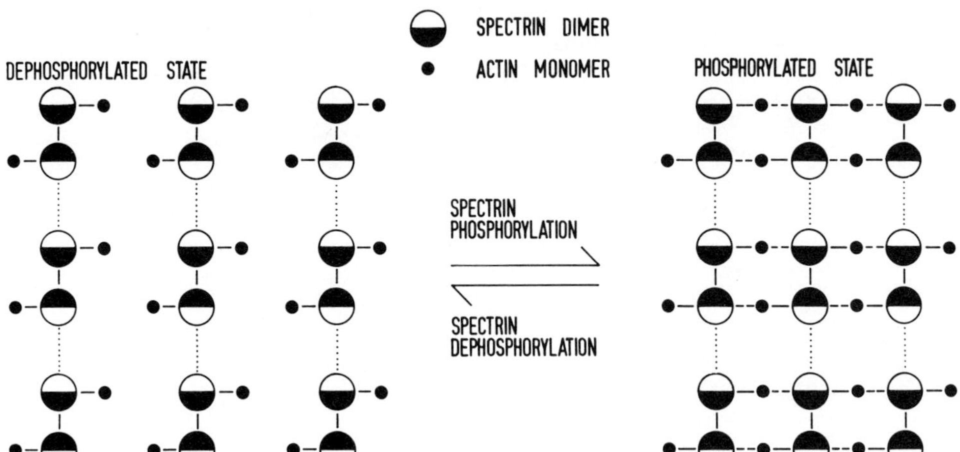

Fig 4. Schematic representation of one possible mechanism for the action of phosphorylation on the structure of the spectrin-actin matrix.

ACKNOWLEDGMENTS

We thank Q.L. Choo for the 2D electrophoretic analysis of erythrocyte actin. E.U. acknowledges the support of a long-term fellowship from the European Molecular Biology Organization.

REFERENCES

1. Makato N, Nakao T, Yamazoe S. Nature, 187:945–946, 1960.
2. Birchmeier W, Singer SJ: J Cell Biol 73:647–659, 1977.
3. Tilney LG, Detmers P: J Cell Biol 66:508–520, 1975.
4. Pinder JC, Bray D, Gratzer WB: Nature 258:765–766, 1975.
5. Pinder JC, Bray D, Gratzer WB: Nature 270:752–754, 1977.
6. Yu J, Fischmann DA, Steck TL: J Supramol Struct 1:233–248, 1973.
7. Hainfeld JF, Steck TL: J Supramol Struct 6:301–311, 1977.
8. Hosey MM, Tao M: Biochim Biophys Acta 482:348–357, 1977.
9. Hitchcock SE, Carlsson L, Lindberg U: Cell 7:531–542, 1976.
10. Bennett V: J Biol Chem 253:2292–2299, 1978.
11. Hulla FW, Gratzer WB: FEBS Lett 25:275–278, 1972.
12. Kasai M, Asakura S, Oosawa F: Biochim Biophys Acta 57:22–31, 1960.
13. Peters R, Peters J, Tews KH, Bähr W: Biochim Biophys Acta 367:282–294, 1974.
14. Wang K, Richards FM: J Biol Chem 250:6622–6626, 1975.
15. Davies GE, Stark GR: Proc Nat Acad Sci USA 66:651–656, 1970.
16. d'Albis A, Gratzer WB: J Biol Chem 251:2825–2830, 1976.
17. Asakura S: Arch Biochem 92:140–149, 1961.
18. Feo C, Mohandas N: Nature 265:166–168, 1977.
19. Guidotti G: Ann Rev Biochem 41:731–752, 1972.
20. Brandon D: FEBS Lett 38:349–352, 1975.
21. Kam Z, Josephs R, Eisenberg H, Gratzer WB: Biochemistry 16:5568–5572, 1977.
22. Garrels JI, Gibson W: Cell 9:793–803, 1976.
23. Choo QL, Bray D: J Neurochem (In press).

Journal of Supramolecular Structure 8:447–453 (1978)
Normal and Abnormal Red Cell Membranes 169–175

Characterization of the Glucose Transporter From Human Erythrocytes

David C. Sogin and Peter C. Hinkle

Section of Biochemistry, Molecular and Cell Biology, Cornell University, Wing Hall, Ithaca, New York 14853

The D-glucose transporter from human erythrocytes has been purified and reconstituted by Kasahara and Hinkle (J Biol Chem 252:7394–7390). Using a similar purification scheme, we have isolated the protein with 65% of the extracted phospholipid at a lipid-protein ratio of 14:1 by weight. The K_D (0.14 μM) and extent (11 nmoles/mg protein) for binding of ^{3}H-cytochalasin B was determined by equilibrium dialysis. Glucose was a linear competitive inhibitor of binding of cytochalasin B, with an inhibition constant of 30 mM. To further characterize the protein, samples were filtered in the presence of sodium dodecyl sulfate (SDS) through Sepharose 6B to remove 95% of the lipid followed by filtration of Sephadex G150 to remove the remaining lipid and a contaminating amount of a minor, lower-molecular-weight protein. This preparation contains only 24% acidic and basic amino acids. The protein also contains 5% neutral sugars (of which 3% is galactose), 7% glucosamine, and 5% sialic acid.

Key words: **membrane proteins, transport proteins, glucose transport, reconstitution of glucose transport, purification of glucose transporter, cytochalasin B**

Recent studies [1, 2] of isolation and reconstitution of the D-glucose transporter from human erythrocytes have shown that it is a glycoprotein with apparent molecular weight of 55,000. Similar conclusions were reached by others using labeling techniques [3, 4]. Now that the protein has been purified, specific questions can be asked about its structure and mechanism using direct chemical measurements. We have begun to answer some of these questions by determining the amino acid and carbohydrate composition of the protein and its ability to bind inhibitors of glucose transport.

METHODS

Materials

Diethylaminoethanol (DEAE) cellulose was purchased from Whatman, phloretin from ICN Pharmaceuticals, cytochalasin B from Aldrich, ^{3}H-cytochalasin from New

Received for publication April 24, 1978; accepted May 15, 1978.

0091-7419/78/0804-0447$01.70

England Nuclear, and Bio Beads from Bio Rad. Outdated human blood was a gift from the American Red Cross, Syracuse, New York.

Analytical Methods

Protein was hydrolyzed [5] and analyzed for amino acids on a Durrum D-500 analyzer. Content of neutral sugars was determined by the phenol-sulfuric acid method [6], and their relative amounts by gas-liquid chromatography of the trimethylsilylated derivatives [7–8]. Sialic acid content was estimated by the resorcinol procedure [9]. Protein was estimated by the method of Lowry et al [10] with bovine serum albumin as a standard and found to agree well with the amount of protein determined from amino acid analysis. Protein fractions were analyzed by sodium dodecyl sulfate (SDS) polyacrylamide gel electrophoresis using the low-ionic-strength system of Fairbanks, Steck, and Wallach [11] or by gradient gels using the buffer system of Laemmli [12] which is similar to that described by Mueller and Morrison [13].

RESULTS

Purification of Glucose Transporter

The procedure reported earlier for purifying the protein has been modified slightly to increase the yield and to decrease the time required to produce amounts of protein required for chemical characterization. Erythrocyte ghosts [14] are washed with 0.1 mM Na EDTA (pH 11.2) [15] rather than the low- and high-salt wash used previously [2, 16]. An extract of these alkaline vesicles at 1 mg protein per milliliter is made from 10 mM Tris-HCl (pH 7.5) and 0.5% Triton X-100. The extract is centrifuged at 100,000g for 45 min, and 90% of the supernatant from each tube is retained. The remaining supernatants are combined and centrifuged again as above. The second centrifugation is required to obtain maximum recovery of protein with minimum contamination from the light pellet. The supernatants are combined and the Tris-HCl concentration is increased to 50 mM. The sample is then applied to a column (45% of the volume of the sample) of DEAE cellulose equilibrated with 50 mM Tris-HCl (pH 7.5) 0.5% Triton X-100. The effluent is applied directly to a column of Bio Beads to remove the Triton [17]. The column of DEAE cellulose was eluted with three sample volumes of the equilibration buffer. The combined cloudy fractions are concentrated sixfold by placing the sample in a dialysis bag and burying in sucrose. The sample is then dialyzed against 2 mM Na MOPS* (pH 7.5) to remove the sucrose, and finally the sample is lyophilized. The fraction obtained has a protein/lipid ratio of 1:14 and contains 65% of the extracted phospholipid. Deviations from the procedure outlined above, or starting with untreated ghosts, usually results in impure preparations or no protein at all. The capacity of the column is much greater than would be required to bind the protein applied. Other proteins, such as band 3, are not completely removed by the column if the flow rate is too fast (protein should be in contact with the resin about 45 min) or if insoluble material from the pellet is included.

Removal of Lipid

To permit chemical characterization of the protein, the lipid was removed by gel filtration of 0.5% SDS as shown in Figure 1. The first column, Sepharose 6B, removed about 90% of the lipid. The protein elutes at a position consistent with a molecular weight much higher than 55,000, which is the value estimated by SDS polyacrylamide gel electrophoresis. Filtration on Sephadex G-150 removes the remaining phospholipid and a small

*MOPS–3-(N-morpholino) propanesulfonate.

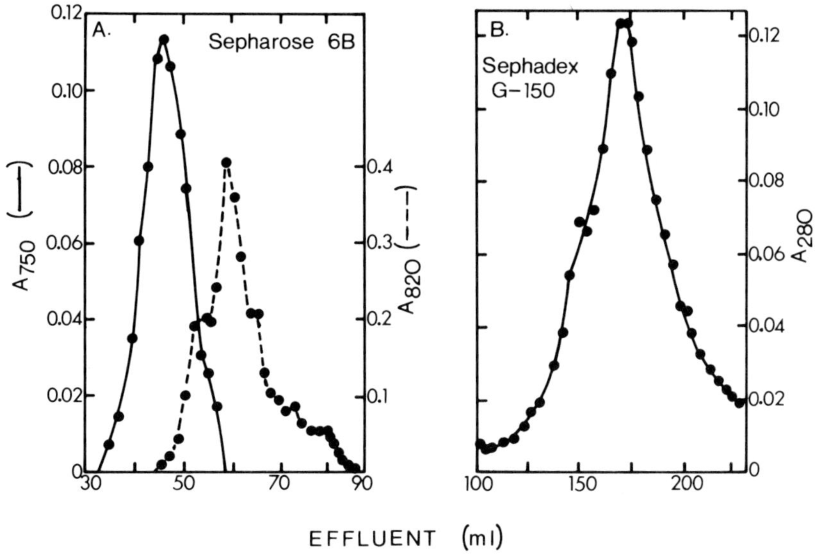

Fig 1. Removal of lipid by gel filtration. A: Purified protein (4 mg with associated lipid) was concentrated to 4 ml and made 5% in SDS and 20 mM in DTT. The sample was centrifuged at 20,000g and applied to a column (1.5 × 42 xm) of Sepharose 6B equilibrated and developed with 0.5% SDS at 37°. The solid is from absorbance at 750 nm after determination of protein of an aliquot (25 μl) in the Lowry procedure [10]. The dashed line is due to absorbance at 820 nm when aliquots (25 μl) were analyzed for phospholipid [28]. The absorbance at 750 nm has been corrected for the contribution of color from the phospholipid. Typically 5–10% of the absorbance at 820 nm is observed at 750 nm during the Lowry procedure even though no protein is shown present. B: The fractions containing protein from A were pooled and concentrated with a Millipore Molecular Separator and then applied to a column (2.5 × 90 cm) of Sephadex G-150 equilibrated and developed with 0.5% SDS at room temperature. The line is for absorbance at 280 nm due to protein. Various regions of the peak were pooled, since the material eluting latest contained protein from band 7.

amount of protein band 7 (Fairbanks' nomenclature [11]) present in the sample. Again the protein behaves as though it were of a molecular weight much greater than 55,000, eluting just after the void volume of the column.

Chemical Composition

The amino acid composition of the purified protein is given in Table I. The protein is relatively hydrophobic, containing 24% charged residues, 39% polar residues, and 37% residues of intermediate polarity. Peaks were detected at the positions of methionine sulfoxide and sulfone. As the peak at the sulfoxide position did not disappear after performic acid oxidation, it is unlikely that this amino acid is responsible for the peak. The peaks may be due to esters formed from the hydrolysis products of the carbohydrate and one or more of the amono acids. The carbohydrate composition for one preparation is also given in Table I.

Gel Electrophoresis

The protein appears as a broad, skewed band on SDS polyacrylamide gel electrophoresis (Fig 2). The broadness of the band might be due to anomolous behavior of the protein on gels or to hetergeneous carbohydrate content. By running the protein in one direction using the discontinuous buffer system of Laemli [12] in SDS on a 7.5% slab gel

TABLE I. Composition of Glucose Transporter*

Amino acid	Mole %	Residues/45,000 MW
Cys	2.0	8.3[a]
Asp	5.44	22.6
Thr	5.4	22.5
Ser	7.56	31.5
Glu	9.67	40.3
Pro	4.78	19.9
Gly	9.35	39.0
Ala	8.0	33.4
Val	8.63	36.0
Met	2.10	8.8
Ile	6.88	28.7
Leu	11.06	46.1
Tyr	2.72	11.0
Phe	7.28	30.3
His	1.18	4.9
Lys	3.57	14.9
Arg	4.10	17.1

Carbohydrate	g/100g Protein
Glucosamine	7
Galactosamine	None detected
Glucose	0.25
Galactose	3.0
Mannose	1.2
Fucose	0.5
Sialic acid	~ 5

*Amino acid composition was determined using a Durrum D-500 after hydrolysis in 6N HCl at 110° for 22, 46, and 72 h. All time points were done in duplicate. The amounts of unstable amino acids were corrected for destruction by extrapolating to time 0. Valine and isoleucine values are those found at the longest hydrolysis period. Total neutral carbohydrate was determined by phenol-sulfuric acid and identity by gas chromatography (after hydrolysis in 1 N H_2SO_4 followed by trimethylsilylation). Amino sugars were determined by amino acid analysis and corrected for destruction. Sialic acid estimated by resorcinol reaction.
[a]Determined as cysteic acid after oxidation with performic acid.

and then rerunning the sample perpendicularly to the original direction of migration on a gradient gel using the same buffer system, we obtained a curved line (not shown), as would be expected if each component in the band remigrates to a position consistent with its apparent molecular weight in the first dimension. With use of the discontinuous buffer system, apparent dimers of the protein were occasionally observed. These dimers were stable as they migrated in the second dimension to a position consistent with their migration in the first dimension. They were usually not seen in the low-ionic-strength system for SDS polyacrylamide gel electrophoresis [11]. The protein would not enter gels of a greater percentage of acrylamide than 7.5% when the discontinuous buffers were used.

Binding of Cytochalasin B

Cytochalasin B is an effective inhibitor of glucose transport in erythrocytes [21–22] and in the reconstituted system [2, 16]. We have measured by equilibrium dialysis the

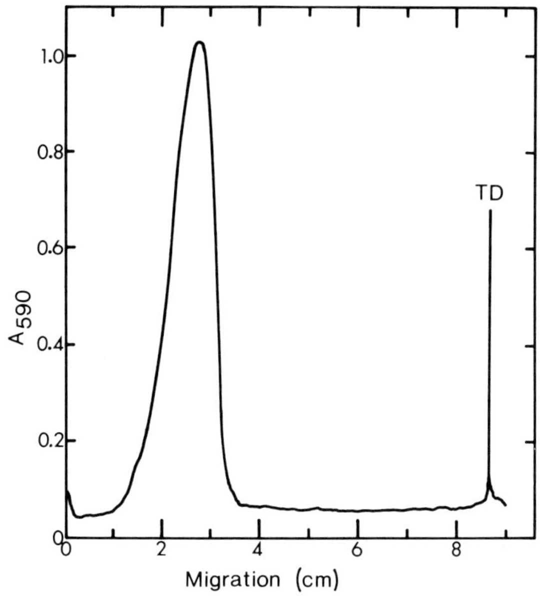

Fig 2. Absorbance scan of SDS polyacrylamide gels. Purifed protein (20 μg) free of lipid and band 7 was applied to a 5.6% polyacrylamide gel [11]. The tracking dye (TD), pyronin Y, was marked with a fine wire. Band 3 migrated about 1.6 cm in a similiar gel.

binding of ^{3}H-cytochalasin B to the purified but not delipidated protein, since removal of lipid requires denaturing conditions. The protein binds 0.5 mole of cytochalasin B per peptide chain (11 nmoles/mg protein) with a dissociation constant of 0.11 μM. About 65% of the total cytochalasin binding sites in the Triton extract are found in the purified protein fraction, which is similar to the recovery of activity for glucose transport measured in the reconstituted system [1, 2].

The binding assay can also be used to determine the inhibition constants for substitutes and inhibitors of glucose transport. By measuring the inhibition of cytochalasin B binding by these compounds, it is possible to determine dissociation constants indirectly which cannot be determined directly due to their low affinities (dissociation constants 2–200 mM [25–27]). As shown in Figure 3, glucose is a linear competitive inhibitor with respect to cytochalasin B and has an inhibition constant of 30 mM. Maltose and phloretin have also been examined and are both linear competitive inhibitors with inhibition constants of 110 mM and 17 μM respectively.

DISCUSSION

Purification

In continuing the work reported earlier [1, 2, 16] we have examined the purification procedure and have improved it while trying to understand why it is successful. Once extracted, the glucose transporter appears to be in a lipid-protein-detergent complex which is depleted of all proteins except the glucose transporter as the Triton extract is passed through the DEAE cellulose column.

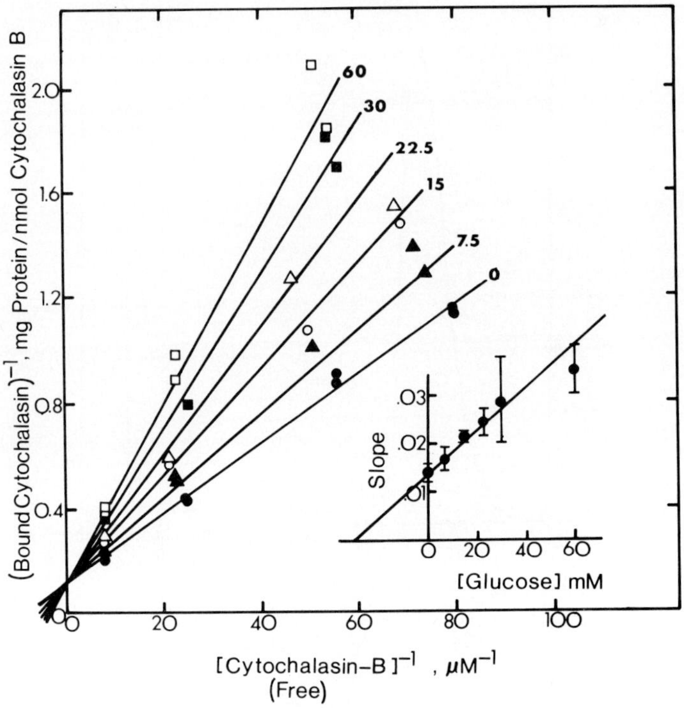

Fig. 3. Inhibition of binding of cytochalasin B by glucose. Protein at 35 μg/ml was placed in one chamber and ^{3}H-cytochalasin B at various concentrations was placed on the other chamber, separated from the first by a dialysis membrane. Glucose was varied from 0 to 60 mM. The chambers were allowed to equilibrate 3 h at 22°. Aliquots were then counted in a liquid scintillation counter to determine the bound and free concentrations of cytochalasin B. The positions of the lines were determined by a least squares fit of the data for each concentration of glucose to equation for a rectangular hyperbola. The standard errors for the slopes for each line are indicated by the error bars in the replot of the slopes.

Physical Characterization

The physical characterization of the protein has been hampered by its insolubility and its tendancy to aggregate even under denaturing conditions. While the amino acid composition is not particularly unusual, it does point toward a relatively hydrophobic molecule. The carbohydrate content may be variable and thus responsible for the broadness of the band on gels. It may also contribute to the anomolous behavior of the protein in gel filtration on Sepharose 6B and Sephadex G-150. The protein also can form dimers on gels, a property which has also been observed with glycophorin [18–20].

Binding of Cytochalasin B

The binding constant for cytochalasin B is similar to those values reported for binding to ghosts [21–23], while the extent per milligram of protein is 15–25 times higher than with ghosts [20, 21–24]. The amount of binding would seem to indicate that either the protein acts as a dimer or our preparation is only 50% pure. An additional indication that the transporter is a dimer was obtained from the freeze-fracture electron microscopy, which showed particles with a diameter of 62 Å, corresponding to a molecular weight of 110,000, twice the estimated molecular weight observed on gels (Telford J, unpublished results). Although it is tempting to conclude that the protein is a dimer in the membrane, additional chemical studies are required to conclusively demonstrate this point.

ACKNOWLEDGMENTS

This work was supported by NIH grant CA-14454 and NS 05667.

We are indebted to Drs William H. Stein and Stanford Moore, in whose laboratory amino acid analyses were performed.

REFERENCES

1. Kasahara M, Hinkle PC: In Semenza G, Carafoli E (eds): "Biochemistry of Membrane Transport." FEBS Symposium. New York: Springer-Verlag, 1977, pp 346–350.
2. Kasahara M, Hinkle PC: J Biol Chem 252:7384, 1977.
3. Batt ER, Abbott RE, Schacter D: J Biol Chem 251:7184, 1976.
4. Lienhard GE, Gorga FR, Orasky JE Jr, Zocolli MA: Biochem 16:4921, 1977.
5. Moore S, Stein WH: Methods Enzymol 6:819, 1963.
6. Dubois M, Gilles KA, Hamilton JK, Rebers PA, Smith F: Anal Chem 28:350, 1956.
7. Sweeley CC, Bentley R, Makita M, Wells WW: J Am Chem Soc 85:2497, 1963.
8. Clamp JR: Biochem Soc Symp 40:3, 1974.
9. Svennerholm L: Biochim Biophys Acta 24:604, 1957.
10. Lowry OH, Rosebrough NJ, Farr AL, Randall RJ: J Biol Chem 193:265, 1951.
11. Fairbanks G, Steck TL, Wallach DFH: Biochem 10:2606, 1971.
12. Laemmli UK: Nature 227:680, 1970.
13. Mueller TJ, Morrison M: J Biol Chem 252:6573, 1977.
14. Dodge JT, Mitchell C, Hanahan DI: Arch Biochem Biophys 100:119, 1963.
15. Steck TL, Yu J: J Supramol Struct 1:220, 1973.
16. Kasahara M, Hinkle PC: Proc Nat Acad Sci USA 73:396, 1976.
17. Holloway PW: Anal Biochem 53:304, 1973.
18. Marton LSG, Gawin JE: Biochem Biophys Res Commun 52:1457, 1973.
19. Furthymayr H, Marchesi VT: Biochemistry 15:1137, 1976.
20. Silverberg M, Marchesi VT: J Biol Chem 253:95, 1978.
21. Taverna RD, Langdon RG: Biochim Biophys Acta 323:207, 1973.
22. Lin S, Santi DV, Spudich JA: J Biol Chem 249:2268, 1974.
23. Jung CY, Rampal AL: J Biol Chem 252:5456, 1977.
24. Juliano RL: Biochim Biophys Acta 300:341, 1973.
25. LeFevre PG, Marshall JK: J Biol Chem 234:3022, 1959.
26. Krupka RM: Biochemistry 10:1143, 1971.
27. Krupka RM: Biochim Biophys Acta 282:326, 1972.
28. Ames BN, Dubin DT: J Biol Chem 235:769, 1960.

Journal of Supramolecular Structure 8:455–463 (1978)
Normal and Abnormal Red Cell Membranes 177–185

Spectrin Binding and the Control of Membrane Protein Mobility

Steven R. Goodman and Daniel Branton

Cell and Developmental Biology, The Biological Laboratories, Harvard University, Cambridge, Massachusetts 02138

Transmembrane proteins of the human erythrocyte show restricted in-plane mobility. Many of the restrictions on mobility are attributable to the molecules of spectrin which are located on the protoplasmic surface of the erythrocyte membrane. These molecules are elongate, form end-to-end heterodimer associations, and bind selectively to protein (or proteins) accessible on inside out, but not right-side out, membrane vesicles.

Key words: protein mobility, spectrin shape, spectrin binding

Our knowledge of the interactions that restrict the mobility of membrane macromolecules is limited for the most part to conclusions drawn from indirect experiments in complex systems. For example, interactions between transmembrane elements and extrinsic fibrous or fiber-forming elements are commonly evoked [1–4] to explain the response of cell surface elements to cytochalasin, colchicine, or polyvalent ligands, but simpler experimental systems are required if underlying biochemical and molecular organization is to be understood. The human erythrocyte membrane, which can be readily purified with a defined orientation, provides an ideal starting point for such studies.

Two kinds of evidence indicate that the transmembrane integral proteins of the human erythrocyte are mobile but that this mobility is restricted. The first kind of evidence comes from experiments [5] in which fluorescently labeled and unlabeled erythrocytes are fused and the movement of fluorescent surface elements is observed by light microscopy. The results (Table I) show that the intrinsic proteins of the red cell membrane exhibit a lateral mobility which is comparable to, but somewhat slower than, that observed for proteins of other plasma membranes measured by similar fusion techniques. The second kind of evidence comes from experiments in which intramembrane particles due to intrinsic proteins are observed by electron microscopy using freeze-fracturing methods [6, 7]. The results of these experiments suggest that the extrinsic protein spectrin, perhaps together with erythrocyte actin, forms a fibrous meshwork that restricts the lateral mobility of the erythrocyte intrinsic membrane proteins.

Received for publication May 5, 1978; accepted May 31, 1978.

0091-7419/78/0804-0455$02.00

TABLE I. Minimum Diffusion Coefficients for Fluorescently Labeled Integral Membrane Proteins

Temperature (°C)	Fused erythrocytes ($cm^2 \cdot s^{-1}$)	Mouse-human heterokaryons ($cm^2 \cdot s^{-1}$)
37	4×10^{-11}	9×10^{-11}
30	3×10^{-11}	–
23	6×10^{-12}	–
0	No movement of label observed	

Diffusion coefficients were calculated from the time required for at least 90% of the initially fused cells to show total intermixing (uniform fluorescence to the human eye) of the labeled membrane proteins. Results for fused erythrocytes are from Fowler and Branton [5]; results for mouse-human heterokaryons are estimated from the data of Edidin and Wei [25].

The notion that spectrin can form a meshwork that restricts or regulates the motion of other membrane macromolecules assumes that spectrin is an elongate molecule that binds to sites at the protoplasmic surface of the erythrocyte membrane [8]. These assumptions can now be confirmed.

SPECTRIN SHAPE

It has been known for some time that spectrin, especially when in the presence of other membrane proteins such as erythrocyte actin, can self-associate to form fibrous aggregates [9]. However, the shape of individual spectrin molecules has been difficult to study. Negative staining for electron microscopy usually aggregates spectrin molecules, and indirect physical methods using analytical ultracentrifugation have produced conflicting results [10–16]. Nevertheless, a consistent picture of the molecule is beginning to emerge from electron microscopy of shadowed molecules [17], light scattering studies [18], and from electrooptical analysis [19]. When the purified, approximately 9S, spectrin heterodimer (one molecule of band 1 and one molecule of band 2; total molecular weight ~460,000) is visualized by low-angle shadowing (Fig 1), it appears as a very flexible molecule approximately 1,000 Å in length. Its constituent monomer polypeptides are often individually visible, lying partially separated from one another or twisting around each other. The purified 12S tetramer is formed by the end-to-end association of two heterodimers, with minimal or no overlap. These electron microscopic results are consistent with the light scattering and birefringence relaxation measurements which show that spectrin heterodimers in solution also have contour lengths in excess of 1,000 Å [18, 19].

SPECTRIN BINDING

The association of spectrin with the red cell membrane has been studied with a binding assay [20] using radiolabeled, purified spectrin and spectrin-depleted vesicles derived from erythrocyte ghosts. Spectrin binds selectively to inside-out but not right-side-out vesicles. The association between spectrin and the vesicles is slow, pH- and salt-

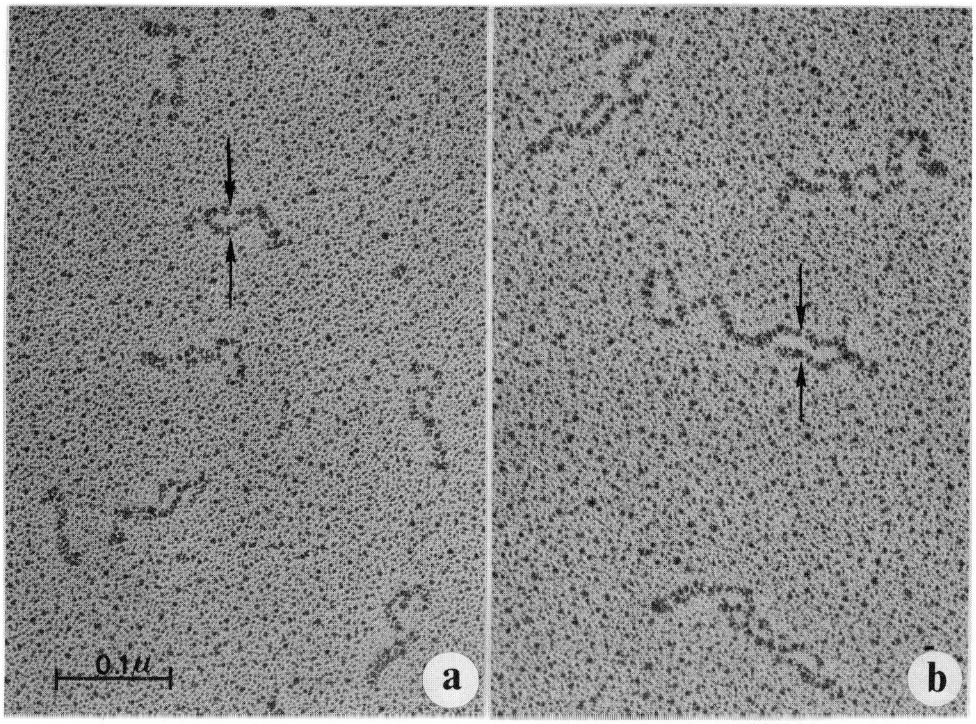

Fig 1. Spectrin heterodimers (a) and tetramers (b). The heterodimers and tetramers were purified on a Sepharose 4-B column according to Ralston, Dunbar, and White [15] and Pt-C replicas of the dried molecules were prepared by low-angle, rotary shadowing. The arrows point to a region of a heterodimer (a) or tetramer (b) where the constituent monomer polypeptides are individually visible (From the work of Shotton, Burke, and Branton [17], with permission. (Magnification: × 170,000, a and b.)

dependent, and saturable. Partial proteolysis of the vesicles indicates that binding depends upon a protein (or proteins) that is attached to the membrane.

These experiments further suggest that under controlled proteolysis, the binding protein can be cleaved so as to release the fragment with which spectrin associates. Indeed, during partial proteolysis with α-chymotrypsin, water-soluble polypeptides are released from the membrane which inhibit binding of spectrin to spectrin-depleted vesicles [20]. Diethylaminoethanol (DEAE) cellulose chromatography of these soluble polypeptides resolves a 72,000-dalton polypeptide which competitively inhibits binding of spectrin to spectrin-depleted vesicles [21]. This 72,000-dalton polypeptide also forms a complex with spectrin in solution and thus appears to be the membrane attachment site for spectrin [21].

This solubilized 72,000-dalton polypeptide has been used to evaluate the role spectrin plays in restricting the lateral mobility of intrinsic membrane proteins [22]. The 72,000-dalton polypeptide causes a rapid and complete dissociation of ^{32}P-spectrin from inside-out vesicles, and when included in the cytoplasmic space of fused erythrocytes, it increases the mobility of their integral membrane proteins [22]. These results confirm that the association of spectrin with its anchorage site plays a role in limiting the lateral mobility of integral membrane proteins. However, when the 72,000-dalton polypeptide was included in the cytoplasmic space of the fused cells, the integral membrane protein mobility was still considerably slower than expected from unrestricted diffusion. Thus, interactions other than those between spectrin and its membrane attachment site may also regulate the mobility of the major integral proteins.

The membrane protein which is the source of the 72,000-dalton attachment site is not known. One way the parent protein is being identified is the preparation of antisera against the solubilized fragment (Bennett V, personal communication). Such antisera should react with the parent protein. Another approach to the identification of the spectrin-binding protein(s) is suggested by the observation [23, 24] that when erythrocytes or erythrocyte ghosts are extracted with nonionic detergents, an insoluble proteolipid "shell" is formed which contains – in addition to lipid, spectrin, and actin – a few other major polypeptides visible on SDS polyacrylamide electrophoresis.

When erythrocytes are extracted with 0.5% Triton X-114 in 10 mM 4-(2-hydroxyethyl)-1-pereazineethanesulfonic acid (Hepes), 2.5 mM reduced glutathione, 0.5 mM ethylene glycol bis(β-aminoethyl ether) N,N′-tetracetic acid (EGTA), and 70 mM KCl, several classes of proteolipid shells are formed which differ in the relative proportions of the major polypeptide species (Goodman, unpublished data). These classes can be separated by sedimentation through a 10–55% sucrose gradient at 120,000g for 15 h. The major class of proteolipid shells sediment to a density of approximately 1.190 g/ml, while most of the free Triton X-114 and unbound protein remain on top of the gradient. These gradient-purified shells have a diameter of 6–8 μ and appear to be composed of small lipid vesicles (1,000–3,000 Å in diameter) clumped within a dense reticulum of filamentous material (Fig 2a). Freeze-fracture of these shells shows the clustered lipid vesicles, some of which contain aggregated intramembrane particles (Fig 2b).

The proteolipid shells purified on the sucrose gradient have a protein composition consisting primarily of spectrin, erythrocyte actin, and polypeptides migrating in the band 3 region and the band 4 region* (Fig 3). The same major bands are found after electrophoresis in sodium dodecyl sulfate (SDS) independently of whether the shells are derived from untreated or chymotrypsin-treated erythrocytes (in which the bulk of band 3 is eliminated). This indicates that the primary component in the band 3 region of the shells is distinct from the bulk of band 3. It has been referred to as band 3′ [24], although its origin and relation to bands existing in the native membrane are unclear. A polypeptide migrating at the same molecular weight as band 3′ is sometimes seen in ghosts derived from chymotrypsin-treated cells, but not if the ghosts are solubilized in SDS as soon as they are produced (as in Fig 3, gel E). Thus, 3′ may itself be derived from some other polypeptide. The fact that the band 3 region of the proteolipid shells contains slightly more protein when derived from untreated rather than chymotrypsin-treated erythrocytes may indicate that a small amount of residual band 3 is also present in shells derived from untreated erythrocytes.

Dialysis of the proteolipid shells against low-ionic-strength buffer at pH 8.2 releases the spectrin and actin, and the vesicles unclump. Electron micrographs of this material

*We do not distinguish bands 4.1 and 4.2 in the proteolipid shells because in some preparations both 4.1 and 4.2 are visualized, while other preparations contain only 4.2. We currently believe that during the triton extraction, band 4.1 is cleaved by an endogenous protease.

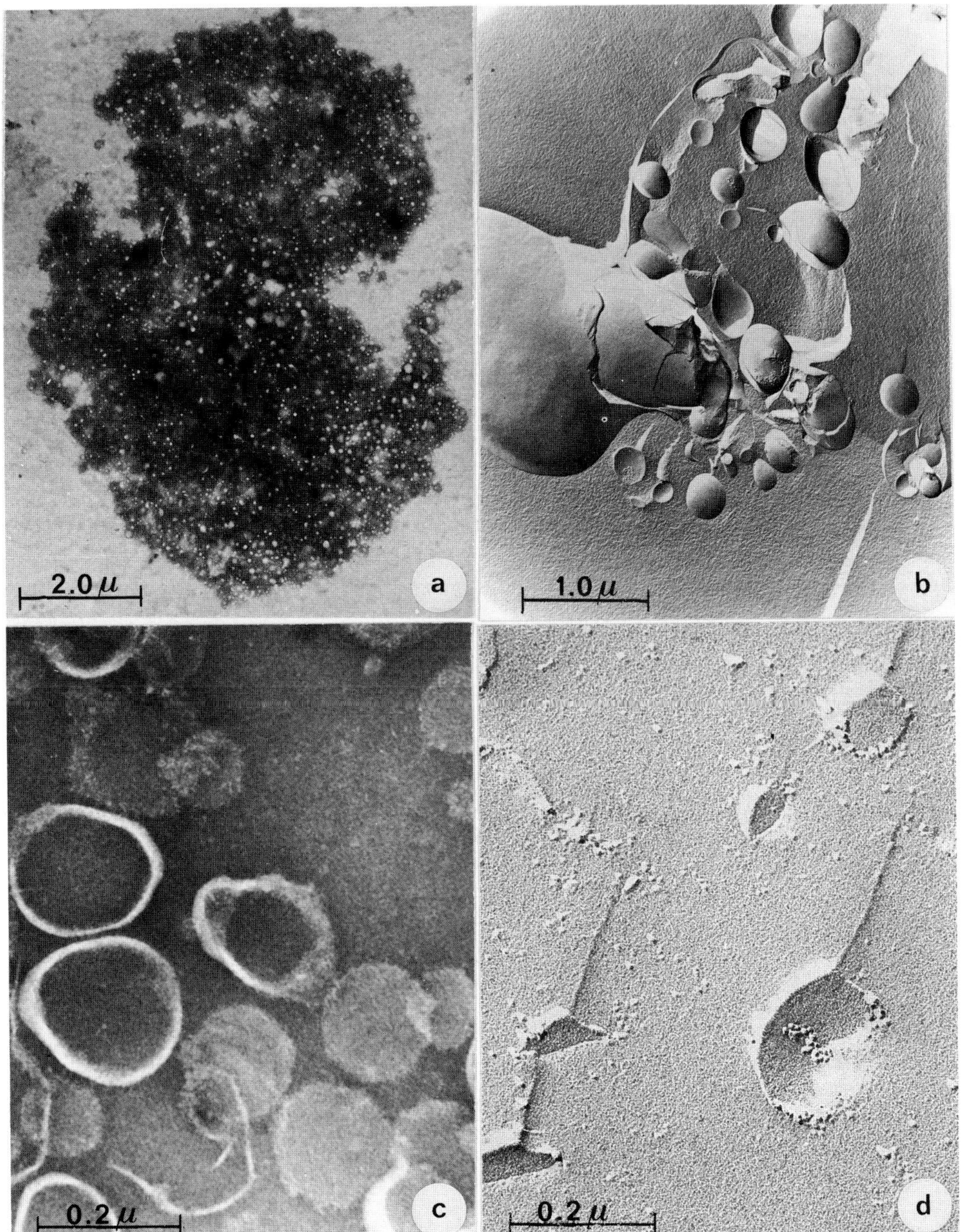

Fig 2. Electron micrographs of the proteolipid shells negatively stained (a and c) or freeze-fractured (b and d). a,b) Proteolipid shells from untreated erythrocytes; c,d) spectrin-depleted proteolipid vesicles obtained by dializing proteolipid shells against 0.3 mM Hepes, 0.2 mM EGTA, 0.2 mM adenosine triphosphate, 0.2 mM dithiothreitol (DTT), pH 8.2, over night at 4°C and sedimented at 120,000g for 60 min. From work in preparation (Goodman et al, 1978). Photographs by D. Anderson. (Magnification: a, × 9,100; b, × 18,200; c,d, × 100,000.)

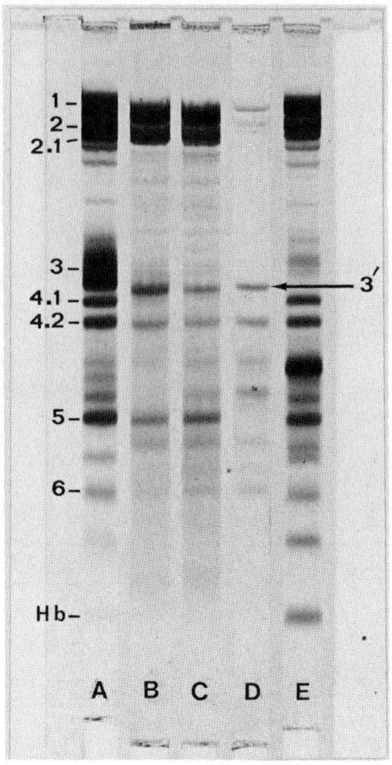

Fig 3. Polyacrylamide gel electrophoresis of ghosts and proteolipid shells. Gel A) ghost protein from untreated erythrocytes; B) proteolipid shells derived from untreated erythrocytes; C) proteolipid shells derived from chymotrypsin-treated erythrocytes (200 μg/ml α-chymotrypsin, 60 min at 37°C); D) spectrin- and actin-depleted proteolipid vesicles derived from chymotrypsin-treated erythrocytes; E) ghost protein from chymotrypsin-treated erythrocytes. Electrophoresis was performed in sodium dodecyl sulphate as in Yu, Fischman, and Steck [23], and the major bands were labeled as in that reference.

reveal a mixture of freely suspended vesicles and amorphous fibrillar material. The large (6–8 μ) structures of clustered vesicles are no longer found. The vesicles can be separated from the spectrin and actin by differential centrifugation at 120,000g for 60 min. The pellet of this centrifugation consists of freely suspended 1,000- to 3,000-Å proteolipid vesicles (Fig 2c). Freeze-fracture of this preparation demonstrates freely suspended vesicles, many of which contain highly clustered intramembrane particles (as in Fig 2d). Electrophoresis of these vesicles after low ionic strength dialysis indicates that at least 95% of the spectrin and all visible actin have been removed. Band 3′, band 4, and traces of residual spectrin are the major components found on SDS acrylamide gels (Fig 3, gel D). The biochemical and morpholigic experiments taken together strongly suggest that the 1,000- to 3,000-Å vesicles contain bands 3′ and 4, while the amorphous filamentous material represents a spectrin-actin complex.

The fact that spectrin, band 3′, band 4, and actin are found complexed in the shells has interesting implications but does not represent proof of their association in vivo. To ask whether bands 3′ and 4 might represent the spectrin attachment site, we isolated ^{32}P-spectrin by the technique of Bennett and Branton [20] and attempted to rebind ^{32}P-spectrin to spectrin-depleted proteolipid vesicles and intact proteolipid shells containing their full complement of spectrin. Binding studies were conducted at 0°C for 90 min under the ionic and pH conditions found to be optimal for spectrin binding to spectrin-depleted inverted vesicles [20]. After the incubation, the components were separated by velocity sedimentation through a 10–50% sucrose gradient at 70,000g for 45 min. Under these conditions, free ^{32}P-spectrin remains at the top, while ^{32}P-spectrin which is bound to vesicles migrates into the gradient. When ^{32}P-spectrin was incubated with the spectrin-depleted proteolipid vesicles, a large peak of ^{32}P-spectrin comigrated on the gradient with the vesicles (Fig 4a), just as when ^{32}P-spectrin was bound to spectrin-depleted inverted vesicles (Fig 4b). If proteolipid shells with their full complement of spectrin are incubated (at a protein concentration which makes the shell spectrin concentration equal to the

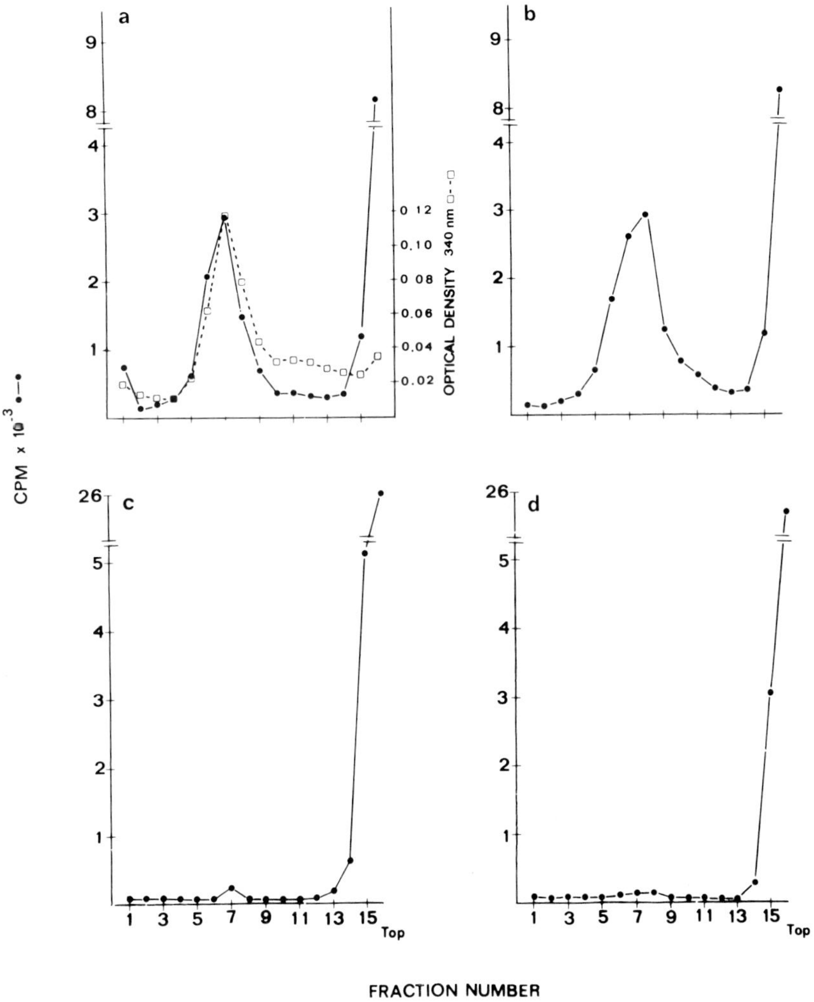

Fig 4. Spectrin binding studies. ^{32}P-spectrin (34 μg; 1,322 cpm/μg) was incubated for 90 min at 4°C in a final volume of 1 ml of buffer containing 0.7 mM $NaPO_4$, 20 mM KCl, 0.6 mM DTT, 0.3 mM $MgCl_2$, 2% sucrose, pH 7.6, with a) spectrin-depleted proteolipid vesicles (1 mg membrane protein), b) spectrin-depleted inverted vesicles (1 mg protein), c) proteolipid shells (100 μg protein), and d) spectrin depleted proteolipid vesicles (1 mg protein), but with heat-denatured (5 min at 55°C) ^{32}P-spectrin. The incubation mixture was layered onto a 13-ml 10–50% sucrose gradient and bound spectrin was separated from free spectrin by centrifuging at 70,000g for 45 min (SW40 rotor, 4°C). Sixteen fractions were dripped directly into counting vials and 10 ml of a counting cocktail of Aquasol containing 80 ml/liter water and 50 ml/liter glacial acetic acid was added. Radioactivity was determined with a Beckman scintillation counter.

residual spectrin concentration in the spectrin depleted triton vesicles) with ^{32}P-spectrin, they bind less than 10% of the ^{32}P-spectrin that binds to spectrin-depleted vesicles (Fig 4c). Therefore, the primary binding of spectrin to the spectrin-depleted proteolipid vesicles is not to the small residue of remaining spectrin in these vesicles. Heat-denatured ^{32}P-spectrin does not bind to the spectrin-depleted vesicles (Fig 4d). Therefore, the binding depends on spectrin's normal quaternary structure and does not seem to be nonspecific. Furthermore, ^{32}P-spectrin will not bind to vesicles which have been pretreated with 1 μg/ml chymotrypsin (30 min, 0°C; data not shown). Therefore, the binding of spectrin appears to be to protein in the vesicles.

These results suggest that in the proteolipid shells the 89,000-dalton polypeptide we call band 3′, perhaps complexed to band 4, is the spectrin-binding site. Although the possibility that a minor protein species present in the shells may actually be involved in the binding of spectrin cannot be ruled out by these experiments, it appears unlikely because only spectrin, bands 2.1 and 3′, and band 4 in the spectrin-depleted vesicles are large enough proteins to give rise to the 72,000-dalton fragment reported to be a water-soluble portion of the binding protein [21]. The provenance of band 3′ remains to be explored. It may itself be a cleavage product of a larger polypeptide. A 72,000-dalton chymotryptic fragment can be generated from spectrin-depleted proteolipid vesicles obtained from untreated erythrocytes or erythrocytes pretreated with 200 μg/ml α-chymotrypsin at 37°C for 2 h (Goodman et al, manuscript in preparation). In addition, the binding of ^{32}P-spectrin to spectrin-depleted vesicles is the same regardless of whether the vesicles are obtained from chymotrypsin-treated or untreated erythrocytes. Therefore, the small residue of band 3 remaining in shells derived from untreated erythrocytes cannot be the binding site (Goodman, unpublished observation).

Although further work is clearly required to complete our understanding of the interactions that control erythrocyte membrane protein mobility, it is evident that this experimental system is one in which a detailed molecular approach is feasible. Solubilization of the 72,000-dalton attachment site for spectrin has led to the first reported isolation of a membrane attachment site for a major cytoskeletal protein [21], but the same approach could be, and no doubt will be, applied to other proteins in other cells.

ACKNOWLEDGMENTS

This study was supported by grants from the National Institutes of Health, the National Science Foundation, and the Department of Energy. S.R. Goodman is supported by a postdoctoral stipend from the National Institutes of Health.

REFERENCES

1. Nicolson G: Biochim Biophys Acta 457:57–108, 1976.
2. Edelman GM: Science 192:218–226, 1976.
3. Korn ED: "Cold Spring Harbor Conference on Cell Proliferation." Cold Spring Harbor, New York: Cold Spring Harbor Laboratories, 1976, vol 3, pp 623–630.
4. Heggeness MH, Wang K, Singer SJ: Proc Nat Acad Sci USA 74:3883–3887, 1977.
5. Fowler V, Branton D: Nature 268:23–26, 1977.
6. Elgsaeter A, Branton D: J Cell Biol 63:395–406, 1974.

7. Elgsaeter A, Shotton DM, Branton D: Biochim Biophys Acta 426:101–122, 1976.
8. Yu J, Elgsaeter A, Branton D: In Marchesi VT, Ginsburg V, Robbins PW, Fox CF (eds): "Cell Shape and Surface Architecture." New York: Alan R Liss, 1978, pp 453–458.
9. Clark M: Biochim Biophys Res Commun 45:1063–1070, 1971.
10. Gratzer WB, Beaven GH: Eur J Biochem 58:403–409, 1975.
11. Schechter NM, Sharp M, Reynolds JA, Tanford C: Biochemistry 15:1897–1904, 1976.
12. Ralston GB: Biochim Biophys Acta 401:83–94, 1975.
13. Ralston GB: Aust J Biol Sci 28:259–266, 1975.
14. Ralston GB: Biochim Biophys Acta 443:387–393, 1976.
15. Ralston G, Dunbar J, White M: Biochim Biophys Acta 491:345–348, 1977.
16. Kam Z, Josephs R, Eisenberg H, Gratzer WB: Biochemistry 16:5568–5572, 1977.
17. Shotton DM, Burke B, Branton D: Biochim Biophys Acta (In press).
18. Elgsaeter A: Biochim Biophys Acta (In press).
19. Mikkelsen A, Elgsaeter A: Biochim Biophys Acta (In press).
20. Bennett V, Branton D: J Biol Chem 252:2753–2763, 1977.
21. Bennett V: J Biol Chem 253:2292–2299, 1978.
22. Fowler V, Bennett V: J Supramol Struct 8:215–221, 1978.
23. Yu J, Fischman DA, Steck TL: J Supramol Struct 1:233–248, 1973.
24. Sheetz MP, Sawyer D, Jackowski S: In Brewer G (ed): "Erythrocyte Metabolism and Function," vol 4. In press (1978).
25. Edidin M, Wei T: J Cell Biol 75:475–482, 1977.

Journal of Supramolecular Structure 8:465–471 (1978)
Normal and Abnormal Red Cell Membranes 187–193

Analysis of the Major Polypeptides of Spectrin by Tryptic Digestion

Alun H. Maddy and Michael J. Dunn

Department of Zoology, University of Edinburgh, Edinburgh, EH9 3JT, Scotland

The two major polypeptides of erythrocyte membrane spectrin have been isolated by preparative polyacrylamide gel electrophoresis in the presence of sodium dodecyl sulfate. The tryptic peptide maps of the two polypeptides have been prepared by thin-layer chromatography and electrophoresis. Radioactive peptides have been prepared by ^{14}C-carboxymethylation and chloramine T-catalysed ^{125}I iodination. Maps of both sets of peptides demonstrate a marked similarity between the two parent polypeptides.

Key words: spectrin, fractionation, trypsin digestion, peptide mapping

The term "spectrin" was originally applied [1] to the protein extracted from erythrocyte ghosts when it was believed that the extract was homogeneous. It is now known that the extract contains three major polypeptides, a pair with molecular weights between 200,000 and 250,000 (P1 and P2 in the terminology of Fairbanks, Steck, and Wallach [2]) and the third with a molecular weight of 43,000. This third component has been identified as actin [3], although it is slightly different from muscle actin [4], and the term "spectrin" is now confined to the two high-molecular-weight chains which probably exist as a P1 + P2 dimer or tetramer in the intact membrane [5–9].

The chemical nature of these two large polypeptides is not yet fully understood and we here report on the peptide maps obtained after trypsin digestion of the polypeptides. Maps show that P1 and P2 share many common peptides, which suggests that they share methylation, or with ^{125}I by iodination under chloramine T catalysis. In both cases the maps show that Pa and P2 share many common peptides, which suggests that they share certain common amino acid sequences: a conclusion consistent with their similar amino acid compositions [10–12] the similarity of their N terminal amino acids [13, 14], and their immunological cross-reactivity [15]. The maps of the two polypeptides also possess peptides unique to themselves, indicating that the two chains are not identical.

Received for publication April 19, 1978; accepted May 27, 1978.

EXPERIMENTAL

Preparation of Ghosts

Fresh cattle (Bos taurus) blood was washed three times with isotonic saline to remove white cells and plasma. The erythrocytes were haemolysed in 5 volumes of 5.0 mM phosphate buffer (pH 6.0) and the ghosts washed several times in this buffer until the supernatant was virtually free of haemoglobin. The remaining haemoglobin was almost completely removed from the ghosts by washing repeatedly in 5.0 mM phosphate buffer at pH 7.5. The final trace of haemoglobin was removed by freezing the ghosts at -20° over night and washing once more in the buffer at pH 7.5 [16].

EDTA Extraction

The ghosts were pelleted by centrifugation at 18,000 g for 20 min and extracted with 4 volumes of 0.5 mM ethylenediaminetetracetic acid (EDTA), at pH 7.5, for 1.5 h at 18°.

Polyacrylamide Gel Electrophoresis

Analytical sodium dodecyl sulfate (SDS) gel electrophoresis was carried out using the buffer system of Fairbanks, Steck and Wallach [2]. The gels, of 7% (w/v) acrylamide and 0.1% bisacrylamide, were polymerised in glass tubes with an internal diameter of 4 mm using ammonium persulphate and N,N,N^1,N^1-tetramethylethylene diamine as catalysts. Protein samples were prepared by addition of dithioerythritol to 20 mM and SDS to 5%, heating at 100° for 5 min, and a final addition of urea to 8.0 M. The gels were electrophoresed for 2 h at 5 mA per gel (10 V/cm).

Preparative electrophoresis was performed in a vertical slab gel of the same composition (200 × 200 × 5 mm) with the same buffer, which was continuously recirculated between the two buffer chambers. P1 and P2 were sufficiently separated after 72 h at 7 V/cm.

Proteins were recovered from the gel by cutting the gel slab into 5 mm horizontal strips and macerating each strip in 10 ml 5 mM sodium bicarbonate, 0.5 mM EDTA, 0.5% SDS. After 16 h the gel was filtered off on a stainless steel sieve and the extract centrifuged at 100,000 g for 1 h to remove small pieces of gel. A second 16-h extraction with 5 ml of bicarbonate yielded a second batch of protein indistinguishable from the first. By this process 70% of a radioactive protein was recovered from a gel.

Carboxymethylation

The method was adapted from Harris and Perham [17]. The protein sample (10 ml EDTA extract at 1 mg/ml) was dialysed over night against 50 mM Tris/HCl, pH 8.0, at 4°; 50 μCi of iodo-(2-^{14}C)-acetic acid (10–25 mCi/ mmole, Radiochemical Centre, Amersham) in 0.5 ml water was added to the protein (12 μCi were used for each protein fraction obtained by preparative gel electrophoresis). Solid urea was added to 8.0 M after 30 min at 18° and 0.1 ml β-mercaptoethanol after a further 90 min; 60 min later the mixture was put to dialyse at 4° for 24 h against three changes of 50 mM Tris/HCl to remove diffusible radioactive material. After dialysis 30 mg of nonradioactive iodoacetic in 0.5 ml water (10 mg for the smaller slab fractions) was added, followed by urea to 8.0 M and dithioerythritol to 20 mM. After 90 min at 18° the mixture was dialysed over night in the cold against the buffer used for trypsinisation.

Purification of the ^{14}C Carboxymethyl Peptides

The peptides were concentrated to 1.0 ml by rotary flash evaporation and passed through a Sephadex G50 column equilibrated with water. Radioactivity was confined to a retarded component which was collected, acidified by the addition of formic acid to 0.1 M, and applied to a sulphoxyethyl (SE) Sephadex column equilibrated with 0.1 M formic acid. All the radioactivity was bound to the column, which was washed with the acid, and then water, before elution of the radioactive peptides with 0.3 M ammonium hydroxide. The peptides were concentrated to a small volume for thin-layer chromatography.

Iodination of Proteins

The method was adapted from Hunter and Greenwood [18]. A 1 mg/ml solution of protein (1 ml) was dialysed against 0.2 M phosphate buffer (pH 7.5) containing 0.5 mM EDTA and 0.1% SDS. Then 1 mCi of ^{125}I (Iodine-125, carrier free, Radiochemical Centre, Amersham) was added followed by 10 μl chloramine T solution (5 mg/Ml). The reaction was stopped after a few seconds by 100 μl sodium metabisulphite solution (2.4 mg/ml) and 100 μl of potassium iodide solution (1 mg/ml). Low-molecular weight radioactivity was removed by an overnight dialysis against 0.5 mM EDTA and finally by an over night dialysis against 10 mM Tris/HCl buffer (pH 8.0).

Trypsinisation

The samples in the 10 mM Tris/HCl buffer (pH 8.0) were trypsinised for 24 h at 37° by the addition of 100 μl of a 1 mg/ml solution of pig trypsin (Miles Laboratories, Ltd) and a second batch after 6 h. Pig trypsin has a very low chymotrypsin activity.

Peptide Mapping

The tryptic digest was fractionated on silica thin-layer plates (Polygram SIL N-HR, Camlab, Cambridge). The mixture was chromatographed in the first dimension in ethanol/ammonia (70:30, v/v) and electrophoresed in the second dimension for 4 h at 15 V/cm in a pyridine/acetic acid/water (5:50:945, v/v) solvent at pH 3.5. The radioactive peptides were finally located by autoradiography.

RESULTS

Peptide maps of tryptic digests of spectrin, P1 and P2 labeled with either ^{14}C carboxymethyl side chains or ^{125}I iodination demonstrate the similarity, but not identity, of the two chains. Many peptides are common to both polypeptides but some are peculiar to P1 and others confined to P2. Some common spots differ in intensity between the two polypeptides. The identification of common spots is based on our interpretation of these maps and similar maps made from replicate preparations. Comparable constellations of spots can be seen, but in complicated iodinated maps the possibility of coincidence of nonidentical peptides must be countenanced (Figs 1–3). The presence of the same peptides in maps of both proteins cannot be due to cross-contamination, for analytical gels of the separated P1 and P2 show no cross contamination. Coomassie blue staining would reveal a contamination of less than 10%, and the similarities between the maps could not result from such low levels of contamination. The presence of peptides peculiar to either of the two fractions is additional evidence against cross-contamination.

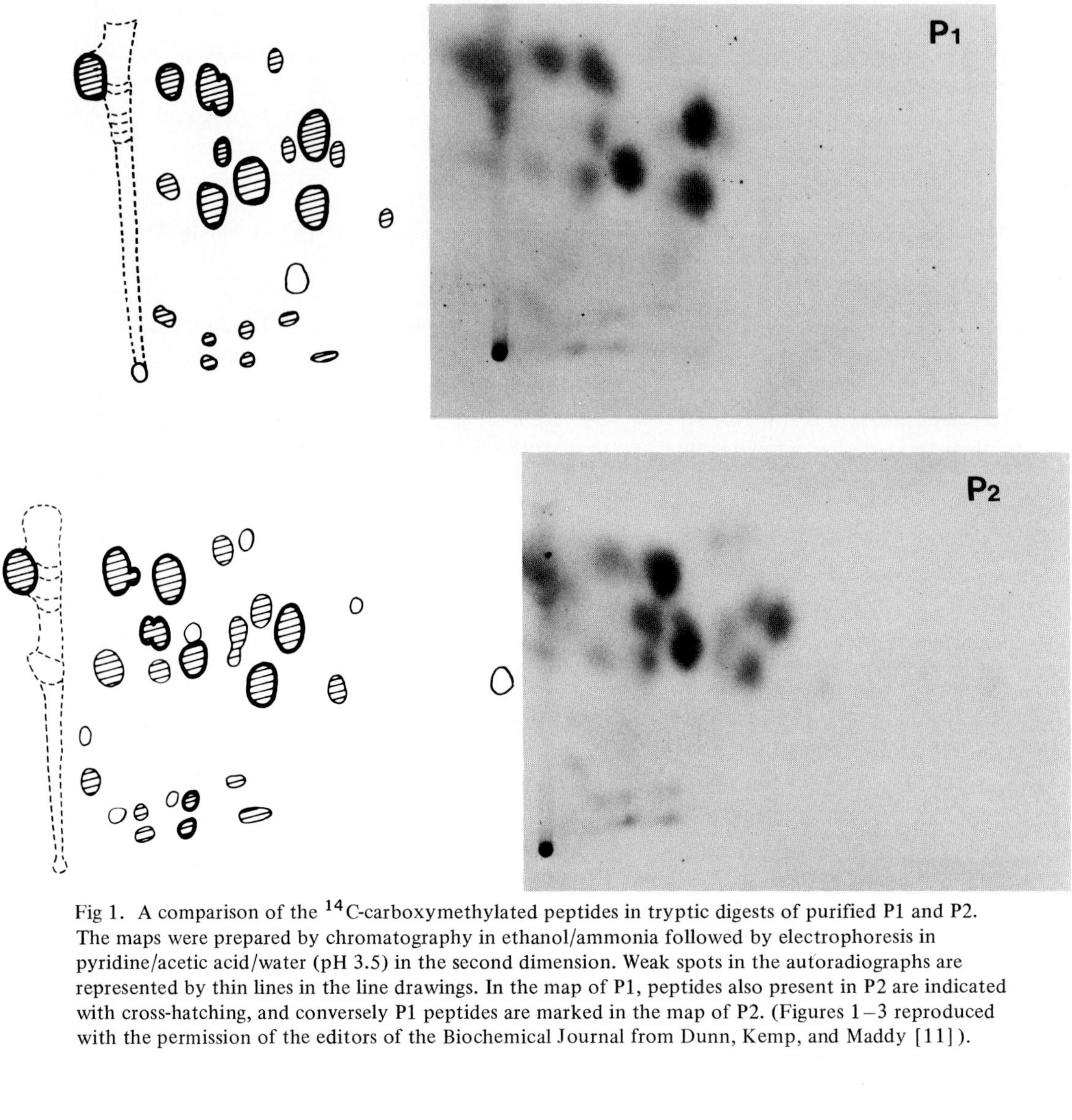

Fig 1. A comparison of the ^{14}C-carboxymethylated peptides in tryptic digests of purified P1 and P2. The maps were prepared by chromatography in ethanol/ammonia followed by electrophoresis in pyridine/acetic acid/water (pH 3.5) in the second dimension. Weak spots in the autoradiographs are represented by thin lines in the line drawings. In the map of P1, peptides also present in P2 are indicated with cross-hatching, and conversely P1 peptides are marked in the map of P2. (Figures 1–3 reproduced with the permission of the editors of the Biochemical Journal from Dunn, Kemp, and Maddy [11]).

No proteolytic activity can be detected in the EDTA extract using standard protein substrates such as azocoll or azoalbumin, but a slow breakdown of P1 and P2 over a period of weeks at 4° may be observed by SDS electrophoresis. Fresh material showing no sign of degradation was always used for the mapping. Maps of polypeptides which had not been digested with trypsin were devoid of radioactivity except at the origin. Cattle red cell ghosts are much less prone to proteolysis from white cells than are those of humans.

The number of peptides (20–25) in the carboxymethyl maps is consistent with the polypeptides being single chains of very approximately 200,000 daltons. (Assuming an average molecular weight of 120 for amino acids, a residue present at 1 mole % would generate around 20 peptides from a 240,000-dalton polypeptide.)

DISCUSSION

Peptide maps of trypsin digests of carboxymethylated and iodinated proteins show the close similarity of P1 and P2. This similarity has previously been inferred from immunologic data, N-terminal analyses, and the amino acid compositions of these same fractions, but the immunology and N-terminal content also led to the conclusion that P1 and P2 were heterogeneous. The relative simplicity of the present maps, particularly carboxymethylated maps, confirm the more widely held belief that P1 and P2 are single polypeptides of high molecular weight.

The immunologic data are ambiguous. Bjerrum et al [15] raised antisera against spectrin which contained antibodies that reacted with P1 and P2, and the P1 and P2 antibodies cross-reacted with each other but not with any other membrane proteins. By contrast the antisera raised by Sheetz, Painter, and Singer [19] against spectrin contained antibody against P1 which did not react with P2.

Comparison of P1 and P2 by their N-terminal end amino acids showed that each had several N-termini and that they both contained the same mixture of N terminal ends [13, 14]. The multiplicity of N termini was found when the usual precautions were taken to minimise proteolytic degradation and the analyses were performed on high-molecular-weight fractions which comigrated with bands P1 and P2 in freshly prepared ghosts, ie, the same type of preparation as used in the present report. The multiplicity of ends is inconsistent with the generally held view that the two fractions consist of single high-molecular-weight polypeptide chains. This apparent anomaly could arise from a limited exopeptidase activity which does not change the molecular weights enough to be detected by gel electrophoresis, or, conceivably, the SDS does not remove some tightly bound small peptides from the long chains [20]. A third possibility which has not been excluded is the formation of covalent cross-links between chains under the influence of the transaminase

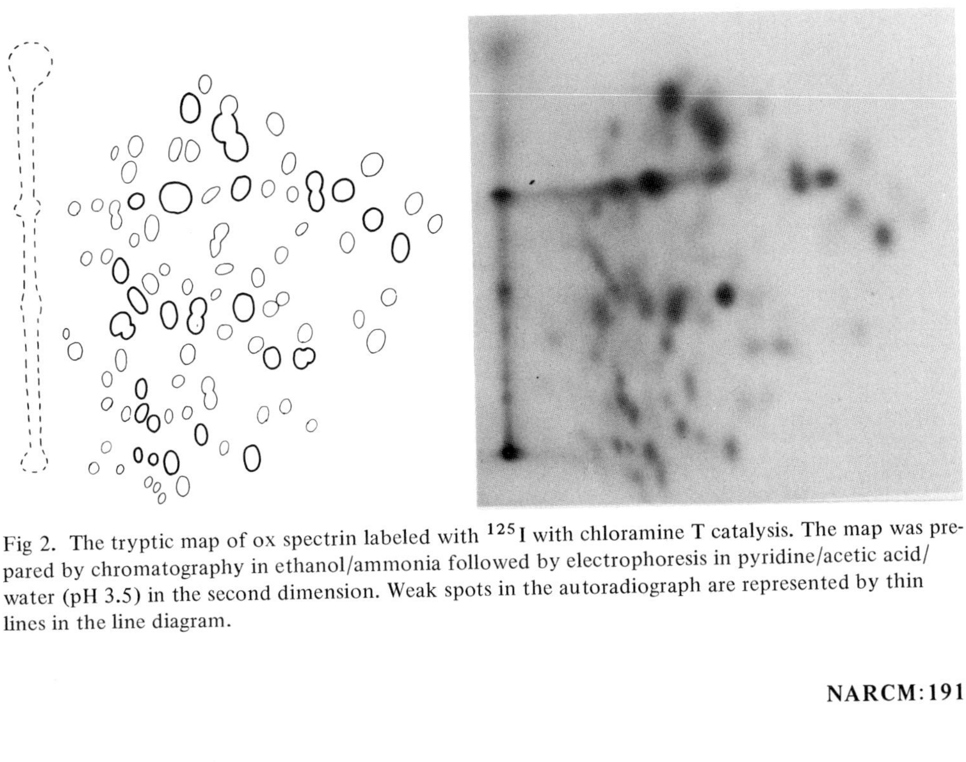

Fig 2. The tryptic map of ox spectrin labeled with ^{125}I with chloramine T catalysis. The map was prepared by chromatography in ethanol/ammonia followed by electrophoresis in pyridine/acetic acid/water (pH 3.5) in the second dimension. Weak spots in the autoradiograph are represented by thin lines in the line diagram.

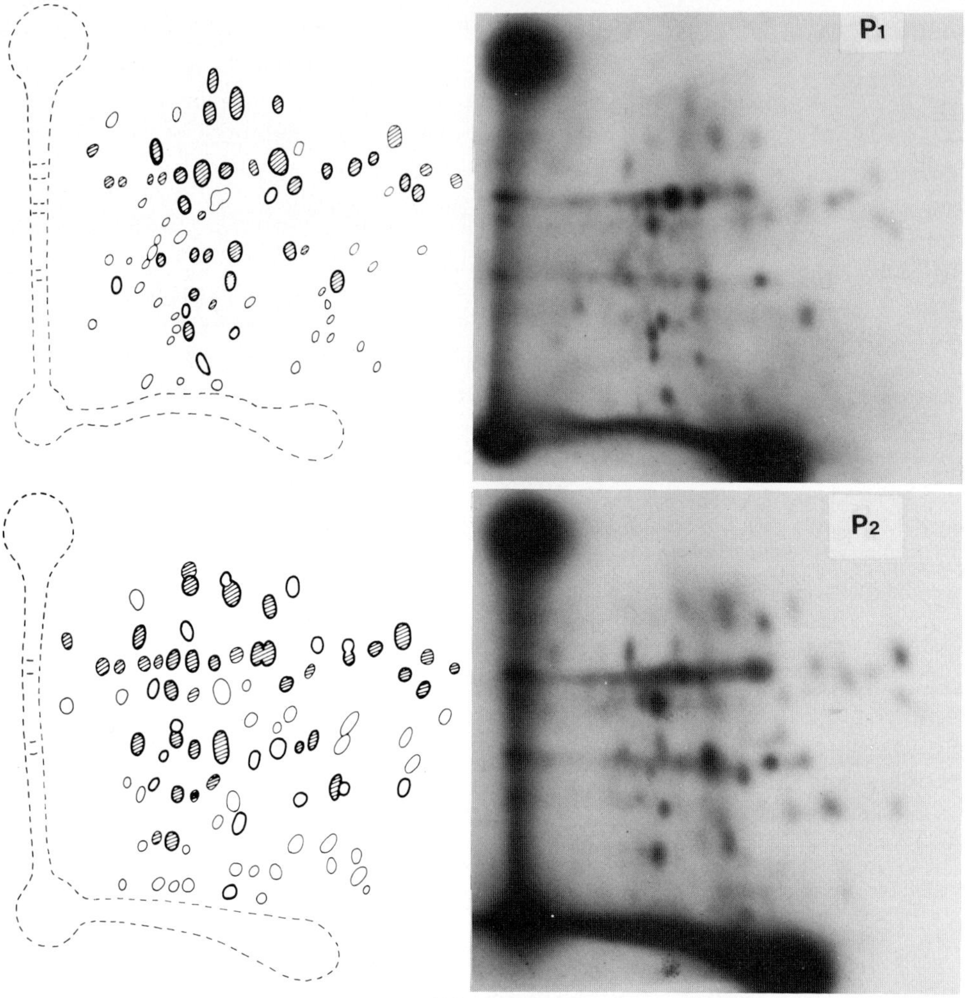

Fig 3. A comparison of the tryptic digests of ^{125}I-iodinated P1 and P2. The large radioactive area spreading from the origin in the second dimension is an iodinated product of the polyacrylamide gel used during the preparation of P1 and P2. In the line drawing of P1, peptides also present in P2 are indicated with cross-hatching and conversely P1 peptides are marked in the map of P2.

present in erythrocytes [21]. Whatever the true explanation for the identical results obtained from both P1 and P2, they point to the similarity of the two polypeptides.

Similarity of the amino acid compositions of P1 and P2 have been reported by three laboratories [10–12]. Too much significance cannot be attached to similarity of amino acid composition, but both fractions possess the high leucine and glutamate contents that characterise the unfractionated spectrin.

The biologic significance of the similarities between the two chains is not obvious. Fukui, Nachbar, and Salton [22] observed common peptides shared by several different proteins extracted from Micrococcus lysodeikticus membranes and concluded that these were derived from segments of proteins which, in vivo, were buried in the lipid hydrocarbon domain and were similar in structure because they all served the same function of anchoring the proteins into the membrane. This explanation is unlikely to apply to the spectrin polypeptides, as spectrin is an extrinsic protein. Another explanation arises out of the model proposed by Ralston [9] for the organization of spectrin in the membrane. Ralston has suggested that the P1 + P2 dimer consists of one P1 chain and one P2 chain at 90° to each other and that these dimers associate as four-armed tetramers. These tetramers are then assembled, with the involvement of actin, into a continuous two-dimensional array on the inner surface of the membrane. It might be argued that the maintenance of symmetry in such an array is achieved by the similarity of the two constituent polypeptide chains. However, the similarities between the chains that have been revealed by the peptide mapping must not be allowed to overshadow the differences. In addition to their differing size and the differences between the peptide maps, P2 can be phosphorylated [23–25] and its phosphorylation affects cell shape [26, 27] and its interaction with actin [4].

ACKNOWLEDGMENTS

This work was carried out under the financial support of the Medical Research Council.

REFERENCES

1. Marchesi VT, Steers E: Science 159:203, 1968.
2. Fairbanks G, Steck TL, Wallach DFH: Biochemistry 10:2606, 1971.
3. Tilney LG, Detmers P: J Cell Biol 66:508, 1975.
4. Pinder JC, Bray D, Gratzer WB: Nature 270:752, 1977.
5. Hulla FW, Gratzer WB: FEBS Lett 25:275, 1972.
6. Ralston GB: Aust J Biol Sci 28:1975.
7. Schechter NM, Sharp M, Reynolds JA, Tanford C: Biochemistry 15:1897, 1976.
8. Kam Z, Josephs R, Eisenberg H, Gratzer WB: Biochemistry 16:5568, 1977.
9. Ralston GB: J Supramol Struct 8:00–00, 1978.
10. Fuller GM, Boughter JM, Morazzani M: Biochemistry 13:3036, 1974.
11. Dunn MJ, Kemp RB, Maddy AH: Biochem J 173:197, 1978).
12. Anderson JM: J Supramol Struct, Suppl 2:191, 1978.
13. Knufermann H, Bhakdi S, Schmidt-Ullrich R, Wallach DFH: Biochim Biophys Acta 330:356, 1973.
14. Dunn MJ, McBay W, Maddy AH: Biochim Biophys Acta 386:107, 1975.
15. Bjerrum OJ, Bhakdi S, Bøg-Hansen TC, Knufermann H: Biochim Biophys Acta 406:689, 1975.
16. Maddy AH: Biochim Biophys Acta 117:193, 1966.
17. Harris JI, Perham RN: J Molec Biol 13:876, 1965.
18. Hunter WM, Greenwood FC: Nature (London) 194:495, 1962.
19. Sheetz MP, Painter RG, Singer SJ: Biochemistry 15:4486, 1976.
20. Maddy AH: J Theor Biol 62:315, 1976.
21. Lorand L: J Supramol Struct, Suppl 2:193, 1978.
22. Fukui Y, Nachbar MS, Salton MRJ: Biochim Biophys Acta 288:65, 1972.
23. Guthrow CE, Allen JE, Rasmussen H: J Biol Chem 247:8145, 1972.
24. Shapiro DL, Marchesi VT: J Biol Chem 252:508, 1977.
25. Wyatt JL, Greenquist AC, Shohet SB: Biophys Biochem Res Commun 79:1279, 1977.
26. Sheetz, MP, Singer SJ: J Cell Biol 73:635, 1977.
27. Birchmeier W, Singer SD: J Cell Biol 73:647, 1977.

Journal of Supramolecular Structure 9:79–95 (1978)
Normal and Abnormal Red Cell Membranes 195–211

Glycophorins A, B, and C: A Family of Sialoglycoproteins. Isolation and Preliminary Characterization of Trypsin Derived Peptides

Heinz Furthmayr

Department of Pathology, Yale University School of Medicine, New Haven, Connecticut 06510

Two new sialoglycoproteins, glycophorin B and glycophorin C, were isolated from erythrocyte membranes by extraction with lithium diiodosalicylate, partition in aqueous phenol, gel filtration in detergent, and preparative polyacrylamide gel electrophoresis in sodium dodecyl sulfate. The two proteins were characterized by amino acid and carbohydrate analysis, separation of tryptic peptides, and isolation and purification of the amino terminal glycopeptide from each polypeptide chain. Glycophorin B is found in two forms in electrophoretograms of normal erythrocyte membranes corresponding to monomer and dimer, as has been similarly described for glycophorin A. By using antibodies to a carboxy terminal determinant of glycophorin A, and direct staining of gels with antibodies and ^{125}I-protein A from Staph. aureus, as well as by two-dimensional immunoelectrophoreis, only the two known forms of glycophorin A are detectable. The data confirm and extend the notion that the sialoglycoproteins in human red cells are dimeric molecules which are either preformed in the membrane or which can readily be generated in vitro. Only glycophorin A and glycophorin C are sensitive to trypsin while in situ in the intact red blood cells.

Key words: **glycophorins A, B, and C, isolation, membrane protein, glycopeptides, erythrocyte**

The sialoglycoproteins of the erythrocyte membrane have been under extensive investigation for many years in different laboratories [1–3]. First isolated and described as a myxovirus receptor substance capable of inhibiting the aggregation of human erythrocytes by influenza virus, then as a blood group substance carrying MN blood group activity, the major sialoglycoprotein became known as glycophorin A. Based on considerable structural work [4–7] it was possible to firmly establish earlier claims [8] that the protein

Abbreviations: ESR – electron spin resonance; SDS – sodium dodecyl sulfate; PAS – periodic acid-Schiff's reagent; Tos-PheCH$_2$Cl or TPCK – L-(1-tosylamido-2-phenyl) ethyl chloromethyl ketone; LIS – lithium diiodosalicylate; AMLO – Ammonyx-LO, N,N-dimethyl laurylamine-N-oxide; Tos-LysCH$_2$Cl – N-p-α-tosyllysyl chloromethyl ketone.

Received April 18, 1978; accepted June 19, 1978.

spans the lipid bilayer and extends into the cytoplasm of the cell with a short carboxy terminal segment of about 35 amino acid residues [9]. As calculated from compositional data, about 80% of the total mass of the glycophorin A subunit is located at the surface of the cell, of which 75% is contributed by a large number of oligosaccharide chains, linked covalently to threonine, serine, and asparagine. It has been suggested that the protein exists in the membrane as a complex due to protein-protein interaction within the hydrophobic region of two or more subunits [10]. Despite the considerable knowledge of its structure, the functional role of glycophorin A for the cell or in membrane organization is virtually unknown. The protein in more or less pure form has been incorporated into artificial lipid bilayer systems and as a result, presumably of interaction with the bilayer, changes in electrical conductance [11] and in translocation of phospholipids across these membranes have been observed [12]. Ideas of implicating the cytoplasmic segment of glycophorin A in the organization and/or anchoring of the submembranous cytoskeleton have not found an experimental basis [3]. Yet while such experiments may well tell us about perturbation of a lipid bilayer by introducing a segment of a membrane protein into its interior, it is questionable that they describe the major functions of this heavily glycosylated protein. Based on ESR spectroscopy data of phosphate-linked, spin-labeled gangliosides and glycophorin incorporated into lipid bilayer vesicles, Sharon and Grant recently suggested that noncovalent, carbohydrate-based interactions between sialic acid bearing molecules may be responsible for the formation of a structural coat at the cell surface [13]. This coat is envisaged to carry a variety of receptors, to be highly deformable, and to allow alterations in the expression of membrane receptors.

Relatively little is yet known about the chemistry of cell surface glycoproteins, their conformation, or the relationship of glycosylated regions to the polar head groups and other structures on the membrane. This study deals with the description of two further species of sialoglycoproteins, glycophorin B and glycophorin C, of which at least one is closely related in a structural sense to glycophorin A.

MATERIALS AND METHODS

Materials

Reagent grade chemicals were used throughout. Dialysis tubing was boiled in EDTA at pH 8–9 and thoroughly rinsed in distilled water before use. The lithium salt of diiodosalicylic acid was prepared from the free acid obtained from Eastman Kodak after 2 × recrystallization from anhydrous methanol. Phenyl methane sulfonyl fluoride was purchased from Calbiochem. Sodium dodecyl sulfate was from Alcolac Chemical Corporation, Ammonyx-LO was obtained from Onyx Chemical Company. Chemicals used to prepare polyacrylamide gels were acrylamide, N,N′-methylene bisacrylamide from Biorad; ammonium persulfate from Canalco; N,N,N′N′-tetramethylethylenediamine from Eastman; Tris and urea, ultrapure, from Schwarz/Mann. Reagents for labeling were dansylchloride from Pierce and fluorescamine from Hoffman-LaRoche.

Methods

Isolation of sialoglycoprotein fractions. Membranes were prepared from human red cells as described by Furthmayr and Marchesi [10] except that for the most part outdated blood (about 20 units) was used. After lyophilization of the white ghosts, the crude glycoprotein fraction was prepared by suspension in a solution of LIS and partition in a phenol-water mixture according to the procedure of Marchesi and Andrews [14]. After extensive dialysis at 4°C against distilled water, the water phase obtained from the two-phase mixture was lyophilized. The dry material was then suspended in ice-cold ethanol and kept stirring for 30 minutes on ice. After centrifugation for 30 minutes at 4,000 rpm in a Sorvall RC-3 centrifuge, the ethanol extraction of the precipate was repeated one more time. The final precipitate was dissolved in water and lyophilized. Glycophorin A was separated from the other sialoglycoproteins by gel filtration in AMLO on Biorad A 1.5 as described [6, 15]. The sialoglycoprotein fraction (80–100 mg) was well resolved into three peaks on a column 100 × 5 cm. After extensive dialysis against distilled water, the three proteins containing pools (AMLO-pool A, B, and C) were lyophilized.

Labeling of sialoglycoprotein fractions. Glycopeptides contained in AMLO-pools A, B, and C (see above) were labeled with dansylchloride or fluorescamine in the presence of SDS. Usually, 20 mg of glycoprotein was dissolved in 1 ml of 0.02 M sodium phosphate, pH 8.0 containing 1% SDS, and 100 μl of fluorescamine at a concentration of 20 mg/ml acetone was added slowly while stirring. After a brief incubation at room temperature, 1 ml of a buffer was added containing 20 mM Tris-HCl, pH 6.8, 4 M urea, 6% SDS, 2 mM EDTA, and the sample was applied onto a polyacrylamide slab gel as described below. Alternatively, 20 mg of glycoprotein was dissolved in 2 ml 0.02 M sodium phosphate, pH 8.0, and 1% SDS and labeled by addition of 1 ml of freshly prepared dansylchloride at a concentration of 0.5% in acetone. After incubation at 37°C for 30 minutes, acetone was added and the precipitate collected by centrifugation. The precipitate was dissolved at a concentration of 10 mg/ml of the buffer given above, mixed with unlabeled protein at a ratio of 1 part labeled to 9 parts unlabeled and was subjected to electrophoresis.

Polyacrylamide gel electrophoresis in dodecyl sulfate. Gels were prepared as described by Furthmayr and Marchesi [10] with slight modifications of the system of Fairbanks et al [16]. Preparative slab gel electrophoresis was done using the gel and buffer system described by Laemmli [17]. Electrophoretic separation was done on polyacrylamide gel slabs (17 × 15 cm or 23 × 15 cm, 5 mm thickness) originally using stacking gels and running times of about 12 hours at 50 mA with or without cooling of the plate. In later experiments the stacking gel was omitted without sacrifice of resolution in separating the various sialoglycopeptide species. Samples for electrophoresis were incubated at 37°C for 30 minutes and 2 minutes at 100°C. Protein loads per slab gel were between 20 mg and 40 mg depending on size. Electrophoresis was stopped after pyronin Y, which was included in the sample before loading, had moved 9–10 cm into the gel bed.

Isolation of labeled sialoglycopeptides from polyacrylamide gels. The labeled protein bands were visualized under UV light and the fluorescent gel strips were cut with razor blades. After thorough homogenization with a Teflon pestle, excess buffer was added to the gel particles containing 50 mM sodium bicarbonate, 0.05% SDS, 0.02% sodium azide, and the protein was extracted by shaking at 37°C overnight. Gel particles were removed by filtration on nylon filters and washed by several additions of water. After dialysis against water, the solution was centrifuged for 30 minutes at 5,000 rpm in a Sorvall RC-3 centrifuge and then lyophilized. Since it was found difficult to remove excess glycine and acrylamide polymers by dialysis, the lyophilized material was subjected to column chromatography on LKB Ultrogel AcA 54 in 0.05% SDS, 5 mM sodium phosphate, pH 8.0 (column dimensions 2.5 × 90 cm). The fractions containing protein were pooled, dialyzed against distilled water, and lyophilized. To remove residual SDS, the lyophilized material was extracted twice with acetone, solubilized in distilled water, and lyophilized.

Proteolytic digestion. Sialoglycoproteins were dissolved at a concentration of 10 mg/ml in 50 mM Tris-HCl, pH 8.0 and after addition of sufficient trypsin (TPCK-treated, Worthington) in 0.001 N HCl, 1 mM $CaCl_2$ to give an enzyme:substrate ratio of 1:30, the sample was incubated at 37°C for 20 hours. Digestion was stopped by acidifying the solution with glacial acetic acid to pH 4.5. A precipitate formed during this step was removed by centrifugation and was found to contain hydrophobic peptide material [cf 7]. The soluble peptides were separated by column chromatography on LKB Ultrogel AcA 54, equilibrated in 50 mM ammonium acetate, pH 6.1, 0.02% sodium azide (2.5 × 150 cm or 1.5 × 182 cm). Column effluents were monitored continuously at 230 nm. Appropriately pooled fractions were concentrated by evaporation and desalted on Biogel P2 columns equilibrated with 0.05 N acetic acid. After lyophilization, some of the peptides were rechromatographed by ion-exchange chromatography on DEAE-cellulose (Whatman DE52), and equilibrated with 50 mM sodium formate, pH 6.1. The peptides were eluted from the column (1.5 × 15 cm) by using a linear gradient from 0 to 0.3 M sodium chloride over a total volume of 400 ml.

Digestion of intact red blood cells with trypsin. Freshly drawn blood was washed several times with excess isotonic phosphate buffered saline, pH 7.2. To 400 ml of packed cells was added 400 ml of 0.2 M sodium phosphate buffer, pH 8.0, containing 0.2 M NaCl as described by Jackson et al [34]. The cells were divided into two parts, and trypsin hydrolysis was initiated by addition of 30 mg and 200 mg of Tos-$PheCH_2Cl$-treated trypsin (Worthington), respectively, and the solutions were shaken gently at 37° for 110 minutes. After this incubation period, the trypsin was inactivated by the addition of a 10-fold molar excess of Tos-$LysCH_2Cl$. The supernate was recovered by centrifugation at 3,000g for 20 minutes. The red cells were washed one more time with phosphate-buffered saline, pH 7.2. Both supernatant and wash were combined and the same volume of 50% phenol was added. After stirring at ice-temperature for 20 minutes, the solution was centrifuged at 5,000 rpm for 1 hour in a Sorvall RC-3 centrifuge. The water phase was extensively dialyzed against distilled water at 4°C and finally lyophilized.

The lyophilized material was then subjected to gel filtration on Sephadex G150 superfine as described above, and the glycopeptides were finally purified by DEAE-cellulose chromatography as described.

Analytical data. Amino acid and carbohydrate analysis was performed as described previously [4, 18]. Norleucine and inositol, respectively, served as internal standards.

Two-dimensional immunoelectrophoresis. Total membrane proteins from freshly prepared human erythrocyte membranes and the isolated crude sialoglycoprotein mixture were analyzed by the technique described by Converse and Papermaster [19]. The protein loads for electrophoresis in the first dimension were 12.5 μg of membrane proteins and 0.5 μg of the isolated glycoprotein mixture. The concentration of the antiserum in the agarose layer was 6%. For a description of the antiserum see text and [9].

Labeling of SDS-polyacrylamide gels with specific antibodies [20]. Erythrocyte membrane proteins or the isolated sialoglycoprotein mixture were separated by SDS-polyacrylamide gel electrophoresis in tube gels, by using the gel and buffer system described by Laemmli [17]. The gels were fixed for 12 hours in 50% methanol, 8% acetic acid, and then rinsed extensively with several changes of buffer containing 50 mM Tris-HCl, pH 7.4, 150 mM sodium chloride, 5 mM EDTA, 0.02% sodium azide, for a period of 12 hours. The gels were then transferred to small test tubes and covered with 3 ml of a 1:50 dilution of antiserum to a C-terminal determinant of glycophorin A [9] or rabbit normal serum, and after a 12-hour incubation nonbound protein was removed by several changes over a 12-hour period of the above buffer. The last step of the procedure consisted of a 12-hour incubation with ^{125}I-labeled Protein A (Staph. aureus, Pharmacia), which had been diluted to 5 × 10^5–10^6 cpm/ml, and extensive washing of the gels with the buffer given above. The gels were sliced into 1-mm slices with a homemade gel slicer and counted in a Beckman Biogamma Counter.

Iodination of protein A [20]. To 50 μg of the protein in 10 μl 0.05 M sodium phosphate buffer, pH 7.5, were added 10 μl 0.2 M sodium phosphate, pH 7.5, 200 μCi in 10–20 μl of ^{125}I-Na (New England Nuclear, Carrier free) and 25 μg Chloramine T in 10 μl 0.05 M sodium phosphate, pH 7.5. After agitation for no longer than 1 minute at room temperature, 100 μl of 8 mM tyrosine was added to quench the reaction. Iodinated protein A was separated from free iodine and tyrosine by gel filtration on Sephadex G25 (1 × 20 cm) equilibrated in 50 mM Tris-HCl, pH 7.4, 150 mM sodium chloride, 5 mM EDTA, 0.02 NaN_3. The iodinated protein was stored at 4°C after 0.25% gelatin or 0.1% ovalbumin (Sigma) had been added.

Radioimmunoassay. The assays used have been described recently and employed the same antisera and reagents [9, 18].

RESULTS

Localization of Glycoprotein A Polypeptides on SDS-Polyacrylamide Gels

From previous work it has been concluded that glycophorin A polypeptides on SDS-polyacrylamide gels occupy two positions, the low-molecular-weight form being about half the size of the high-molecular-weight form [10, 21, 22]. Since these two electrophoretic forms were found to be interconvertible [10] and the high-molecular-weight form could be completely converted to the low-molecular-weight form by chemical modification [22] or by lowering the protein concentration [10], it has become clear that glycophorin, at least under the conditions of SDS-gel electrophoresis or gel filtration in SDS, is present as a complex. The data were consistent with the idea that a dimeric complex was dissociable into monomeric subunits. However, it has been impossible thus far to obtain reliable absolute molecular weights for these glycoconjugates by these techniques. Although no other PAS-stainable bands of molecular weight lower than the presumptive monomer have been observed, it is not clear how many subunits the glycophorin A complex contains.

Glycophorin A amounts to 1.6% of the total membrane protein as determined by radioimmunoassay (Fig. 1). We have used antibodies to a C-terminal protein determinant of glycophorin A in order to locate glycophorin A polypeptides on SDS-gels and with the hope to detect with this rather sensitive tool small amounts of glycophorin A subunits. In two-dimensional immuno-electrophoresis only two precipitin arcs are observed corresponding to the two known positions occupied by glycophorin A on the gel (Fig.2). The total amount of glycophorin A seen here is 200 ng. Since the formation of a visible antigen-antibody complex is dependent on optimal concentrations of both antigen and antibody, this technique may have missed additional products. Despite our attempts to cover a range of different concentrations, no additional precipitin arcs were observed.

The second technique we have used, namely direct staining of glycophorin A with antibodies on the gel, does circumvent this problem. In order to do the experiment, the gels have to be fixed to retain the protein during the somewhat lengthy procedure. The C-terminal antigenic determinant on glycophorin A is still reactive despite treatment with SDS and fixation with methanol-acetic acid and two radioactively labeled bands are seen

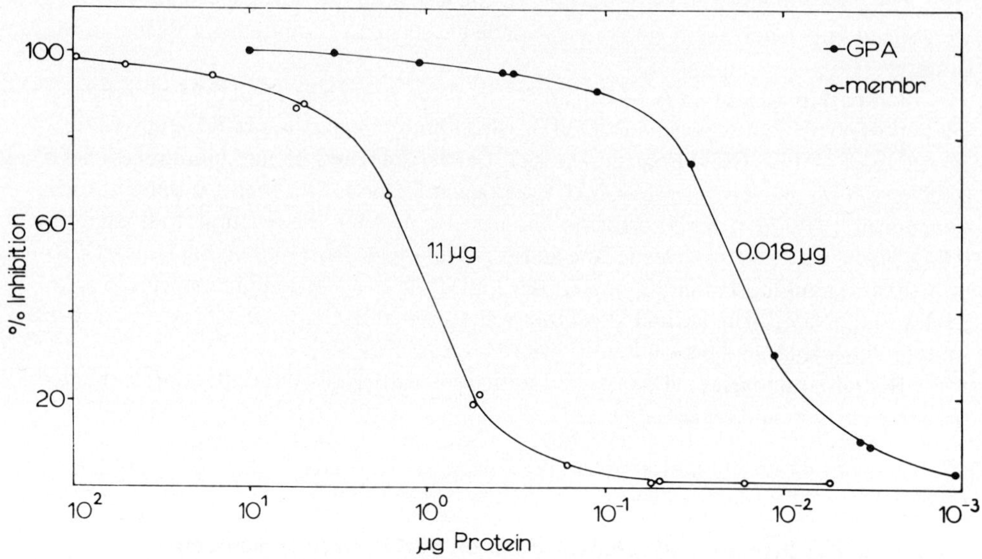

Fig. 1. Quantitation of glycophorin A in normal human erythrocytes by radioimmunoassay. Erythrocyte membranes (–○–) and isolated glycophorin A (–●–) were used as competitive inhibitors in the radioimmunoassay as described elsewhere [9, 18]. Inhibitor concentrations were determined by amino acid analysis and Lowry using norleucine and bovine serum albumin, respectively, as internal standards.

corresponding to the two positions known to contain glycophorin A (Fig. 3B). By varying the protein load on the gel, the amount of radioactive protein A bound to these regions was found to be nonlinear (data not shown) and starts to reach a plateau at a certain protein concentration. Since excess of antibody and ^{125}I-labeled protein A is used, the limitation seems to come from the fact that the protein has been fixed and that the rather large ligands do not penetrate sufficiently into the protein bands. The technique thus appears to be relatively more sensitive for smaller amounts of antigen in the gel. When membrane samples were heated at 100°C for 3 minutes at concentrations of 1 mg membrane protein per ml and loaded onto gels, 200 ng of glycophorin A was easily detectable. Heat treatment causes a considerable change in the amount of radioactivity found in the two positions on the gel, but apparently does not dissociate the low-molecular-weight form of glycophorin A further. If this form were still a dimer, it cannot be further reduced in size by simple manipulation. This conclusion is not invalidated by the fact that the technique of detection is not strictly quantitative.

Isolation of Glycophorin B and Glycophorin C

Several laboratories have shown that human red cell membrane proteins give a much more complex pattern in the SDS-gel system described by Laemmli [23, 24]. The sialoglycoprotein bands in particular are distinctly different from previously observed analysis. After isolation of the sialoglycoprotein fraction by the LIS-phenol method [14], the PAS-stainable pattern of this fraction on SDS-polyacrylamide gels was nearly identical to that of the original membrane protein mixture (Fig. 4T). The relative staining intensities of

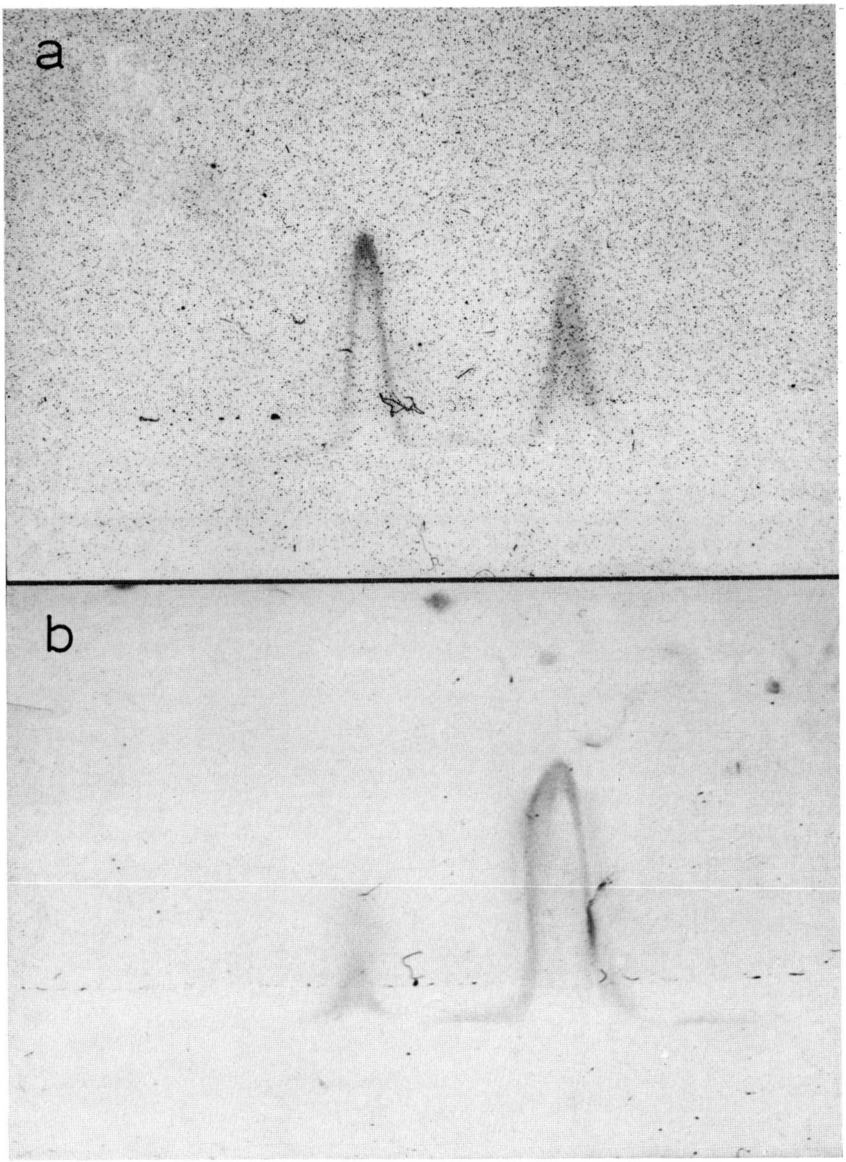

Fig. 2. Two-dimensional immunoelectrophoresis of human erythrocyte membranes. The antiserum was developed in rabbit against a fragment of glycophorin A and contains antibodies specific for a carboxy terminal protein determinant [9]. Red cell ghosts were dissolved in sample buffer and incubated for 30 minutes at 37°C (a) and for additional 3 minutes at 100°C (b) before loading on an SDS-polyacrylamide slab gel for separation in the first dimension (from left to right). Electrophoresis in the second dimension (from bottom to top) of the proteins into the antibody containing layer shows precipitin arcs formed at the two position where glycophorin A is found on gels in the first dimension.

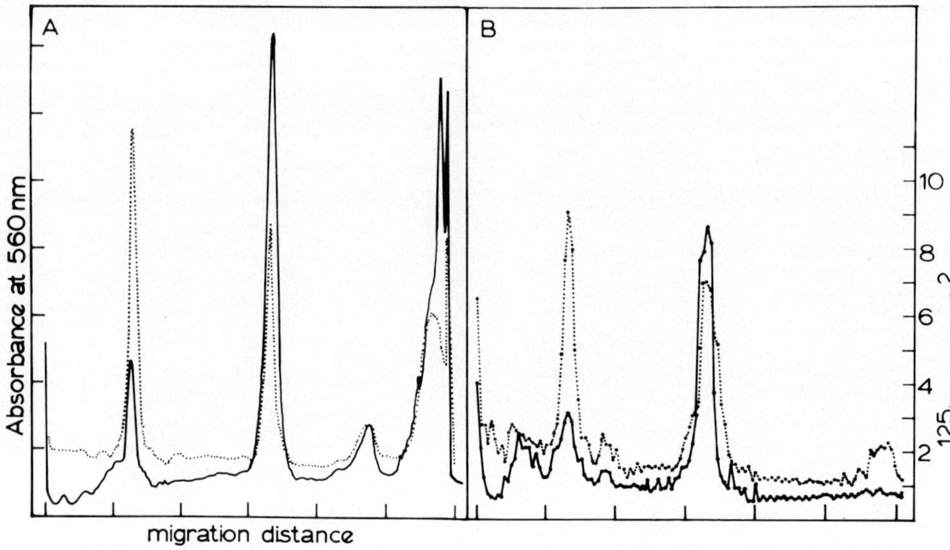

Fig. 3. Labeling of glycophorin A polypeptides on SDS-polyacrylamide gels with specific antibodies. 10-μl samples of erythrocyte membranes dissolved in SDS-loading buffer and containing approximately 25 μg protein were incubated at 37°C for 30 minutes (dotted line) and an additional 3 minutes at 100°C (solid line) before being subjected to electrophoretic separation on Laemmli tube gels. The gels in A were stained with PAS reagent and scanned at 560 nm. The absorbance is given in arbitrary units. In B the gels were treated with antiserum and ^{125}I-labeled protein A, as described in the Methods section, sliced and counted.

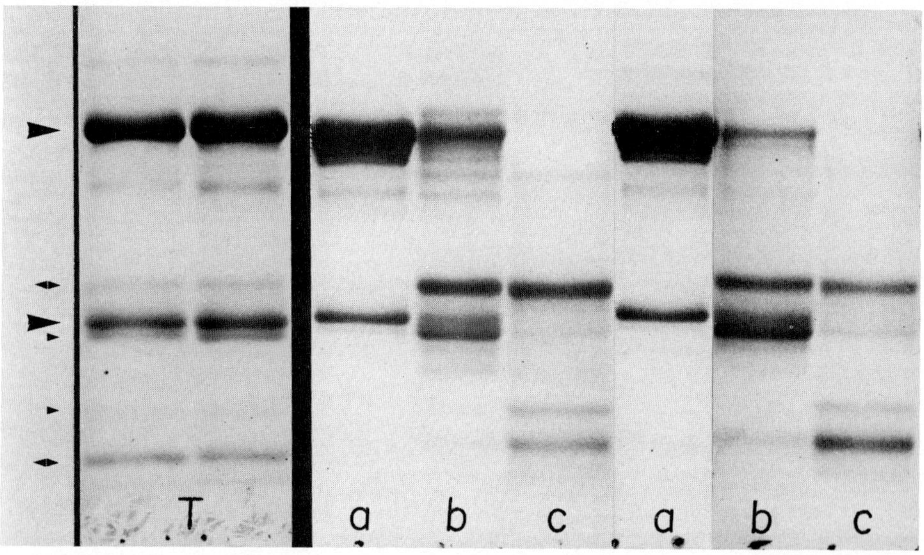

Fig. 4. SDS-polyacrylamide gel electrophoresis of sialoglycoprotein fractions obtained by gel filtration in the detergent Ammonyx-LO (cf [6, 15]). The gel system was as described by Laemmli [17] and about 50 μg of each sialoglycoprotein mixture was loaded. The gel was stained with PAS reagent. T designates two different sialoglycoprotein samples before fractionation; abc correspond to protein pools A, B, and C (in [6, 15]) from two separate gel filtration experiments.

TABLE I. Distribution of Glycophorins on SDS-Polyacrylamide Gels

Glycophorin	Band	%
A	1	51
	2, 2A	12
B	3	6
A	4	17
C	5	6
C	6	1
B	7	7

some of the bands changes to some extent in comparison to the membrane protein profile and a small amount of material of higher molecular weight is observed (Table I, cf [23].

It was shown previously that the major sialoglycoprotein species, glycophorin A, can be isolated in pure form and separated from other glycopeptide components by gel filtration in nonionic and other detergents [15]. When the glycopeptide pools A, B, and C, obtained by gel filtration on Biorad A 1.5 in the detergent Ammonyx-LO was analyzed by SDS-polyacrylamide gel electrophoresis according to Laemmli, the patterns shown in Figure 4a,b,c are obtained (for a more detailed description of the chromatogram see [6] and [15]). The first and major protein peak eluting from the column contains glycophorin A, seen as two bands on the gel indicated by large arrowheads. Small amounts of other bands are seen contaminating the preparation. This contamination can be avoided by pooling fractions of the major peak without including the fractions from the trailing shoulder which is frequently observed and presumably is caused by aggregation of the minor glycoproteins. The second peak eluting from the column which originally has been described to contain tryptophan as measured by its fluorescence [15], gives the peptide pattern shown in Figure 4b. Most of the peptide material indicated by the small arrowhead in the original sialoglycopeptide mixture is found in this fraction in addition to the high-molecular-weight form of peptides indicated by the double arrowhead. AMLO-pool C from the column contains mostly peptides indicated by double arrowheads in addition to small amounts of lower-molecular-weight peptides. As can be seen from the figure, the amount of individual peptides found in these positions varies from preparation to preparation.

The preparative step of gel filtration in detergents to remove glycophorin A and to enrich in a relatively efficient way for the minor components made it feasible to isolate adequate amounts of these polypeptides for chemical characterization. Conventional separation techniques like gel filtration in SDS or ion-exchange chromatography in nonionic detergents failed to further separate these glycoproteins and to produce proteins homogeneous as judged by SDS-electrophoresis. Since only the Laemmli gel system seems to distinguish these minor sialoglycoproteins we decided to isolate the proteins from polyacrylamide slab gels. In order to visualize the peptides, part of the AMLO-pool B and C material was chemically modified by dansylation; and after mixing with unlabeled protein and electrophoresis, fluorescent bands were cut from regions of slab gels as indicated in Figure 5. Although traces of fluorescent bands at other positions were observed for both fractions (cf Fig. 4 b,c), we made no attempt to recover these minute amounts. Re-electrophoresis of the isolated sialoglycopeptides demonstrated their remarkable tendency to aggregate and to form oligomers (Fig. 6). As judged from these gel patterns, peptides

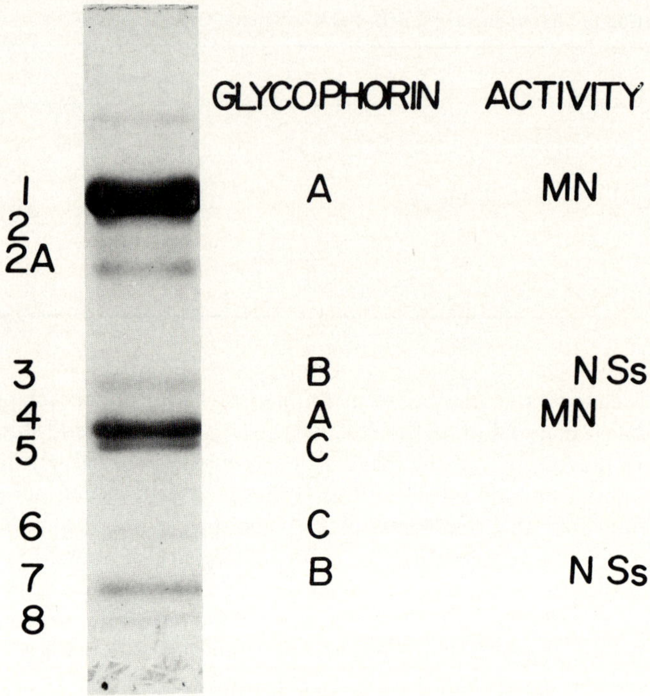

Fig. 5. Dansylated sialoglycoprotein mixture on SDS-polyacrylamide gels after staining with PAS reagent. The fluorescent profile (not shown) as identical to the stained gel shown here. The numbers on the left indicate positions 1–8 on the gel, from which fluorescent labeled proteins were isolated (cf Fig. 6). A, B, and C designate the glycophorin species, and on the far right, serological activities associated with glycophorin A and B are indicated.

isolated from regions 3–7 appear homogeneous by forming oligomers at distinct positions while those from regions 1 and 2 are mixtures of all the components from the original mixture. Although the data are shown only for AMLO-pool B material, identical findings were obtained for the pool C polypeptides. The original gel filtration in detergent thus appears to separate complexes of different size and does not distinguish between different molecules. Since the same polypeptides are found in both peaks, apparently these molecules can be incorporated into an aggregate of variable composition, which is either preformed in the membrane or is generated during the isolation technique. It is not clear if such sialoglycoprotein complexes contain only one species of protein.

Chemical Characterization of Glycophorin B and Glycophorin C

Amino acid analysis of the peptides isolated from the gels indicates that three proteins account for the complex electrophoresis pattern. We have named these proteins glycophorin A, B, and C (Table II). Glycophorin A is found, as expected, in positions 1 and 4, glycophorin B in 3 and 7, and glycophorin C was identified in positions 5 and 6 (cf Fig. 5). The three proteins lack cysteine, but are distinguished by considerable differences particularly in the values for aspartic acid, proline, glycine, alanine, valine, and isoleucine. Glycophorin C contains tryptophan, which is absent in the other two proteins, and glycophorin B lacks N-acetyl glucosamine and mannose (see below), markers for the com-

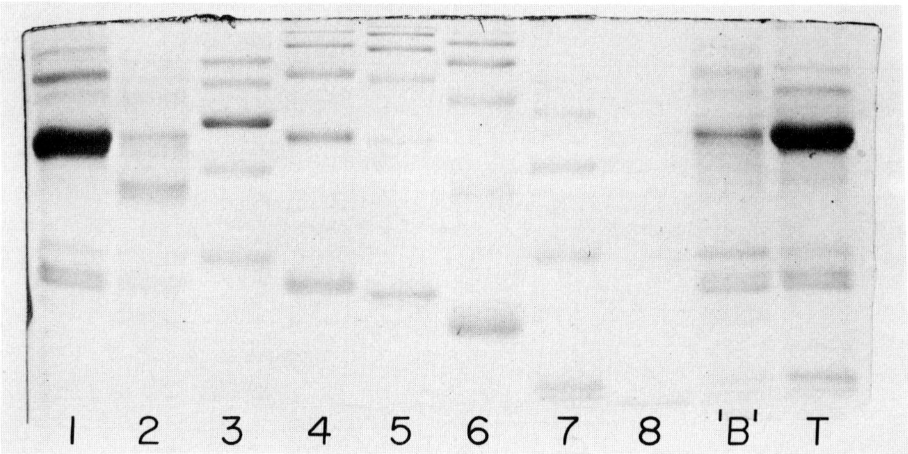

Fig. 6. Re-electrophoresis of sialoglycopeptides isolated from positions 1–8 (cf Fig. 5) of AMLO-pool B peptides ("B," of Fig. 4b), T indicates total sialoglycoprotein mixture and is used as an internal marker. The gel system was that of Laemmli and staining was done with the PAS reagent.

TABLE II. Amino Acid Composition of Human Erythrocyte Membrane Glycophorins*

	Glycophorin A				
	mole/mole			Glycophorin B	Glycophorin C
	Expected	Found	Mole %	Mole %	Mole %
Asp	8	8.9	6.8	3.9	8.9
Thr[a]	15	14.5	11.1	14.5	10.6
Ser	18.5	17	13.0	13.8	10.5
Glu	14.5	15.6	11.9	9.4	9.7
Pro	10	10	7.7	4.0	7.9
Gly	5.5	5.5	4.2	5.2	9.2
Ala	6	6.7	5.1	7.3	11.5
Cys	–[b]		–	–	–
Val	11	11.3	8.6	7.2	2.8
Met[c]	2	1.3	1.0	1.8	3
Ile	11	9.8	7.5	8.0	3.3
Leu	7.5	7.7	5.9	8.0	5.5
Tyr	4	3.8	2.9	3.1	3
Phe	2	2.1	1.6	2.1	2.3
His	5	4.6	3.5	3.3	3.2
Lys	5	5.1	3.9	3.3	2.9
Arg	6	6	4.6	5.1	4.6
Trp[d]		–		–	+
GalNAc[e]			+	+	+
GlcNAc[e]			+	–	+

*Amino acid analysis was done on a Durrum D500 analyzer. The values were calculated from duplicate analyses obtained for two preparations.

[a]Values for Thr and Ser are corrected for losses during hydrolysis by extrapolation to zero time after 24, 36, and 48 hours hydrolysis.

[b]Dash denotes 0.1 or less.

[c]Uncorrected values for Met.

[d]Determined spectrofluorometrically.

[e]Determined only semiquantitatively after acid hydrolysis on the amino acid analyzer.

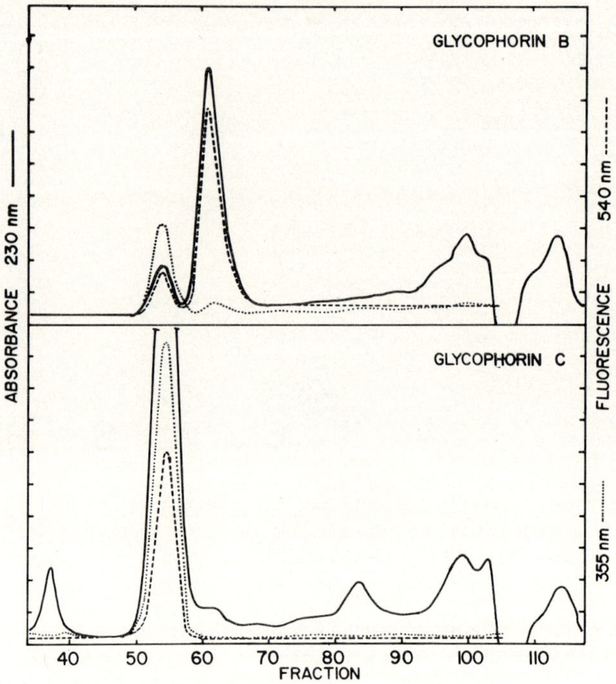

Fig. 7. Separation of soluble tryptic peptides of glycophorin B and glycophorin C by gel filtration on Aca 54. The column dimensions were 2.5 × 150 cm, flow rate 35 ml/hour, fraction volume 7 ml. ——) Absorbance at 230 nm in arbitrary units; ·········) tryptophan fluorescence (excitation 290 nm, emission 355 nm); - - - - -) dansyl chloride fluorescence (excitation 380 nm, emission 540 nm).

plex oligosaccharide linked N-glycosidically to an asparaginyl residue in glycophorin A and probably glycophorin C.

To confirm these findings the proteins isolated from the eight positions indicated in Figure 5 were treated with trypsin and after removal of insoluble peptide material, generated as a result of proteolysis, the soluble peptides were applied to a column of AcA 54. The elution of peptide material was monitored at 230 nm and by fluorescence measurements. In Figure 7 representative chromatograms for glycophorin B and C are given. Both proteins contain one major peptide, which carries the dansylchloride label and thus is derived from the amino terminal end of each of the polypeptide chains. The peptide in glycophorin C contains tryptophan as an additional marker, which is absent from the major peptide in glycophorin B. The small amount of peptide material in glycophorin B also containing tryptophan is present in nonstoichiometric amounts, elutes in the same position as the glycophorin C glycopeptide, and presumably is derived from contaminating material. These major peptides elute in exactly the same positions as the two amino terminal peptide products T1 and T2 from glycophorin A [5, 6, 15, 18], but they can be distinguished by ion-exchange chromatography on DEAE-cellulose [5]. Rechromatography of the amino terminal glycopeptides of glycophorin B and C on DEAE-cellulose gave uniform peaks (not shown), and the purity of the peptides was confirmed by amino acid analysis, by amino terminal analysis, and partial amino acid sequence studies [18 and unpublished].

TABLE III. Amino Acid and Carbohydrate Analysis of N-Terminal Peptides of Glycophorin A, B and Glycophorin C*

	A^{MN}-T1[a]	A^{M}-T1	A^{N}-T1	A^{MN}-T2	A^{M}-T2	A^{N}-T2	B^{MN}-T2	C^{MN}-T1[b]
Asp	3 (3)	2.9 (3)	3 (3)	2.2 (2)	2 (2)	2 (2)	1.3 (1)	3.1
Thr[c]	9 (9)	9 (9)	9 (9)	7.3 (7)	7 (7)	7.1 (7)	7.2 (7)	5.3
Ser	8.7 (8.5)	8.7 (9)	7.7 (8)	8.5 (8.5)	8.5 (9)	7.9 (8)	8.3 (8)	5
Glu	1.7 (1.5)	1.1 (1)	2.3 (2)	1.7 (1.5)	1.2 (1)	2.3 (2)	4 (4)	1.9
Pro	.9 (1)	.8 (1)	1 (1)	– (-)	–	–	.2 (-)	4.8
Gly	.6 (.5)	1.1 (1)	– (-)	.6 (.5)	1 (1)	–	2.2 (2)	2.7
Ala	2.9 (3)	2.7 (3)	2.9 (3)	1.2 (1)	1.1 (1)	1.1 (1)	1.2 (1)	3.2
Cys	–[d]	–	–	–	– (-)	–	– (-)	–
Val	2.2 (2)	2.1 (2)	2.1 (2)	2 (2)	2 (2)	2.1 (2)	2.7 (3)	–
Met[e]	.8 (1)	.9 (1)	.7 (1)	.4 (1)	.4 (1)	.4 (1)	.6 (1)	.6
Ile	1 (1)	1 (1)	1 (1)	1 (1)	.9 (1)	1 (1)	.9 (1)	1
Leu	.5 (.5)	– (-)	1.1 (1)	.6 (.5)	– (-)	1.1 (1)	2 (2)	1.4
Tyr	1.7 (2)	2 (2)	2 (2)	.8 (1)	.7 (1)	.8 (1)	.6 (1)	–
Phe	–	–	– (-)	–	– (-)	– (-)	– (-)	–
His	2.1 (2)	2 (2)	2.1 (2)	2 (2)	2 (2)	2 (2)	1.7 (2)	1
Lys	2.1 (2)	2 (2)	2.1 (2)	2 (2)	2 (2)	1.9 (2)	1.2 (1)	–
Arg	1.7 (2)	1.6 (2)	1.8 (2)	.5 (-/1)	.5 (-/1)	.6 (/1)	.7 (1)	1.2
Total	39	39	39	30	30	30	35	
Carbohydrate composition[f]								
Fuc	.41	.5	.55	.4	.6	.2	–	.7
Man	2.7	2.8	3	3.2	2.8	2.6	–	2.4
Gal	13.5	12.3	12.4	11.1	11.9	10.5	10.7	10.6
GalNAc	10	9.8	10.1	7.9	8.3	7.6	13.8	8.1
GlcNAc	6.9	6.8	6.8	6.3	5.4	5.1	–	5.4
NANA	12.7	13	12	10.7	9.8	10	15.8	11.2

*Amino acid analysis was done on a Durrum D500 analyzer, using Nle as an internal standard. The values are given in moles/mole peptide with expected values in brackets.

[a]Superscripts M, N, and MN indicate the MN blood group type of the red cells, from which the glycophorin molecules were isolated.

[b]Contains tryptophan which was determined spectrofluorometrically only. The exact size of the peptide has not been determined.

[c]Values for Thr and Ser are corrected for losses during hydrolysis by extrapolation to zero time after 24, 36, and 48 hours hydrolysis.

[d]Dash denotes 0.1 or less

[e]Uncorrected values for Met.

[f] Moles/mole peptide. Carbohydrates were determined as trimethylsilyl derivatives of methyl glycosides by gas-liquid chromatography, on a Hewlett-Packard 5110 B gas chromatograph, using inositol as an internal standard [27].

Yields were obtained only for the purified peptides from glycophorin B and C and were in the order of 1 μmole from 20 units of blood. The amino acid and carbohydrate composition of the peptides derived from glycophorin B and glycophorin C (B^{MN}T2 and C^{MN}T1) is given in Table III in addition to the amino terminal peptides derived from glycophorin A^{M}, A^{N}, and A^{MN} [18]. Because of their chromatographic behavior, characteristic amino acid and carbohydrate composition these peptides thus provide reliable markers for the presence of the type of glycophorin in any given position on the SDS-gels. Isolation of these glycopeptides by the methods outlined above, confirm the scheme presented in Figure 5, namely that both, glycophorin B and C, occur in two positions on SDS-polyacrylamide gels. Incomplete cleavage was observed only for glycophorin C isolated from position 6 and may be due to modification of lysyl groups by dansylchloride.

Although the chromatograms of the tryptic digests of glycophorin B and C contain at least one other soluble peptide in stoichiometric amounts of low molecular weight which has not been further purified yet, the peptide patterns are strikingly different from that obtained for glycophorin A [5, 15, 18]. The abscence of peptides in the 3,000–4,000 dalton range may suggest that both glycophorin B and C are yet smaller than glycophorin A and do not contain an extended cytoplasmic segment.

Release of Sialoglycopeptides From Intact Human Erythrocytes With Trypsin

To determine which of the three glycophorins were accessible and susceptible to protease while in situ, intact red cells were treated with high concentrations of trypsin to release glycopeptides. Two different concentrations of enzyme were used at enzyme: substrate ratios of 1:20 and 1:3 when calculated on the basis of total membrane proteins of the red cells. The relative concentration of the enzyme is much higher, however, since only a fraction of the membrane proteins is accessible. The major sialoglycopeptides of glycophorin A partition into the water phase of a phenol-water mixture [Furthmayr, unpublished]. When the supernatant fluids after digestion of the intact cells and after phenol-partitioning were analyzed for glycopeptides by gel filtration, only two peptide peaks are obtained for both digests corresponding to the elution position of peptides T1 and T2 of glycophorin A [18]. Chromatography of the peptides from the first peak separated two peptides (T1A and T1B), as shown by Tomita et al [5]. The second peak was found homogeneous in this system. The amino acid composition of these three fragments was identical to the composition of peptides T1 and T2 of glycophorin A and peptide T1 of glycophorin C. These results indicate that even at high protease concentrations only glycophorin A and glycophorin C are sensitive and accessible to trypsin to release amino terminal peptides.

DISCUSSION

We have shown in this study that human erythrocyte membranes contain at least three different sialoglycoproteins, for which we propose the names glycophorin A, B, and C. Glycophorin A amounts to 1.6% of the total membrane protein as determined by radioimmunoassay. By using the figures on the relative abundance of red cell membrane proteins given by Fairbanks et al [16], the number of polypeptides per ghost is 420,000, corresponding to about 200,000 dimers of glycophorin A. Since glycophorin B and C contain similar amounts of sialic acid, the number of polypeptide copies per cell can be estimated as 70,000 and 35,000, respectively. There are possibly other glycoprotein species present in the crude sialoglycoprotein fraction, but the minute quantities of these peptides seen by PAS-stain or after dansylation made isolation unwarranted at this time. Admittedly, these minor components could be variants of the known proteins, which are separated in the gel system because of heterogeneity in carbohydrate structure. Small amounts of glycophorin C are found mainly in AMLO-pool C and migrate differently from the bulk of the glycophorin C polypeptides on SDS-gels for reasons which are unexplained at present. This component does not appear to be a subunit of a higher-molecular-weight complex of glycophorin C, since the electrophoretic mobilities of its oligomeric form differed from glycophorin C. On the other hand, glycophorin A and B apparently can readily undergo associations to form oligomers. These aggregates obviously are artifacts of the isolation

GLYCOPHORIN A^M	SER - SER - THR - THR - GLY -
A^N	LEU - SER - THR - THR - GLU -
GLYCOPHORIN B^{MN}	LEU - SER - THR - THR - GLU -

Fig. 8. Amino terminal sequences of glycophorin A^M, A^N and glycophorin B^{MN}. Superscripts M, N, and MN indicate the MN blood group type of the red cells, from which the glycophorin molecules were isolated. Residues in boxes indicate sites of glycosylation.

since they are not seen in membrane samples to the same extent. In fresh ghosts glycophorin A and B are always found in two electrophoretic forms which possibly correspond to monomers and dimers. With the exception of the high-molecular-weight form of glycophorin A, these complexes are stable in SDS and cannot be dissociated. Isolation of the sialoglycoprotein fraction by the method used causes some rearrangement, since higher amounts of glycophorin B dimers are found as compared to the ghost in addition to small amounts of aggregates of mixed composition.

Previous attempts to isolate the minor glycoproteins have dealt with impure preparations due to lack of separation on SDS-gels [15, 25]. Analytical data on amino acid and carbohydrate composition were significantly different from the results presented here. The compositional data on glycophorin A isolated from SDS-gels are comparable to those reported earlier on the column-purified protein [15]. Although the values for some amino acids deviate somewhat from the expected values, this seems to be a property of this highly glycosylated membrane protein rather than due to the fact that the proteins were isolated from SDS-gels. More accurate data can be obtained on smaller peptides, and in fact the isolation of sialoglycopeptides from the polypeptide mixtures has proven to yield reliable data, since the peptides obtained previously from AMLO-pool B [18] can now be shown to be derived from the amino terminal ends of glycophorin B and C.

Glycophorin B is related to glycophorin A in structure and antigenicity. It is, however, not a proteolytic degradation product of glycophorin A. The C-terminal peptide and antigenic determinant located in this region of glycophorin A [9] is apparently absent in glycophorin B, which could suggest shortening of the protein at the C-terminal end by proteases. However, peptide T3, located in the amino terminal half of glycophorin A (residues 40–61), is also not found in glycophorin B. These findings in addition to differences in amino acid sequence [18] make it rather unlikely that glycophorin B is derived from glycophorin A by post-translational modification or artificial degradation, but rather that it is the product of a different gene. The amino terminal sequence of B is identical to one form of glycophorin A, called A^N, in the first 22 amino acid residues (Fig. 8). In addition, the same sites are occupied by oligosaccharides in glycophorin B with the exception of N-glycosylation in position 26 of the sequence [18]. Correlated with this structural similarity or identity are serological characteristics. Glycophorin B carries the N antigen regardless of the MN type of the red cell which is determined predominantly by glycophorin A [18, 26]. Structural information on glycophorin C is limited and the relationship to the two other glycoproteins, if any, has to be defined yet.

The three proteins are integral membrane proteins [27] since portions of the polypeptide are interacting with the hydrophobic core of the lipid bilayer and hydrophobic peptides have been isolated which serve this function ([7] and Furthmayr, unpublished).

It is difficult at present to determine the molecular weight of glycophorin B and glycophorin C. The data presented here suggest however, that the polypeptide chains are considerably shorter than glycophorin A and may not exceed 100 amino acid residues. Further structural studies on the isolated peptides will be required to answer this question. The data available thus far also suggest that glycophorin B and glycophorin C lack the cytoplasmic segment of about 35 amino acid residues found in glycophorin A. The proteins may still span the entire thickness of the membrane with only rather short segments extending out of the inner face of the membrane. Alternatively, the hydrophobic segment is entirely buried within the membrane.

Analysis of membranes prepared from trypsinized intact cells by SDS-gel electrophoresis has indicated that glycophorin B is not digested in intact cells and that the cells retain their Ss activity [31]. Several groups have analyzed in some detail the glycopeptides released from cells by trypsin [32–34], but the fragments which have been described are only marginally related to the glycopeptides isolated here, since amino acid and carbohydrate compositions are rather different from those reported here. Presumably, these studies were dealing with insufficiently purified proteolytic fragments. It is interesting that in situ only glycophorin A and glycophorin C are sensitive to trypsin despite the high concentration of enzyme employed. The differential sensitivity of these proteins to proteases may be an indication for a definite arrangement of these molecules on the surface of the red cell.

In the red cells of certain individuals, some of the sialoglycoproteins are absent without apparent deficiencies for the individual, for red cell survival in the circulation, or red cell function. Such genetic variants have been described for glycophorin A and glycophorin B, either of which can be totally absent in homozygotes [18, 28]. This loss is associated with serologically recognizable changes of the red cell and lack of expression of MN and Ss antigens [29]. From this data it also has been concluded that glycophorin B (Fig. 5) carries the Ss determinants since both bands are absent in S-s-U-cells [28]. Combined absence of glycophorin A and B has been found only in heterozygotes with genetically determined loss of 50% of these proteins [18]. Variations with respect to glycophorin C have not been described and it is not known whether it carries determinants of any known antigenic system.

These latter findings put some strain on any hypothesis to explain the function of these complex glycoconjugates. Although they do not address the question, whether these proteins are synthesized at all at any stage during cell differentiation in these individuals, or at which stage of differentiation this loss occurs, these observations may indicate that a certain minimal amount of sialic acid conjugated to protein is required for normal function of the red cell. Reduction of the surface charge even lower than the "critical potential" [30] at which nonspecific aggregation of red cells occurs with specific ligands, may result in agglutination of cells in vivo in the presence of normal serum components. Alternatively, these proteins play a role much more important earlier during differentiation and genetic events which interfere with the expression of the proteins may result in nonviable conditions.

ACKNOWLEDGMENTS

This work was supported by grant BC-102C from the American Cancer Society and PHS grant GM AM 21714-01C09.

I am grateful to Gail Dunbar, Manyee Tang, Wolfgang Furthmayr, and Bruce Proctor who during the course of this work at one time or another have contributed their skilled technical help.

REFERENCES

1. Winzler RJ: In Jamison GA, Greenwalt TJ (eds): "Red Cell Membrane: Structure and Function." Philadelphia: JB Lippincott, 1969, p 157.
2. Springer GF, Nagai Y, Tegtmeyer H: Biochemistry 5:3254, 1966.
3. Marchesi VT, Furthmayr H, Tomita M: Annu Rev Biochem 45:667, 1976.
4. Tomita M, Marchesi VT: Proc Natl Acad Sci USA 72:2964, 1975.
5. Tomita M, Furthmayr H, Marchesi VT: Biochemistry. In press.
6. Furthmayr H: J Supramol Struct 7:121, 1977.
7. Furthmayr H, Galardy RE, Tomita M, Marchesi VT: Arch Biochem Biophys 185:21, 1978.
8. Bretscher MS: Nature (London) New Biol 231:229, 1971.
9. Cotmore SF, Furthmayr H, Marchesi VT: J Mol Biol 153:539, 1977.
10. Furthmayr H, Marchesi VT: Biochemistry 15:1137, 1976.
11. Tieffenberg Tosteson M: J Membr Biol 38:291, 1978.
12. VanDeenen LLM: J Supramol Struct (Abstr) Suppl 2:187, 1978.
13. Sharon FJ, Grant CWM: Biochim Biophys Acta 507:280, 1978.
14. Marchesi VT, Andrews EP: Science 174:1247, 1971.
15. Furthmayr H, Tomita M, Marchesi VT: Biochem Biophys Res Commun 65:113, 1975.
16. Fairbanks G, Steck TL, Wallach DFH: Biochemistry 10:2606, 1971.
17. Laemmli UK: Nature (London) 227:680, 1970.
18. Furthmayr H: Nature (London) 271:519, 1978.
19. Converse CA, Papermaster DS: Science 189:469, 1975.
20. Cotmore SF: Personal communication.
21. Marton LSG, Garvin JE: Biochem Biophys Res Commun 52:1457, 1973.
22. Silverberg M, Furthmayr H, Marchesi VT: Biochemistry 15:1448, 1976.
23. Dahr W, Uhlenbruck G, Janssen E, Schmalisch R: Blut 32:171, 1976.
24. Mueller TJ, Dow AW, Morrison M: Biochem Biophys Res Commun 72:94, 1976.
25. Fujita S, Cleve H: Biochim Biophys Acta 382:172, 1975.
26. Wasniowska K, Drzeniek Z, Lisowska E: Biochem Biophys Res Commun 76:385, 1977.
27. Singer SJ, Nicolson GL: Science 175:720, 1972.
28. Dahr W, Uhlenbruck G, Issitt PD, Allen FM: J Immunogenet 2:249, 1975.
29. Race RR, Sanger R: "Blood Groups in Man." Blackwell: Oxford, 1975, p 463.
30. Pollack W, Hagen HJ, Reckel R, Toren DA, Singher HO: Transfusion 5:158, 1965.
31. Dahr W, Uhlenbruck G, Knott H: J Immunogenet 2:87, 1975.
32. Winzler RJ, Harris ED, Pekas DJ, Johnson CA, Weber P: Biochemistry 6:2195, 1967.
33. Jackson LJ, Seaman GVF: Biochemistry 11:44, 1972.
34. Jackson RL, Segrest JP, Kahane I, Marchesi VT: Biochemistry 12:3131, 1973.

Journal of Supramolecular Structure 9:97–112 (1978)
Normal and Abnormal Red Cell Membranes 213–228

Phosphorylation and Dephosphorylation of Spectrin

Grant Fairbanks, Joseph Avruch, Judith E. Dino, and Vikram P. Patel

Worcester Foundation for Experimental Biology, Inc., Shrewsbury, Massachusetts 01545 (G.F., J.E.D., V.P.P.); and Diabetes Unit, Massachusetts General Hospital, Boston, Massachusetts 02114 (J.A.)

The phosphorylation of spectrin polypeptide *2* is thought to be involved in the metabolically dependent regulation of red cell shape and deformability. Spectrin phosphorylation is not affected by cAMP. The reaction in isolated membranes resembles the cAMP-independent, salt-stimulated phosphorylation of an exogenous substrate, casein, by enzyme(s) present both in isolated membranes and cytoplasmic extracts. Spectrin kinase is selectively eluted from membranes by 0.5 M NaCl and co-fractionates with eluted casein kinase. Phosphorylation of band *3* in the membrane is inhibited by salt, but the band *3* kinase is otherwise indistinguishable operationally from spectrin kinase. The membrane-bound casein (spectrin) kinase is not eluted efficiently with spectrin at low ionic strength; about 80% of the activity is apparently bound at sites (perhaps on or near band *3*) other than spectrin. Partitioning of casein kinase between cytoplasm and membrane is metabolically dependent; the proportion of casein kinase on the membrane can range from 25% to 75%, but for fresh cells is normally about 40%. Dephosphorylation of phosphorylated spectrin has not been studied intensively. Slow release of ^{32}Pi from [^{32}P]spectrin on the membrane can be demonstrated, but phosphatase activity measured against solubilized [^{32}P] spectrin is concentrated in the cytoplasm. The crude cytoplasmic phosphospectrin phosphatase is inhibited by various anions – notably, ATP and 2,3-DPG at physiological concentrations. Regulation of spectrin phosphorylation in intact cells has not been studied. We speculate that spectrin phosphorylation state may be regulated 1) by metabolic intermediates and other internal chemical signals that modulate kinase and phosphatase activities per se or determine their intracellular localization and 2) by membrane deformation that alters enzyme–spectrin interaction locally. Progress in the isolation and characterization of spectrin kinase and phosphospectrin phosphatase should lead to the resolution of major questions raised by previous work: the relationships between membrane-bound and cytoplasmic forms of the enzymes, the nature of their physical interactions with the membrane, and the regulation of their activities in defined cell-free systems.

Key words: **dephosphorylation, spectrin, protein kinase, cAMP-independent, phosphoprotein phosphatase, phosphorylation**

Received May 18, 1978; accepted July 5, 1978.

0091-7419/78/0901-0097$02.90

The phosphorylation of spectrin was observed initially in the context of descriptive red cell membrane biochemistry, but it is now studied with increasing intensity because of its probable importance in cellular regulation. The enzymes involved – protein kinase(s) and phosphoprotein phosphatase(s) – are of intrinsic interest because they are relatively accessible and present intriguing problems in regulation. However, the main impetus for the work has been the idea that phosphorylation and dephosphorylation direct major changes in the physical state of spectrin and that these effects account in part for the metabolic dependence of cell shape and membrane deformability. The development of this perspective was strongly influenced by Weed et al [1], who in 1969 presented a refined description of the effects of metabolic depletion on cell and membrane properties and inferred that protein organization at the membrane–cytoplasm interface undergoes major changes as ATP levels decline. The first direct evidence for spectrin phosphorylation in human erythrocytes appeared two years later in another context [2]. During the same period, the fractionation and characterization of soluble protein kinases from rabbit reticulocytes [3, 4] and mature red cells [4, 5] was undertaken. This work ultimately contributed to the development of general criteria that distinguish the three major classes of protein kinases [6]. Both cAMP-dependent and cAMP-independent activities were detected in hemoglobin-free human erythrocyte ghosts [7]. And endogenous, or "autophosphorylation," reactions in which the membrane-bound enzymes utilize [γ-^{32}P] ATP in phosphorylating spectrin and other membrane proteins were described by several laboratories [8–13].

Most studies of spectrin phosphorylation have been confined to phenomenology and have yielded little insight into its functional significance. There have been several attempts to demonstrate altered phosphorylation in association with abnormal membrane function in hemolytic disease, but no convincing evidence for such a relationship has yet appeared [14, 15]. Recent work does, however, implicate spectrin phosphorylation directly in the regulation of protein organization in normal membranes: Singer and associates [16, 17] presented evidence that spectrin phosphorylation is required in the MgATP-dependent shape change of ghosts from crenated spheres to smooth biconcave discs. Another important contribution was made by Pinder et al [18–20], who examined the interaction between spectrin and skeletal muscle actin in solution and observed that phosphorylation of spectrin both increases its binding to actin and greatly enhances its capacity to induce actin polymerization. These results have been elaborated in the form of a working hypothesis: that the spectrin array on the membrane is cross-linked by actin monomers or very short filaments and that these associations are regulated by spectrin phosphorylation [20, 21].

A simplified diagram of the spectrin phosphorylation–dephosphorylation system is shown in Figure 1. Some of its components and interactions are known, but many are hypothetical. Because spectrin is multiply phosphorylated [15, 22], the equilibrium between phosphorylated and dephosphorylated forms may be much more complex than indicated. The phosphorylation sites are clustered on polypeptide *2* [23], but need not be functionally equivalent; the possibility that multiple enzymes are involved also remains to be tested. We envision that changes in the level of spectrin phosphorylation modulate actin–spectrin cross-linking on the membrane, and that this cross-linking (together with other factors) regulates cell shape, membrane deformability, and lateral mobility of integral proteins [1, 24]. In this scheme, turnover of spectrin-bound phosphate could

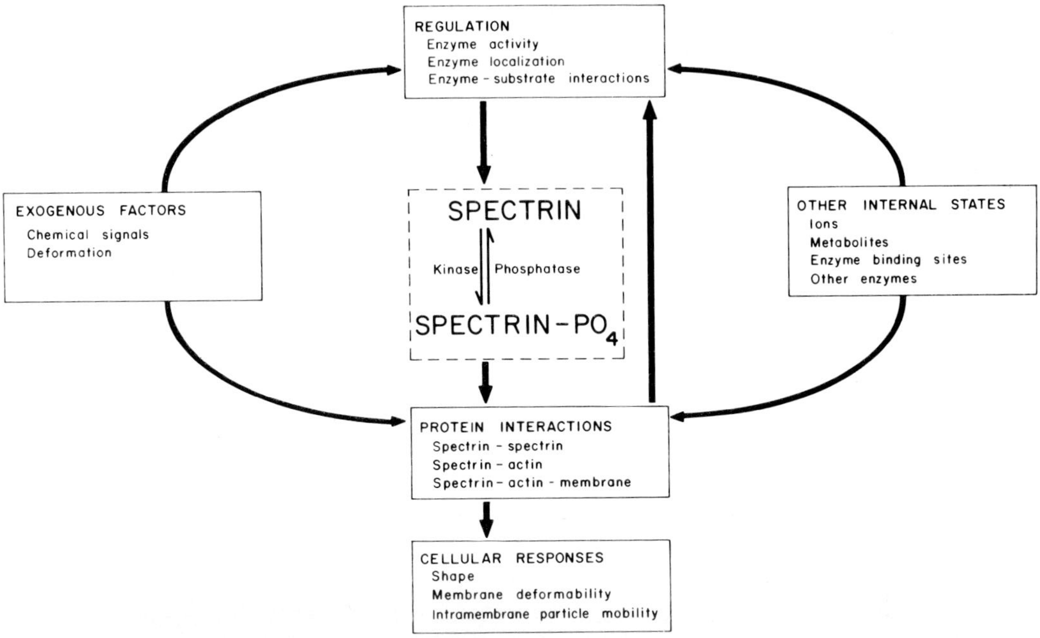

Fig. 1. The spectrin phosphorylation–dephosphorylation system. This heuristic model embodies the hypothesis that cell shape and membrane material properties are determined by the organization of peripheral proteins on the cytoplasmic face of the membrane and that spectrin phosphorylation modulates the protein interactions involved. Hypothetical factors in the regulation of interconversion of phosphorylated and dephosphorylated spectrin are 1) external influences, 2) various internal states, and 3) direct feedback from the spectrin–actin meshwork.

have the critical function of allowing reordering of the spectrin–actin meshwork after derangement by hemolysis or other trauma.

Virtually nothing is known about the regulation of spectrin phosphorylation except for its MgATP requirement. As indicated in Figure 1, it is conceivable that both external signals and internal states influence the interconversion rates. Furthermore, it is important to observe that the actions of these factors are not necessarily restricted to modulation of protein kinase or phosphoprotein phosphatase activity per se. Spatial disposition may play a major role if enzyme(s) bind to the membrane at sites other than their substrate, spectrin, or if enzyme partitioning between membrane and cytoplasm is variable. In Figure 1, possibilities for regulation at the level of enzyme–substrate interaction are shown as 1) direct feedback from the spectrin–actin meshwork, 2) deformation as an external stimulus, and 3) enzyme-binding sites on the membrane as internal regulatory elements.

Our primary objective in this paper is to review briefly the phenomenology of spectrin phosphorylation and dephosphorylation and to describe the current status of research on the properties of spectrin kinase and phosphospectrin phosphatase. We conclude with further speculation on modes of regulation that are consistent with the data available and are sufficiently attractive in principle to stimulate further investigation.

SPECTRIN PHOSPHORYLATION

As illustrated in Figure 2, both cytoplasmic and membrane proteins are labeled in intact red cells incubated with ^{32}Pi in a physiological buffer system. Sodium dodecyl sulfate–polyacrylamide gel electrophoresis of the whole hemolysate resolves about 20 phosphopeptides with molecular weights above 18,000. The labeling patterns of the cytoplasmic and membrane fractions show no significant overlaps, demonstrating that each phosphopeptide is apportioned uniquely to one of the two cellular compartments. These data also suggest that, among all high molecular weight phosphoproteins in the cell, spectrin *2* bears the largest pool of exchangeable phosphate groups.

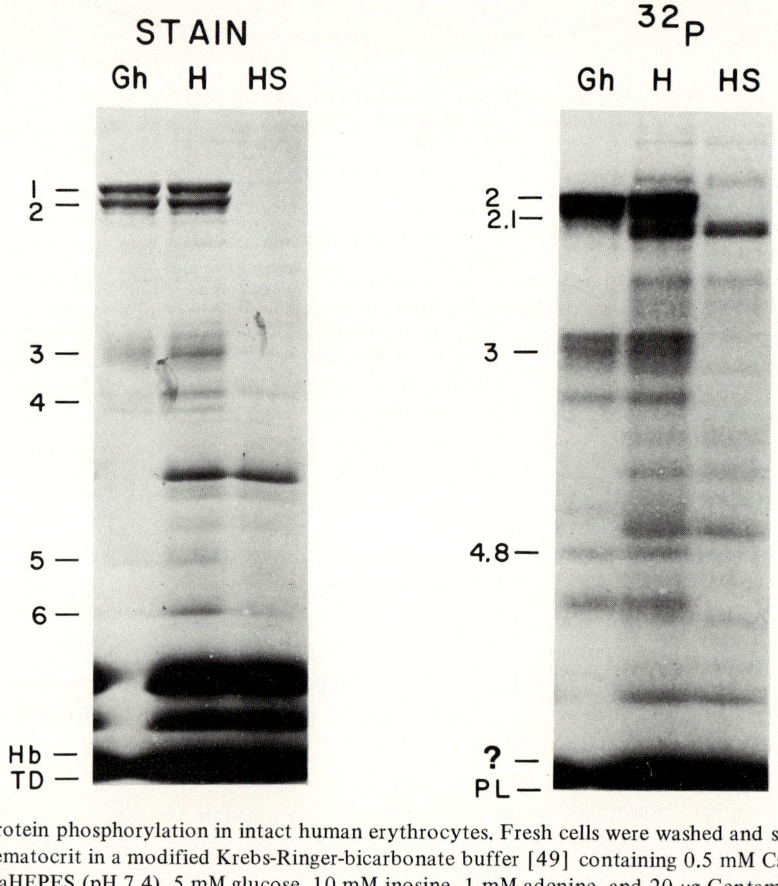

Fig. 2. Protein phosphorylation in intact human erythrocytes. Fresh cells were washed and suspended at 10% hematocrit in a modified Krebs-Ringer-bicarbonate buffer [49] containing 0.5 mM $CaCl_2$, 20 mM NaHEPES (pH 7.4), 5 mM glucose, 10 mM inosine, 1 mM adenine, and 20 μg Gentamicin/ml plus carrier-free ^{32}Pi at approximately 400 μCi/ml. The suspension was incubated at 37°C with gentle shaking and continuous gassing with humidified 5% CO_2/95% N_2. After 18 h, the cells were washed and hemolyzed [50] for membrane preparation. Samples of the hemolysate (H), hemolysate supernatant (cytoplasmic extract – HS), and washed membranes (Gh) were subjected to electrophoresis in Maizel/Laemmli slab gels [51]. The Coomassie blue staining patterns (left panel) are compared with the [^{32}P] distributions in the same lanes revealed by autoradiography (right panel). Protein from approximately 2.3 μl packed cells was applied to each lane; in H and Gh, this represented 8 μg membrane protein. Methods used in sample preparation and autoradiography of slices from stained slabs will be described in a future report.

Phosphorylation of endogenous substrates in isolated membranes requires addition of Mg^{++} and nucleoside triphosphate (either ATP or GTP, with the γ-^{32}P-labeled nucleotide as tracer). Incubation conditions have varied greatly in many respects, but, in all published labeling patterns, [^{32}P] spectrin is prominent [8–13]. The nature of the phosphorylation sites has not yet been investigated extensively, but it is known that most of the ^{32}P in labeled membranes can be recovered in the stable esters, phosphoserine and phosphothreonine [9, 10]. Our own contributions [11, 12, 26] have stressed the effects of cations and cAMP. Based on high-resolution fractionation of the substrates and the observation of differential responsiveness to cAMP, monovalent ions, and Ca^{++}, we suggested that at least two protein kinase activities are expressed independently in isolated membranes [11, 12]. The principal finding was that phosphorylation of spectrin *2* and band *3* is unaffected by cAMP, which selectively stimulates incorporation into several minor components, including *2.1* (mol. wt. ~ 200,000) and *4.5* (mol. wt. ~ 50,000), as indicated in Figure 3. Because band *2.1* migrates at the leading edge of *2*, resolution of the cAMP-dependent and cAMP-independent components of labeling in that zone requires selective elution of spectrin [12] or extended running time in electrophoresis [27]. Hosey and Tao [13, 27, 28] have contributed the useful observation that [γ-^{32}P] GTP can be utilized in the cAMP-independent phosphorylation of bands *2* and *3*, but not in the cAMP-dependent reactions.

Spectrin phosphorylation is stimulated by increasing the ionic strength up to an optimum in the range 0.1–0.2 M NaCl or KCl [11, 15]. This distinguishes it from all the other phosphorylation reactions (including those with band *3* and lipid), which are progressively inhibited with increasing ionic strength. In our early experiments we observed that addition of 1 mM Ca^{++} stimulated spectrin *2* phosphorylation 50–150% [12]. The

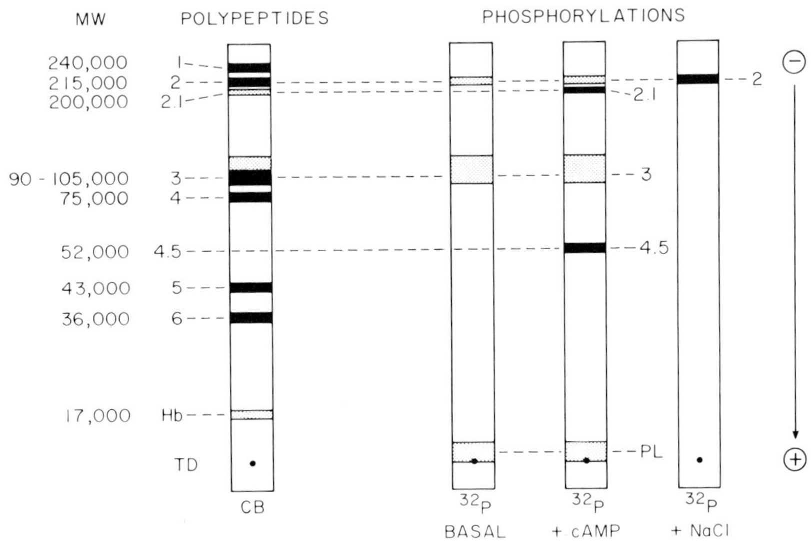

Fig. 3. Schematic representation of endogenous phosphorylation reactions. The band patterns shown are obtained by electrophoretic fractionation of membranes in sodium dodecyl sulfate–polyacrylamide gels after phosphorylation in 10-second reactions with 2 μM [γ-^{32}P] ATP in 1 mM $MgCl_2$ – 20 mM imidazole chloride (pH 7.4) [11, 12]. Addition of 20 μM cAMP or 0.2 M NaCl to the basal reaction mixture alters phosphorylation as diagrammed. Band *4.5* corresponds to the band labeled *4.8* in reports by Hosey and Tao [13, 28] and in Figure 2. [From ref. 26].

reactions were initiated by adding ghosts (to 1 mg/ml protein) to the mixture of Mg[γ-^{32}P] ATP, salts, and buffer. We suspect that Ca^{++} stimulation under these conditions is a transient effect resulting from Ca^{++}-spectrin interaction. Other laboratories have reported only inhibition by Ca^{++} [8, 9]; when we regulated the concentration of free Ca^{++} using an EGTA buffer system, the ion exerted inhibition of spectrin phosphorylation over the entire range tested – 10^{-7}–10^{-3}M [unpublished observations]. Because increased internal Ca^{++} is associated with dramatic alterations of shape in both metabolically depleted cells and reconstituted ghosts [1], the interactions of Ca^{++} with the spectrin phosphorylation–dephosphorylation system need to be examined in greater detail.

PROPERTIES OF SPECTRIN KINASE

The interpretation of the endogenous phosphorylation reactions is fraught with ambiguities because both protein kinases and substrates are semi-immobilized in the membrane, where their interactions may be subject to complex control. The isolation and characterization of spectrin kinase, the analysis of its regulation in a defined system, and the study of its mode(s) of binding to the membrane all require a quantitative assay of enzyme activity. Histone and casein kinase activities have been detected in both the cytoplasmic and membrane fractions of human erythrocytes [7, 13, 26, 29, 30]. These exogenous reactions have properties that correspond in general with the major distinguishing features of the endogenous reactions [26]. The cAMP-dependent histone kinases have not been studied extensively, because their function in a cell lacking significant levels of adenylate cyclase [31–33] is obscure. Our attention is directed to the cAMP-independent, salt-stimulated casein kinase, which appears to represent the enzyme phosphorylating spectrin *2* and, possibly, band *3* [26, 28].

Hosey and Tao have reported [29] that the membrane-associated casein kinase is unaffected by purified regulatory subunit of cAMP-dependent protein kinase under conditions that abolish activity directed against histone. We have made similar observations using the heat-stable inhibitor protein of rabbit skeletal muscle [34], which inhibits only the histone kinase activity [unpublished observations]. Both results establish that the casein kinase of the membrane is a true cAMP-independent, or type III [6], protein kinase.

Attempts to purify this enzyme have so far met with limited success. This is attributable, at least in part, to the capricious instability of the casein kinase, its tendency to aggregate at low ionic strength, and the fact that it is a minor component of the membrane. (Electrophoretic analysis of salt extracts indicates that the molar excess of spectrin over spectrin kinase must be at least 10:1 [unpublished observations].) Other laboratories have encountered the same frustrations [28, 29].

The observations that 1) spectrin phosphorylation is stimulated by salt and that 2) spectrin kinase is not eluted efficiently with spectrin at low ionic strength [11] led us to investigate systematically the effects of salt on enzyme–membrane interaction. Some results of this line of work are presented in Figure 4. As demonstrated earlier [26, 29], the casein kinase of the human red cell membrane is rapidly and selectively eluted by washing with 0.5 M NaCl at 0–4°C. It is evident in Figure 4 that the salt-elution profile for the enzyme is quite broad compared to that for glyceraldehyde-3-phosphate dehydrogenase. There is no evidence to suggest that the enzyme itself is heterogeneous, but its environment on the membrane may vary significantly. (The "tail" on the elution profile at low salt concentrations may reflect the presence of some readily dissociated aggregates, like

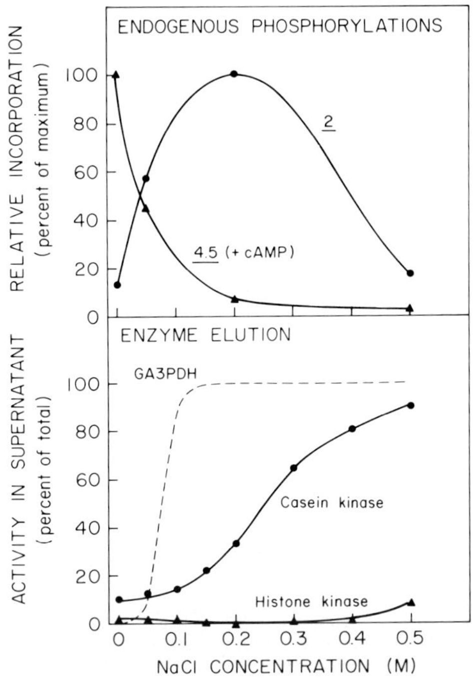

Fig. 4. Salt concentration dependence of endogenous phosphorylation reactions and protein kinase elution. Upper curves are derived from published data on the phosphorylation of spectrin *2* and band *4.5* (Fig. 3) [11]. Lower curves are enzyme elution profiles obtained in 20-min extractions of ghosts diluted 1/10 in ice-cold 5 mM sodium phosphate (pH 8) – 1 mM dithioerythritol plus salt at the indicated final concentrations. Protein kinase activities were measured as described previously [26]. Elution is expressed as percent of total activity released to the 3.5×10^5 g-min supernatants.

those demonstrated in Figure 5. However, it is unlikely that aggregation is responsible for the retention of casein kinase by membranes, because lysis in isotonic $NaHCO_3$–NH_4Cl does not alter partitioning between membrane and cytoplasm [unpublished observations].) It is of interest that salt concentrations that are effective in eluting casein kinase are inhibitory in the endogenous phosphorylation of spectrin *2* (Fig. 4). This suggests that the salt optimum for phosphorylation [11] may be attributed to local enhancement of enzyme–substrate interaction rather than the release of enzyme to the solution phase.

Extraction with 0.5 M NaCl has been the basis for resolving the cAMP-independent and cAMP-dependent protein kinases of the membrane [26, 28, 29]. We have extracted over 85% of the casein kinase activity while leaving at least 85% of the histone kinase in the membranes [26]. After removal of salts, the extracted membranes exhibited unimpaired phosphorylation of bands *2.1* and *4.5* in the cAMP-dependent endogenous reactions, but spectrin phosphorylation was reduced to about 15% of the original level. Significantly, when the dialyzed extract was restored to the membranes in its original proportion, spectrin *2* phosphorylation was elevated to about 50% of the level in unextracted membranes, whereas none of the cAMP-dependent reactions was altered [unpublished observations]. Selective phosphorylation by a salt extract was also demonstrated in semi-quantitative experiments by Hosey and Tao [28]. These findings constitute the best evidence available that the salt-extractable casein kinase is identical to spectrin kinase. Clearly, however, the

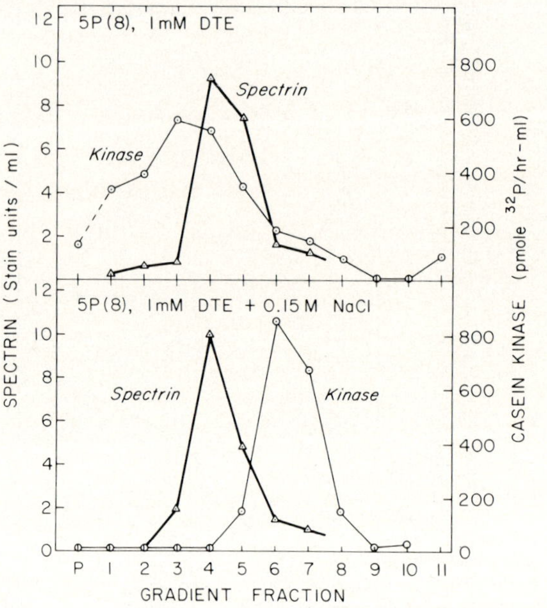

Fig. 5. Zone sedimentation analysis of spectrin and casein kinase in a low ionic strength extract. Ghosts were prepared from fresh red cells as described previously [50], except that hemolysis was carried out by 1/30 dilution into stirred 5 mM sodium phosphate (pH 8)–1 mM EDTA–0.25 mM dithioerythritol at 37°C. The extract was prepared by 1/5 dilution of packed washed ghosts into 0.1 mM EDTA (pH 8) at 37°C followed by homogenization and centrifugation for 6×10^6 g-min [50]. Samples (0.5 ml) were layered on 20–40% glycerol gradients (4.2 ml) containing 5 mM sodium phosphate (pH 8)–1 mM dithoerythritol, with or without saline as indicated, and centrifuged for 20 h at 50,000 rpm using a Spinco SW56Ti rotor. Gradient fractions were assayed for casein kinase activity [26]. Spectrin concentrations were determined by densitometric scanning of stained sodium dodecyl sulfate–polyacrylamide gels.

possibility that spectrin kinase simply cofractionates with other cAMP-independent protein kinase(s) cannot be excluded until the enzyme is purified to homogeneity.

In our experiments, we noted that salt extraction and reconstitution depleted and restored the capacity to phosphorylate band *3* just as described above for spectrin. Hosey and Tao [28] also noted that the salt-extracted enzyme selectively phosphorylated both spectrin *2* and band *3* in membranes in which the endogenous enzymes were inactivated by prior treatment with heat or 2,3-dimethylmaleic anhydride. The possibility that the salt-stimulated spectrin kinase phosphorylates band *3* in a salt-*inhibited* reaction is thus raised; resolution of the question awaits progress in the isolation and characterization of the salt-extracted enzyme(s).

Selective elution of spectrin, actin, and minor membrane proteins at low ionic strength has also been helpful in analyzing the organization of the spectrin phosphorylation system [11]. In repeated measurements we have determined that only about 20% of the membrane-associated casein kinase is eluted with spectrin [unpublished observations]. This correlates perfectly with the low spectrin phosphorylation in the extracts [11] and strongly suggests that most spectrin kinase is not bound to its substrate in the membrane but occupies separate sites nearby. There is no evidence that more than one enzyme is involved: The eluted and retained enzymes have the same salt optimum in the reaction with casein; and both the enzyme eluted at low ionic strength and the total salt-extracted enzyme sediment as a single peak (apparent mol. wt. 30,000–45,000) in sucrose gradients containing salt [Fig 5, ref 29 and unpublished observations]. When spectrin eluates are fractionated by zone sedimentation in low salt, as shown in Figure 5 (upper panel), the casein kinase sediments much more rapidly and appears heterogenous. In this respect also it resembles the salt-extracted enzyme, which aggregates variably when the ionic strength is reduced [29; unpublished observations]. The sedimentation profiles of spectrin and casein kinase differ markedly, suggesting that specific interactions between the two are minimal in the low ionic strength eluate.

Table I summarizes the available information on the properties of the putative spectrin kinase present in isolated membranes. The extent to which the properties of casein kinase faithfully reflect those of spectrin kinase is a fundamental question that must be addressed in the future. Other important issues to be considered are the utilization of [γ-^{32}P]GTP by spectrin kinase and the relationship between the membrane-bound and cytoplasmic forms of cAMP-independent protein kinase.

In their analysis of the endogenous phosphorylation reactions, Hosey and Tao [13] observed that [γ-^{32}P]GTP would serve as a phosphate donor only in the cAMP-independent phosphorylation of spectrin *2* and band *3*. These results are consistent with the distinctions derived from experiments on enzyme extraction and reconstitution [26, 28]. The use of [γ-^{32}P]GTP with crude red cell fractions is problematic because of the high activity of nucleoside diphosphokinase [35], which rapidly forms [γ-^{32}P]ATP from endogenous ADP. However, labeled ATP is not produced in this fashion in assays of purified reticulocyte protein kinase [4] or in incubation of isolated membranes [28; unpublished observations]. According to Hosey and Tao [28, 29], the cAMP-independent casein kinase of the membrane cannot utilize [γ-^{32}P]GTP in phosphorylating casein but readily accepts GTP as a phosphate donor in the endogenous reaction and in the phosphorylation of heat-inactivated membranes by extracted enzyme. The mechanism by which interaction with the membrane confers the ability to accept GTP as phosphate donor is unkonwn.

Because of the metabolic dependence of casein kinase partitioning [26] (see below), the relationship between the membrane-bound and cytoplasmic forms is of great interest. The casein kinases from the two cellular compartments exhibit similar properties in zone sedimentation and gel filtration [29, 36; unpublished observations]. However, neither form

TABLE I. Properties of Membrane-Bound Casein (Spectrin) Kinase*

cAMP-independent
Salt-stimulated
Extracted by 0.5 M NaCl
Aggregates in < 0.1 M NaCl
MW 30-45,000 in > 0.1 M NaCl
Optimum pH ~ 7.5
Optimum [Mg^{++}] 2–5 mM
K_m(ATP) ~ 65 μM
GTP utilization?
Relationship to cytoplasmic casein kinase?

*K_m(ATP) and optimums for pH and Mg^{++} are data of Hosey and Tao [29] on the rabbit enzyme. The most rigorous mol. wt. estimate was also made by Hosey and Tao [29]: the value of 30,000 is based on their results in gel filtration and zone sedimentation.

has yet been isolated in high purity, so definitive information on possible heterogeneity is lacking. Hosey and Tao [27] partially purified cytoplasmic casein kinase and used it to phosphorylate membranes with [γ-^{32}P] GTP as phosphate donor. This led to the phosphorylation of several minor components in addition to spectrin *2* and band *3* and suggested that the cytoplasmic casein kinase lacks the strict specificity for the two major substrates that is characteristic of the membrane-bound enzyme. It will be important to repeat this experiment using highly purified enzyme.

SPECTRIN DEPHOSPHORYLATION

Dephosphorylation of [^{32}P] spectrin has been observed with both isolated membranes and intact cells subjected to metabolic depletion [17, 37–39]. In general, the dephosphorylation reaction has not been studied with the intensity it merits considering its co-equal status with protein kinase-mediated phosphorylation. In analyzing the kinetics of phosphorylation at 2 μM ATP, we noted that incorporation reached a plateau within 5 min and declined only slightly between 5 and 10 min [11]. As shown in Figure 6, dephosphorylation in isolated membranes is more readily demonstrated with prolonged incubation. However, in the experiment shown, [^{32}P] was released from spectrin *2* and band *3* at an initial rate of only about 50% per hour – less than one-twentieth the rate at which the proteins were phosphorylated prior to continuing incubation.

We have also explored some of the properties of red cell phosphoprotein phosphatase using isolated [^{32}P] spectrin as the substrate [40]. Very high levels of phosphospectrin phosphatase activity were detected in diluted crude cytoplasmic extracts, whereas less

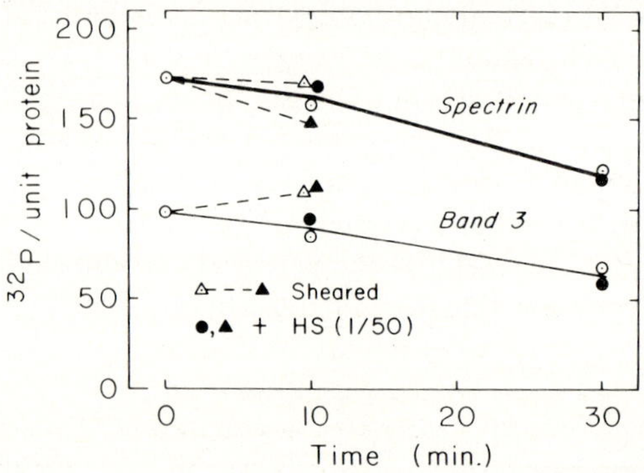

Fig. 6. Dephosphorylation of major membrane phosphopeptides. Ghosts were prepared by 1/100 dilution of washed cells in 10 mM Tris-HCl (pH 7.4)–0.25 mM dithioerythritol, washed once with the same buffer, and once with 20 mM Tris-HCl (pH 7.4)– 0.25 mM dithioerythritol. Phosphorylation of ghosts at 70/106 dilution was performed in 4.7 mM magnesium acetate–22.5 μM [γ-^{32}P] ATP. After incubation for 5 min at 37°C, the suspension was diluted with 30 volumes of cold 20 mM Tris-HCl. The ghosts were sedimented and washed once with the same buffer. Reaction mixtures for dephosphorylation contained 85 μl packed [^{32}P]-labeled ghosts plus 15 μl buffer or dialyzed hemolysate (final concentration 1/50 relative to packed cells). Incubations at 37°C were terminated by rapid addition of 1 ml 10 mM sodium borate (pH 8.3)–1 mM EDTA–5 mM N-ethylmaleimide–0.25 M sucrose–1.6% sodium dodecyl sulfate and heating for 2 min at 95°C. Two samples were sheared during the 10-min incubation using a motor-driven homogenizer with Teflon pestle rotating at 1,400 rpm. After reduction with 40 mM dithioerythritol (pH 8) for 2 min at 95°C, the samples were applied to Maizel/Laemmli [51] cylindrical gels. Counts in the spectrin and band *3* zones were normalized to corresponding areas in densitometer tracings of the stained gels.

than 1% of the total cellular activity was recovered in hemoglobin-free membranes (Table II). Triton X-100 did not significantly activate dephosphorylation of exogenous [^{32}P] spectrin by membranes. Interestingly, dialyzed cytoplasm had no effect on spectrin dephosphorylation in situ under standard conditions but appeared to accelerate dephosphorylation in suspensions that were homogenized during the first 10 min of incubation (Fig. 6). The physical basis of this effect is under study: Shearing appears to enhance the accessibility of [^{32}P] bound to spectrin on the membrane; it might act by expanding holes in the membrane to admit the added enzyme or by changing the conformation of the [^{32}P] spectrin *2* chain in the region of the phosphorylation sites. The data extant leave open the possibility that the cytoplasmic phosphatase is a nonspecific enzyme inactive against native spectrin, while a membrane-bound enzyme not detected in our assay catalyzes dephosphorylation of spectrin in the membrane. Further characterization of the enzyme(s) should resolve this question.

Some potentially significant responses to red cell metabolites were observed in our study of the cytoplasmic phosphatase (Table III). Like other phosphoprotein phosphatases [41], the enzyme is inhibited by fluoride ions. In addition, it is strongly inhibited by inorganic and organic phosphates, particularly those containing multiple phosphate groups. The effects of these compounds have so far been tested only in the absence of Mg^{++}, which in other systems moderates inhibition strikingly [42]. The effect of Mg^{++} may account for the apparent discrepancy between the ATP inhibition we observed in the reaction with solubilized [^{32}P] spectrin and the reported dephosphorylation of spectrin in membranes incubated with MgATP [37–39]. In any case, the concentrations of free 2,3-DPG and ATP in oxygenated red cells are sufficiently high [43] to suppress phosphospectrin phosphatase completely if its regulation in vivo resembles that in the cell-free assay system.

REGULATION

There is no direct evidence that either spectrin kinase or phosphospectrin phosphatase in the human red cell changes activity in response to extracellular signals. Hence, our discussion of regulation is confined to potential roles of metabolic intermediates in modulating enzyme activity and localization and to possible effects of local deformation on enzyme–substrate interaction.

TABLE II. Properties of Human Erythrocyte Phosphospectrin Phosphatase*

Assay conditions		
Substrate:	[^{32}P] spectrin, 1 mg/ml (~ 1X re packed cells)	
Crude enzyme:	Hemolysate supernatant, 0.1 mg/ml protein (~ 1/6000X re packed cells)	
Activity:	Initial rate ~ 60% [^{32}P] release/h at 37°C	
Optimum milieu		
pH ~ 7		
Salt ~ 0.1 M NaCl or KCl		
Subcellular distribution		
Hemolysate super + 1st wash		100%
2nd wash		0
Ghosts		~0.04

*Data from ref 40 and unpublished observations.

Changes in the oxygenation state of hemoglobin alter levels of free ATP, 2,3-DPG and Mg^{++} [43] and may be reflected in the state of spectrin phosphorylation. On the venous side of the circulation, binding of 2,3-DPG to deoxyhemoglobin sharply reduces the level of free 2,3-DPG while elevating the concentration of free Mg^{++}. Under this condition, the casein (spectrin) kinase would be activated due to the increase in Mg^{++} below its optimum concentration (Table I) [29] and, possibly, release from modest inhibition by 2,3-DPG [29]. At the same time, the phosphospectrin phosphatase activity would also be sharply activated as free ATP and 2,3-DPG were sequestered and prevented from exerting their strong inhibition (Table III). The net result could be sharply accelerated turnover of spectrin-bound phosphate. This prediction has yet to be tested, but is of interest because a plausible function for this mode of regulation can be put forth. The necessary assumptions are 1) that spectrin phosphorylation promotes its binding to actin, thereby contributing to the establishment of long-range order in the spectrin–actin lattice [19–21]; and 2) that passage through capillaries is sufficiently traumatic to cause perturbations in membrane organization that require periodic repair. The acceleration of spectrin phosphate turnover in the low-shear environment of the venous circulation would then allow the rearrangement of the spectrin–actin lattice and a realignment of its elements with underlying proteins [25, 44, 45] to establish the optimal state for the maintenance of membrane integrity and deformability under subsequent shear deformation.

We have suggested elsewhere [26] that spectrin phosphorylation might be regulated by translocations of spectrin kinase between membrane and cytoplasm. This speculation was based on the observation that partitioning of casein kinase in the red cell is apparently under metabolic control. Membranes isolated from fresh red cells normally contain about 40% of the total cellular casein kinase activity. However, overnight metabolic depletion elevates membrane retention of casein kinase to a maximum of 75%, whereas incubation with adenine, inosine, and glucose, which elevates intracellular ATP levels [46], reduces the fraction of total enzyme on the membrane to about 25% [26; unpublished observations]. When the incubations are done in a nitrogen atmosphere, these shifts in enzyme localization occur without change in total cellular casein kinase activity.

TABLE III. Inhibitors of Phosphospectrin Phosphatase*

> 75% Inhibition	25–75% Inhibition	< 25% Inhibition
ATP, GTP (0.1 mM)		
ADP, GDP (1 mM)	AMP, GMP (1 mM)	Adenosine (1 mM)
2,3-DPG (5 mM)	2,3-DPG (1 mM)	2,3-DPG (0.5 mM)
PPi (0.1 mM)		
Pi (10mM)	Pi (1 mM)	Pi (0.1 mM)
F^- (10 mM)		F^- (0.1 mM)
	Mg^{++} (10 mM)	Mg^{++} (1 mM)
	Mn^{++} (10 mM)	Mn^{++} (1 mM)
	Ca^{++} (10 mM)	Ca^{++} (1 mM)
		EGTA (1 mM)
		EDTA (1 mM)

*Erythrocyte cytoplasm diluted 1/12000 was incubated at 37°C with 42 μg [^{32}P]spectrin in 0.05 ml mixtures containing 20 mM NaHEPES (pH 7.0)–0.1 M KCl–4 mM dithiothreitol–1 mM EDTA plus additions at the concentrations indicated (EDTA omitted in tests of EGTA and divalent cations). Inhibition was calculated as percent reduction in [^{32}Pi] release relative to controls incubated without additions.

Figure 7 shows the results of two attempts to correlate the endogenous phosphorylation reactions in isolated membranes with the increase in protein kinase activity induced by metabolic depletion. Because the membranes from depleted cells contain higher levels of casein kinase, and because the acceptor capacity of the substrate, spectrin, is presumably elevated due to progressive dephosphorylation [37,38], we expected to observe a significant increase in the rate of spectrin phosphorylation in the endogenous reaction. In fact, we consistently produce the paradoxical finding illustrated – a slight reduction in spectrin phosphorylation in the face of a 40–70% increase in membrane-bound casein kinase [unpublished observations]. The accessibility of a membrane inner surface marker, glyceraldehyde-3-phosphate dehydrogenase, is nearly 100% for both membrane preparations, so the results cannot be attributed to preferential resealing of membranes from depleted cells.

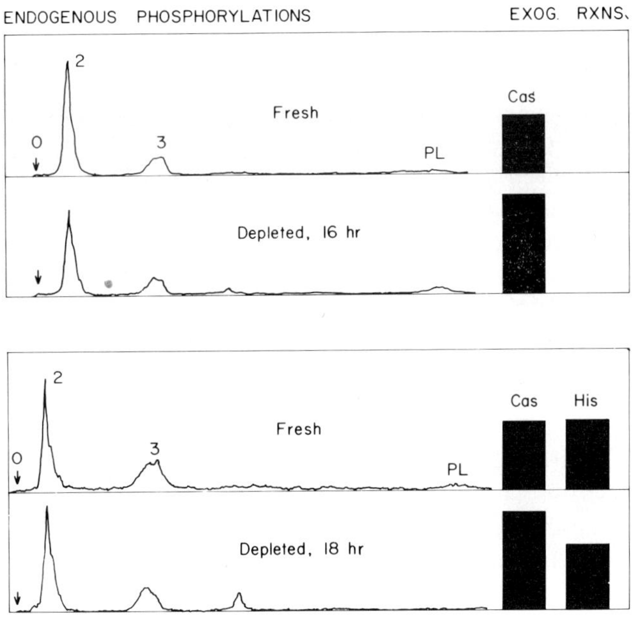

Fig. 7. Endogenous phosphorylation reactions in membranes from fresh and metabolically depleted cells. Red cells were depleted metabolically by overnight incubation in modified Krebs–Ringer–bicarbonate as described in Figure 2, but in the absence of adenine, inosine, and glucose. Fresh cells were drawn from the same donor on the second day and washed in the same medium. Leaky ghosts were prepared from the washed cells by hemolysis in 5 mM sodium phosphate–1 mM EDTA–0.25 mM dithioerythritol at 37°C, as described in Figure 5. The membranes were phosphorylated in 20-sec reactions with 2 μM [γ-^{32}P]ATP in 5 mM magnesium acetate–20 mM NaHEPES (pH 7.5). The reactions were terminated by adding 1.1% sodium dodecyl sulfate–5.6 mM EDTA–0.24 M sucrose–14 mM dithioerythritol (final concentrations) and incubating in a boiling water bath for 2 min. The solubilized proteins were resolved by electrophoresis in Tris-acetate-EDTA gels at pH 7.4 [50]. The [^{32}P] labeling patterns are densitometer scans of autoradiographs of dried longitudinal slices [11]. Casein and histone kinase activities (Cas and His, respectively, at the right) in the membranes were measured as described previously [26] and are displayed as vertical bars with arbitrary units.

These findings raise questions that cannot be answered on the basis of current knowledge of the spectrin phosphorylation–dephosphorylation system:

1. Is the extra membrane-bound casein kinase a distinct enzyme that is unable to utilize spectrin or other major membrane proteins as its substrate? This would imply that the cytoplasmic form of casein kinase is not identical to spectrin kinase.
2. Is the extra enzyme bound in a fashion that renders it nonfunctional? Possibilities include aggregation or localization at sites remote from the phosphorylated segment of spectrin *2*.
3. Does metabolic depletion induce membrane alterations that hinder the normal interaction between spectrin and its kinase? Palek and associates [47, 48] have demonstrated changes in susceptibility to oxidative cross-linking in membranes of cells depleted under nitrogen. We postulate that membrane reorganization under these conditions leads to a state in which phosphate acceptor sites on the protein are less accessible to the kinase.

Clearly, the ultimate resolution of the apparent paradox of Figure 7 will require further comparative studies of the membrane and cytoplasmic casein kinase(s) together with a definitive analysis of enzyme binding to the membrane under various conditions.

Both models considered above involve chemical signals that modify enzyme activity or localization. The schemes relegate spectrin phosphorylation to a secondary role in relation to other cellular functions because they do not envision a mechanism for feedback regulation. In fact, if spectrin phosphorylation indeed controls red cell shape and membrane material properties, the regulatory apparatus should have the capacity to sense deviations from optimal shape or alterations in membrane organization induced by deformation. We find it intriguing that most of the membrane-bound spectrin kinase activity is apparently not associated with spectrin itself but is bound to some other site on the membrane. Given this mode of organization, it is conceivable that physical stress on the membrane alters the intermolecular distance between spectrin and spectrin kinase or shifts spectrin conformation to promote or inhibit the phosphorylation reaction. Such local effects would permit the spectrin-phosphorylation system to serve as a sensor for membrane deformation and would provide feedback regulation without the elaboration of chemical signals.

Although much progress has been made in describing some properties of the enzymes involved in phosphorylation and dephosphorylation, as well as in defining membrane elements that respond to alterations in phosphorylation state, most of the data are indirect and compromised by major ambiguities. As we have repeatedly stated above, isolation and characterization of membrane and cytoplasmic forms of casein kinase and phosphospectrin phosphatase is indispensable. Ultimately, this will lead to definitive identification of the enzymes involved and will permit the analysis of enzyme regulation in defined systems in which metabolite interconversion is precluded. Work in our laboratories is directed at the characterization of casein (spectrin) kinase binding sites on the membrane and at analysis of effects of membrane deformation on spectrin phosphorylation. Further knowledge of these may clarify our ideas concerning regulation at the level of enzyme–substrate interaction. We are hopeful that, just as the study of the red cell membrane has contributed greatly to present understanding of membrane structure in general, continued investigation of the spectrin phosphorylation–dephosphorylation system may lead to useful insights into the more complex mechanisms of cAMP-independent regulation of protein phosphorylation in nucleated cells.

ACKNOWLEDGMENTS

This work was supported by NIH grants AM 16914, HL 15157 (Boston Sickle Cell Center) and HL 19933; and by NCI grant P30 12708. G.F. was aided by a Cancer Research Scholar Award from the American Cancer Society, Massachusetts Division, Inc., and by the Mimi Aaron Greenberg Cancer Research Institute. J.A. was the recipient of a Research and Development Award from the American Diabetes Association and is an Investigator of the Howard Hughes Research Institute.

REFERENCES

1. Weed RI, LaCelle PL, Merrill EW: J Clin Invest 48:795, 1969.
2. Palmer FBStC, Verpoorte JA: Can J Biochem 49:337, 1971.
3. Tao M, Salas ML, Lipmann F: Proc Natl Acad Sci USA 67:408, 1970.
4. Traugh JA, Traut RR: J Biol Chem 249:1207, 1974.
5. Tao M, Hackett P: J Biol Chem 248:5324, 1973.
6. Traugh JA, Ashby CD, Walsh, DA: Meth Enzymol 38:290, 1974.
7. Rubin CS, Erlichman J, Rosen OM: J Biol Chem 247:6135, 1972.
8. Guthrow CE, Allen JE, Rasmussen H: J Biol Chem 247:8145, 1972.
9. Roses AD, Appel SH: J Biol Chem 248:1408, 1973.
10. Rubin CS, Rosen OM: Biochem Biophys Res Comm 50:421, 1973.
11. Avruch J, Fairbanks G: Biochemistry 13:5507, 1974.
12. Fairbanks G, Avruch J: Biochemistry 13:5514, 1974.
13. Hosey MM, Tao M: Biochemistry 15:1561, 1976.
14. Valentine WN: Blood 49:241, 1977.
15. Wolfe LC, Lux SE: J Biol Chem 253, In press.
16. Sheetz MP, Singer SJ: J Cell Biol 73:638. 1977.
17. Birchmeier W, Singer SJ: J Cell Biol 73:647, 1977.
18. Pinder JC, Bray D, Gratzer WB: Nature 258:765, 1975.
19. Pinder JC, Bray D, Gratzer WB: Nature 270:752, 1977.
20. Pinder JC: J Supramol Struct 8:439–446, 1978.
21. Ralston GB: J Supramol Struct 8:361–379, 1978.
22. Harris HW Jr, Wolfe LC, Lux SE: J Supramol Struct Suppl 2:204, 1978.
23. Anderson JM, Tyler JM: In Lux S, Marchesi VT, Fox CF (eds): "Normal and Abnormal Red Cell Membranes." New York: Alan R Liss, (In press).
24. Fowler V, Branton D: Nature 268:23, 1977.
25. Goodman SR, Branton D: J Supramol Struct 8:455–463, 1978.
26. Avruch J, Fairbanks G, Crapo LM: J Cell Physiol 89:815, 1976.
27. Hosey MM, Tao M: J Biol Chem 252:102, 1977.
28. Hosey MM, Tao M: Biochemistry 16:4578, 1977.
29. Hosey MM, Tao M: Biochim Biophys Acta 482:348, 1977.
30. Rubin CS: J Biol Chem 250:9044, 1975.
31. Wolfe SM, Shulman NR: Biochem Biophys Res Commun 35:265, 1969.
32. Sheppard H, Burghardt CR: Biochem Pharmacol 18:2576, 1969.
33. Rodan SB, Rodan GA, Sha'afi RI: Biochim Biophys Acta 428:509, 1976.
34. Walsh DA, Ashby CD, Gonzalez C, Calkins D, Fischer EH, Krebs G: J Biol Chem 246:1977, 1971.
35. Mourad N, Parks RE Jr: J Biol Chem 241:271, 1966.
36. Fairbanks G, Avruch J, Dino JE, Bober K: J Cell Biol 70:243a, 1976.
37. Greenquist AC, Shohet AB: In Brewer G (ed): "Erythrocyte Structure and Function." New York: Alan R Liss, 1975, p 515.
38. Greenquist AC, Shohet SB: Blood 48:877, 1976.
39. Beutler E, Guinto E, Johnson C: Blood 48:887, 1976.
40. Graham C, Avruch J, Fairbanks G: Biochem Biophys Res Commun 72:701, 1976.
41. Mayer SE, Krebs EG: J Biol Chem 245:3153, 1970.
42. Nakai C, Thomas JA: J Biol Chem 249:6459, 1974.
43. Bunn HF, Ransil BJ, Chao A: J Biol Chem 246:5273, 1971.
44. Sheetz MP, Sawyer D: J Supramole Struct 8:399–412, 1978.

45. Litman D, Chen JH, Marchesi VT: J Supramol Struct Suppl 2:209, 1978.
46. Warrendorf EM, Rubenstein D: Blood 42:637, 1973.
47. Palek J, Liu SC, Snyder LM: Blood 51:385, 1978.
48. Palek J, Liu D: J Supramol Struct (In press).
49. Umbreit WW, Burris RH, Stauffer JF: Manometric Techniques. Minneapolis: Burgess, p 132, 1957.
50. Fairbanks G, Steck TL, Wallach DFH: Biochemistry 10:2606, 1971.
51. Laemmli UK: Nature 227:680, 1970.

Journal of Supramolecular Structure 9:113–124 (1978)
Normal and Abnormal Red Cell Membranes 229–240

Actin—Membrane Interactions: Association of G-Actin With the Red Cell Membrane

Carl M. Cohen, Pamela L. Jackson, and Daniel Branton

Cell and Developmental Biology, The Biological Laboratories, Harvard University, Cambridge, Massachusetts 02138

Chemically tritiated actin from rabbit skeletal muscle was used to investigate the association of G-actin with the red cell membrane. The tritiated actin was shown to be identical to unmodified actin in its ability to polymerize and to activate heavy meromyosin ATPase. Using sealed and unsealed red cell ghosts we have shown that G-actin binds to the cytoplasmic but not the extracellular membrane surface of ghosts. Inside-out vesicles which have been stripped of endogenous actin and spectrin by low-ionic-strength incubation bind little G-actin. However, when a crude spectrin extract containing primarily spectrin, actin, and band 4.1 is added back to stripped vesicles, subsequent binding of G-actin can be increased up to 40-fold. Further, this crude spectrin extract can compete for and abolish G-actin binding to unsealed ghosts. Actin binding to ghosts increases linearly with added G-actin and requires the presence of magnesium. In addition, actin binding is inhibited by cytochalasin B and DNAase I. Negative staining reveals an abundance of actin filaments formed when G-actin is added to reconstituted inside-out vesicles but none when it is added to unreconstituted vesicles. These observations indicate that added G-actin binds to the red cell membrane via filament formation nucleated by some membrane component at the cytoplasmic surface.

Key words: spectrin, actin, actin binding to red cell membrane

The filamentous proteins actin and myosin are thought to be responsible for most types of eukaryotic cell motility and frequently form extensive trans-cellular networks which seem to determine and stabilize cell shape by a direct or indirect association with the plasma membrane [1–3]. Actin has been found in association with plasma membranes from a variety of cells [2, 4–7] and has also been shown to associate with membranes of

Dr. Cohen's present address is St. Elizabeth's Hospital, Dept of Research 736 Cambridge St, Boston, MA 02135.

Received April 11, 1978; accepted July 3, 1978.

secretory vesicles [8, 9]. In addition, there is suggestive evidence for a transmembrane linkage of cell surface receptors and integral membrane proteins with submembrane actin filaments [10, 11]. While such morphological and biochemical studies provide strong evidence that some fraction of a cell's actin complement is associated with its plasma membrane, the molecular nature of this association is not understood.

The red cell is known to contain membrane-associated actin [12, 13], and although this cell is nonmotile, its membrane serves as an important model for those of more complex cells. Further, its mechanochemical properties are interesting in their own right, since it is now recognized that red cell shape and deformability both in normal and disease states are primarily determined by the cell membrane [14–16]. Even in diseases where the initial lesion is not of membrane origin, such as sickle cell anemia, the final result can be loss of intrinsic membrane flexibility [16]. Since these properties of the membrane may determine the in vivo fate of both abnormal red cells and normal aged cells, an understanding of molecular interactions in the membrane is of interest from both a medical and a biochemical viewpoint.

Although it has been repeatedly suggested that the mechanical properties of the red cell membrane are controlled by its interaction with red cell actin and the high-molecular-weight protein spectrin, only recently has a specific association of spectrin with the membrane been demonstrated [17]. While actin is present in nearly a 1:1 molar ratio with spectrin, much less is known about its association with the membrane. The fact that actin and spectrin appear to coelute from the membrane at low ionic strength [18] and form a self-associating filamentous network upon solubilization of membrane lipids by detergent [19] has led to the proposal that these molecules may interact with each other in vivo [13]. Although recent work [20, 13] has provided some evidence of a spectrin–actin interaction, its nature and physiological relevance is far from clear.

To study how actin associates with membranes, we have begun an investigation of actin binding to the red cell membrane using ^{3}H-G-actin. The use of radioactive actin in these experiments offers several advantages: 1) It allows the quantification of membrane-associated actin; 2) it permits the study of actin binding to membranes at very low concentrations of either G- or F-actin, minimizing possible nonspecific associations. We describe here some preliminary studies of the associations formed when G-actin is added to the red cell membrane; a report of similar studies with F-actin is in preparation [C.M. Cohen, P.L. Jackson, and D. Branton, in preparation].

MATERIALS AND METHODS

Preparation of ^{3}H-Actin

Actin was extracted from rabbit skeletal muscle by the method of Spudich and Watt [21] and stored as a powder after colyophilization with 2 mg sucrose/mg actin. Prior to labeling, 2–6 mg of actin powder was suspended at a protein concentration of 2–3 mg/ml in 3 mM imidazole, pH 7.5, 0.1 mM $CaCl_2$, 0.5 mM ATP, homogenized gently in a Teflon–glass Dounce homogenizer, and dialyzed for 18 hours against this same buffer at 4°C. Sulfhydryl reducing agents were omitted from the buffer so as not to interfere with the labeling reaction. The G-actin was then centrifuged at 150,000g for 30 minutes at 4°C to remove aggregated material, after which the protein concentration was determined by the Lowry method.

An amount of ^{3}H-N-ethylmaleimide (in pentane, New England Nuclear Corp., Boston, Mass) calculated to be 3.5 × the amount of actin to be labeled, on a molar basis, was added to the bottom of a 5-ml glass test tube. The tube was then rotated, to allow the N-ethylmaleimide (NEM)–pentane to coat the sides, until all visible pentane had evaporated. G-Actin (typically 2 ml of a 2 mg/ml solution) was then added to the tube and incubated with the ^{3}H-NEM at room temperature with gentle agitation for 0.5 hours, after which the reaction was terminated by the addition of 2 mM β-mercaptoethanol (final concentration). Additional experiments demonstrated that lengthening the time of labeling beyond 0.5 hour or increasing the amount of ^{3}H-NEM added did not significantly increase the amount of ^{3}H-NEM incorporated into the actin. The G-actin was clarified by centrifugation at 150,000g for 30 minutes to remove any aggregated material which may have formed, polymerized by the addition of 0.1 M KCl and 2 mM $MgCl_2$ (final concentration), and incubated at 25°C for 1.5 hours. The F-actin was collected by centrifugation at 150,000g for 2.5 hours and resuspended to about 2 ml in 3 mM imidazole, pH 7.5, 0.1 mM $CaCl_2$, 0.5 mM ATP, and 0.75 mM β-mercaptoethanol. The resuspended actin was gently dispersed in a Teflon–glass Dounce homogenizer and dialyzed for 2 days at 4°C against 1 liter of the above buffer. Repeating this polymerization and dialysis had no effect upon the final properties of the labeled actin. After dialysis, the G-actin was again clarified by centrifugation at 150,000g for 30 minutes, made 0.02% w/v in Na azide, and assayed for protein and radioactivity. The ^{3}H-actin was stored in solution either in the G or F form at 4°C for no more than 10 days before use.

Preparation of Red Cell Membranes and Crude Spectrin

Whole blood obtained from donors was stored in plasma at 4°C and used within 1 week. Red cells were washed four times in 140 mM NaCl, 5 mM $NaPO_4$, pH 7.6, and lysed by rapid dilution into 30 volumes of ice-cold 20 mOsm $NaPO_4$, pH 7.6. The ghosts were washed 3–4 times in this buffer until they were white, each time removing the pellet of contaminating white cells [18]. For some experiments, fragmented ghosts were prepared by forceful passage of concentrated white ghosts 4–6 times through a ½ inch 27-g hypodermic needle on a 1-ml syringe until the ghosts had broken down into small vesicles as seen in the phase contrast microscope. The vesicles are morphologically right side out [17] and are unsealed, as shown by 100% accessibility of their cytoplasmic surface by glyceraldehyde 3-phosphate dehydrogenase assay [22; data not shown].

Unsealed spectrin–actin depleted inside-out vesicles were prepared as described by Bennett and Branton [17]. Briefly, ghosts were resuspended in 30 volumes of 0.3 mM $NaPO_4$, pH 7.6, and incubated at 37°C for 30 minutes. The small vesicles resulting from this incubation were centrifuged at 34,000g for 30 minutes and washed once in the same way with ice cold 0.3 mM $NaPO_4$, pH 7.6. In some experiments these vesicles were used directly for actin-binding studies while in others the vesicles were centrifuged on a 10% w/v Dextran T 110 shelf as described [17], and the pellet was used for binding studies. No major differences were observed between the two methods of preparation.

Resealed ghosts were prepared by incubating freshly prepared white ghosts in 20 mOsm $NaPO_4$, pH 7.6, plus 2 mM $MgCl_2$ at 37°C for 40 minutes followed by centrifugation on an equal volume of 1.03 g/ml dextran (160,000 mol wt, Sigma) in an SW 40 rotor at 40,000 rpm for 2 hours. Sealed ghosts were collected from the buffer–Dextran interface and washed twice in 20 mOsm $NaPO_4$, pH 7.6, 2 mM $MgCl_2$, prior to use. Sealed ghosts were generally 85–95% sealed as measured by the glyceraldehyde 3-phosphate dehydrogenase assay [22].

Crude spectrin, containing primarily spectrin (bands 1 and 2), actin (band 5), and band 4.1 (nonmenclature of Fairbanks et al [18]) was prepared from white ghosts made from blood on the same day it was drawn. Ghosts were washed once in ice-cold 0.3 mM $NaPO_4$, pH 7.6, and then resuspended in a volume of this buffer approximately equal to that of the packed ghosts and incubated at 37°C for 25 minutes. The suspension was centrifuged at 150,000g for 30 minutes and the supernatant, containing the crude spectrin, was carefully extracted and the following components were added (final concentrations): 20 mM KCl, 0.7 mM $NaPO_4$, pH 7.6, 1 mM DTT, 0.1 mM $MgCl_2$, 0.05 mM ATP. After these additions, the pH was readjusted to 7.6.

Assay of ^{3}H-Actin Binding to Membranes

^{3}H-G-Actin at concentrations specified in the figure legends was incubated in a volume of 0.8 ml with membranes at a protein concentration of 0.25 mg/ml in 20 mM KCl, 5 mM $NaPO_4$, pH 6.5, 2 mM $MgCl_2$, 1 mM ATP, and 0.75 mM β-mercaptoethanol (actin-binding buffer). Incubations were done on ice for 1 hour, and three 0.2-ml samples were withdrawn and layered on 0.2 ml 20% w/v sucrose (made in actin-binding buffer) in 0.5-ml polyethylene microfuge tubes. The tubes were centrifuged at 18,000 rpm for 25 minutes in a Sorvall SS 34 rotor; and the tips, containing the membrane pellet, were frozen in liquid nitrogen, cut off, and placed into 10 ml of scintillation fluid [toluene: Protosol:Liquefluor (New England Nuclear Corp., Boston, Mass); 1 liter:50 ml:40ml]. The tubes were shaken vigorously and counted for ^{3}H. Control experiments demonstrated that the presence of sucrose from the clipped tube had no effect on counting efficiency. To further test the efficiency of ^{3}H counting by this method, samples containing ghost membranes and ^{3}H-G-actin were centrifuged as described, but the supernatant and sucrose were completely removed by aspiration and the ghost pellet resuspended in 0.4 ml of 1% SDS which was then transferred to scintillation fluid. The counts in these samples and in the clipped tube tips from identical incubations were equivalent to within 15%. No ^{3}H-G-actin sedimented through the sucrose in the absence of membranes under any of the conditions used. Recovery of ghost or vesicle membrane in the pellet was 70–100% (measured by membrane-bound ^{125}I-labeled wheat germ agglutinin) depending upon the conditions of incubation. Corrections for this were applied where appropriate.

Additional Methods

Heavy meromyosin (HMM) was prepared by the method of Lowey and Cohen [23]. Activation of HMM ATPase by F-actin was measured by incubating 50 μg of HMM in the presence or absence of 40 μg F-actin in a volume of 0.5 ml containing (final concentrations) 25 mM Tris, pH 7.0, 2.2 mM $MgCl_2$, 0.8 mM ATP. Incubations were carried out at 25°C for 5 minutes and terminated by the addition of 200 λ of 30% TCA. After centrifugation to remove the precipitate, the supernatant was assayed for inorganic PO_4.

SDS polyacrylamide gel electrophoresis was done by the method of Fairbanks et al [18]. For counting ^{3}H, the gels were frozen and sliced into 1.2-mm sections, each slice was then soaked in 5 ml scintillation fluid (see above) overnight, and counted for ^{3}H. By this procedure, 97–100% of the ^{3}H counts electrophoresed were recovered.

RESULTS

Several properties of the ^{3}H-actin are listed in Table I. The molar ratio of incorporated ^{3}H-NEM to actin varied between 0.7 and 0.95 in 20 separate preparations. This ratio is consistent with observations by others that nondenaturing sulfhydryl reagents such as NEM react rapidly with only one, or possibly two, of actin's six sulfhydryl groups [24–27] and that stoichiometric labeling (1 mole/mole) of actin with either ^{14}C-NEM or spin-labeled NEM can be easily achieved [25, 28]. Table I also shows that the labeled actin is functionally identical to native actin since its ability to activate HMM-ATPase, and to form filaments (as assayed by sedimentation) is not affected by labeling. When ^{3}H-actin was electrophoresed in an SDS polyacrylamide gel (Fig. 1), approximately 97% of the ^{3}H added to the gel comigrated with actin as a single band.

Table II shows the results obtained when various red cell membrane preparations were tested for their ability to bind ^{3}H-G-actin. Resealed ghosts bound little or no ^{3}H-G-actin at the low actin concentration used in this experiment (35 μg/ml). G-Actin binding was generally done at low concentrations and at 0°C to reduce the possibility of spontaneous polymerization. Unsealed ghosts, however, under the same conditions, bound 25.8 μg of the added ^{3}H-G-actin/mg membrane protein. Since these unsealed ghosts already contain ~ 45 μg endogenous actin/mg protein (based on integrated staining intensity of band 5 [29]), the amount of ^{3}H-G-actin bound represents a 50% increase over the endogenous membrane actin. Table II also shows that actin binding to ghosts requires the presence of MgATP in the binding medium. While Mg can cause ghosts to reseal, this generally occurs only at elevated temperatures (these experiments were done at 0°C) so that the MgATP dependence of actin binding is unlikely to result from trapping of actin inside ghosts. In addition, estimation of the internal volume of the ghosts showed that

TABLE I. Properties of (^{3}H)-N-Ethyl Maleimide Actin

Moles N-ethyl maleimide/mole actin	0.7–0.95
Specific activity of ^{3}H-actin	1300–1800 CPM/μg
Activation of HMM-ATPase by ^{3}H-F-actin (% relative to unmodified F-actin)	90–100%
Recovery of ^{3}H-F-actin in 2.3 × 10^{7}g × min pellet (% relative to unmodified F-actin)	100–109%

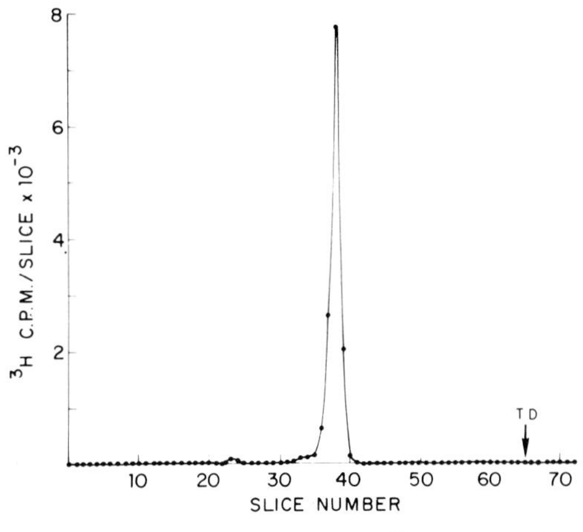

Fig. 1. SDS-polyacrylamide gel electrophoresis of 10 μg of ^{3}H-G-actin. The gel was sliced and counted for ^{3}H as described in Methods. The peak of radioactivity comigrated with the coomassie blue stained actin band (not shown). T D: Tracker Dye.

TABLE II. G-Actin Binding to Red Cell Membranes

	Actin bound $\mu g/mg$ membrane protein
Resealed ghosts	0.05
Unsealed ghosts	
Control	25.8
Minus MgATP	0.4
Plus crude spectrin[a]	3.2
Plus heat-denatured crude spectrin[b]	24.2
Inside-out vesicles	
Control	0.5
Minus MgATP	0.4
Reconstituted with crude spectrin[c]	20.8
Reconstituted:minus MgATP[d]	0.3

Red cell membranes at a protein concentration of 0.25 mg/ml were incubated with ^{3}H-G-actin at a concentration of 35 μg/ml in actin-binding buffer (see Methods) for 1 hour at 0°C. ^{3}H-G-Actin binding was measured as described in Methods. All values are the mean of three determinations; the standard deviation was generally less than 15% of the values shown.

[a]Unsealed ghosts plus ^{3}H-G-actin were incubated as described above with the addition of 50 μg/ml crude spectrin.

[b]Crude spectrin was denatured by heating to 70° C for 5 minutes before inclusion in the assay as described in (a).

[c]Inside-out vesicles (0.3 mg/ml) were incubated with 12.5 μg/ml crude spectrin in actin-binding buffer (see Methods) for 1 hour at 4°C, washed once, resuspended to 0.25 mg/ml, and assayed for actin binding.

[d]Same as (c) except actin binding was done in the absence of MgATP.

actin entrapment could account for less than 20% of the actin bound. The fact that MgATP also greatly stimulates binding to reconstituted inside-out vesicles (see below and Table II) but has little effect on unreconstituted vesicles further demonstrates that factors other than membrane sealing are responsible for actin binding.

Since spectrin is the major protein at the cytoplasmic membrane surface and has been reported to interact with actin [20, 13], we tested the ability of a crude spectrin extract [Fig. 2, gel C), obtained from a separate batch of fresh ghosts, to compete for or inhibit actin binding to unsealed ghosts. Table II shows that when unsealed ghosts were incubated with ^{3}H-G-actin plus a small amount of crude spectrin, actin binding to the ghosts was reduced by nearly 90%. If, however, the crude spectrin was first denatured by heating to 70°C for 5 minutes, it did not inhibit binding to ghosts. These results suggest either that actin bound to some component of free crude spectrin and was prevented from binding to the ghost or that the crude spectrin associated with the ghost in such a way as to prevent actin binding.

To further examine these possibilities, we studied actin binding directly to the cytoplasmic membrane surface by using inside-out vesicles. These vesicles are depleted of most of their endogenous spectrin and actin (Fig. 2, gel B) compared to ghosts (Fig. 2, gel A) and are morphologically inside-out as judged by intramembrane partical distribution seen by freeze fracture [17]. Table II shows that these vesicles bind only a small amount of G-actin. However, if they are first reconstituted with crude spectrin (Fig. 2, gel D) their ability to bind G-actin is increased more than 40-fold, and is close to that of unsealed ghosts. ^{3}H-G-Actin binding to these reconstituted vesicles is also dependent upon the

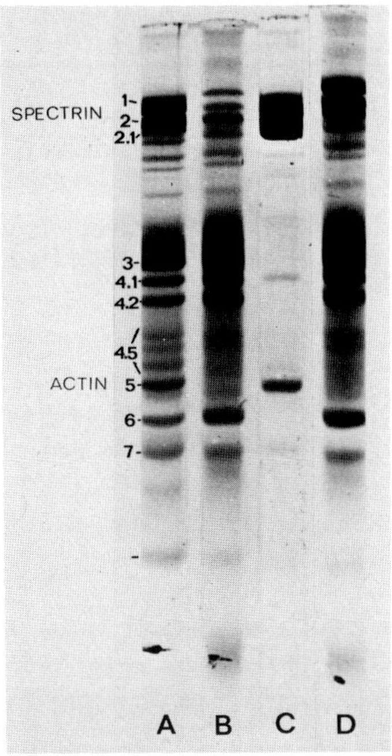

Fig. 2. SDS-polyacrylamide gels of red cell membranes and crude spectrin: a) Unsealed ghosts; b) inside-out vesicles; c) crude spectrin; d) inside-out vesicles reconstituted with crude spectrin (see legend, Table II).

presence of MgATP and is abolished when this is omitted. These experiments show that the inhibition of actin binding to ghosts by crude spectrin described above must be due to actin binding to some component of the free crude spectrin, since if the crude spectrin had associated with the ghost actin binding would have been stimulated rather than inhibited.

Figure 3 shows the concentration dependence of ^{3}H-G-actin binding to the various membrane preparations described above. For these experiments, fragmented ghosts were used (see Methods) since it was found that they bound more ^{3}H-G-actin under all conditions tested than intact ghosts. Fragmented ghosts have a polypeptide composition identical to intact ghosts but are presumably more permeable to G-actin. Figure 3 shows a linear dependence of bound actin on added ^{3}H-G-actin for fragmented ghosts, while the curve for inside-out vesicles reconstituted with crude spectrin is slightly concave. The crude spectrin varied in its ability to stimulate binding of actin to inside-out vesicles (eg compare the stimulation of G-actin binding to inside-out vesicles by crude spectrin in Table II and Fig. 3). The reason for this variability is unclear, but it may be related to the state of phosphorylation of spectrin upon extraction [20] or to the variable presence of F-actin in the crude spectrin (see Discussion). At very low actin concentration ($<$20 μg/ml), the fragmented ghosts bind a small but nearly constant amount of actin, which then increases sharply above 20 μg/ml actin. This transition, along with the concave binding curve for reconstituted inside out vesicles, suggests that actin binding may result from induced polymerization of actin on the membrane above a certain critical concentration.

To explore further the possibility that filament formation is involved in actin binding, we tested the effects of DNAase I which depolymerizes F-actin and forms a highly

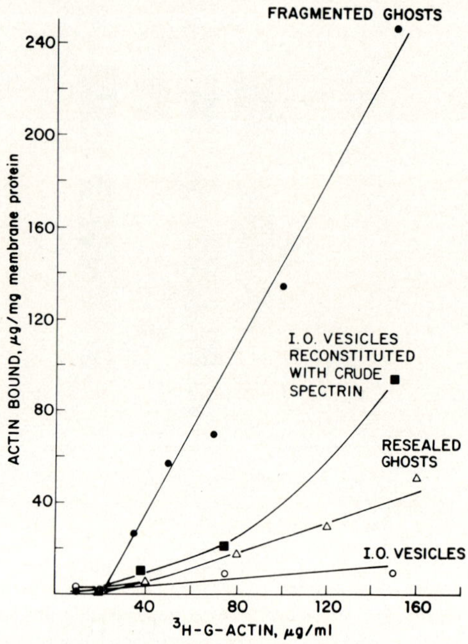

Fig. 3. Concentration dependence of ^{3}H-G-actin binding to red cell membranes. Vesicles or ghosts at a protein concentration of 0.25 mg/ml were incubated in actin binding buffer for 1 hour at 0°C with ^{3}H-G-actin at the concentrations indicated. Inside-out vesicles were reconstituted with crude spectrin as described (see legend, Table II). In this experiment the sealed ghosts bound more ^{3}H-G-actin than the unreconstituted inside-out vesicles (compare with Table II), probably due to contamination of sealed ghosts with unsealed ghosts. All points are the mean of three determinations; the standard deviation was less than 15% of the values shown.

stable 1:1 complex with G-actin [30] and cytochalasin B which has a wide variety of disruptive effects on actin filament-related cellular phenomena [2] and is thought to affect actin filament–actin binding protein interactions [31, 32]. Figure 4a shows that 5 μM cytochalasin B virtually eliminates actin binding to reconstituted inside-out vesicles (dimethyl sulfoxide alone, in which the cytochalasin was added, had no effect) and Figure 4b shows that 50 μg/ml DNAase I (which is 1.6 × molar excess over the G-actin present) completely prevents actin binding. These results suggest that filament formation and filament membrane association are required for binding. This observation was confirmed by negative staining of inside-out vesicles which were reconstituted with crude spectrin and then incubated with G-actin. Figure 5b shows that these vesicles clearly have a large number of actin filaments associated with them, whereas unreconstituted inside-out vesicles treated in the same way had no actin filaments. (Fig. 5a).

DISCUSSION

We have demonstrated that G-actin from rabbit skeletal muscle is capable of forming a specific association with the cytoplasmic surface of the red cell membrane. A similar result has also been reported recently by Birchmeier and Singer [33]. Our data suggest that G-actin binding results from an association of actin with some membrane component present in crude spectrin, which consists primarily of spectrin, actin, and band 4.1. This

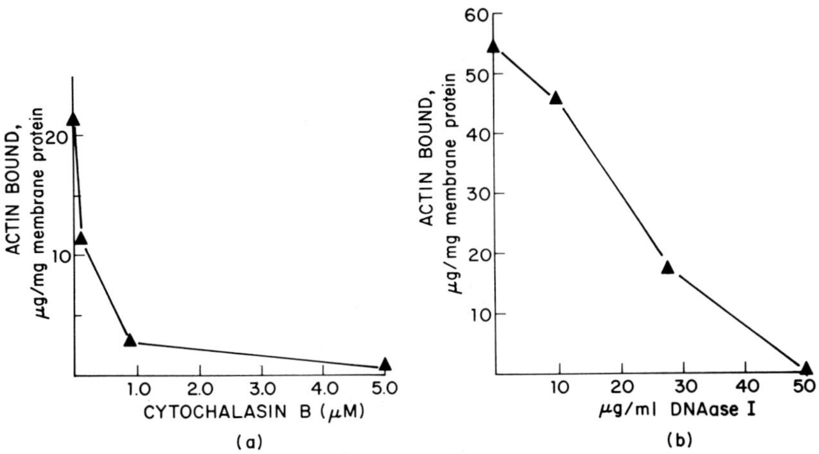

Fig. 4. a) Effect of cytochalasin B on G-actin binding to reconstituted inside-out vesicles. Inside-out vesicles reconstituted with crude spectrin, as described in Table II, were incubated with 48 μg/ml ^{3}H-G-actin in the presence of the indicated concentrations of cytochalasin B obtained by adding 5 μl of 20 μM, 130 μM, 1 mM cytochalasin B in DMSO to a 1 ml incubation. b) Effect of DNAase I on G-actin binding to reconstituted inside-out vesicles. DNAase I in binding buffer was added as a concentrate to vesicles plus 48 μg/ml G-actin. In a) and b) actin binding was measured as described in Methods except that the incubations were only 40 minutes. All points are the mean of three determinations; the standard deviation was less than 15% of the values shown.

conclusion is supported by several observations: 1) Red cell ghost membranes lose their capacity to bind G-actin when converted into inside-out vesicles, a process which results in the specific release from the membrane of spectrin, actin, and some of band 4.1; 2) when inside-out vesicles are reconstituted with crude spectrin, they regain their ability to bind G-actin; 3) crude spectrin in solution will inhibit the binding of G-actin to unsealed ghosts presumably by binding G-actin in solution and preventing it from binding to the ghost membrane. Since this inhibition does not occur after crude spectrin is denatured by heating, it probably represents a specific interaction of actin with some component of the crude spectrin.

The nature of the association between actin and the red cell membrane remains unclear. Although we have shown that G-actin binding is greatly enhanced by the presence of MgATP, ATP itself does not appear to play a role since Mg alone can stimulate binding to the same extent (data not shown). The linear dependence of bound actin on added actin suggests a nonsaturable type of association. While such a feature is generally thought to indicate nonspecific association, this would be hard to reconcile with the high degree of specificity of binding to the cytoplasmic surface and the marked dependence upon Mg. While we cannot rule out the possibility that some of the binding we observe is due to G-actin which binds to the membrane and remains there as monomeric actin, the lack of saturability and dependence on the presence of a divalent cation is consistent with the interpretation that actin binding proceeds by polymerization of G-actin on or from the cytoplasmic membrane surface. This conclusion is supported by our observation that reconstituted inside-out vesicles which have been incubated with G-actin can clearly be seen to have F-actin filaments associated with them (Fig. 5b). Since actin binding is prevented by DNAase I which disrupts or prevents filament formation and cytochalasin B, which may act by inhibiting actin binding protein–actin filament interactions, it is clear

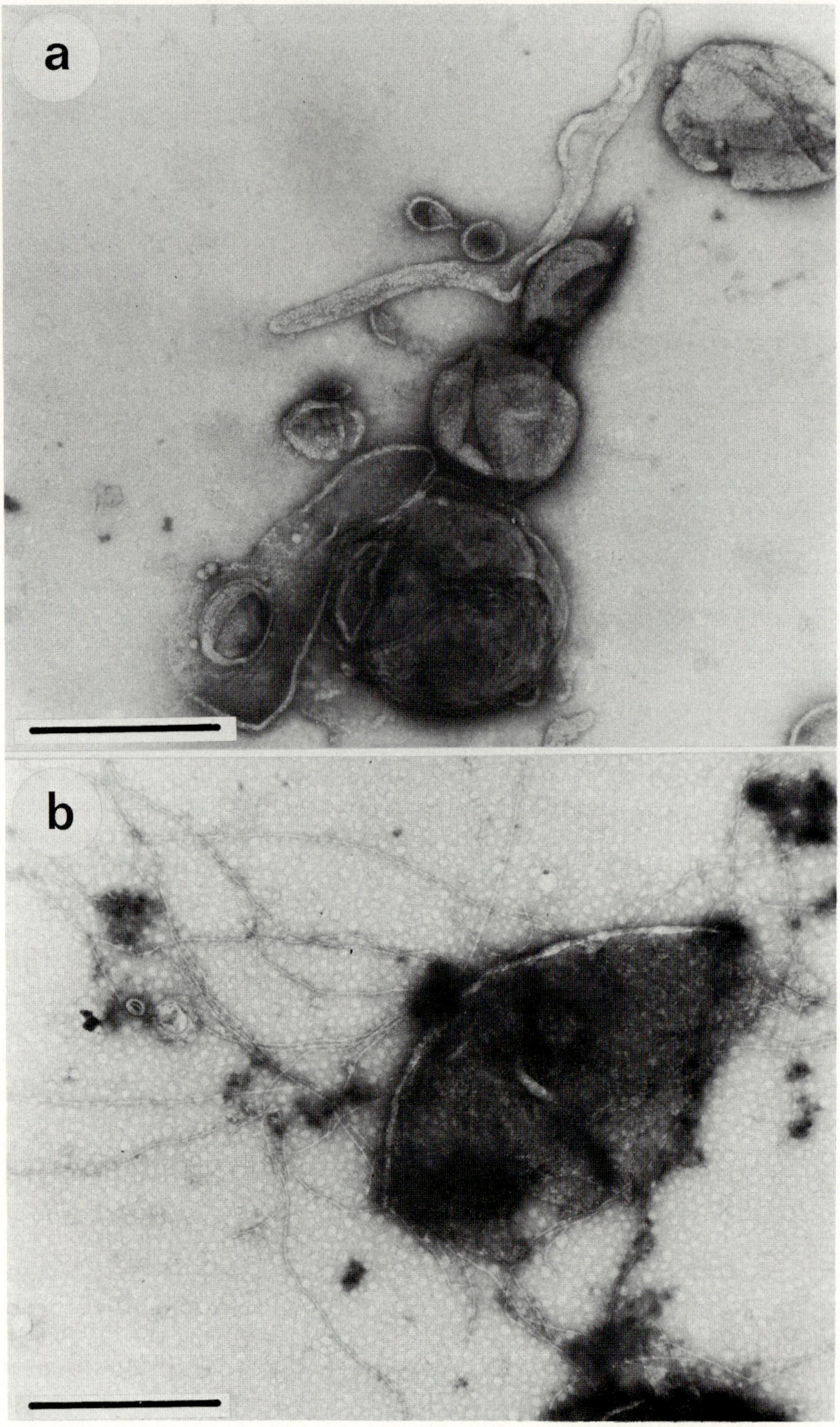

Fig. 5. Inside-out vesicles (a) or inside-out vesicles reconstituted with crude spectrin as described in Table II (b) were incubated for 60 minutes with 50 μg/ml ^{3}H-G-actin, and sedimented into 20% w/v sucrose as described in Methods. The vesicle pellet was gently resuspended, applied to a Formvar coated grid and stained with 1% uranyl acetate. Bar is 0.5 μm; magnification = × 54,000.

that the actin–membrane association is a direct result of actin filament formation. This implies that some component or components at the cytoplasmic surface, present in crude spectrin, serve as a nucleation site or initiator of actin polymerization.

Spectrin itself seems a likely candidate for this function particularly in view of recent observations [20] showing that purified phosphorylated spectrin (bands 1 and 2) can initiate polymerization of G-actin in solution. However, we have found that purified spectrin (bands 1 and 2, prepared by the method of Bennett and Branton [17], from freshly drawn blood) does not have the ability to stimulate G-actin binding to inside-out vesicles or to inhibit binding to ghosts [C.M. Cohen, P.L. Jackson, and D. Branton, in preparation] in the way that crude spectrin does. While it is possible that preparation of pure spectrin from crude spectrin induces subtle alterations in phosphorylation or conformation which abolish the spectrin–actin interaction, it is equally plausible that proteins in the crude spectrin (Fig. 2C) other than bands 1 and 2 are responsible for the observed effects. Such a protein could be red cell actin, some fraction of which could already exist in the F form in crude spectrin. We consider this to be a real possibility since we have found that preformed F-actin will bind to inside-out vesicles and, when bound, will stimulate the subsequent binding of G-actin in a manner analogous to that seen with crude spectrin [C.M. Cohen, P.L. Jackson, and D. Branton, in preparation]. This suggests that there may be F-actin present in the crude spectrin which binds to the membrane and is responsible for the stimulation of G-actin binding, possibly by acting as a nucleation site for filament elongation in the same way as F-actin fragments in solution can induce the explosive polymerization of G-actin [34, 35]. Although the protein composition of reconstituted inside-out vesicles prior to incubation with G-actin (Fig. 2d) reveals no apparent increase in actin content, the amounts of F-actin involved may be too low to detect above the high background staining in this region of the gel.

The relationship of the observations presented here to the state of endogenous actin on the red cell membrane is difficult to assess, especially since it is still unknown whether actin on the red cell membrane is filamentous or monomeric. While Tilney and Detmers [13] have proposed that red cell actin exists in a nonfilamentous form in vivo, it has also been shown that phosphorylated spectrin can induce filament formation of skeletal muscle actin in vitro [20]. Nevertheless, our demonstration that ghost membranes can bind large amounts of actin over and above that already present on the membrane and that this bound actin is in the filamentous form indicates that several types of actin–membrane association may be possible. Further, our observation that ghosts may possess nucleation sites for actin polymerization suggests that they may serve as a valuable model system for the study of actin–membrane associations. Similar studies should be possible with more complex cells using methods specifically designed to expose their cytoplasmic membrane surface [36, 37].

REFERENCES

1. Pollard TD: In Inoue S, Stephens RE (eds): "Molecules and Cell Movement." New York: Raven, 1975, p 259.
2. Pollard TD, Weihing RR: CRC Crit Rev Biochem 2:1, 1974.
3. Clarke M, Spudich J: Ann Rev Biochem 46:797, 1977.
4. Gruenstein E, Rich A, Weihing RR: J Cell Biol 64:223, 1975.
5. Clarke M, Schatten G, Mazia D, Spudich JA: Proc Natl Acad Sci USA 72:1758, 1975.
6. Pollard TD, Korn ED: J Biol Chem 248:448, 1973.
7. Wickus G, Gruenstein E, Robbins PW, Rich A: Proc Natl Acad Sci USA 72:746, 1975.
8. Burridge K, Phillips JH: Nature (London) 254:526, 1975.

9. Ostlund RE, Leung JT, Kipnis DM: J Cell Biol 73: 78, 1977.
10. Ash JF, Louvard D, Singer SJ: Proc Natl Acad Sci USA 74:5584, 1977.
11. Bourguignon LY, Singer SJ: Proc Natl Acad Sci USA 74:5031, 1977.
12. Sheetz MP, Painter RG, Singer SJ: Biochemistry 15:4486, 1976.
13. Tilney LG, Detmers P: J Cell Biol 66:508, 1975.
14. Weed RI, LaCelle P, Merrill EW: J Clin Invest 48:795, 1969.
15. Sheetz MP, Singer SJ: J Cell Biol 73:638, 1977.
16. Lux SE, John KM, Karnovsky M: J Clin Invest 58:955, 1976.
17. Bennett V, Branton D: J Biol Chem 252:2753, 1977.
18. Fairbanks G, Steck TL, Wallach DFH: Biochemistry 10:2606, 1971.
19. Yu J, Fischman DA, Steck TL: J Supramol Struct 1:233, 1973.
20. Pinder JC, Bray D, Gratzer WB: Nature (London) 270:752, 1977.
21. Spudich JA, Watt SJ: J Biol Chem 246:4866, 1971.
22. Steck TL, Kant JA: Methods Enzymol 31:172, 1974.
23. Lowey S, Cohen C: J Mol Biol 4:293, 1962.
24. Lusty CJ, Fasold H: Biochemistry 8:2933, 1969.
25. Martonosi A: Arch Biochem Biophys 123:29, 1968.
26. Bridgen J: Biochem J 126:21, 1972.
27. Katz AM, Mommaerts WFHM: Biochim Biophys Acta 65:82, 1962.
28. Burley RW, Seidel JC, Gergely J: Arch Biochem Biophys 146:597, 1971.
29. Steck TL: J Cell Biol 62:1, 1974.
30. Hitchcock SE, Carlsson L, Lindberg V: Cell 7:531, 1976.
31. Hartwig J, Stossel TP: J Cell Biol 71:295, 1976.
32. Weihing RR: J Cell Biol 71:303, 1976.
33. Birchmeier W, Singer SJ: Biochem Biophys Res Commun 77:1354, 1977.
34. Nakaoka Y, Kasai M: J Mol Biol 44:319, 1969.
35. Oosawa F, Kasai M: In Timasheff SN, Fasman GD (eds): "Subunits in Biological Systems." New York: Marcel Deckker, 1971, p 261.
36. Cohen CM, Kalish DI, Jacobson BS, Branton D: J Cell Biol 75:119, 1977.
37. Cohen CM, Branton D: J Cell Biol 75:216a, 1977.

Journal of Supramolecular Structure 9:125–130 (1978)
Normal and Abnormal Red Cell Membranes 241–246

Erythrocyte Membrane Alterations in Huntington Disease: Effects of γ-Aminobutyric Acid

D. A. Butterfield, M. L. Braden, and W. R. Markesbery

Department of Chemistry, University of Kentucky, Lexington, Kentucky 40506 (D.A.B., M.L.B.); and Departments of Neurology and Pathology, University of Kentucky Medical Center, Lexington, Kentucky 40506 (W.R.M.)

The interaction of the inhibitory neurotransmitter γ-aminobutyric acid (GABA) with erythrocyte membranes from patients with Huntington disease and normal controls has been studied by electron spin resonance. GABA affects the physical state of erythrocyte membrane proteins in control and Huntington disease differently. In addition, after exposure of spin-labeled Huntington disease erythrocyte membranes to 0.1 mM GABA, the relevant electron spin resonance parameters reflecting the physical state of membrane proteins are indistinguishable from those of untreated control membranes. These findings support the concept that this disease is associated with a generalized membrane defect.

Key words: GABA, Huntington disease, spin labeling, erythrocyte membranes, protein alterations

Huntington disease (HD), inherited in an autosomal dominant manner, is characterized clinically by progressive involuntary movements and dementia [1], pathologically by cell degeneration in the neostriatum and cerebral cortex [2], and biochemically by decreased levels of γ-aminobutyric acid (GABA) [3] and decreased activities of glutamic acid decarboxylase and choline acetyltransferase in the basal ganglia [4].

Although HD has been considered a defect of the basal ganglia, recent biophysical and biochemical experiments from our laboratory have suggested that this disease may be associated with a generalized membrane abnormality. Electron spin resonance (ESR) studies of erythrocyte membranes have demonstrated alterations in the physical state of membrane proteins in HD erythrocytes [5]. Scanning electron microscopic investigations of unmanipulated erythrocytes revealed an increased number of stomatocytes in HD compared to controls [6], with a slight exacerbation of this effect when the cells were processed in fixative of lower pH. These findings probably result from an altered response to fixation by an altered membrane in HD and support the ESR results. We have also observed the activity of the erythrocyte membrane sodium plus potassium-stimulated adenosine triphosphatase to be increased in HD [7].

Address all correspondence to D. A. Butterfield.

Received March 3, 1978; accepted July 10, 1978.

The molecular basis for the clinical manifestations of Huntington disease is unknown. One hypothesis to explain the presence of choreiform movements in HD involves the decreased amount of GABA [3], an inhibitory neurotransmitter in the basal ganglia. In the current report we present the results of ESR studies of the interaction of GABA with erythrocyte membranes from patients with Huntington disease and normal controls.

MATERIALS AND METHODS

GABA and β-alanine were purchased from Sigma Chemical Company and the spin label employed, 2,2,6,6-tetramethylpiperidin-1-oxyl-4-maleimide (MAL-6), was obtained from Syva. All other reagents were of the highest purity available.

Heparinized blood was obtained by venipuncture from twelve different individuals from eleven different families with well-documented Huntington disease. All patients had involuntary movements and/or dementia and a positive family history for HD. Twenty-five percent of the subjects were in the early stages of the disease, 42% in the mid stages, and 33% in the late stages. Seventy-five percent of the patients were ambulatory and active, and the majority were on a regular at-home diet; the others were on a regular hospital diet. One-third of the HD patients were on no medication while the remainder were on phenothiazines or a butyrophenone, or on an assortment of medication. A different, healthy, sex- and age-matched, drug-free individual with no family history of inherited neurologic disease served as a control for each HD subject.

Intact erythrocytes and erythrocyte membranes (ghosts) were prepared and the spin labeling performed using MAL-6 as previously described [5]. Magnetic resonance experiments were performed on a Magnion-Ventron MVR-9X or a Varian E-109 electron spin resonance spectrometer.

Membrane protein content was estimated according to the method of Lowry et al [8]. The GABA incubation was performed as follows: 50 μl of a solution of GABA dissolved in 5 mM sodium phosphate buffer, pH 8.0 was incubated with 200 μl of control or HD ghost membranes to a final concentration of 0.1 mM GABA for 15 minutes at room temperature and the ESR spectra recorded. Control experiments in which 200 μl of ghosts was incubated with 50 μl of the buffer without GABA were also performed. In experiments in which the ESR signal intensity of membrane-bound MAL-6 per mg membrane protein was determined, NaOH was added to a final concentration of 0.2 M. This procedure is known to convert all MAL-6 binding sites to weakly immobilized ones [10, 11]. The line shapes of the resulting spectra were the same in all such experiments. SDS-polyacrylamide gel electrophoresis of erythrocyte membranes was performed as previously described [9].

RESULTS

The spin label used in the present study is covalently bonded principally to sulfhydryl (SH) groups of membrane proteins, although fewer than 5% of the labeled sites may be amino groups [12]. The principal proteins of the erythrocyte membrane labeled by MAL-6 are thought to be the set of large (> 200,000 dalton) peripheral proteins (spectrin), the higher-molecular-weight proteins present in smaller amounts, and a group of transmembrane proteins (Band 3) [11]. A typical ESR spectrum of MAL-6 incorporated into control erythrocyte membranes is shown in Figure 1. Spectra similar to that in Figure 1 have been previously described [10–15] as having ESR parameters reflective of at least two different classes of SH group sites in the red blood cell membrane: one strongly immobilized and the other weakly immobilized. The ratio of the ESR spectral amplitude of MAL-6 attached to weakly immobilized SH groups (W) to that of MAL-6 attached to strongly immobilized SH groups (S) is a convenient monitor of protein organizational and/or conformational changes in membranes [10–15].

The mean W/S values of control and subject experiments were compared by a two-way analysis of variance [16] (Table I). This two-tailed method of statistical analysis minimizes the effects of possible fluctuations from day to day that may occur with biological samples. P is the significance of the mean values of $(W/S)_{control}$ and $(W/S)_{subject}$ calculated from the two-way analysis of variance. $(W/S)_{HD}$ is significantly increased compared to $(W/S)_{control}$ ($P < 0.025$, Table IA), suggesting alterations in the physical state of membrane proteins in erythrocytes in Huntington disease. These data confirm our previous ESR results [5].

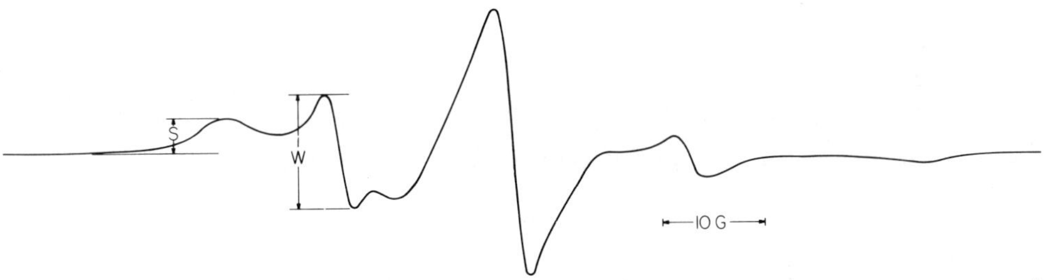

Fig. 1. Typical electron spin resonance spectrum of MAL-6 attached to membrane proteins in control erythrocytes. The ESR spectral amplitudes of MAL-6 attached to weakly immobilized sulfhydryl groups (W) and that of MAL-6 attached to strongly immobilized sulfhydryl groups (S) are indicated.

TABLE I. Effect of GABA on the W/S Ratio of ESR Spectra of MAL-6 in Erythrocyte Membranes in Normal (N) and Huntington Disease (HD)*

A) No GABA added			
$(W/S)_N$		$(W/S)_{HD}$	
4.13 ± 0.19		4.53 ± 0.20	
$P^a < 0.025$			
B) Differential effect of 0.1 mM GABA in normal and Huntington disease			
$(W/S)_N$	$(W/S)_{N + GABA}$	$(W/S)_{HD}$	$(W/S)_{HD + GABA}$
4.13 ± 0.19	4.77 ± 0.26	4.53 ± 0.20	4.22 ± 0.23
$P < 0.005$		$0.05 < P < 0.1$	
C) Equalization of MAL-6 W/S ratio in HD after addition of 0.1 mM GABA			
$(W/S)_N$		$(W/S)_{HD + GABA}$	
4.13 ± 0.19		4.22 ± 0.23	
$P > 0.8$			

*Mean ± SEM for 12 different samples in each case are presented.

[a]P value calculated by a two-way analysis of variance [16].

GABA has a differential effect on control and HD erythrocyte membranes as reflected by the W/S ratio of MAL-6 (Table IB). This ratio is highly significantly increased in control membranes upon incubation of 0.1 mM GABA ($P < 0.005$); however, upon GABA incubation, a reduction of this ratio in Huntington disease erythrocytes compared to untreated HD membranes is suggested, although the significance is borderline ($0.1 \; P < 0.05$). However, after addition of GABA to erythrocyte membranes from patients with Huntington disease, the W/S ratio of MAL-6 attached to membrane proteins is not altered from that of untreated normal controls ($P > 0.8$, Table IC), indicating that this ESR parameter has been lowered by GABA treatment (compare Table IA and IC). Moreover, the results shown in Table IC suggest that on the basis of ESR parameters GABA has made the physical state of proteins in HD erythrocyte membranes indistinguishable from that of controls.

Initial experiments in which control and HD erythrocytes were incubated with GABA followed by centrifugation at 27,000g for 30 minutes and recentrifugation of the resulting supernatant under the same conditions were performed. Aliquots of the second supernatant were subjected to SDS-polyacrylamide gel electrophoresis and ESR spectroscopy. Some of the peripheral protein, spectrin, is released into the supernatant from control membranes under these conditions as observed on gels and by the presence of a noticeable ESR signal. The W/S ratio of this signal detected at high spectrometer gain was approximately one-third that of MAL-6 attached to untreated erythrocyte ghosts, a value that is typical for spectrin [D.A.B., unpublished results]. Approximately 89% of the total MAL-6 signal intensity remained in the membrane pellet after GABA treatment. In contrast, the HD supernatant either demonstrated no spectrin ESR signal or at extremely high instrument gain settings, one of much lower intensity than that observed in control samples. In addition, under the conditions employed no HD protein was observable on SDS-polyacrylamide gels, suggesting that GABA has interacted differently with control and HD erythrocyte membranes and supporting the ESR data in Table IB and IC.

Preliminary evidence for the specificity of GABA has been obtained. Four different experiments were performed in which control and HD erythrocyte membranes were incubated with β-alanine (3-aminopropionic acid), a compound differing from GABA only in that it has one less CH_2 group. No definitive differences in the W/S ratio of MAL-6 could be demonstrated in either control or HD erythrocyte membranes upon incubation with β-alanine.

DISCUSSION

A differential effect of 0.1 mM GABA, an inhibitory neurotransmitter, on the physical state of membrane proteins in Huntington disease and control erythrocytes has been suggested in the present experiments. The relevant ESR parameter, the W/S ratio, was increased in control samples upon GABA incubation, whereas this parameter was apparently decreased in Huntington disease (compare Table IA, IB, and IC). After treatment with GABA, no statistically significant difference in the W/S ratio in Huntington disease erythrocytes compared to untreated controls could be demonstrated (Table IC). This last result suggests that GABA has caused a change in the physical state of membrane proteins in erythrocytes in HD such that the original ESR differences (Table IA) are no longer present. Our previous studies [5–7] have suggested that HD may be associated with a generalized membrane defect. If the phenomenon observed in the present experiments with erythrocytes were to occur in the basal ganglia, it would suggest that increasing GABA levels in the neostriatum in HD may cause remaining neuronal membranes to revert to a normal physical state. This suggestion lends support for the pharmacological strategy of inhibiting GABA transaminase activity [17, 18] and replacing GABA [18] in HD. Moreover, by monitoring the effects on the physical state of membrane proteins in erythrocytes induced by various drugs potentially useful in HD therapy, the relative effectiveness and usefulness of these pharmacological agents may be discerned. Experiments employing these concepts are currently in progress.

GABA is thought to act as an inhibitory neurotransmitter by increasing Cl^- conductance [19]. In the erythrocyte the major anion transporting protein is located in Band 3 [20], a set of 100,000-mw transmembrane proteins. It may be pertinent to the present study that we recently found in HD erythrocytes an increased activity of the $Na^+ + K^+$-stimulated adenosine triphosphatase [7], the phosphorylated intermediate of which is located in Band 3 [21].

Although our initial experiments with β-alanine suggest a specific GABA effect, it is still uncertain whether there exist GABA receptors in the erythrocyte membrane. However, the discovery of acetylcholine [22] and opiate [23] receptors, and the presence of acetylcholinesterase [24] in the erythrocyte membrane lend support for such a possibility. Experiments using GABA antagonists are currently in progress to resolve the specificity of GABA interaction observed in the present study.

Spectrin, the large, filamentous, myosin-like peripheral protein located on the cytoplasmic side of the erythrocyte membrane, is thought to be important in the equilibrium conformation adopted by several membrane proteins partially by serving as an "anchor" to which these other proteins are attached [25]. The loss of some spectrin from control erythrocyte membranes exposed to 0.1 mM GABA might be expected to allow these other proteins to become more free to move, resulting in a higher W/S ratio consistent with the present results.

The molecular mechanisms of the interaction of GABA with erythrocyte membranes are as yet unclear, but the differential response of this neurotransmitter on the physical state of extraneural membranes in HD and controls lends support to the concept that Huntington disease is a diffuse membrane disease.

ACKNOWLEDGMENTS

We thank Donna Kersey, Marcia Butterfield, and Kim Hisle for technical assistance. This work was supported in part by the National Institute of Neurological and Communicative Disorders and Stroke, National Institutes of Health (grants NS13791-01A1 [D.A.B. and W.R.M.] and NS14221-01 [W.R.M.]), the Muscular Dystrophy Association of America (D.A.B.), and the Graduate School of the Univeristy of Kentucky (D.A.B.).

REFERENCES

1. Merritt HM: "A Textbook of Neurology." Philadelphia: Lea and Febiger, 5th ed, 1973, pp 458–462.
2. Dreese MJ, Netsky MG: In Minkler J (ed): "Pathology of the Nervous System." New York: McGraw-Hill, 1968, pp 1186–1193.
3. Perry TL, Hansen S, Kloster M: N Engl J Med 288:337, 1973.
4. Bird ED, Iversen LL: Brain 97:457, 1974.
5. Butterfield DA, Oeswein JQ, Markesbery WR: Nature (London) 267:453, 1977.
6. Markesbery WR, Butterfield DA: Biochem Biophys Res Commun 78:560, 1977.
7. Butterfield DA, Oeswein JQ, Prunty ME, Hisle KC, Markesbery WR: Annals Neurol 4:60, 1978.
8. Lowry OH, Rosebrough NJ, Farr AC, Randall RJ: J Biol Chem 193:265, 1959.

9. Fairbanks G, Steck TL, Wallach DFH: Biochemistry 10:2606, 1971.
10. Schneider H, Smith ICP: Biochim Biophys Acta 219:73, 1970.
11. Butterfield DA, Roses AD, Appel SH, Chesnut DB: Arch Biochem Biophys 177:226, 1976.
12. Chapman D, Barratt MD, Kamat VB: Biochim Biophys Acta 173:154, 1969.
13. Kirkpatrick FH, Sandberg HE: Arch Biochem Biophys 156:653, 1973.
14. Holmes DE, Piette LH: J Pharmacol Exp Ther 173:78, 1970.
15. Butterfield DA: Biochim Biophys Acta 470:1, 1977.
16. Brownlee K: "Statistical Theory and Methodology in Science and Engineering." New York: John Wiley, 1960.
17. Perry TL, MacLeod PM, Hansen H: N Engl J Med 297:840, 1977.
18. Shoulson I, Kartzinel R, Chase TN: Neurology 25:61, 1976.
19. Cooper JR, Bloom FE, Roth RH: "The Biochemical Basis of Neuropharmacology." New York: Oxford University Press, 2nd ed, 1974
20. Wolosin JM, Ginsburg H, Cabantchik ZI: J Biol Chem 252:2419, 1977.
21. Avruch J, Fairbanks G: Proc Nat Acad Sci USA 69:1216, 1972.
22. Huestis WH, McConnell HM: Biochem Biophys Res Commun 57:726, 1974.
23. Abood LG, Atkinson H, MacNeil: J Neurosci Res (In press).
24. Ellman GL, Courtney KD, Andres V, Featherstone RM: Biochem Pharmacol 7:88, 1961.
25. Singer SJ: Ann Rev Biochem 43:805, 1974.

Journal of Supramolecular Structure 9:131–141 (1978)
Normal and Abnormal Red Cell Membranes 247–257

Erythrocyte Troponin Inhibitor-Like Protein: Isolation and Characterization

Jonathan Maimon and Saul Puszkin

Department of Pathology, Mount Sinai School of Medicine of The City University of New York, 1 Gustave L. Levy Place, New York, New York 10029

A protein was isolated from a human erythrocyte lysate with an apparent molecular weight of 23,000–24,000 daltons. This protein was purified by batch DEAE cellulose followed by column DEAE cellulose chromatography and a gradient of NaCl. On sodium dodecyl sulfate acrylamide electrophoresis, the erythrocyte protein comigrated with muscle troponin inhibitor. An isoelectric precipitation (pH 9.25) was used for the separation of muscle troponin inhibitor from a complex with another troponin component. Both the erythrocyte protein and the muscle troponin inhibitor partially inhibited muscle myosin Ca^{2+} and K^+-EDTA ATPase activity. Furthermore, they inhibited actin-activated Mg^{2+}-ATPase of muscle myosin. The inhibitory effects were absent in the presence of muscle troponin calcium-binding component. Muscle troponin inhibitor and the erythrocyte troponin inhibitor-like protein bound to muscle myosin when myosin was precipitated twice at low ionic strength. The presence of a troponin inhibitor-like protein in erythrocytes suggests that it may be a component in the regulation of contractile activity.

Key words: **human erythrocyte troponin inhibitor-like protein, muscle troponin inhibitor purification, muscle myosin binding, inhibition of myosin ATPase activity**

The regulatory proteins of nonmuscle contractile systems have received a great deal of attention in recent years [1]. The isolation from several nonmuscle tissues of a protein of low molecular weight possessing Ca^{2+}-binding ability and the capacity to confer Ca^{2+} sensitivity to nonmuscle contractile protein interactions has given new insight into the mode by which contractile events are regulated in nonmuscle tissues [2–6]. This new group of Ca^{2+}-modulator proteins, as they are called, are similar to troponin-C (TN-C), the troponin Ca^{2+}-binding protein from skeletal muscle, and are isolated from a variety of tissues including brain [2], platelets [7], erythrocytes [8], and adrenal medulla [9].

Received April 11, 1978; accepted July 3, 1978.

However, a complex system of proteins similar to that of the troponin complex from skeletal muscle has been reported present in platelets [10, 11] and in brain [12]. In human platelets, brain, and smooth muscle, the troponin system probably coexists with another regulatory mechanism associated with the phosphorylation and dephosphorylation of a light chain of myosin [13, 14]. In erythrocytes, the presence of an actin myosin complex has not been established. In its place, an erythrocyte actin-spectrin complex was shown and believed responsible for maintaining the characteristic shape of erythrocytes [15–17].

It was deemed important to determine if other proteins in erythrocytes could regulate contractile activity. We report here the isolation and partial characterization of a protein from erythrocytes which exhibits similarities to those of striated muscle troponin inhibitor (TN-I).

MATERIALS AND METHODS

Purification of Human Erythrocyte TN-I

Red cells were sedimented from whole blood at 5,000g for 6 minutes and the plasma was removed by three washes with 0.154 M NaCl, 1 mM EDTA, and 5 mM Tris-HCl buffer, pH 7.5. Washed erythrocytes were hemolyzed for 20 minutes with two volumes of 5 mM Tris-HCl, pH 7.5, containing 14 mM 2-mercaptoethanol, 5 mM EDTA, and 5 mM EGTA (Buffer-A). The hemolysate was centrifuged at 40,000g for 30 minutes to sediment membranes. The supernatant was used for batch DEAE cellulose chromatography (Whatman Laboratories, Mass.) and equilibrated with Buffer-A in a proportion of 25 gm of dry cellulose/liter of hemolysate and left standing for 24 hours at 4°. The fluid was separated by filtration and the DEAE cellulose fibers washed with three volumes of 1.4 mM 2-mercaptoethanol in 50 mM Tris-HCl, pH 7.5, (Buffer-B). The resin was washed with 0.2 M NaCl in Buffer-B followed by another wash of 0.3 M NaCl in Buffer-B. Proteins were eluted with 0.4 M NaCl in Buffer-B, and the 30–70% $(NH_4)_2SO_4$ saturation pellet dissolved in Buffer-B. The protein solution was dialyzed overnight against Buffer-B and chromatographed on a DEAE cellulose column of 1.5 × 30 cm, equilibrated with Buffer-B. A protein peak was eluted within 0.3 and 0.6 M NaCl in Buffer-B. The 40–70% $(NH_4)_2SO_4$ precipitate was dissolved and dialyzed against Buffer-B. The protein was clarified at 40,000g for 30 minutes and the supernatant used as the erythrocyte TN-I preparation. Biological activity was tested within 48 hours.

Purification of Rabbit Muscle Troponin Components

Rabbit muscle troponin was fractionated by a modification of a previously described method [18]. The protein solution of TN-I and troponin-tropomyosin (TN-T) binding component that emerged unadsorbed from the DEAE cellulose column was adjusted in its pH to 9.25. The resulting precipitate was pelleted at 5,000g for 5 minutes. The protein pellet contained TN-T as the major protein and traces of TN-I. The supernatant consisted of a homogeneous solution of TN-I. Both protein solutions were dialyzed against 0.1 mM $CaCl_2$, 5 mM Tris-HCl, pH 8.0, and stored frozen at −20°.

Preparation of Other Muscle Proteins

Muscle myosin and actin were prepared from fresh rabbit muscle as described elsewhere [19]. Protein concentration was measured by the method of Lowry et al [20], using bovine serum albumin as the standard.

Determination of ATPase Activity

ATPase activities of proteins were determined by the release of inorganic phosphate (Pi) from ATP according to the method of Marsh [21], modified to detect 0.3 nmoles of Pi [22]. Mixtures of gamma-labeled [^{32}P] ATP and nonradioactive ATP were employed. One-half-milliliter aliquots of the butanol layer were counted in a scintillation spectrophotometer. ATPase assays were performed in volumes of 5 ml. Proteins and reagents were mixed initially in a volume of 0.9 ml, incubated at room temperature for 10 minutes, diluted to 5 ml with 50 mM Tris-HCl, pH 7.5, and incubated with ATP at 37° for 10 minutes. For assay purposes, the quantity of protein was 0.01 mg of muscle myosin per ml and 0.01 to 0.02 mg of actin per ml. $CaCl_2$ (10 μM) was added when mixtures of actin and myosin were used. The reaction was initiated by the addition of 0.1 ml of 5 mM gamma-labeled [^{32}P] ATP, 10 mM $MgCl_2$, or 10 mM $CaCl_2$ and allowed to proceed at 37° for 10 minutes. Aliquots of 1 ml were removed at various time intervals. Reactions were stopped by the addition of 0.4 ml 20% trichloroacetic acid. ATPase was estimated as the difference between Pi at zero time and Pi at the end of the reaction.

Sodium Dodecyl Sulfate (SDS) Polyacrylamide Gel Electrophoresis

SDS electrophoresis was performed at room temperature (Buchler Instruments, Inc., New Jersey) on single 7% or 10% polyacrylamide gels containing 10 mM phosphate buffer and 1 gm of SDS per liter [23].

Binding of Proteins to Muscle Myosin

For the determination of binding of muscle and erythrocyte TN-I proteins to muscle myosin, appropriate concentrations of muscle myosin (2 mg/ml) and the inhibitors (2 mg/ml) were mixed and incubated at 37° for 15 minutes in a solution of 0.5 M KCl, 20 mM Tris, pH 7.2. Myosin-inhibitor mixtures were diluted 10 times with distilled water at 4° and the protein precipitate allowed to form by standing 30 minutes at 4°. Proteins were sedimented by centrifugation at 15,000g for 10 minutes. The pellets were dissolved in 0.5 M KCl, 20 mM Tris buffer, pH 7.2, and precipitated again as above. This final precipitate was dissolved in 0.5 M KCl, 20 mM Tris, pH 7.2, and the newly bound protein to myosin molecules was visualized by SDS acrylamide electrophoresis. Binding of TN-I to myosin also was carried out in the presence of TN-C.

RESULTS

For the purification of the human erythrocyte TN-I (see flow chart 1), batch DEAE cellulose chromatography was found suitable to process large volumes of red cell hemolysates. DEAE cellulose adsorbed large amounts of various proteins from the red cell hemolysate. Three washing steps of the DEAE cellulose with Buffer-B and 0.2 and 0.3 M NaCl removed most of the hemoglobin. Several proteins were eluted by 0.4 M NaCl, among them 2 major bands in the 100,000 and 24,000 molecular-weight regions. By DEAE cellulose column chromatography, most of the proteins eluted as one peak (Fig. 1). The inhibitor emerged in the tail portion of the peak as illustrated in Figure 2, when NaCl concentration ranged from 0.35 to 0.6 M.

A 40–70% $(NH_4)_2SO_4$ cut permitted concentration of this protein by precipitation and solubilization at a higher protein concentration, about 2–3 mg/ml. The TN-I preparation showed a 24,000 molecular-weight band. Attempts to isolate TN-I from erythrocyte membranes gave negative results.

PURIFICATION PROCEDURES OF HUMAN ERYTHROCYTE TROPONIN INHIBITOR

WHOLE BLOOD

PACKED ERYTHROCYTES
- WASH 3 X WITH SALINE
- CENTRIFUGE

WASHED ERYTHROCYTES
- HEMOLYZE WITH 2 VOLUMES
- 5 mM TRIS-HCL, 5 mM EDTA, 5 mM EGTA (pH 7.5)
- CENTRIFUGE 40,000 x G FOR 30 MINUTES

HEMOLYZATE
- BATCH DEAE CELLULOSE (25 GR/L)
- STAND FOR 24 HOURS
- 1) WASH WITH 50 mM TRIS-HCL (pH 7.5)
- 2) WASH WITH 0.2 M NACL, 50 mM TRIS-HCL (pH 7.5)
- 3) WASH WITH 0.3 M NACL, 50 mM TRIS-HCL (pH 7.5)
- 4) ELUTE WITH 0.4 M NACL, 50 mM TRIS-HCL (pH 7.5)

0.4 M NACL ELUATE
- 30-70% AMMONIUM SULFATE CUT
- DISSOLVE IN 50 mM TRIS-HCL (pH 7.5)
- DIALYZE, COLUMN DEAE CELLULOSE CHROMATOGRAPHY
- WASH WITH 50 mM TRIS (pH 7.5)
- ELUTE WITH 0-0.6 M NACL, 50 mM TRIS-HCL (pH 7.5)

0.3-0.6 M NACL FRACTION
- 40-70% AMMONIUM SULFATE CUT
- DIALYZE AGAINST 50 mM TRIS-HCL (pH 7.5)
- CENTRIFUGE 40,000 x G FOR 30 MINUTES

RBC-TN-I SUPERNATANT SOLUTION

Flow chart 1.

Purification of The Troponin Components From Muscle

The purification procedure used for muscle troponin is similar to that described previously [18] (see flow chart 2). It was found, however, that by DEAE cellulose chromatography equilibrated with 8 M urea and 50 mM Tris-HCl, only TN-C can be separated as a purified protein, while TN-I eluted as a complex with TN-T. When the complex of TN-I and TN-T was adjusted to pH 9.25, a precipitate was formed within 1–2 seconds which consisted of TN-T with small amounts of TN-I. Most of the TN-I remained in the supernatant. Solubilization and precipitation at pH 9.25 for a second time gave a purer TN-T protein solution. Figure 2 shows the purity and electrophoretic mobility of the erythrocyte inhibitor and muscle TN-I.

Binding of Troponin to Muscle Myosin

To determine the affinities of TN-I for myosin, myosin was precipitated at low ionic strength after 15 minutes of incubation with the inhibitor proteins. It was found that for

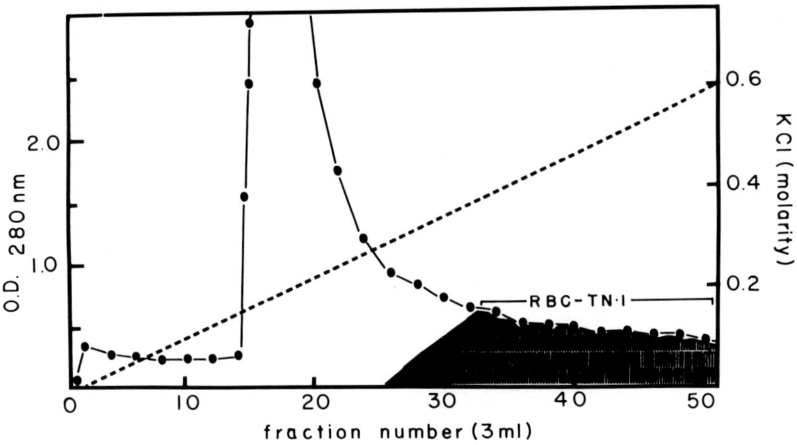

Fig. 1. DEAE-cellulose column chromatography for the purification of the erythrocyte troponin inhibitor-like protein. The 0.4 M NaCl eluate from batch DEAE cellulose (approximately 75 mg of proteins) was loaded on a 1.5 × 30 cm column. The column was washed with 200 ml of buffer and eluted with 150 ml of a continuous gradient of 0–0.6 M NaCl. The shaded area is where the erythrocyte inhibitor eluted.

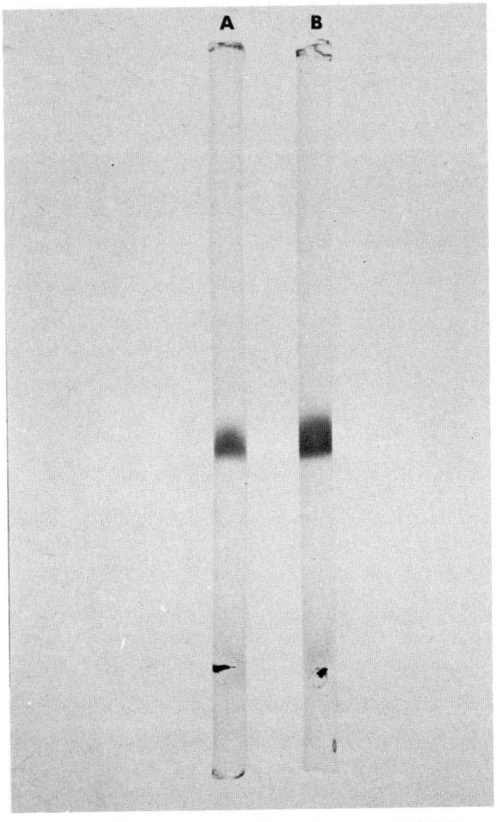

Fig. 2. SDS acrylamide electrophoresis of muscle and erythrocyte TN-I-like protein. Gel A: Muscle TN-I (25 μg). Gel B: Erythrocyte TN-I-like protein (45 μg). Both proteins were loaded on top of single 10% polyacrylamide gels.

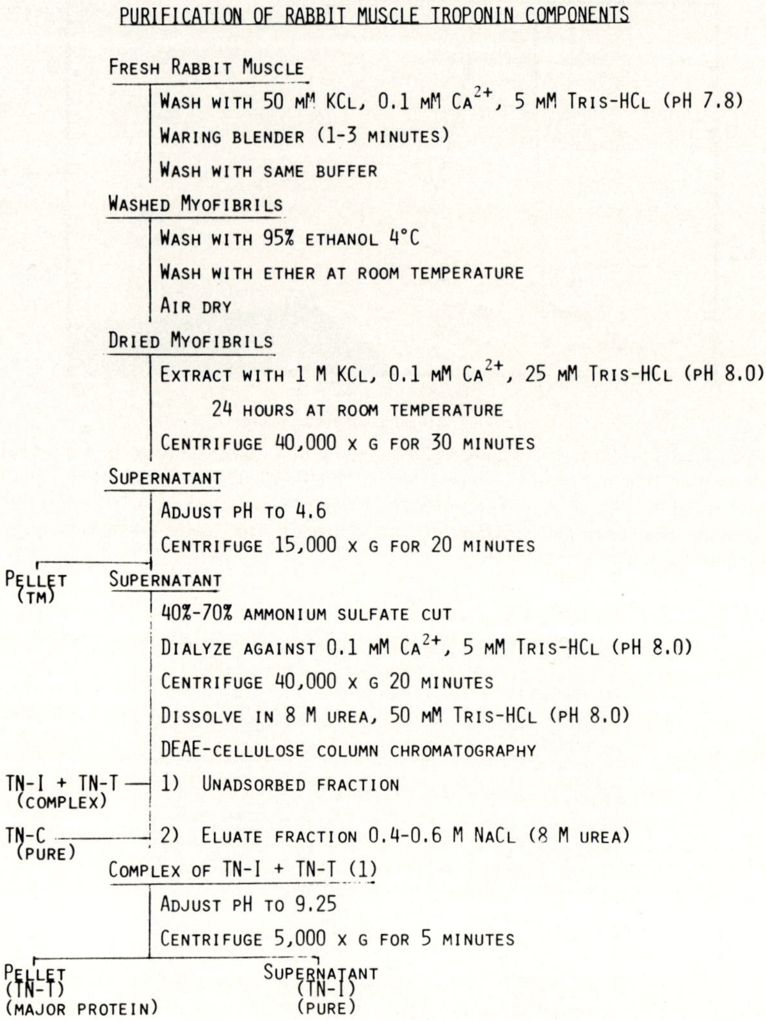

Flow chart 2.

myosin, after solubilization, a second precipitation and solubilization again contain a new band bound at equimolecular amounts with that of myosin light chains. By densitometry, the area of the new band bound to myosin was the same as the sum of myosin light chains. Figures 3 and 4 illustrate the binding of the muscle and erythrocyte inhibitors of muscle myosin. Gel A of Figure 3 shows TN-I. Gel B illustrates myosin heavy chains and its three light chains (LC-1, LC-2 and LC-3). Gel C illustrates the polypeptide composition of myosin after allowing muscle TN-I to bind. The muscle TN-I exhibited a relative mobility slightly greater than the LC-1 of myosin. Figure 4 shows similar results obtained with the erythrocyte TN-I. Gel A contains myosin; Gel B contains the erythrocyte TN-I; and Gel C contains bound inhibitor to myosin. The band of TN-I migrated immediately below the LC-1 of myosin. TN-I did not bind in the presence of TN-C.

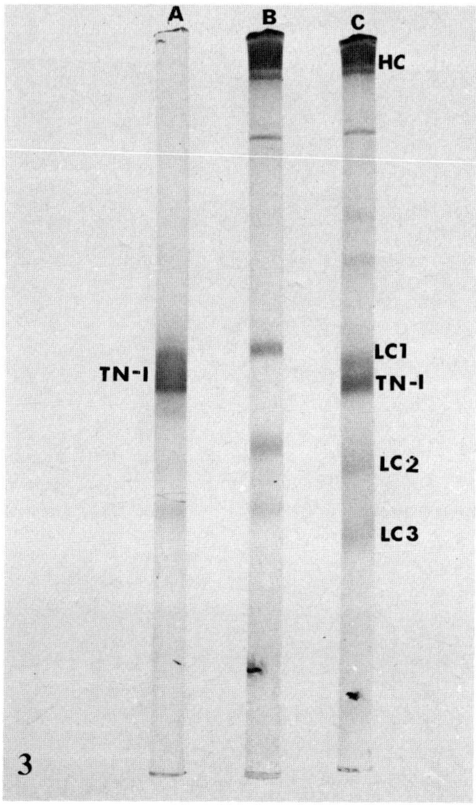

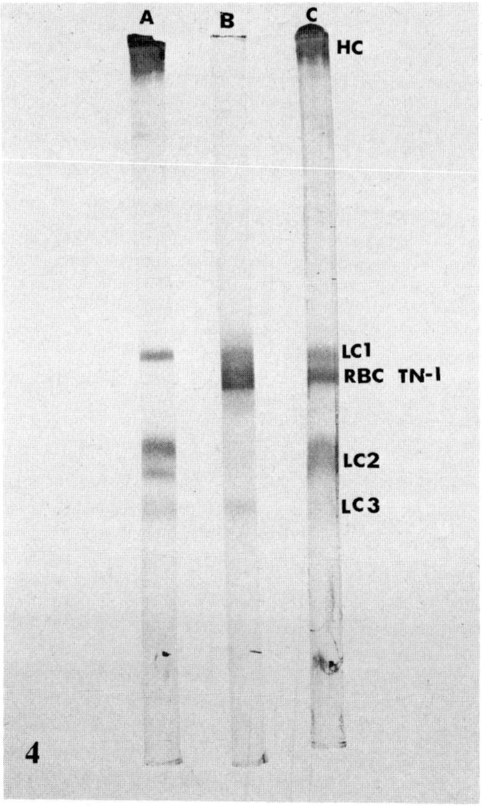

Fig. 3. SDS acrylamide electrophoresis of muscle TN-I bound to muscle myosin. All proteins were loaded on top of single 10% polyacrylamide gels. Gel A: Muscle TN-I. Gel B: Muscle myosin. Gel C: Twice-precipitated muscle myosin after preincubation with muscle TN-I. Bound TN-I migrated slightly below the LC-1 of myosin.

Fig. 4. SDS acrylamide electrophoresis of muscle myosin and erythrocyte TN-I-like protein bound to muscle myosin. All proteins were loaded on top of single 10% polyacrylamide gels. Gel A: Muscle myosin. Gel B: Erythrocyte TN-I-like protein. Gel C: Twice-precipitated muscle myosin after preincubation with erythrocyte inhibitor. Bound erythrocyte inhibitor migrated slightly below the LC-1 of muscle myosin.

ATPase Activity

The three types of cation-activated ATPase activities exhibited by myosin were tested with and without the inhibitor. It was found that myosin Ca^{2+}-ATPase activity at low KCl concentrations was inhibited 30–60% when the inhibitor was present. Figure 5 illustrates the results of such experiments. ATPase activity at 0.5 M KCl and 1 mM EDTA (K^+-EDTA) is inhibited 50% in the presence of TN-I. The Mg^{2+}-ATPase activity of myosin activated by actin was inhibited up to 60% in the presence of TN-I even when 10 μM Ca^{2+} was present in the medium. Figure 6 shows similar effects obtained by the red cell inhibitor on Ca^{2+}-, K^+-EDTA-, and Mg^{2+}-ATPase activities of muscle myosin. Inhibition ranged from 30–50% on myosin Ca^{2+}- and K^+-EDTA-ATPase activities and up to 70% on the Mg^{2+}-ATPase activity of myosin stimulated by actin.

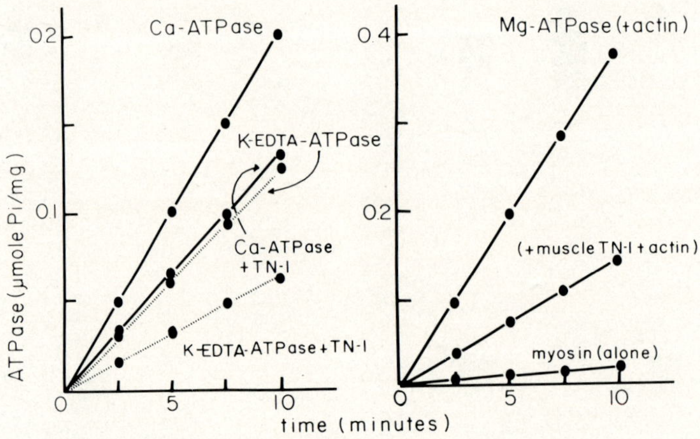

Fig. 5. Effect of muscle TN-I on Ca^{2+}- and K^+-EDTA-ATPase activity of muscle myosin (left) and on the muscle actin-activated Mg^{2+}-ATPase of muscle myosin (right). The TN-I was preincubated with myosin at 37°C for 15 minutes before addition of gamma-labeled [^{32}P] ATP. For further details see text. Representative experiment (n = 10).

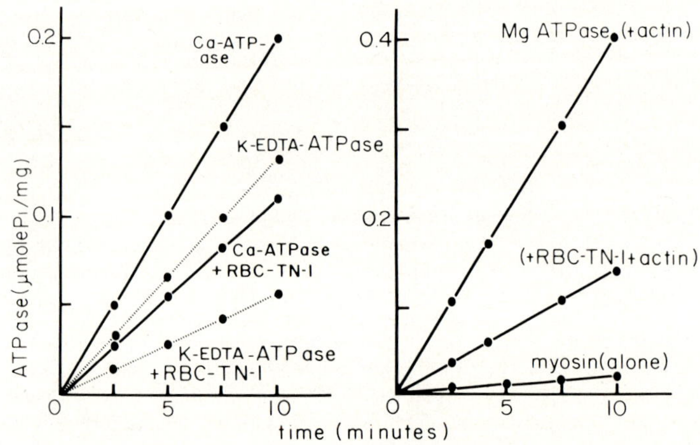

Fig. 6. Effect of erythrocyte TN-I on Ca^{2+}- and K^+-EDTA-ATPase activity of muscle myosin (left) and on the muscle actin-activated Mg^{2+}-ATPase of muscle myosin (right). Experimental conditions were the same as those described in legend for Figure 5. Representative experiment (n = 10).

Effects of TN-C on Inhibitor Proteins

In order to determine if erythrocyte TN-I possessed affinities for TN-C similar to those reported for muscle troponin, ATPase activities were performed with mixtures of TN-I and TN-C on myosin and on myosin-actin mixtures containing 10 μM Ca^{2+}. Muscle TN-C and the erythrocyte inhibitor were allowed to react in solution for 10 minutes before starting ATPase activity by the addition of Mg^{2+}-ATP. Figure 7 illustrates the results of such experiments. Myosin shows little Mg^{2+}-ATPase activity. Upon addition of actin, Mg^{2+}-ATPase activity is increased. TN-C produced a small increase in the rate of ATPase activity while addition of TN-I, as expected, showed inhibition. When both proteins,

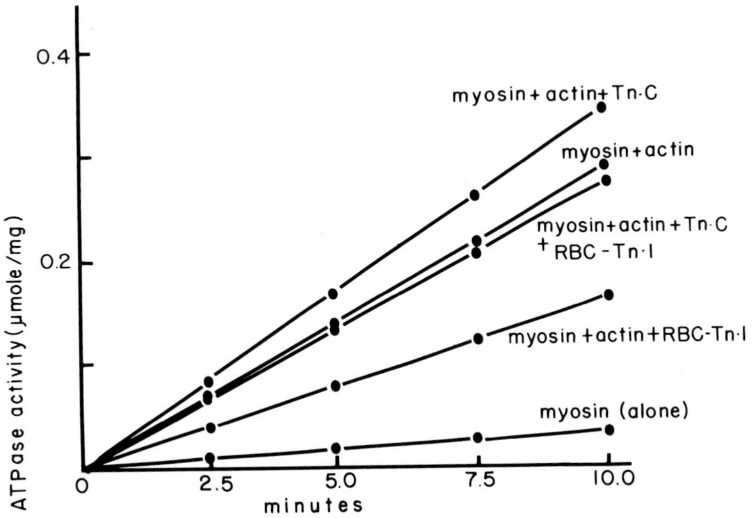

Fig. 7. Effect of muscle TN-C and erythrocyte TN-I-like protein on the muscle actin Mg^{2+}-activated ATPase of muscle myosin. Experimental conditions were the same as those described in legend for Figure 5 except that muscle TN-C was added together with the erythrocyte inhibitor. Representative experiment (n = 10).

TN-C and TN-I, were added the rate of ATPase activity was similar to that of myosin and actin. Both the inhibitory activity of TN-I or the slight activation by TN-C were found cancelled.

DISCUSSION

From human erythrocytes a protein has been isolated with characteristics similar to those of TN-I of muscle. This protein apparently is present in the red cell cytoplasm. Upon rupture of the erythrocyte membrane the inhibitor protein appeared in the hemolysate. The inhibitor – after purification by batch and column DEAE cellulose chromatography – was found to bind to myosin, to inhibit myosin ATPase activity, and to migrate like muscle TN-I on SDS acrylamide gels. Furthermore, it prevented actin from fully stimulating the Mg^{2+}-ATPase activity of myosin. In the presence of muscle TN-C and 10 μM Ca^{2+}, the erythrocyte protein did not show inhibitory activity.

Binding of the erythrocyte inhibitor protein was evident after solubilizing and precipitating myosin at low ionic strength. This effect of muscle TN-I has not been reported previously. In myofibrils it is known that TN-I modulates actin and myosin interaction while attached to the thin filaments of actin through the TN-T component of troponin and tropomyosin [24]. On the other hand, evidence has been presented that actin-myosin interaction in vitro can be modulated by a Ca^{2+}-modulator protein from brain and a muscle TN-I in the absence of TN-T [4]. The effects of TN-I reported in this work may be due to an affinity expressed by TN-I for myosin sites, ie for its light chains, in the absence of TN-T and tropomyosin. In the presence of TN-T and tropomyosin, the inhibitory activity of troponin most likely would occur through the thin filaments.

Although unlikely, the possibility that TN-I binds unspecifically to myosin should be considered. Binding was performed with myosin precipitated from solution at low ionic strength. In the presence of TN-I, both proteins were found in the precipitate. However, a solution of TN-I showed no precipitation at low ionic strength. These considerations together with the effects of TN-I on myosin ATPase suggest that true binding of the inhibitor to the myosin molecule is the most likely explanation for the inhibitor activity.

The muscle TN-I was separated from TN-T by isoelectric precipitation because the elution of troponin components from DEAE cellulose column chromatography equilibrated with 8 M urea resolved only TN-C while TN-I and TN-T emerged together. Similar results were reported by other investigators [18,24]. An earlier report [25] found that washes of actomyosin gels with low ionic strength buffers and alkaline pH resulted in desensitized actomyosin, probably by removing the components of troponin or by denaturation. When a solution of TN-I and TN-T – dialyzed to remove most of the urea – was adjusted to pH 9.25, a precipitate formed within 1–2 seconds. The supernatant contained TN-I of high purity. The precipitate dissolved easily in neutral pH buffers and contained TN-T with small amounts of TN-I. A second precipitation at pH 9.25 yielded a homogeneous TN-T preparation.

Since erythrocytes apparently do not contain a protein with characteristics similar to those of TN-T of muscle, it was unnecessary to perform DEAE chromatography in the presence of 8 M urea. To resolve the troponin-like inhibitor of erythrocytes from other proteins of the red cell hemolysate, regular DEAE cellulose column chromatography was used with a low ionic strength buffer followed by a NaCl gradient. DEAE chromatography rendered a single peak containing most of the protein present in the erythrocyte hemolysate and permitted elution of erythrocyte TN-I in the tail portion of the peak.

The erythrocyte protein showed inhibitory activity over a wide range of concentration. At molecular ratios of inhibitor to myosin of 0.5 to 5, inhibitory activity was observed. ATPase activity was reduced from 30–60% to that exhibited by muscle myosin alone. Preincubation of the protein for 10 minutes at 37° was sufficient to detect inhibitory activity. It is possible that a relationship exists between the inhibitor protein and the Ca^{2+}-modulator protein since in the presence of TN-C from muscle and 10 μM Ca^{2+}, the inhibitor protein shows no effect on myosin ATPase. Attempts made to isolate the erythrocyte Ca^{2+}-modulator protein have yielded preparations contaminated with other proteins and inadequate at present to test its biological activity.

The physiological role of the protein inhibitor present in erythrocytes remains to be elucidated. A Ca^{2+}-modulator protein with characteristics similar to those of TN-C – or C^{2+}-modulator proteins from other tissues – has been reported present in erythrocyte [8]. These proteins not only modulated the Ca^{2+} sensitivity of actomyosin mixtures, but also activated phosphodiesterase activity [5]. The erythrocyte inhibitor may interact with the modulator protein in vivo for certain red cell functions.

Erythrocytes have been found not to possess an actin myosin system similar to that found in other nonmuscle tissues; however, erythrocytes contain spectrin attached to the cytoplasmic side of the membrane, which to a certain degree exhibits properties similar to those of smooth muscle myosin [15]. Spectrin has been found to complex with actin [15, 26], to influence the polymerizing activities of erythrocyte actin [16, 27], and to possess antigenic determinants common to smooth muscle myosin [15]. It is possible that the erythrocyte inhibitor may play a role in the interaction between erythrocyte actin and spectrin and indirectly regulate specific properties of the erythrocyte membrane; this aspect is being investigated currently. It is significant, however, that erythrocytes contain a protein capable of altering the interacting activity of muscle proteins. Presently, it is not known if the erythrocyte inhibitor exists in the intact erythrocyte, free in its cytoplasm or attached to actin or spectrin polymers. Likewise, it is not known if, during the separation of proteins, during the formation of a hemolysate, and in the presence of divalent cation chelator, conditions are such that release of this protein from a given site at or near the membrane allows its isolation from the erythrocyte hemolysate.

Recently it was reported [17] that actin plays an important role in the integrity of the erythrocyte membrane and in the shape of the erythrocyte resealed ghosts. Such an inhibitor could provide regulation of actin attachment to membrane sites. Undoubtedly, further study should elucidate its role in red cell functions.

ACKNOWLEDGMENTS

Supported in part by NIH grants NS 12467, HL 20718, and AHA Grant-in-Aid 75-811. S.P., to whom correspondence may be addressed, is an Established Investigator of the AHA.

REFERENCES

1. Perry SV, Margreth A, Adelstein RS (eds: "Contractile Systems in Non-muscle Tissues." Amsterdam: Elsevier/North-Holland Biomedical Press, 1976.
2. Fine RE, Lehman W, Head J, Blitz A: Nature (London) 258:260, 1975.
3. Watterson DM, Harrelson WG Jr, Keller PM, Sharief F, Vanaman TC: J Biol Chem 251:4501, 1976.
4. Amphlet GW, Vanaman TC, Perry SV: FEBS Lett 72:163, 1976.
5. Vanaman TC, Sharief F, Awramik JL, Mendel PA, Watterson DM: In Perry SV et al (eds): "Contractile Systems in Non-muscle Tissues." Amsterdam: Elsevier/North-Holland Biomedical Press, 1976, p 165.
6. Stevens FC, Walsh TM, Ho HC, Teo TC, Wang JH: J Biol Chem 251:4495, 1976.
7. McGowan EB, Speiser S, Stracher A: J Cell Biol 70:79a, 1976.
8. Gopinath RM, Vincenzi FF: Biochem Biophys Res Comm 77:1203, 1977.
9. Kuo IY, Coffee CJ: J Biol Chem 251:6315, 1976.
10. Cohen I, Kaminski E, DeVries A: FEBS Lett 34:315, 1973.
11. Puszkin S, Lin E, Kochwa S, Rosenfield RE: Fed Proc Fed Am Soc Exp Biol 35:299a, 1976.
12. Puszkin S, Kochwa S: J Biol Chem 249:7711, 1974.
13. Adelstein RS, Chacko S, Barylko B, Scordilis SP, Conti MA: In Perry SV et al (eds): "Contractile Systems in Non-muscle Tissues." Amsterdam: Elsevier/North-Holland Biomedical Press, 1976, p 153.
14. Hartshorne DJ, Abrams L, Aksoy M, Dabrowka R, Driska S, Sharkey E: In Stephens NL (ed): "The Biochemistry of Smooth Muscle." Baltimore: University Park Press, 1977.
15. Sheetz MP, Painter RG, Singer SJ: Biochemistry 15:4486, 1976.
16. Pinder JC, Bray D, Gratzer WB: Nature (London) 258:765, 1975.
17. Birchmeier W, Singer SJ: Biochem Biophys Res Comm 77:1354, 1977.
18. Greaser ML, Gergely J: J Biol Chem 248:2125, 1973.
19. Puszkin S, Puszkin E, Maimon J, Rouault C, Schook W, Ores C, Kochwa S, Rosenfield RE: J Biol Chem 252:5529, 1977.
20. Lowry OH, Rosebrough NJ, Farr AL, Randall RJ: J Biol Chem 193:265, 1951.
21. Marsh BB: Biochim Biophys Acta 32:357, 1959.
22. Puszkin S, Kochwa S, Puszkin E, Rosenfield RE: J Biol Chem 250:2085, 1975.
23. Weber K, Osborn M: J Biol Chem 244:4406, 1969.
24. Potter JD, Gergely J: Biochemistry 13:2697, 1974.
25. Stewart JM, Levy H: J Biol Chem 245:5764, 1970.
26. Tilney LB, Detmers P: J Cell Biol 66:508, 1975.
27. Puszkin S, Maimon J, Puszkin E: (In preparation).

Journal of Supramolecular Structure 9:269–274 (1978)
Normal and Abnormal Red Cell Membranes 259–264

Modulator Binding Protein Antagonizes Activation of (Ca^{2+} + Mg^{2+})-ATPase and Ca^{2+} Transport of Red Blood Cell Membranes

Fred L. Larsen, Beat U. Raess, Thomas R. Hinds, and Frank F. Vincenzi

Department of Pharmacology, School of Medicine, University of Washington, Seattle, Washington 98195

Red blood cells contain a protein that activates membrane-bound (Ca^{2+} + Mg^{2+})-ATPase and Ca^{2+} transport. The red blood cell activator protein is similar to a modulator protein that stimulates cyclic AMP phosphodiesterase. Wang and Desai [Journal of Biological Chemistry 252:4175–4184, 1977] described a modulator-binding protein that antagonizes the activation of cyclic AMP phosphodiesterase by modulator protein. In the present work, modulator-binding protein was shown to antagonize the activation of (Ca^{2+} + Mg^{2+})-ATPase and Ca^{2+} transport by red blood cell activator protein. The results further demonstrate the similarity between the activator protein from human red blood cells and the modulator protein from bovine brain.

Key words: **modulator-binding protein, (Ca^{2+} + Mg^{2+})-ATPase, calcium transport, red blood cell membrane, calcium-dependent regulator protein**

The Ca^{2+} pump of the human red blood cell (RBC) membrane has been linked to membrane-bound (Ca^{2+} + Mg^{2+})-ATPase activity [1–3]. A proteinaceous activator of the (Ca^{2+} + Mg^{2+})-ATPase activity is present [4] and can be isolated [5] from RBC hemolysates. Hemolysates [6] as well as purified activator protein increase the rate of uptake of $^{45}Ca^{2+}$ into inside-out vesicles of RBC membranes [7]. Because of the close association of ATPase activity and transport [3], and because of reversible Ca^{2+}-dependent binding of the activator protein to RBC membranes [8, 9], it has been suggested that the activator protein acts as a "switch" for the Ca^{2+}pump.

RBC activator protein is similar, if not identical, to a modulator protein that has been reported to activate cyclic nucleotide phosphodiesterase [10] and adenylate cyclase [11]. Modulator protein, as it will be referred to here, is also known as calcium-dependent regulator (CDR) [11]. Modulator protein also activates the (Ca^{2+} + Mg^{2+})-ATPase activity of isolated RBC membranes [12, 13] and stimulates active Ca^{2+} uptake into inside-out vesicles [7], presumably by a similar mechanism. In addition, RBC activator protein

Received April 25, 1978; accepted June 22, 1978.

0091-7419/78/0902-0269$01.40

activates phosphodiesterase [12]. Thus, the two proteins appear to be functionally similar. Modulator protein, and/or activator protein, or the family of Ca^{2+}-binding proteins they represent, may mediate a number of intracellular actions of Ca^{2+} [14], but elucidation of these remains to be determined.

Recently, Wang and co-workers described the isolation from bovine brain of a protein that antagonizes the activation of cyclic AMP phosphodiesterase by a modulator protein [15]. This protein was named modulator-binding protein (MBP) because it antagonizes the activation of phosphodiesterase by binding the modulator protein-Ca^{2+} complex, thereby antagonizing the activation of phosphodiesterase. Thus, MBP and phosphodiesterase can "compete" for the protein modulator–Ca^{2+} complex. The activity of phosphodiesterase in vitro thus depends on the relative amounts of MBP and phosphodiesterase (as well as protein modulator and Ca^{2+}) [15]. We reasoned that if RBC protein activator and the protein modulator are closely related or identical and if activation of (Ca^{2+} + Mg^{2+})-ATPase and Ca^{2+} transport is analogous to phosphodiesterase activation, then modulator-binding protein should antagonize the activation of the ATPase and transport by RBC protein activator. Present results demonstrate that MBP antagonizes the activation of both (Ca^{2+} + Mg^{2+})-ATPase and Ca^{2+} transport by RBC activator protein.

METHODS

RBC membrane ghosts were prepared [16] from outdated human cells and assayed at 37° for ATPase activity as previously described [13], with modifications noted herein. The (Ca^{2+} + Mg^{2+})-ATPase assay medium contains, in a final incubation volume of 3.0 ml, approximately 0.2 mg membrane protein; 18 mM–18 mM histidine–imidazole buffer, pH 7.1; 3 mM ATP; 3 mM $MgCl_2$; 80 mM NaCl; 15 mM KCl; 0.1 mM ouabain; 0.2 mM $CaCl_2$ and 0.1 mM EGTA. Mg^{2+}-ATPase activity was determined in tubes in which $CaCl_2$ was omitted. Purified RBC activator protein and/or MBP were included in some tubes as noted. Tubes were incubated for 60 or 90 min, and the reaction was terminated by addition of sodium dodecyl sulfate (SDS, final concentration 6.67%).

The activator protein from RBCs was isolated by a method developed in our laboratory. The method will be reported elsewhere [Jung, Hinds and Vincenzi, in preparation]. In brief, the RBC hemolysate from outdated human RBCs was subjected to DEAE-Sephadex and gel filtration (G-75) chromatography (apparent mol wt ~ 30,000). The resulting protein gives a single band on isoelectric focusing (pI = 4.0) and SDS-polyacrylamide gel electrophoresis (apparent mol wt = 20,000). MBP from bovine brain was a gift from Dr. Jerry Wang, University of Manitoba, Canada.

Inside-out RBC membrane vesicles were prepared from fresh RBCs according to the method of Steck and Kant [17], with minor modifications in order to remove phosphate. Purified inside-out vesicles were washed once in 10 mM Tris-glycylglycine buffer (pH 7.4) with 0.025 mM $MgCl_2$, once in 20 mM Tris-glycylglycine buffer (pH 7.4) with 0.05 mM $MgCl_2$, and once in 40 mM Tris-glycylglycine (pH 7.4) with 0.1 mM $MgCl_2$. Vesicles were stored in a small volume of 40 mM Tris-glycylclycine buffer and were used within two days.

The percent inside-out vesicle concentration was assessed by the previously described method [17] of measuring acetylcholinesterase activity in the absence and presence of Triton X-100. Our preparation typically contained 75–80% inside-out vesicles. $^{45}Ca^{2+}$ uptake experiments were conducted at 25°C in 25 mM Tris-glycylglycine (pH 7.4), 50.0 mM NaCl, 1.0 mM $MgCl_2$, 1.0 mM ATP, 0.1 mM $CaCl_2$ ($^{45}CaCl_2$ specific activity, 1.799

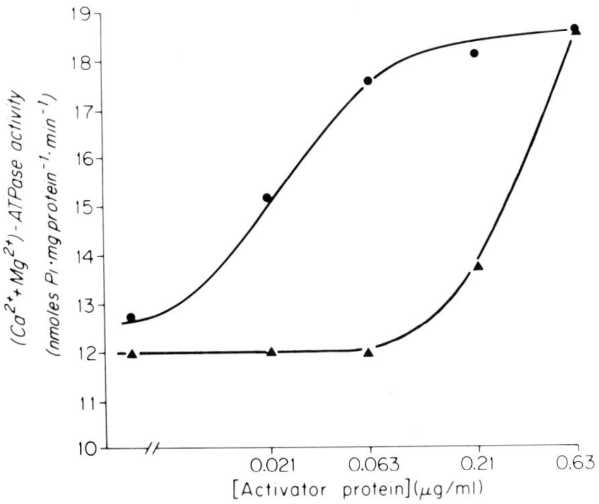

Fig. 1. Modulator-binding protein antagonism of $(Ca^{2+} + Mg^{2+})$-ATPase activation by RBC activator protein. ATPase activity was determined as described in Methods. In the absence of modulator-binding protein (●—●), the ATPase activity increased above "basal" (approximately 12.5 nmoles Pi·mg protein^{-1}·min^{-1}). In the presence of 1.67 µg/ml modulator-binding protein (▲—▲), the curve of activation was shifted.

$\times 10^6$ cpm/µmole), and about 0.2 mg inside-out vesicle protein in a total volume of 0.6 ml. Vesicles were preincubated for 30 min prior to addition of ATP. Beginning 10 min after the addition of ATP, 100 µl samples were removed at 20-min intervals (total 5 samples) and quenched in 1.5 ml of ice-cold 40 mM tris-glycylglycine (pH 7.4) and 0.1 mM $MgCl_2$. Inside-out vesicles were collected by vacuum filtration on Amicon microporous filters (0.45 µm) and were washed once with 1.5 ml of the Tris-glycylglycine buffer. Filters were dissolved in 10 ml of Aquasol and counted for $^{45}Ca^{2+}$ activity. Transport rates were determined by linear regression of the five data points.

RESULTS

As previously reported, $(Ca^{2+} + Mg^{2+})$-ATPase activity of RBC membranes is stimulated by activator protein [12, 13]. Average values for maximal activation are usually about twofold or threefold above the "basal" activity (in the absence of added activator). Data in Figure 1 were obtained from membranes in which the magnitude of activation was somewhat less than aveage. As a function of activator protein concentration, $(Ca^{2+} + Mg^{2+})$-ATPase activity increased from approximately 12 to 19 pmoles Pi·mg protein^{-1}·min^{-1} (Fig. 1, solid circles). Half-maximal activation was obtained at an activator concentration of approximately 0.027 µg/ml; 1.35×10^{-9}M assuming a molecular weight of 20,000 or 0.40 µg activator·mg membrane protein^{-1}. MBP antagonized activation of $(Ca^{2+} + Mg^{2+})$-ATPase by activator. In the presence of modulator-binding protein (1.67 µg/ml, 1.75×10^{-8}M, assuming mol wt 95,000), the curve of ATPase activation was shifted approximately tenfold in an apparently competitive fashion (1.41×10^{-8}M activator for ½ maximal).

MBP inhibited the activated $(Ca^{2+} + Mg^{2+})$-ATPase in a concentration-dependent fashion. Figure 2 shows $(Ca^{2+} + Mg^{2+})$-ATPase activity of a different membrane prepara-

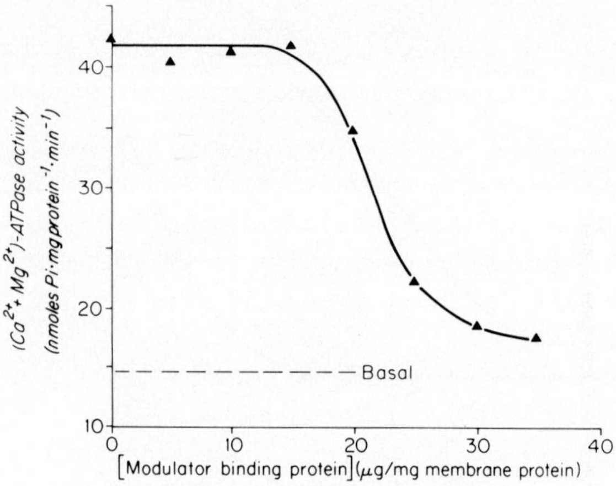

Fig. 2. Inhibition of activated (Ca^{2+} + Mg^{2+})-ATPase by modulator-binding protein. ATPase activity was assayed as described in Methods, except that all tubes contained 0.18 μg/ml of activator protein. "Basal" indicates activity present in the same membranes without activator. Addition of modulator-binding protein produced a dose-dependent inhibition of the activated (Ca^{2+} + Mg^{2+})-ATPase. As in Figure 1, modulator-binding protein did not inhibit the basal (Ca^{2+} + Mg^{2+})-ATPase activity.

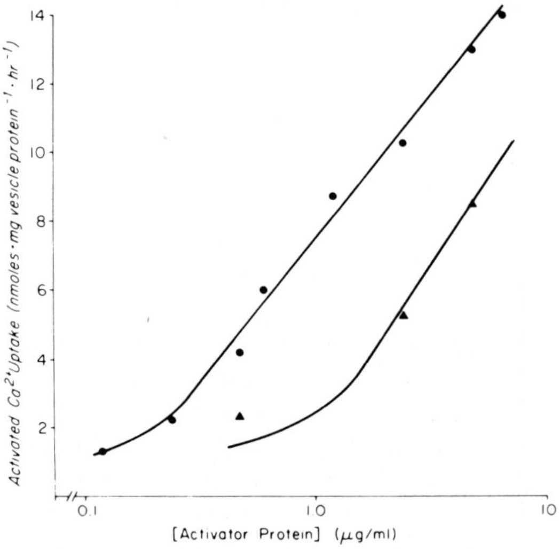

Fig. 3. Modulator-binding protein antagonism of Ca^{2+} transport activation by RBC activator protein. Activator stimulated uptake of $^{45}Ca^{2+}$ into inside-out vesicles of RBC membrane was measured as described in Methods. Both in the absence (●—●) and presence (▲—▲) of modulator-binding protein (3.25 μg/ml), $^{45}Ca^{2+}$ uptake was increased as a function of the concentration of activator protein. The curve was shifted to higher activator concentrations in the presence of modulator-binding protein.

tion as a function of MBP concentration in the presence of activator (1.02×10^{-8}M). The molar ratio of activator/MBP ranged from 2.63 (8% inhibition) to 0.38 (88% inhibition). Even at the highest concentration, MBP did not inhibit the activity below the basal level.

The Ca^{2+}pump normally transports Ca^{2+} from inside the cell to outside and Ca^{2+}, Mg^{2+}, and ATP are required at the inner membrane surface [3]. Because the transport is directional, and because the activator protein interacts with the inner membrane surface [9], it is convenient to use inside-out vesicles of RBC membrane for such studies. As reported previously [7], Ca^{2+} impermeable inside-out vesicles of RBC membrane actively take up Ca^{2+}. In the absence of added activator the vesicles took up 1.75 nmoles $Ca^{2+}\cdot$mg vesicle protein$^{-1}\cdot$h^{-1}. The rate of active transport of Ca^{2+} across the RBC membrane was increased by the activator protein. Activator-stimulated uptake (Fig. 3) was taken as the uptake rate above "basal" occurring in the presence of added activator protein. In the presence of activator (6.5 μg/ml) activated uptake was 14.95 nmoles $Ca^{2+}\cdot$mg vesicle protein$^{-1}\cdot$hr^{-1}, which corresponds to an eightfold activation. The stimulatory effect was antagonized by modulator-binding protein in an apparently competitive fashion (Fig. 3), although saturation was not obtained. A double reciprocal plot of these data yielded an apparent K_d for activator of 4.16×10^{-8}M. Even considering the influence of temperature, the rate of transport into inside-out vesicles is considerably less than the rates reported for RBCs or right-side out resealed RBC ghosts [18]. The specific activity of the (Ca^{2+} + Mg^{2+})-ATPase of inside-out vesicles is also markedly reduced. At 37° in the presence of 1 μg/ml of activator protein, inside-out vesicles exhibited an ATPase activity of 0.25 nmoles Pi$\cdot$mg protein$^{-1}\cdot$min. By contrast, isolated RBC membranes usually exhibit ATPase activities in the range of about 30–40 nmoles Pi$\cdot$mg protein$^{-1}\cdot$min^{-1} (activator present).

DISCUSSION

The present results demonstrate that MBP from bovine brain can antagonize the activation of membrane-bound (Ca^{2+} + Mg^{2+})-ATPase by RBC activator protein. It was also shown that MBP antagonizes activation of Ca^{2+} transport by the activator protein. From the work of Wang and Desai, it is known that MBP antagonizes activation of phosphodiesterase by protein modulator [15]. Given the similarities between modulator protein and RBC activator protein [12, 13], it seems likely that a similar mechanism of antagonism is operative in each case. Modulator protein activates phosphodiesterase by binding Ca^{2+} and then binding to the enzyme. Wang and Desai [15] showed that the modulator protein–Ca^{2+} complex can also bind to MBP. The result is that activation of phosphodiesterase can be competitively antagonized by modulator-binding protein, depending on the relative amounts of the two proteins. Similar findings were obtained in this study. Thus, modulator-binding protein appears to antagonize RBC activator protein competitively, both in the activation of ATPase and in transport. The model described by Wang and Desai would appear to be applicable and sufficient to interpret the present results.

Although MBP did antagonize the effects of activator protein, it did not inhibit "basal" (Ca^{2+} + Mg^{2+})-ATPase activity. This probably means that the basal ATPase activity is not due to endogenous activator protein bound to the membrane. The basal (Ca^{2+} + Mg^{2+})-ATPase activity that is present in the absence of activator (or presence of sufficient MBP) may represent the activity of an enzyme not related to Ca^{2+} transport. The apparent K_d for activator protein determined by uptake experiments is considerably larger than the same value obtained from ATPase activities in isolated RBC membranes.

From this and the relatively low rate of transport in inside-out vesicles, we assume that some damage to the membrane and/or transport system occurs under the rather drastic conditions necessary to prepare inside-out vesicles. In spite of these limitations, active uptake of Ca^{2+} does occur, and the rate of uptake is increased as a function of activator protein concentration.

The present results provide another illustration of the similarities between RBC activator protein and protein modulator. It is not yet known whether RBC activator and protein modulator are identical. It is also not known whether modulator-binding protein exists in the RBC. If activator protein and/or similar proteins stimulate plasma membrane $(Ca^{2+} + Mg^{2+})$-ATPase and Ca^{2+} transport, then, where present, they may influence Ca^{2+} transport as well as cyclic AMP metabolism.

ACKNOWLEDGMENTS

Dr. Jerry Wang of the University of Manitoba, Canada, kindly supplied the modulator-binding protein. This work was supported in part by US Public Health Service grants AM 16436 and GM 00109 and by a grant from the Cystic Fibrosis Foundation. B.U.R. was supported by a National Research Service Award from the National Institutes of Health (GM 07270).

REFERENCES

1. Schatzmann HJ, Vincenzi FF (1969): J Physiol (Lond) 201:369–395.
2. Olson EJ, Cazort RJ (1969): J Gen Physiol 53:311–322.
3. Schatzmann HJ (1975): In Bronner F, Kleinzeller A (eds): "Current Topics in Membranes and Transport," Vol. 6, New York: Academic, pp 125–168.
4. Bond GH, Clough DL (1973): Biochim Biophys Acta 323:592–599.
5. Luthra MG, Hildenbrandt GR, Hanahan DJ (1976): Biochim Biophys Acta 419:164–179.
6. Macintyre JD, Green JW (1977): Fed Proc (Abstr) 36:271.
7. Hinds TR, Larsen FL, Vincenzi FF (1978): Biochem Biophys Res Commun 81:455–461.
8. Farrance ML, Vincenzi FF (1977): Biochim Biophys Acta 471:59–66.
9. Vincenzi FF, Farrance ML (1977): J Supramol Struct 7:301–306.
10. Cheung WY (1970): J Biol Chem 246:2859–2869.
11. Brostrom MA, Brostrom CO, Breckenridge BM, Wolff DJ (1975): Proc Natl Acad Sci USA 72:64–68.
12. Jarrett HW, Penniston JT (1977): Biochem Biophys Res Commun 77:1210–1216.
13. Gopinath RM, Vincenzi FF (1977): Biochem Biophys Res Commun 77:1203–1209.
14. Vanaman TC, Sharief F, Watterson DM (1977): In Wasserman RH, Carradino RA, Carafoli E, Kretsinger RH, MacLennan DH, Siegal FL (eds): "Calcium-Binding Proteins and Calcium Function." New York: North-Holland, pp 107–116.
15. Wang JH, Desai R (1977): J Biol Chem 252:4175–4184.
16. Farrance ML, Vincenzi FF (1977): Biochim Biophys Acta 471:49–58.
17. Steck TL, Kant JA (1974): In Fleischer S, Packer L (eds): "Methods in Enzymology," Vol. 31, New York: Academic, pp 172–180.
18. Larsen FL, Hinds TR, Vincenzi FF (1978): J Membrane Biol 41:361–376.

Journal of Supramolecular Structure 9:275–288 (1978)
Normal and Abnormal Red Cell Membranes 265–278

Membrane Effects of Imidoesters in Hereditary Stomatocytosis

W. C. Mentzer, G. K. H. Lam, B. H. Lubin, A. Greenquist, S. L. Schrier, and W. Lande

From the Departments of Pediatrics and the Cancer Research Institute, University of California, San Francisco, CA 94143; Department of Medicine, Stanford University, Stanford, CA 94305; and the Bruce Lyon Memorial Research Laboratories, Children's Hospital of the East Bay, Oakland, CA 94609

The marked increase in cation (Na^+, K^+) permeability that results in swollen, cup-shaped red cells in the hereditary stomatocytosis syndrome can be corrected in vitro with a bifunctional crosslinking reagent, dimethyl adipimidate (DMA). ^{45}Ca influx in intact RBC, ^{45}Ca efflux in red ghosts, and ^{45}Ca retention in red ghosts are normal and not influenced by DMA. Endocytosis in resealed red ghosts is strikingly impaired but becomes normal if cells are first treated with 2 mM DMA. Protein kinase mediated phosphorylation of membrane proteins by AT^{32}P – only 20–40% of normal control values in both short-term (5 min) and more extended (60 min) incubations – is not improved by DMA. After reaction of ^{14}C-DMA with stomatocytes, radiolabel is found associated with phosphatidyl serine and phosphatidyl ethanolamine and is also widely distributed among membrane proteins. Cation permeability of stomatocytes is corrected at DMA concentrations (1 mM) that result in barely detectable crosslinking of aminophospholipids or proteins, suggesting that either crosslinking of a minor component present in only small quantities or intramolecular (rather than intermolecular) crosslinking is responsible for the permeability effects. DMA, whose maximal crosslinking dimension is 7.3–9 Å, is the most effective bifunctional imidoester of those tested. Shorter (dimethyl malonimidate) or longer (dimethylsuberimidate) reagents are either less effective than DMA or totally without effect.

Key words: endocytosis; abnormality in stomatocytosis; hemolytic anemia, associated with hereditary stomatocytosis; stomatocytosis, hereditary; imidoesters, effects in stomatocytosis

Stomatocytes, or cup-shaped red cells, are the primary morphologic abnormality in the blood of individuals with hereditary stomatocytosis, a congenital and sometimes familial form of moderate to severe hemolytic anemia.

Although several earlier reports commented on the association between stomatocytes

Received April 24, 1978; accepted July 26, 1978.

0091-7419/78/0902-0275$02.60

and hemolytic anemia, Zarkowsky and his co-workers were the first to describe this disorder in biochemical terms [1]. They, and others subsequently, found a near-complete reversal of the usual monovalent cation composition of the erythrocyte [1–4]. Such abnormalities have proved to be the result of remarkable increases in passive cation permeability. Potassium permeability is increased 3- to 20-fold, and sodium permeability is even higher. These increases are, to some extent, counterbalanced by equally remarkable increases in active transport supported by markedly accelerated erythrocyte glycolysis. However, when optimal conditions for glycolysis do not exist, the rate of active transport diminishes, the cation permeability lesion becomes predominant, and there may be rapid passive movement of sodium into the cell and efflux of potassium. Since the rate of sodium movement exceeds that of potassium, there is a net increase in cell cation content, leading to an obligate osmotic increase in cell water, cell swelling, and eventually cell lysis [2].

We have previously shown that the cation permeability defect can be repaired in vitro by chemical modification of stomatocytes with imidoesters [5]. In one patient with severe hemolytic anemia, reaction of stomatocytes with dimethyl adipimidate (DMA) reduced ouabain-associated potassium loss from 15 to 1.7 and sodium gain from 22 to 2.5 mEq per liter of red cells per hour. Red cell volume, cation concentration, and deformability, previously abnormal, rapidly became normal after stomatocytes were reacted with DMA. Instead of stomatocytes, normal red cells and target cells were noted on both light microscopy and scanning electron microscopy. The survival (half-time) of ^{51}Cr-labeled DMA-treated stomatocytes infused into rats rendered tolerant to human erythrocytes by pretreatment with ethyl palmitate and cobra-venom factor was double that of untreated stomatocytes. Thus, chemical modification of the defect in vitro allowed stomatocytes to regain many properties of normal erythrocytes and favorably influenced the subsequent survival of these cells in vivo.

The studies of endocytosis and calcium metabolism described in this report further characterize the effect of imidoesters on intact cells or membrane ghosts. In addition, attempts to determine the location and nature of the reaction between imidoesters and the stomatocytic erythrocyte membrane are described. These observations confirm the potential of imidoesters as chemical probes, of value in defining the nature of the membrane defect in hereditary stomatocytosis.

METHODS

After informed consent was obtained, heparinized blood was drawn from an eight-year-old splenectomized boy [2, 5] with hereditary stomatocytosis and persistent hemolytic anemia. Blood was also obtained from normal controls and patients with reticulocytosis due to sickle cell anemia, glucose phosphate isomerase deficiency, or glucose-6-phosphate dehydrogenase deficiency. The reaction between red cells and imidoesters was carried out as previously described [5]. Imidoester was added in dry powder form to heparinized, washed cells which were then incubated at 37° in Krebs-Henseleit buffer, pH 7.4, with added 10 mM glucose and 1% bovine serum albumin at a hematocrit of 5% for six hours. After incubation the cells were washed in isotonic Tris-Mg Cl_2, and red cell Na^+ and K^+ content were determined by flame photometry [5]. Shorter incubation periods were used in some experiments. Endocytosis was studied in red ghosts prepared from cells incubated with or without imidoester. The ghosts were resealed with 2.5 mM ATP, 2.5 mM Mg^{++}, and 1.0 mM Ca^{++} present in the hemolyzing solution [6]. After resealing, ghosts were incubated for 15 min and then fixed for transmission electron microscopy [6]. Calcium influx (^{45}Ca) was measured in red cells that had been metabolically depleted by incubation for 90 min with 1 mM iodoacetate. The procedure used was that described by Wiley et al [7], except that 5 mM adenosine was substituted for 5 mM inosine in the initial metabolic depletion step and the final concentration of Ca^{++} was 1.0 mM instead of 1.5 mM. Efflux of ^{45}Ca was measured in resealed red ghosts, as described by Schrier and his co-workers [6]. At the conclusion (total incubation time, 20 min) of each efflux experiment, residual ^{45}Ca in the ghost pellet was also determined [6]. To evaluate the stability of the permeability effect of DMA, red cells were first incubated with imidoester (2 mM DMA) for 6 h (using the standard conditions described above) to restore normal cation and water content. As a control, cells were also incubated under identical conditions with sucrose (2 mM) instead of DMA. After incubation, the buffer was removed; the red cells were resuspended in fresh autologous plasma with added acid citrate dextrose (NIH formula "A" 0.6 cc/4 cc plasma), penicillin (12.5 μ/ml blood), and streptomycin (12.5 μgm/ml blood); and the cell-plasma mixture (hematocrit 20–25%) was stored at 4°C. At intervals, aliquots were removed for measurement of cell size, cation (Na^+, K^+) content, and water content [5]. At the end of two weeks of storage, hemolysis of normal red cells or stomatocytes was less than 1%.

To determine relative binding of imidoester to the cell membrane or to hemoglobin, red cells were incubated for 6 h with ^{14}C-DMA (specific activity 2.52 mCi/mM). After lysis, radioactivity present in ghosts or hemoglobin obtained from 1 ml of packed red cells was measured. Samples were thoroughly solubilized (Protosol) and bleached with H_2O_2 prior to analysis by B scintillation spectrometry.

Red cell ghosts were prepared using 5 mM phosphate buffer, pH 8.0, as described by Fairbanks and his associates [8]. For lipid analysis, ghosts were extracted with chloroform-methanol 1:1 v/v [9] and back extracted with 0.02 M KCl. The resulting extract was spotted on silica gel thin layer chromatography (TLC) plates. The usual developing solvent consisted of chloroform:methanol:ammonium hydroxide:water (35:15:2.5:1). In some experiments, another solvent, chloroform:methanol:acetic acid:water (50:15:4:1.5) was used. The location of each major phospholipid was determined by exposure of the TLC plate to iodine vapor. Comparisons were made with simultaneously chromatographed purified phospholipid standards obtained from bacterial membranes (Sigma Chemical Co). In addition, amidinated and crosslinked phospholipid standards were prepared with DMA for use in subsequent TLC analyses. Phosphatidyl ethanolamine and phsophatidyl serine were sonicated with Hepes-salt buffer (pH 7.84) in separate tubes. The resulting emulsions were transferred to tubes containing dry 1,6-^{14}C-DMA dihydrochloride (ICN Pharmaceuticals) and resonicated. The DMA concentration was 5 mM and the DMA to phospholipid molar ratio was 3.7 to 1. The lipid was extracted with 2:2:1.8 chloroform–methanol–0.02 M KCl as described by Bligh and Dyer [33] and then concentrated under a stream of dry nitrogen. The identity of amidinated or crosslinked phospholipids was verified by determining the molar ratio of DMA:phosphorus after elution and concentration of each abnormally migrating phospholipid found after reaction with DMA. Total lipid phosphorus was determined by the method of Lowry et al [34], and the amount of DMA present was calculated from its known specific activity after suitable corrections for counting efficiency. Molar ratios obtained were: PE-DMA = 1.01, PE-DMA-PE = 2.07, PS-DMA = 0.78. PS-DMA-PS could not be determined because it migrated with cold PS in the systems we used. In some experiments, measured segments of the silica gel were removed from the TLC plate by scraping, and the amount of radioactivity in each segment was determined by B scintillation spectrometry.

Red cell ghosts were solubilized in 0.5% SDS plus 0.5 mM EDTA and 0.02 M dithiothreitol, incubated 1 h (37°), then analyzed by 4% polyacrylamide gel electrophoresis, as described by Fairbanks et al [8]. The resulting gels were stained for protein with Coomassie blue and for glycoproteins with PAS [8]. Alternatively, the gels were sliced (2-mm segments), heated to 60° with 30% H_2O_2 for 1–2 h, then analyzed for radioactivity using B scintillation spectrometry.

The phosphorylation of membrane proteins was evaluated in ghost preparations using methods described by Greenquist and Shohet [11]. The incorporation of ^{32}P from $AT^{32}P$ was determined after both 5 and 60 min of incubation. In some experiments, casein (10 mg/ml) was added to the system in order to detect the rate of phosphorylation of an exogenous (nonmembrane) protein substrate by membrane protein kinase [12].

Imidoesters were obtained from Pierce Chemical Company, $^{45}Ca\ Cl_2$ from New England Nuclear, and ^{14}C-DMA from ICN Pharmaceuticals, Inc. $AT^{32}P$ was prepared according to the method described by Glynn and Chappell [13]. Precast 4% polyacrylamide gels were supplied by Bio Rad.

RESULTS

Endocytosis and Calcium Metabolism

Endocytic vacuole formation induced in resealed red ghosts by ATP in the presence of calcium and magnesium is shown in Figure 1. Endocytosis was virtually absent in stomatocyte ghosts. If stomatocytes were treated with 2 mM DMA, intense, rather than impaired, endocytosis was subsequently noted in ghost preparations. The active endocytosis present in untreated normal control ghosts was not altered by DMA.

Because alterations in the incorporation of calcium into red cell membranes or in Ca^{++} efflux may modify endocytosis [6], several aspects of calcium metabolism were evaluated. As shown in Table I, ^{45}Ca uptake by metabolically depleted stomatocytes was twice that observed in normal cells and was further increased slightly in DMA-treated stomatocytes. The efflux of $^{45}Ca^{++}$ from resealed red ghosts was slightly higher in stomatocytes than in normal control cells, consistent with the large number of reticulocytes present [14]. DMA had no effect on calcium efflux of either normal or stomatocytic red cells. Measurement of residual $^{45}Ca^{++}$ within the ghosts at the conclusion of the efflux study revealed increased Ca^{++} in stomatocytes, once again probably consistent with reticulocytosis [14]. DMA did not affect residual $^{45}Ca^{++}$ in normal cells or stomatocytes.

Duration of the Effect of DMA Upon Stomatocyte Cation Permeability

Under the incubation conditions employed, uptake of ^{14}C-DMA was rapid and was virtually complete after 30 min of incubation [15]. The continued presence of imidoester in the incubation medium after 30 min was not required for the complete correction of the permeability defect in stomatocytes.

The duration of the effect upon permeability was evaluated in red cells stored at 4° in acid citrate dextrose (Fig 2). Under these conditions, normal erythrocytes gradually gained sodium. In contrast, stomatocytes rapidly gained sodium, reaching an equilibrium value within the first day of incubation. However, if stomatocytes were first treated with DMA and allowed to reestablish normal levels of potassium and sodium, the subsequent gain of sodium by such cells after two weeks of storage was no greater than that observed

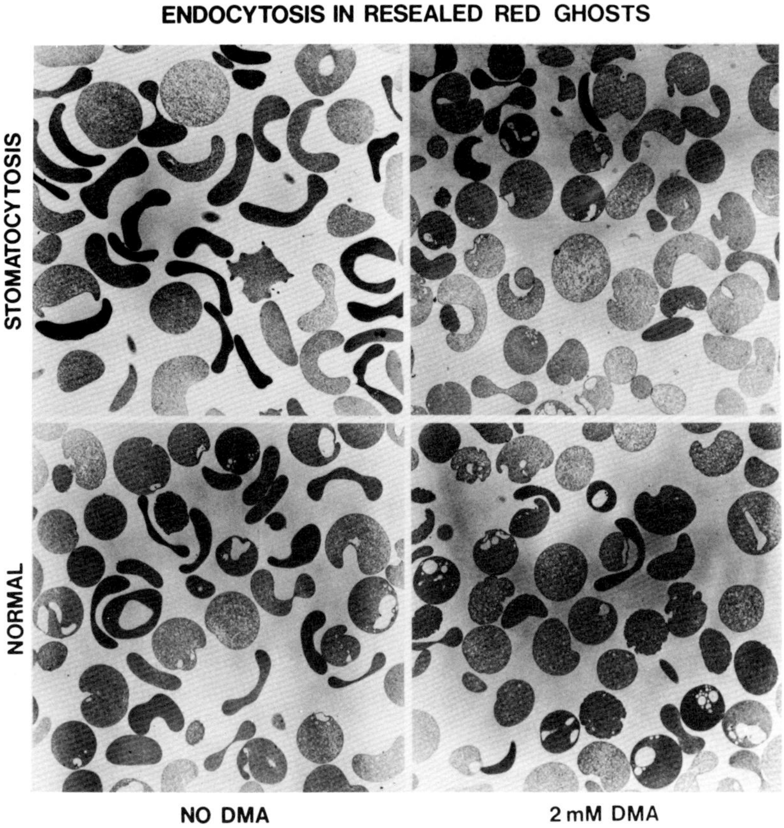

Fig 1. Electron micrographs of erythrocyte ghosts hemolyzed with 2.5 mM ATP, 1.0 mM Ca, and 2.5 mM Mg and then incubated for 15 min at 37° [6]. Top left – stomatocytes, no DMA; top right – stomatocytes + 2 mM DMA; bottom left – normal red cells, no DMA; bottom right – normal red cells + 2 mM DMA. (original magnification, × 1,900).

TABLE I. Calcium Metabolism in Stomatocytosis

	No DMA	2 mM DMA
^{45}Ca Uptake[a] by red cells		
Stomatocytosis	5.59	9.95
Normal control	2.61	–
^{45}Ca Efflux[b] from resealed red ghosts		
Stomatocytosis	98	102
Normal control	75	68
Residual ^{45}Ca[c] in resealed red ghosts		
Stomatocytosis	77	62
Normal control	22	20

[a]Nanomoles Ca/ml RBC/2 h.
[b]Nanomoles Ca/10^{10} ghosts/min
[c]Nanomoles Ca/10^{10} ghosts (after 20 min)

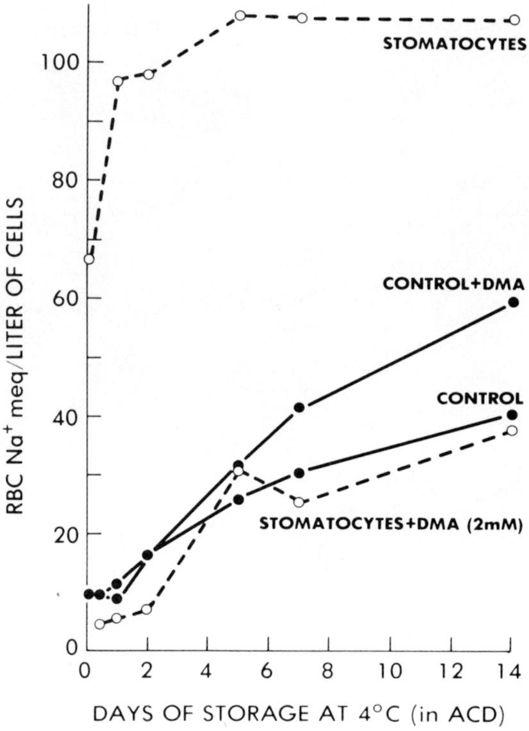

Fig 2. Stability of DMA effect on Na^+ permeability. ○- - -○ Stomatocytes. ●—● Control.

for normal cells. Favorable effects of DMA on potassium and water content, as well as on cell size, were also stable over a two-week period of storage. The prolonged duration of these effects is consistent with the expected formation of stable covalent bonds between imidoester and membrane-free amino groups.

Sites of Reaction of DMA With the Erythrocyte Membrane

It has previously been shown that DMA rapidly enters the erythrocyte and reacts with free amino groups on hemoglobin, resulting in intermolecular crosslinking and the formation of high molecular weight hemoglobin aggregates [16, 17].

In stomatocytes, at the concentrations of DMA that alter permeability, considerably more radioactive DMA is bound to hemoglobin than is bound to the membrane. The ratio of binding to hemoglobin and to membrane (calculated from total radioactivity associated with each component/ml of packed red cells) varies from 69.4:1 at 5 mM DMA to 44.3:1 at 0.5 mM DMA. At the lower DMA concentration, 4.26 nmoles of DMA are bound per milligram of membrane protein.

Under the reaction conditions we employed, approximately 80% of all membrane-associated ^{14}C-DMA was associated with lipid (stomatocytes 80%, normal cells 82%) and approximately 20% with protein. The lipid extracts obtained from ghosts prepared from red cells reacted with DMA (1–10 mM) were analyzed by TLC. In the absence of DMA, no difference between the phospholipid pattern of stomatocyte or normal red cell membranes was detected. Crosslinked and amidinated aminophospholipids, prepared by reacting purified phosphatidyl ethanolamine or phosphatidyl serine with DMA, were used to define the position of imidoester reaction products on TLC. As shown in Figure 3, both amidinated and crosslinked aminophospholipids were evident in membranes prepared from red cells reacted with DMA. To determine the extent to which aminophospholipids had reacted with DMA, the amidinated and crosslinked products were removed from the TLC plate by scraping. Their phosphate content was then determined and compared to the total amount of lipid phosphorus applied to the plate. Approximately 30% (range 28–31%) of membrane aminophospholipids reacted with imidoester at a DMA incubation concentration of 10mM. At lower (2mM) DMA concentrations no visable amidination or crosslinking was evident on TLC. However, with ^{14}C-DMA it was possible to detect trace amounts of both amidinated and crosslinked aminophospholipids. Calculations based on the known specific activity of ^{14}C-DMA indicated that less than 3% of the total membrane phospholipid (8% of membrane aminophospholipid) had reacted with DMA, assuming that all

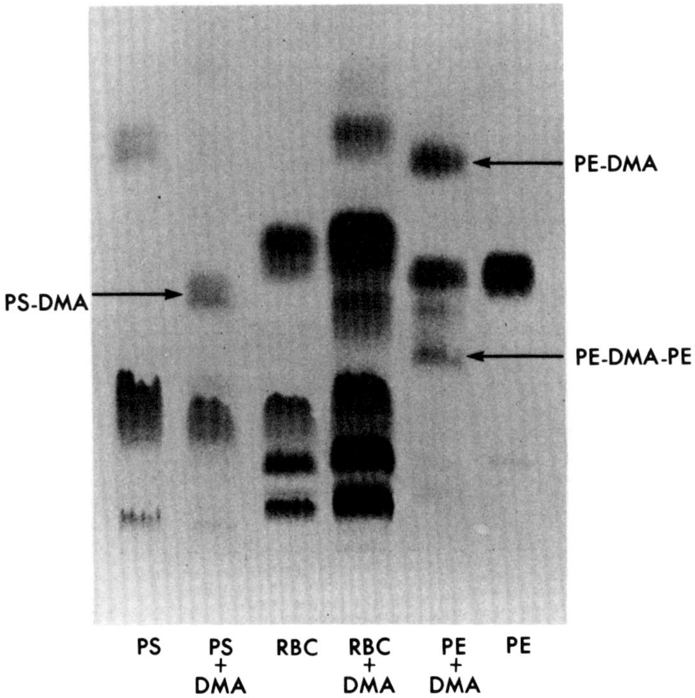

Fig 3. Effect of DMA on RBC membrane phospholipids. A membrane lipid extract obtained from red cells treated with 10 mM DMA or from untreated cells was subjected to thin layer chromatography on silica gel using chloroform:methanol:acetic acid:water (50:15:4:1.5) as the developing solvent. Aminophospholipid standards (PE = phosphatidyl ethanolamine, PS = phosphatidyl serine) were prepared (see Methods) to identify the positions of amidinated (PE-DMA, PS-DMA) and crosslinked (PE-DMA-PE) phospholipids. The slower migration of PE standard when compared to RBC PE was attributed to differences between bacterial and human PE. Crosslinked PS (PS-DMA-PS) was also probably present since ^{14}C-DMA radioactivity was found in the region of normal PS (in the DMA treated specimen), but the TLC system used did not separate PS from PS-DMA-PS. The impurities migrating ahead of and behind untreated PS standard were also usually seen in DMA-treated PS standard specimens. Although their migration was slightly altered by DMA, they did not contribute to the region labeled PS-DMA.

reactions represented crosslinking (ie, 1 mole of DMA equivalent to 2 moles of crosslinked phospholipid). The actual amount of reacted phospholipid was even lower, however, since a portion of the radioactive aminophospholipid was amidinated (1 mole of DMA equivalent to 1 mole of phospholipid) rather than crosslinked. The minimal effective concentration of DMA that corrects the membrane permeability defect (0.05 mM) is far lower than the concentration used in these studies. At these lower concentrations of DMA one would expect little or no amidination or crosslinking of aminophospholipids to occur.

No major differences between stomatocyte and control membrane proteins were detected on SDS-PAGE, although it was noted that band 7 was considerably less intense in stomatocyte membranes than in normal (Fig 4). SDS polyacrylamide gel electrophoresis of membranes prepared from erythrocytes treated for 1 h with 2 mM DMA (stained with Coomassie blue for proteins) revealed the presence of small amounts of high molecular weight aggregates and of globin. The remainder of the pattern was identical to that of the untreated specimen. Incubation of erythrocytes for 6 h instead of 1 h did not appreciably increase the amount of high molecular weight aggregates. If higher concentrations of DMA were employed, the pattern was considerably more altered. Carbon-14 DMA was used in an attempt to locate any preferential reaction of DMA with certain membrane proteins. However, there was no selective accumulation of radioactivity in any one component. Instead, small amounts of radioactivity were dispersed among the various bands. Gels were also stained with PAS to detect glycoproteins. The glycoprotein pattern was normal in stomatocytosis and was not altered in membranes prepared from cells reacted with 2 mM DMA.

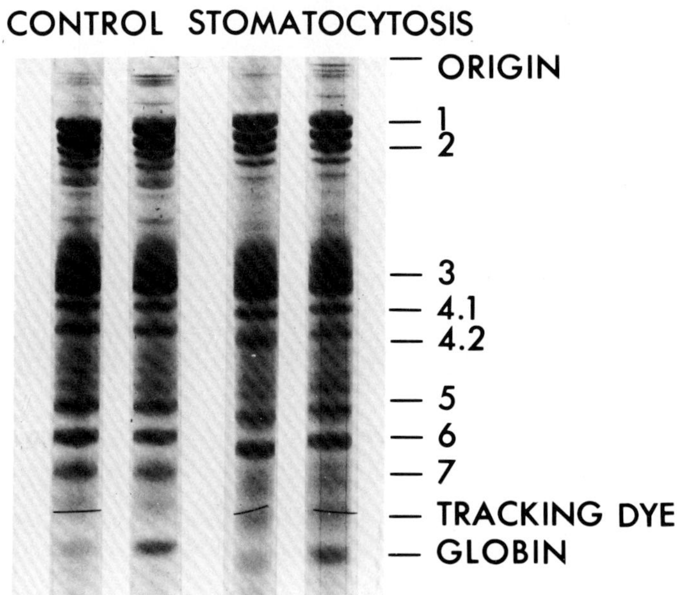

Fig 4. Effect of DMA on RBC membrane proteins.

The extent of phosphorylation of membrane proteins was evaluated in ghost preparations (Fig 5) after 1 h of incubation with $AT^{32}P$. The results were compared to those obtained with normal ghosts and ghosts from hereditary spherocytosis red cells. Phosphorylation of band 2 in hereditary stomatocytes was only 20% of normal, and treatment with 2 mM DMA had no favorable effect upon phosphorylation. The addition of cyclic AMP failed to normalize membrane protein phosphorylation in stomatocytes. The extent of phosphorylation of band 3 was also reduced in stomatocytes and was not improved by treatment with DMA.

Membrane protein phosphorylation was also evaluated in short-term incubations (Table II). The phosphorylation of an endogenous membrane protein, spectrin, in stomatocytosis was 79 pmoles per mg per 5 min, a value only 40% that of a simultaneously run control. Prior incubation of stomatocytes with 2 mM DMA had little influence on these results. In contrast, phosphorylation of an exogenous substrate, casein, by membrane protein kinase was similar in control and stomatocytic red cells. Again, DMA had little influence upon the rate of phosphorylation.

A variety of both monofunctional and bifunctional imidoesters was used in an attempt to determine whether crosslinking is a prerequisite for the effect on stomatocyte cation permeability or whether, alternatively, the effect is due to chemical modification alone (Table III). If no imidoester were employed, stomatocytes remained high in sodium and low in potassium after 6 h of incubation. Use of as little as 0.1 mM DMA, a bifunctional reagent, converted these cells into high-potassium, low-sodium cells, and a partial effect was noted at the even lower concentration of 0.05 mM. In contrast, the mono-

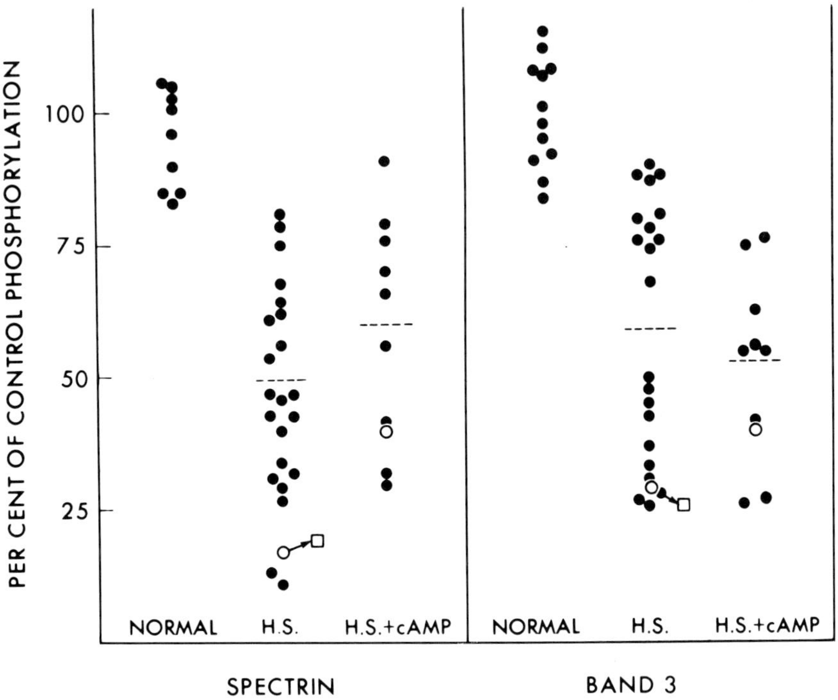

Fig 5. Membrane protein phosphorylation in hereditary stomatocytosis. ● – Normal or hereditary spherocytosis (H.S.). [Data reprinted from Greenquist, A., and Shohet, S.G., Blood Cells 3:122, 1977.] ○ – Stomatocytosis. ■ – Stomatocytosis + 2 mM DMA.

TABLE II. Protein Phosphorylation in Red Cell Ghosts

	Spectrin[a]	Casein[b]
Control	197 ± 4	19.2 ± 1.2
Stomatocytosis	79 ± 9	17.8 ± 0.2
Stomatocytosis + 2 mM DMA	101 ± 9	17.3 ± 1.3

[a]Picomoles/mg/5 min
[b]Nanomoles

TABLE III. Correction of the Abnormal Cation Content of Stomatocytes by Monofunctional and Bifunctional Imidoesters

Reagent	Concentration (mM)	RBC Cation K^+	Content[a] Na^+
None	–	28.9	99
Bifunctional			
Dimethyl adipimidate	0.1	107	10.1
Dimethyl adipimidate	0.05	84.1	34.1
Monofunctional			
Methyl acetimidate	5	20.2	118.6
Ethyl acetimidate	5	25.7	101.8
Ethyl acetimidate	20	48.6	45.7
Methyl butyrimidate	5	45	83.6
Methyl butyrimidate	20	72.8	26.7
Isothionyl acetimidate	5	14.3	124.9
Normal values	–	90–110	6–12

[a]mEq/liter Cells after 6 h incubation in vitro with indicated reagent. T 37°, pH 7.4, Hct 5%.

functional reagents methyl acetimidate and ethyl acetimidate were without effect at 5 mM, although, at a concentration of 20 mM, a partial correction was seen with ethyl acetimidate. The most effective monofunctional agent evaluated was methyl butyrimidate but, on a concentration basis, this reagent was 400 times less effective than the bifunctional reagent DMA. Isothionyl acetimidate, a monofunctional imidoester that reacts primarily at the external surface of the erythrocyte membrane, had no influence upon stomatocyte cation permeability.

Using imidoesters of differing chain length allowed a tentative estimate to be made of the distance between the crosslined free amino groups responsible for alternation in cation permeability (Table IV). A short imidoester, dimethyl malonimidate, whose maximal crosslinking dimension is approximately 3.7–5 Å, was without effect on cation permeability. The maximal effect on permeability was noted with dimethyl adipimidate, and a slightly lesser effect was seen with the larger imidoester dimethyl suberimidate.

DISCUSSION

The impaired endocytosis noted in resealed red ghosts prepared from stomatocytes highlights the difference between stomatocytosis and other membrane disorders such as spherocytosis [20] or pyropoikilocytosis [21] where ghost endocytosis is normal. Endocytosis is a complex and incompletely understood process variably involving energy, Ca^{++},

TABLE IV. Effect of Chain Length on the Correction of Stomatocyte Cation Content by Crosslinking Reagents

Reagent	Maximal crosslink dimension (Å)	RBC Cation content[a] K^+	Na^+
None	–	28.9	99
Dimethyl malonimidate	3.7–5.0	28.9	83.9
Dimethyl adipimidate	7.3–9.0	87.2	14.4
Dimethyl suberimidate	9.7–11	51.2	58.5
Normal values	–	90–110	6–12

[a] mEq/liter Cells after 6 h incubation in vitro with indicated reagent (at a concentration of 5 mM). T 37°, pH 7.4, Hct 5%.

and the membrane processes of invagination and fusion [6, 14, 20]. Although the specific defect responsible for impaired endocytosis in stomatocytes has not yet been defined, an increase in membrane rigidity would be consistent with previous observations on the abnormal rigidity of intact red cells [5]. The restoration of both whole cell deformability [5] and ghost endocytosis to normal by DMA would then be the consequence of a reduction in membrane rigidity induced by the imidoester. Because of the well-known relationships between red cell rigidity and membrane calcium [22], as well as those between Ca^{++}, Ca^{++}–Mg^{++} ATPase, and endocytosis [6], we evaluated several aspects of Ca^{++} metabolism. The severalfold increases in calcium influx into metabolically depleted stomatocytes, calcium efflux from ghosts, and calcium retention by red ghosts are all consistent with the high reticulocyte content of the blood sample used for analysis [7, 14]. Wiley and co-workers [23] have also found normal calcium uptake by metabolically depleted cells, normal membrane calcium content, and a normal rate of calcium extrusion in the red cells of other individuals with the hereditary stomatocytosis syndrome who, in some respects, resemble the patient we studied. The lack of any effect of DMA on ^{45}Ca efflux or ^{45}Ca retention make it unlikely that the enhanced endocytosis induced by DMA is a consequence of altered calcium metabolism. Furthermore, if the favorable effect of DMA on endocytosis involved calcium, one would expect a reduction in calcium influx rather than the increase actually observed.

The dramatic effects of DMA on stomatocytes led us to investigate the nature and location of the reaction between imidoesters and the stomatocytic erythrocyte membrane. The persistence of normal cation permeability during several weeks of storage of imidoester-treated stomatocytes is consistent with the expected formation of stable covalent bonds between imidoester and membrane-free amino groups. In view of the ubiquity of free amino groups on proteins, glycoproteins, and aminophospholipids, imidoesters would be expected to react with a variety of membrane constituents. In normal red cell membranes, reactions have been demonstrated with proteins [18], glycoproteins [19], and aminophospholipids [9]. The present study has confirmed that such reactions also occur in stomatocyte membranes and has attempted to define which reaction is responsible for the correction of cation permeability.

A number of investigators have failed to demonstrate any major abnormality in stomatocyte membrane lipids. Total membrane lipids are increased on a per cell basis, reflecting the larger size and increased membrane surface area of such cells [1, 2, 4, 24]. However, calculated per liter of cells, the amount of membrane lipids is normal in stomatocytes. There is no abnormality in the distribution of phospholipids [2, 4] and no undue loss of phospholipids on incubation for periods of up to 24 h [1]. Pathways of membrane lipid renewal also appear to be normal [1].

On the other hand, several observations suggest that there may be an abnormality of membrane proteins in stomatocytosis. First, amino reactive reagents can completely correct the permeability defect in vitro [5]. Second, Bienzle and co-workers [25] have tentatively identified an abnormal membrane protein with a molecular weight of about 25,000 daltons in red cells from one patient. Although we have not yet subjected the membrane proteins from our case of stomatocytosis to analysis by the two directional electrophoretic techniques employed by Bienzle, the appreciable diminution in band 7 (mol wt = 29,000 daltons [32]) we noted on SDS-PAGE (Fig 3) certainly underscores the possibility of an abnormality in one or more low molecular weight membrane proteins. Finally, the defective phosphorylation of spectrin and band 3 in the subject of the current study implies a general disturbance in regulatory mechanisms important in the maintenance of normal cell shape (Fig 5) [11, 27]. That this disturbance is not unique to stomatocytosis is evident from previous reports of similar defects in hereditary spherocytosis [11] and in sickle cell anemia [26]. Furthermore, any inference that membrane protein phosphorylation is defective in intact stomatocytic red cells would be premature, since the measurements were made in ghosts and not in whole cells. In this regard it is important to note, as recently shown by Wolfe and Lux [31], that in hereditary spherocytosis membrane protein phosphorylation, although abnormal in ghost preparations, is normal in intact cells. In stomatocytosis, the abnormal phosphorylation seems to involve an altered interaction between the substrate proteins and the protein kinase, rather than a defect in protein kinase, since protein kinase-mediated phosphorylation of an exogenous substrate, casein, by ghost preparations is normal. Abnormal phosphorylation is not repaired by imidoesters, but it is conceivable that they may stabilize membrane proteins in an optimal conformation, perhaps substituting, in this regard, for a process normally requiring phosphorylation by protein kinase.

Whether chemical modification or crosslinking of free amino groups is required for the permeability effects is not yet completely clear. When red cells were reacted with 2 mM DMA, intermolecular crosslinking of membrane aminophospholipids was limited to a maximum of 8% of the available PE & PS. A barely detectable amount of high molecular weight material, evident on SDS gel electrophoresis, was the only indication of intermolecular crosslinking of membrane proteins. These results suggest that, if crosslinking is essential, it must involve a minor membrane component, present in low concentration, or be predominantly intramolecular rather than intermolecular. The experiments with bifunctional reagents of differing chain length support the premise that crosslinking is required for the permeability effects observed in stomatocytes. If chemical modification, rather than crosslinking, of free amino groups were required to alter permeability, the entire family of bifunctional reagents employed should be equally effective, since they differ only in chain length. The clear superiority of DMA, compared to larger or smaller bifunctional reagents, suggests that crosslinking is essential and that the dimensions of the critical crosslink are approximately 7–9 Å.

It is of interest that isothionyl acetimidate, a monofunctional imidoester that reacts primarily at the external surface of the erythrocyte membrane, has no influence upon stomatocyte cation permeability, implying that the effect of imidoesters upon permeability may occur deeper within the membrane. Although the effects of monofunctional reagents seemingly demonstrate that chemical modification also can influence permeability, these effects may, in fact, be the result of crosslinking, since Browne and Kent have noted that, at the pH range we employed for these studies, monofunctional reagents may form transient intermediates that have crosslinking capabilities [28]. That monofunctional reagent are, indeed, capable of crosslinking reactions in red cells and other tissues has been confirmed by several investigators [29, 30]. The relatively small amount of such transient intermediates available for crosslinking would then explain the much larger concentration requirement for monofunctional reagents noted in the present study.

The potential of imidoesters as probes, useful in defining the nature of the membrane abnormality in stomatocytosis, is apparent from the studies described here. It can be anticipated that their continued use will provide additional insight into the nature of these fascinating cells.

ACKNOWLEDGMENTS

We gratefully acknowledge the editorial assistance of Ms. Terry Tschopp. Ms. Susan Emmons, Irene Junga, and Muriel Johnson provided experienced technical help, and Dr. Klaus Bensch was responsible for the electron microscopy of endocytosis. Dr. Dan Chiu advised us regarding the phospholipid studies.

This work was supported by grants from the National Foundation (649) and the USPH (1 K04 HL00086) (HL17357) (AM16095) (AM13682). (HL 20985)

REFERENCES

1. Zarkowsky HS, Oski FA, Sha'afi R, Shohet SB, Nathan DG: N Engl J Med 278:593, 652, 1968.
2. Mentzer WC, Smith WB, Goldstone J, Shohet SB: Blood 46:659, 1975.
3. Bienzle U, Niethammer D, Kleeberg U, Ungefehr K, Kohne E, Kleihauer E: Scand J Haematol 15:339, 1975.
4. Schroter W, Ungefehr K: "Membrane and Disease." New York: Raven Press, 1976, p 95.
5. Mentzer WC, Lubin BH, Emmons S: N Engl J Med 294:1200, 1976.
6. Schrier SL, Bensch KG, Johnson M, Junga I: J Clin Invest 56:8, 1975.
7. Wiley JS, Gill FM: Blood 47:197, 1976.
8. Fairbanks G, Steck TL, Wallach DFH: Biochemistry 10:2606, 1971.
9. Marinetti GV, Baumgarten R, Sheeley D, Gordesky S: Biochem Biophys Res Commun 53:302, 1973.
10. Marfey SP, Tsai KH: Biochem Biophys Res Commun 65:31, 1975.
11. Greenquist A, Shohet S: Blood 48:887, 1976.
12. Greenquist A, Wyatt J, Guatelli J, Shohet S: "Erythrocyte Membranes: Recent Clinical and Experimental Advances." New York: Alan R Liss. In press.
13. Glynn Chappell: Biochem J 90:147, 1964.
14. Schrier SL, Bensch KG: "Membranes and Disease." New York: Raven Press, 1976, p 31.
15. Lubin B, Bradley T, Mentzer W, Messer M, McRae J: INSERM 44:291, 1975.
16. Lubin BH, Pena V, Mentzer WC, Bymun E, Bradley TB, Packer L: Proc Natl Acad Sci USA 72:43, 1975.
17. Waterman MR, Yamaoka K, Chuang AH, Cottam GL: Biochem Biophys Res Commun 63:580, 1975.
18. Ji TH: Proc Natl Acad Sci USA 71:93, 1974.
19. Wang K, Richards FM: J Biol Chem 249:8005, 1974.
20. Schrier SL, Ben-Bassat I, Bensch K, Seeger M, Junga I: Br J Haematol 26:59, 1974.
21. Walter T, Mentzer W, Greenquist A, Schrier S, Mohandas N: Blood 50:98, 1977.
22. Weed RL, LaCelle PL, Merrill EW: J Clin Invest 48:795, 1969.
23. Wiley JS, Ellory JC, Shuman MA, Shaller CC, Cooper RA: Blood 46:337, 1975.
24. Wiley JS: "Membranes and Disease." New York: Raven Press, 1976, p 89.
25. Bienzle U, Bhadki S, Knufermann H, Niethammer D, Kleihauer E: Klin Woschr 55:569, 1977.

26. Beutler E, Guinto E, Johnson C: Blood Cells 3:135, 1977.
27. Shohet SB, Greenquist AC: Blood Cells 3:115, 1977.
28. Browne DT, Kent SBH: Biochem Biophys Res Commun 67:126, 1975.
29. Chao TL, Berenfeld MR, Gabuzda TG: FEBS Lett 62:57, 1976.
30. Packer L, Bymun EN, Tinberg HM, Ogunmola GB: Arch Biochem Biophys 177:323, 1976.
31. Wolfe LC, Lux SE: Blood 48:963, 1976.
32. Steck TL: J Cell Biol 62:1, 1974.
33. Bligh EG, Dyer WJ: Can J Biochem Physiol 37:911, 1959.
34. Lowry OH, Roberts NR, Leiner K, Wu ML, Fan AL: J Biol Chem 207:1, 1954.

Journal of Supramolecular Structure 9:427–440 (1978)
Normal and Abnormal Red Cell Membranes 279–292

Formation of γ-Glutamyl-ϵ-Lysine Bridges Between Membrane Proteins by a Ca^{2+}-Regulated Enzyme in Intact Erythrocytes

L. Lorand, G. E. Siefring, Jr, and L. Lowe-Krentz

Department of Biochemistry and Molecular Biology, Northwestern University, Evanston Illinois 60201

A rise in the intracellular concentration of Ca^{2+}-ions in human erythrocytes causes the formation of high-molecular-weight membrane protein polymers, cross-linked by γ-glutamyl-ϵ-lysine side chain bridges. Cross-linking involves proteins at the cytoplasmic side of the membrane (band 4.1, spectrin, and band 3 materials) and the reaction is catalyzed by the intrinsic transglutaminase. This enzyme is regulated by Ca^{2+}-ions and it exists in a latent form in normal cells. The protein polymer, isolated from the membranes of Ca^{2+}-loaded intact human red cells, is heterogeneous in size and may contain as many as 6 moles of γ-glutamyl-ϵ-lysine cross-links per 100,000 gm of protein.

Synthetic compounds, which either compete against the ϵ-lysine cross-linking functionalities of the protein substrates (eg, histamine, aminoacetonitrile, cystamine) or directly inactivate the transamidase (eg, cystamine), inhibit the membrane polymerization reaction in intact human erythrocytes.They also interfere with the Ca^{2+}-induced irreversible shape change from discocyte to echinocyte and inhibit the irreversible loss of membrane deformability. Thus, the transamidase-catalyzed production of γ-glutamyl-ϵ-lysine cross-links in the membrane may be a common denominator in these cellular manifestations.

Key words: fibrin cross linking, erythrocyte transamidase, spectrin, cytoskeleton

SOME CHARACTERISTICS OF Ca^{2+}-LOADED ERYTHROCYTES

The experimental approach of rapid loading of erythrocytes with Ca^{2+} by using the specific ionophore A23187 proved to be of considerable advantage in our efforts to assess the molecular basis of the Ca^{2+}-induced irreversible alterations of shape and loss of membrane deformability. Inasmuch as general terms such as "Ca^{2+}-loaded" or "energy-depleted"

Received May 12, 1978; accepted July 28, 1978.

cells may have different meanings for different investigators, it may be best to specify conditions at the outset. Experiments were performed with freshly washed human red blood cells (hematocrit 10–70%), typically over periods of 30 min to 18 h at 37°C, with 10–20 μM ionophore and 0–1.5 mM added concentration of Ca^{2+}. Controls always contained Mg^{2+}, equimolar to the Ca^{2+} employed. Loss of K^+ from the cells was counteracted by using a buffer containing 0.1 M KC1, 0.06 M NaC1, 10 mM glucose, and 5 mM Tris-HC1 (pH 7.4). It should be pointed out that in spite of inclusion of glucose the intracellular adenosine triphosphate (ATP) concentration dropped to less than 20% of normal by 2 h of incubation with 1.5 mM Ca^{2+}. Thus, it is important to bear in mind that within the context of the experiments described Ca^{2+}-loaded cells are also low in ATP. The loss of ATP is attributable to the presence of Ca^{2+}, because cells incubated with ionophore and Mg^{2+} had essentially normal levels of ATP.

For purposes of the present discussion, attention should be directed to three important manifestations resulting from the intracellular accumulation of Ca^{2+}-ions in human erythrocytes: irreversible echinocytic transformation [1, 2], irreversible loss of membrane deformability [3, 4], and formation of membrane protein polymers cross-linked by γ-glutamyl: ε-lysine peptide bridges [5–9]. These nondisulfide-linked polymers can be readily detected by electrophoresis of the membrane constituents after reduction with dithiothreitol (DTT) and solubilization in sodium dodecyl sulfate (SDS) (Fig. 1), and their formation may be a common denominator in the irreversible cellular manifestations referred to above. In most experiments the polymers are so large ($\geqslant 10^6$, as in Fig. 1, marked by X) that they can barely penetrate polyacrylamide (4.5%) gels. As judged by

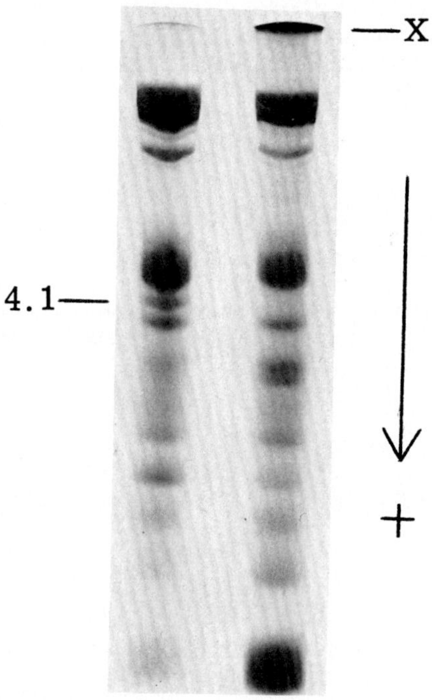

Fig. 1. Polyacrylamide (4.5%) SDS (0.2%) gel electrophoresis of membrane proteins obtained from fresh erythrocytes following incubation (3 h, 37°C) with ionophore (20 μM) and 1.5 mM $CaCl_2$ (gel on right) and 1.5 mM $MgCl_2$ (gel on left).

Coomassie blue staining, polymer production is accompanied by the disappearance of the 4.1 band, and by a lowering of the amount of proteins in the spectrin and band 3 regions (for nomenclature, see Fairbanks et al [10]), suggesting that polymerization involves at least these three membrane protein constituents. Polymer formation was observed at added concentrations of Ca^{2+} as low as 0.15 mM.

The chemical nature of the nondisulfide cross-links in the membrane polymer and the manner in which they arise are obviously of great interest. Past research in our laboratory on blood clotting [11–14] provided the conceptual as well as the technical framework for the erythrocyte studies presented here, and a brief review of the enzyme chemical background might be helpful in appreciating various aspects of the problem.

TRANSAMIDASE-CATALYZED CROSS-LINKING OF PROTEINS

In its simplest form, the dimerization of two protein molecules (P and P′) by a transamidase (transglutaminase*) of the endo-γ-glutamine:ϵ-lysine transferase type [14] may be outlined as follows:

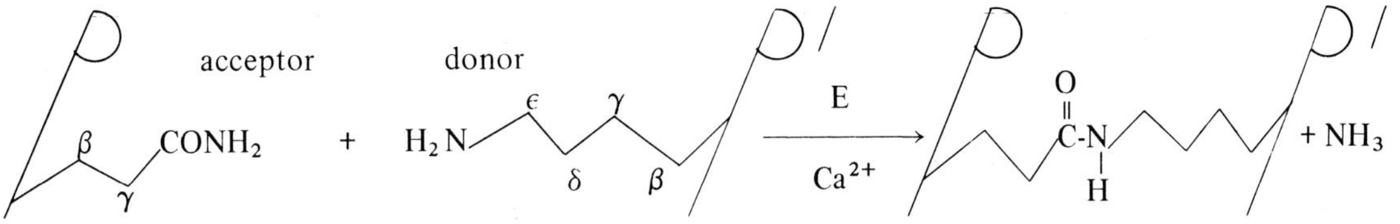

If P and P′ represent molecules belonging to the same protein species, a homologous dimer is obtained, whereas if they are of different types, a hybrid dimer ensues. From a thermodynamic point of view, as written, the amide exchange reaction would be expected to be readily reversible, but in reality – as in clot formation, where polymerization leads to a phase transition – reversibility may be hard to demonstrate. There is clear evidence from studies on fibrin that, of the large number of glutaminyl and lysyl residues of the protein, only a select few react with the specific enzyme [15] and are involved in the actual cross-linking event as acceptor and donor functionalities, respectively. It is also interesting to recall that relatively minor alterations of the protein substrate, as occurring in the fibrinogen ⟶ fibrin transformation, can affect reactivity towards the cross-linking enzyme.

A given protein is considered bifunctional if it carries enzyme-specific acceptor as well as donor cross-linking functionalities. If in shorthand notation a bifuctional protein is symbolized as 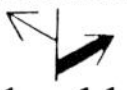 [where the | vertical line, regardless of the protein species, represents the polypeptide backbone, the  heavy arrow represents the acceptor glutamine, and the  light arrow represents the electron donor lysine side chains], the possibility of an infinite degree of linear polymerization by γ-glutamyl-ϵ-lysine bridges may be indicated as:

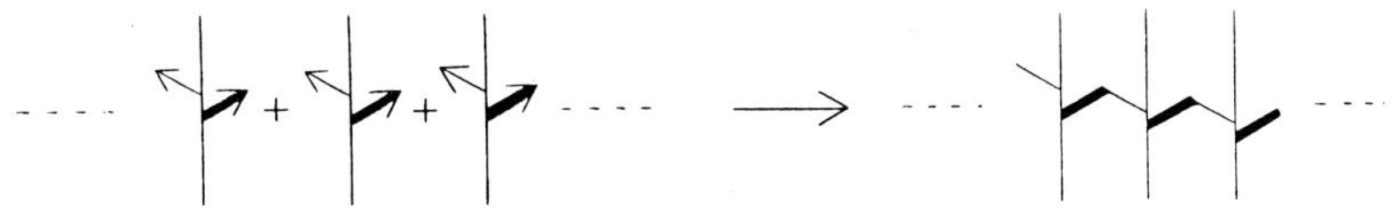

*The name "transglutaminase" (given by Clarke et al, Arch Biochem Biophys 79:338, 1958) is actually a misnomer because glutamine (with its α-NH_2 group free) is not even a substrate for these types of enzymes.

There might be proteins which carry acceptor or donor functionalities exclusively. Accordingly, they could only serve either as chain initiators or terminators, and their presence in a mixture might give rise to the following possibilities:

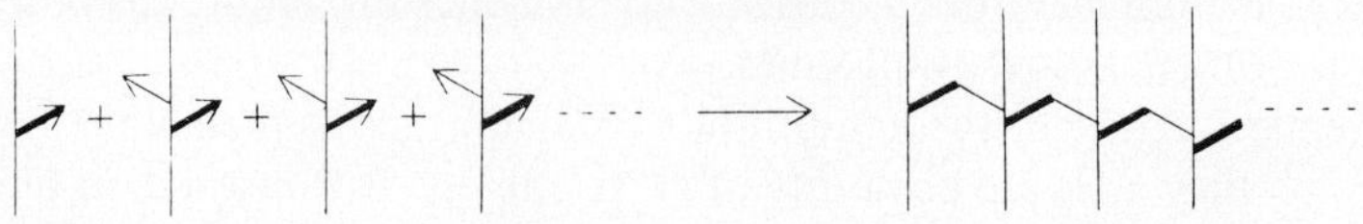

or

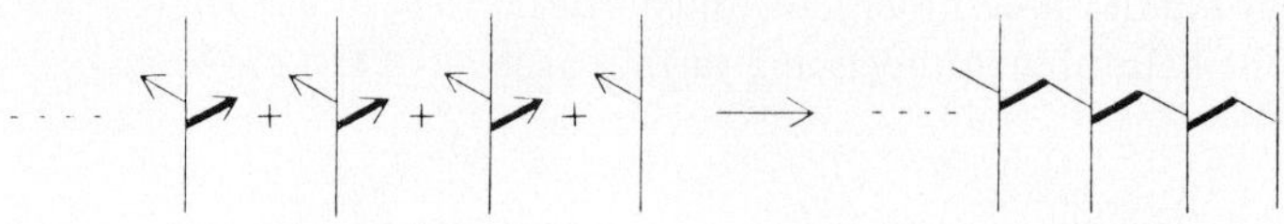

or even

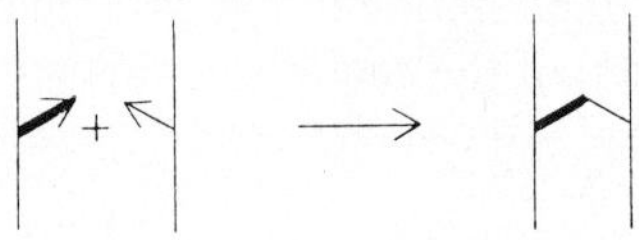

The minimum requirement for branching would be that a reacting protein substrate be present either with two acceptor or two donor functionalities:

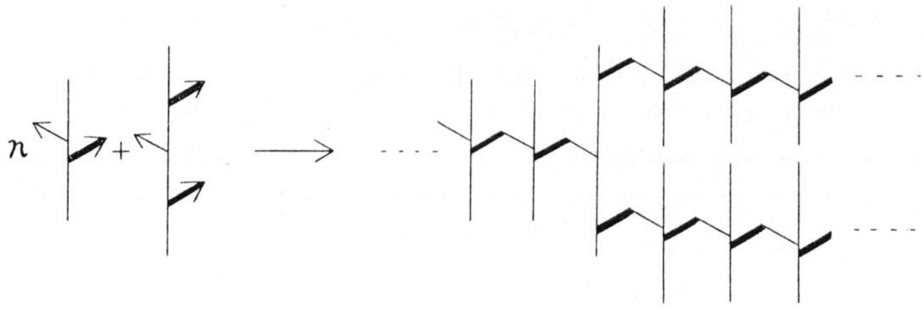

or

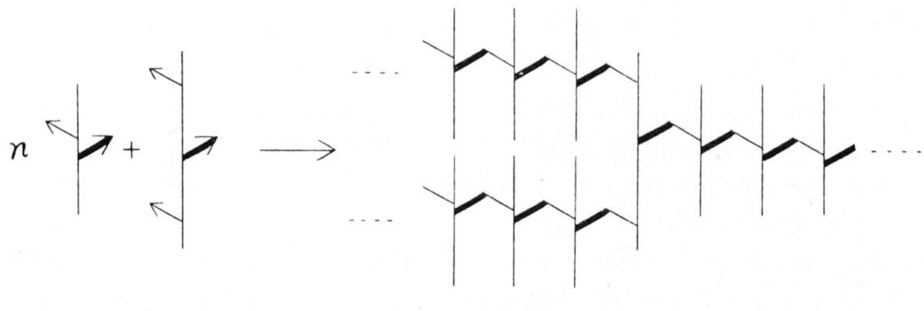

This brief analysis may suffice to show that the pattern of fusion can be varied and that cross-linked proteins of the type formed in the erythrocyte membrane during accumulation of intracellular Ca^{2+} (Fig. 1) may in fact represent diverse populations of growing polymers of not very well definable size and composition.

The enzymic reaction pathway is far more complex than could be inferred from the simple presentation of a nucleophilic displacement, written for dimerization as:

$$P\text{-}CONH_2 + H_2N\text{-}P' \longrightarrow P\text{-}CONH\text{-}P' + NH_3$$

As suggested for the cross-linking of fibrin, the reaction is thought to proceed through an acylenzyme intermediate which is formed between the γ-carbonyl group of the glutamine in P and the cysteine thiol center of the enzyme (HS-E). The thiolester intermediate (P-COS-E) then undergoes an aminolytic deacylation by reacting with the ϵ-NH_2 function of lysine in P′. Specific binding steps operate with regard to both protein substrates and involve the formation of Michaelis complexes between E and P prior to acylation of the enzyme, and between P′ and the acylenzyme intermediate prior to deacylation:

$$\text{Acylation: } \text{P-CONH}_2 + \text{HS-E} \rightleftharpoons [\text{P-CONH}_2\text{; HS-E}] \rightarrow \text{P-COS-E} + \text{NH}_3$$

$$\text{Deacylation: } \text{P-COS-E} + \text{H}_2\text{N-P}' \rightleftharpoons [\text{P-COS-E; H}_2\text{N-P}'] \rightarrow \text{P-CONH-P}' + \text{HS-E}$$

$$\text{Net reaction: } \text{P-CONH}_2 + \text{H}_2\text{N-P}' \rightarrow \text{P-CONH-P}' + \text{NH}_3$$

In addition to chelating Ca^{2+} with ethelenediaminetetraacetic acid disodium salt (EDTA) or ATP, or inactivating the enzyme by Zn^{2+} [16], mercurials, or disulfides [17], the above type of formulation of the pathway suggests that primary amines – if they satisfy the specificity requirements of the enzyme – might interfere with the formation of the P-CONH-P′ product. Indeed, we found that such synthetic compounds could inhibit cross-linking rather effectively even in the complex biological system of clotting in whole blood [13, 18]. The inhibitory amine (H_2NR) competes against H_2N-P′ in the deacylation step by virtue of the fact that it serves as an alternate substrate:

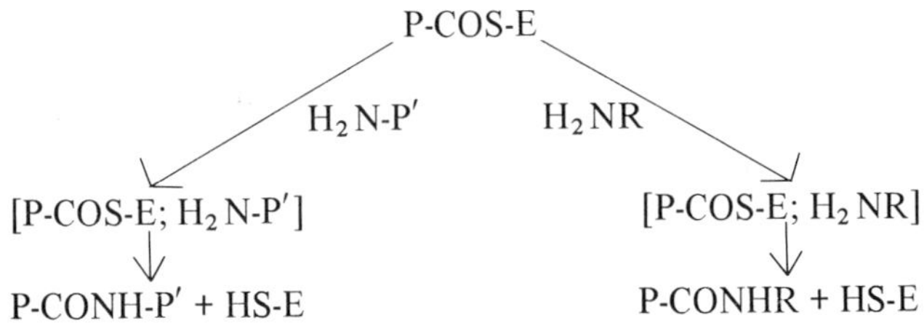

The more efficiently the acylenzyme intermediate can be diverted towards forming P-CONHR (on the right), the less cross-linked protein product P-CONH-P′ is formed (on the left). It should be emphasized that the inhibitor becomes incorporated into P, specifically blocking and (with appropriate labeling of R) uniquely identifying its reactive glutamine sites.

IDENTIFICATION OF γ-GLUTAMYL-ϵ-LYSINE CROSS-LINKS IN THE MEMBRANE POLYMER OF Ca^{2+}-LOADED CELLS

The protein polymer formed as a result of intracellular accumulation of Ca^{2+}-ions in erythrocytes was isolated by means of gel filtration chromatography following reduction of the membrane materials in 0.025 M dithiothreitol and dispersion in 1% SDS. The appearance of peaks emerging early from the Sepharose 4B CL column (represented by fractions emerging before 46 in Fig. 2) is a characteristic feature of the chromatographic profile of cells exposed to Ca^{2+}. As inferred from considerations of particle size, this region contained the polymeric products and this was confirmed by electrophoretic analysis of the various fractions using either SDS-polyacrylamide (4.5%) or SDS-agarose (2%). Both of these techniques, but particularly the latter, indicated that "the polymer"

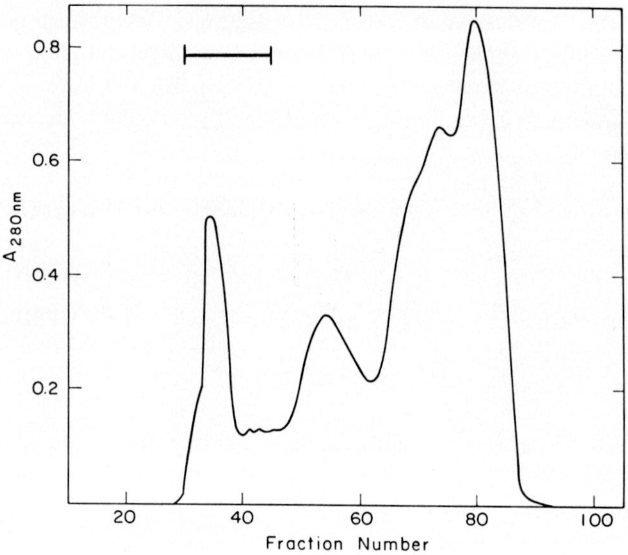

Fig. 2. Elution profile of membrane proteins from Sepharose 4B CL following incubation of red blood cells with 1.5 mM $CaCl_2$ and 20 μM ionophore for 18 h at 37°C. For details, see Siefring et al [9]. Horizontal bar represents polymer-containing fractions.

comprised several distinct components of different molecular weights and that probably even each component itself was somewhat heterogeneous in size. As discussed above, such a heterogeneity was not unexpected and it suggested that polymerization was a graded rather than a concerted, fusion of membrane proteins proceeding by way of a number of oligomeric intermediates. The identification of γ-glutamyl-ϵ-lysine dipeptide bridges in the isolated bulk polymer was carried out by procedures first developed in our laboratory for measurements of this isodipeptide in cross-linked fibrin [13, 19]. Advantage was taken of the fact that the γ-peptide linkage is resistant to hydrolysis by known proteolytic enzymes. Thus the protein could almost totally be digested by sequential treatment with proteases (subtilisin, leucine aminopeptidase, prolidase, and carboxypeptidase A) without impairing the γ-glutamyl-ϵ-lysine structure. The direct isolation, identification, and quantitation of this unique dipeptide could then be performed using the Beckman 120 C chromatographic system in the manner previously described, so that the isopeptide emerged between leucine and tyrosine (Fig. 3). From the measured ninhydrin color value of a synthetic reference peptide and from the amino acid composition of the polymeric protein, a γ-glutamyl-ϵ-lysine cross-bridge content of about 6 per 100,000 gm of protein could be calculated. This value represents a relatively high average cross-linking frequency involving approximately 10% of all lysines in the protein material. It should be mentioned in passing that the enzymic cross-linking of fibrin, though producing a much lower frequency of γ-glutamyl-ϵ-lysine bridging, contributes significantly to the viscoelastic stiffening of the clot structure [20, 21].

EFFECT OF TRANSAMIDASE INHIBITORS ON MEMBRANE PROTEIN POLYMERIZATION IN INTACT ERYTHROCYTES

Earlier work from this laboratory showed that the transamidase-catalyzed cross-linking of fibrin could be effectively inhibited by primary amines. Inhibition by such compounds is so specific that the "clotting time," which is a reflection on the overall process

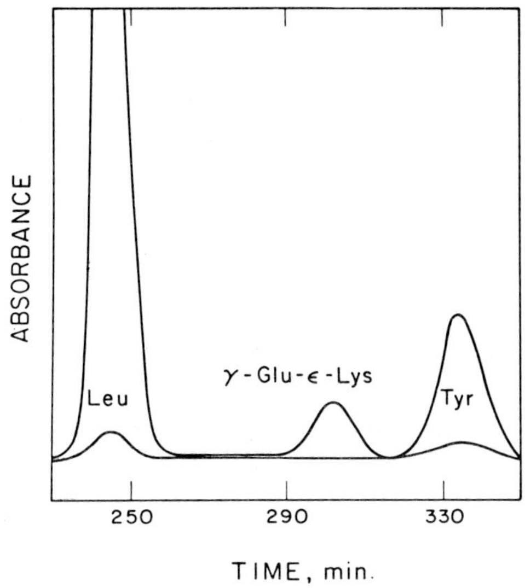

Fig. 3. Isolation of γ-glutamyl-ε-lysine isodipeptide from the enzymic digest of the polymer obtained from the membranes of Ca^{2+}-loaded erythrocytes. For details, see Siefring et al [9]. The lower tracing represents the pattern obtained when the enzymes used for digestion were incubated without addition of polymer. The γ-Glu-ε-Lys peak obtained from 0.72 mg of polymer corresponds to a recovery of 40 nmoles of the isodipeptide. The equimolar Glu and Lys content of the material in this peak was confirmed by further acid hydrolysis and amino acid analysis.

of fibrin aggregation, is not even delayed. The best synthetic inhibitors carry a bulky substituent attached to an aminoalkane residue essentially the equivalent of a lysine side chain in proteins. This type of amine specificity, exemplified by the structural features in dansylcadaverine, seems to be a common requirement for all endo-γ-glutamine:ε-lysine transferases. Though there are several amines which inhibit fibrin cross-linking at concentrations less than 10^{-4}M and which also yield K_i's of about 10^{-5}M with liver transglutaminase, their use with whole erythrocytes is fraught with difficulties. Apart from enzyme specificity, inhibition in this system would also depend on whether the amine could pass through the cell membrane to the cytoplasmic interface and whether it could gain access to the acylenzyme intermediate during the process of the intrinsic cross-linking of presumably organized membrane protein components. Compounds with large hydrophobic constituents (such as the dansyl group in dansylcadaverine) would hardly be suitable. Nevertheless, in an apparent compromise between the specificity requirement of the transamidase and passage through the cell membrane, it was still possible to select some amines which inhibited the Ca^{2+}-triggered cross-linking in intact erythrocytes. Aminoacetonitrile, glycine methyl or ethylester, histamine, cysteamine and cystamine serve as typical examples and Figure 4 provides some illustrations. At 10 mM concentrations, all of these amines prevented polymer formation for periods of up to 2 h during loading of cells with 1.5 mM Ca^{2+} at 37°C. Neither sarcosine methylester (ie, N-methylglycine methylester), an analogue of glycine methylester, nor $^{\alpha}$N-dimethylhistamine, an analogue of histamine, inhibits membrane protein polymerization. Thus the presence of a primary amino group seems to be essential.

Cystamine is obviously in a special category and inhibition by this compound cannot be ascribed to its primary amino groups alone. It is known from studies with pure transamidating enzymes (C.-M. Svahn and L. Lorand, unpublished results) that cystamine

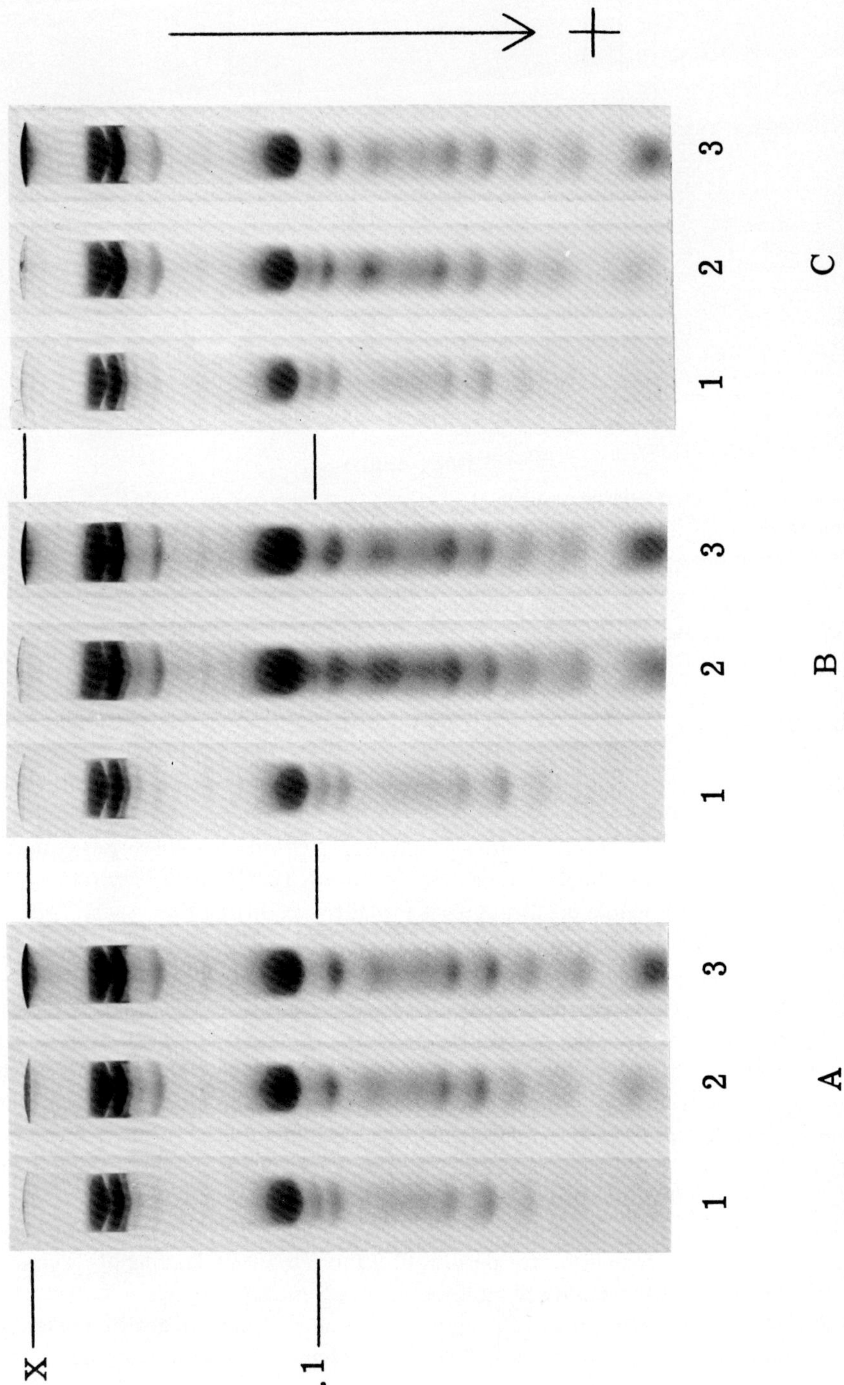

Fig. 4. Inhibition of membrane protein polymerization by amines. Fresh erythrocytes were incubated for 3 h at 37°C with 20 μM A23187 ionophore and 1.5 mM $MgCl_2$ (gel 1), 1.5 mM $CaCl_2$ (gel 2) in presence of 10 mM of an amine (histamine in panel A, aminoacetonitrile in B, and cystamine in C), or 1.5 mM $CaCl_2$ only (gel 3). Following incubation, membranes were isolated, solubilized in 1% SDS–40 mM DTT and subjected to polyacrylamide gel (4.5%) electrophoresis. Polymer is denoted as X.

undergoes a specific disulfide exchange reaction with the active center cysteine of these enzymes, causing their inactivation as:

$$E\text{-}SH + H_2NCH_2CH_2S\text{-}SCH_2CH_2NH_2 \longrightarrow E\text{-}S\text{-}SCH_2CH_2NH_2 + HSCH_2CH_2NH_2$$

Thus there is reason to believe that inhibition of polymer formation by cystamine is due in large extent to its direct inactivating effect on transglutaminase itself.

The disappearance of band 4.1 seems to be the most sensitive sign of the changes occurring in the membrane protein profile of cells during the intracellular accumulation of Ca^{2+}-ions. Of the inhibitors tested, at 10 mM concentration, thus far cystamine was the most effective in preventing the disappearance of the 4.1 band.

When the Ca^{2+}-loading of erythrocytes is carried out in the presence of a radioactive amine (^{14}C-histamine), selective labeling of membrane proteins occurs, in agreement with the postulated mode of action of amine type inhibitors as discussed before. Thus far, we have been able to demonstrate the covalent incorporation of the labeled amines into spectrin and band 3 material, as well as the growing polymer itself.

Ca^{2+}-REGULATION OF ERYTHROCYTE TRANSAMIDASE

The transglutaminase activity of red cell hemolysates can be conveniently assayed by the filter paper technique developed in our laboratory for measuring the covalent incorporation of radioactive amines (eg, ^{14}C-putrescine) into casein derivatives [22]. Regarding the latter, N,N-dimethylcasein is very useful [23] because the ϵ-lysine groups are blocked and the protein substrate can only function as an acceptor in the enzymic reaction:

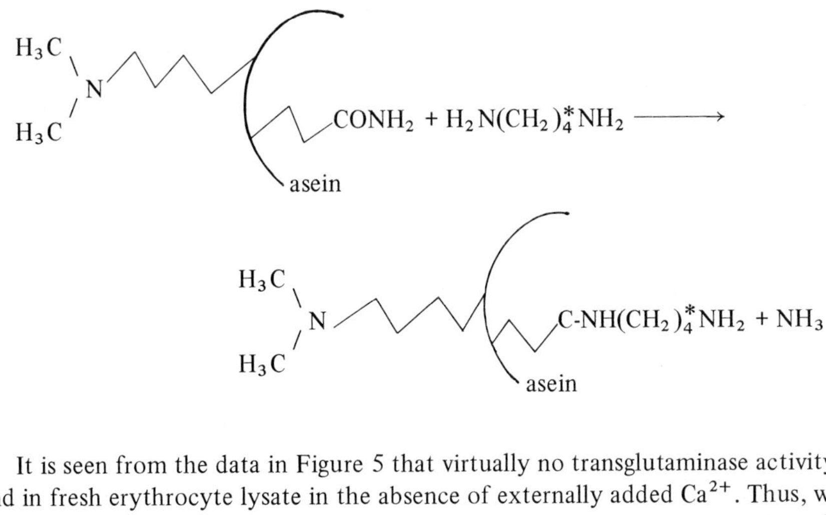

It is seen from the data in Figure 5 that virtually no transglutaminase activity can be found in fresh erythrocyte lysate in the absence of externally added Ca^{2+}. Thus, within the normal red cell milieu, the enzyme may be assumed to exist in a "latent form." However, transamidase activity becomes easily detectable by raising the Ca^{2+} concentration to about 5×10^{-5}M and the enzyme exhibits half-maximal velocity at about 3×10^{-4}M of Ca^{2+}. It should be mentioned that the Ca^{2+} dependence of the "latent-to-active transglutaminase" transition coincides with Ca^{2+} concentrations found in old cells [24], sickle cells [25, 26], or cells with impaired metabolism [27].

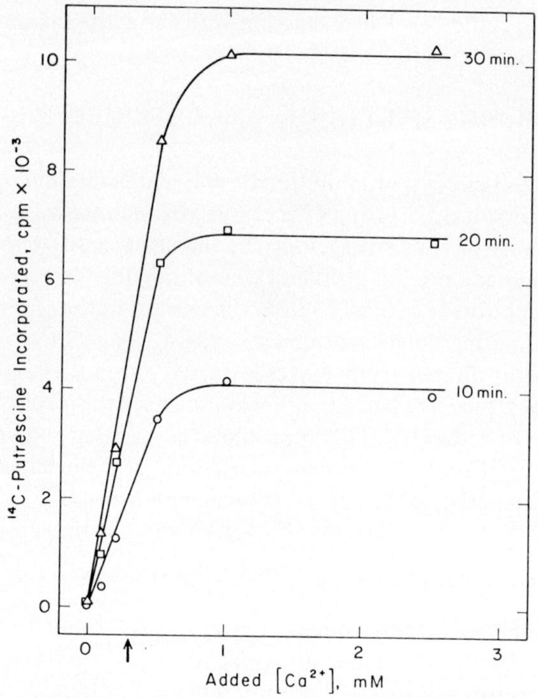

Fig. 5. Ca^{2+} dependence of transglutaminase activity in fresh erythrocyte lysate obtained from an individual donor. For details see Siefring [9]. Arrow indicates Ca^{2+}-requirement for half-maximal activity of the enzyme.

EFFECT OF TRANSAMIDASE INHIBITORS ON THE Ca^{2+}-INDUCED LOSS OF MEMBRANE DEFORMABILITY AND ECHINOCYTIC TRANSFORMATION IN ERYTHROCYTES

With specific transglutaminase inhibitors as primary tools, efforts are being directed towards examining the relationship of the enzyme-dependent cross-linking of membrane proteins to the cellular phenomena of irreversible membrane rigidification and irreversible echinocytic transformation. Though the results are still quite preliminary, a connection emerges already as a strong possibility.

In collaboration with Dr Paul LaCelle and Mr Brian Smith of the University of Rochester Medical School, the effect of histamine was examined on the Ca^{2+}-dependent irreversible loss of membrane deformability [28] using the micropipette methodology. The elastic membrane extension for cells incubated for 1 h in 0.05 M $CaCl_2$ (in the presence of 10 μM ionophore A23187) was only about 32% of control, whereas still 93% extension was obtained in the presence of histamine (80 mM). $^{\alpha}$N-dimethylhistamine, which as mentioned before does not contain a primary amino group and is not a transamidase inhibitor, did not interfere with the loss of membrane deformability.

Transglutaminase inhibitors also appear to have a rather dramatic effect on the Ca^{2+}-induced irreversible shape change in erythrocytes [29]. It is shown in Figure 6 that the echinocytic transformation is irreversible in the sense that the majority of the cells (as documented in Table I) retain this shape even after the removal of Ca^{2+} and of ionophore by washing with serum albumin and EDTA according to Sarkadi et al [30]. If fixation of the echinocytic shape took place by cross-linking of membrane proteins through

γ-glutamyl-ϵ-lysine bonds, the presence of a suitable transglutaminase inhibitor during the echinocytic transformation should allow the shape change to become reversible. Indeed, the results (Fig. 6 and Table I) clearly show that if an inhibitory amine is added before loading of the cells with Ca^{2+}, although the echinocytic shape prevails as long as Ca^{2+} is present, once this ion and the ionophore are removed a significant proportion of the cells return to a form which approximates that of normal discocytes and cupped cells. It is interesting to note that this apparent reversal of shape occurs without a need for augmenting the intracellular concentration of ATP.

CONCLUSIONS

The intracellular accumulation of Ca^{2+}-ions in human erythrocytes initiates a cascade of events by activating a latent transamidating enzyme of the endo-γ-glutamine:ϵ-lysine transferase type. Following the Ca^{2+}-dependent conversion into the active form, this enzyme causes the fusion of certain membrane proteins (P, P′. . .) by γ-glutamyl-ϵ-lysine cross-bridges (X):

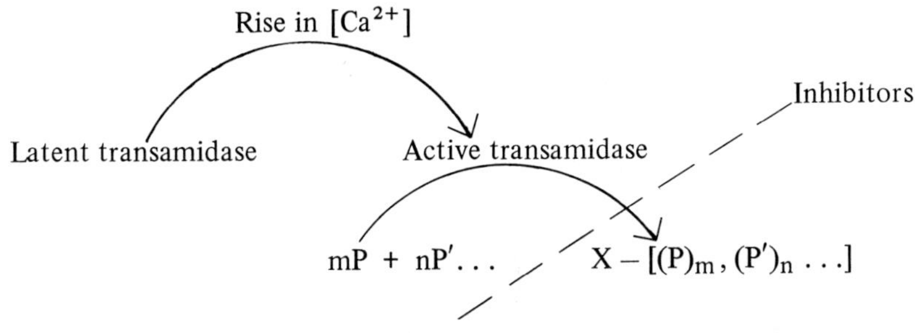

TABLE I. Effect of Transamidase Inhibitors on the Reversibility of Ca^{2+}-Induced Shape Change

I[a]	II	Before wash		After wash with BSA-EDTA[b]	
2 h, 37°C	2 h, 37°C (20 μM A23187, 0.4% DMSO)	Echinocytes[c] (%)	ATP[d] (nmoles/gm Hb)	Echinocytes[c] (%)	ATP[d] (nmoles/gm Hb)
	Plus 1.5 mM $MgCl_2$	15	2,885	5	2,830
	$CaCl_2$	90	460	77	500
Plus 20 mM H_2NCH_2CN	$CaCl_2$	90	230	40	200
$H_2NCH_2CH_2$– 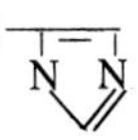	$CaCl_2$	85	490	38	620
$H_2N(CH_2)_2SS(CH_2)_2NH_2$	$CaCl_2$	88	285	30	50

[a]Incubation with buffer A: 0.1 M KCl, 0.06 M NaCl, 10 mM glucose, 5 mM Tris-HCl, pH 7.4. Hematocrit 50%.

[b]Wash: 40 volumes of 0.4% BSA–1 mM EDTA in buffer A for 5 min at 4°C, then 2 h at 37°C, followed by 40 volumes of 0.05% BSA–1 mM EDTA in buffer A for 2 × 1 h at 37°C.

[c]Monitored by counting ca. 2,000 cells and refers to echinocytes type II-IV and spheroechinocytes (for classification, see Bessis [31]).

[d]ATP was measured as described by Beutler [32].

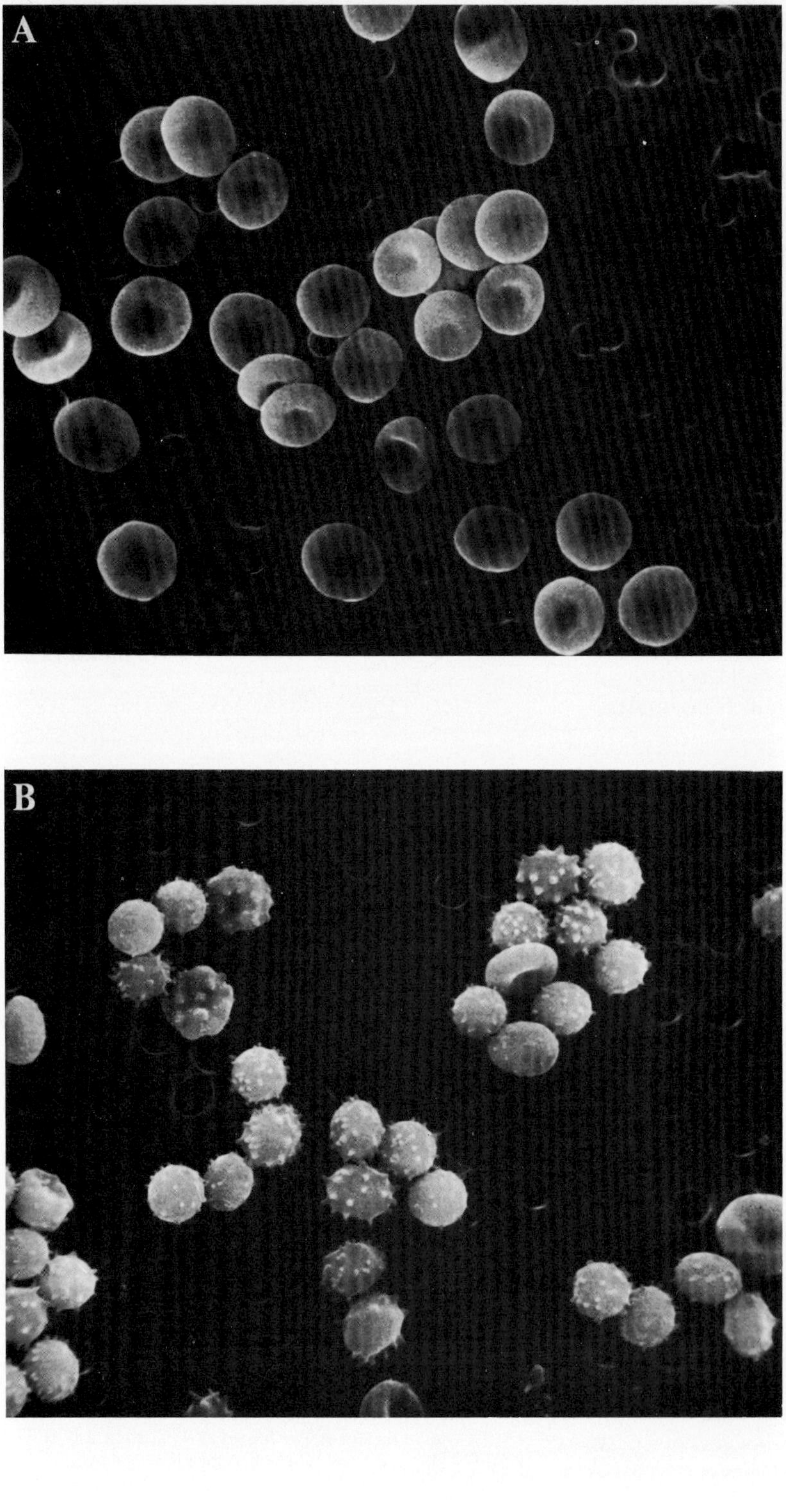

6

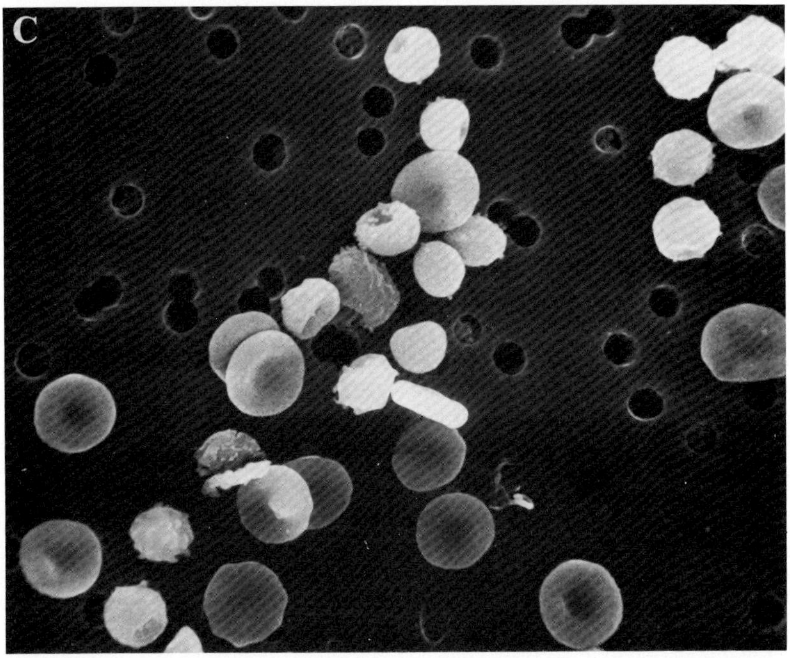

Fig. 6. Scanning electron microscopic photographs of human erythrocytes incubated at 37°C for 2 h with 20 μM ionophore and 1.5 mM $MgCl_2$ (top, left), 1.5 mM $CaCl_2$ (bottom), or 1.5 mM $CaCl_2$ plus 20 mM cystamine (above). Electron microscopic examination was performed on the cells after washing in bovine serum albumin (BSA) [28] and EDTA on Nucleopore membrane N300CPR with holes of 3-μ diameter. For details see Table I.

The demonstration that specific transamidase inhibitors can interfere with the Ca^{2+}-induced irreversible loss of membrane deformability and with the irreversible fixation of echinocytic shape underscores the possible significance of this enzymic cross-linking mechanism.

ACKNOWLEDGMENTS

This work was supported by US Public Health Service Career Award 5 K06 HL 03512 and by National Heart, Lung and Blood Institute grant HL 02212.

We thank Mrs Pauline Velasco and Miss Alma Apostol for their assistance.

REFERENCES

1. Weed RI, Chailley B: In Bessis M, Weed RI, Leblond PF (eds): "Red Cell Shape." New York: Springer Verlag, 1973, p 55.
2. White JG: Sem Hematol 13:121, 1976.
3. Kirkpatrick FH, Hillman DG, LaCelle PL: Experientia 31:653, 1975.
4. Kuettner JF, Dreher KL, Rao GHR, Eaton JW, Blackshear TL Jr, White JG: Am J Path 88:81, 1977.
5. Lorand L, Weissmann LB, Bruner-Lorand J, Epel DL: Biol Bull 151:419, 1976.

6. Lorand L, Weissmann LB, Epel DL, Bruner-Lorand J: Proc Natl Acad Sci USA 73:4479, 1976.
7. Siefring GE Jr, Lorand L: Fed Proc 36:747, 1977 (Abstract No. 2498).
8. Siefring GE Jr, Lorand L: In Kruckeberg WC, Eaton JW, Brewer GJ (eds): "Erythrocyte Membranes: Recent Clinical and Experimental Advances." New York: Alan R. Liss, 1978, p 25.
9. Siefring GE Jr, Apostol AB, Velasco PT, Lorand L: Biochemistry 17:2598, 1978.
10. Fairbanks G, Steck TL, Wallach DFH: Biochemistry 10:2606, 1971.
11. Lorand L: Ann NY Acad Sci 202:6, 1972.
12. Lorand L: In Kaminer B (ed): "Search and Discovery, a Tribute to Albert Szent-Gyorgyi." New York: Academic, 1977, p 177.
13. Lorand L, Rule NG, Ong HH, Furlanetto R, Jacobsen A, Downey H, Oner N, Bruner-Lorand J: Biochemistry 7:1214, 1968.
14. Lorand L, Stenberg P: In Fasman GF (ed): "Handbook of Biochemistry and Molecular Biology." Proteins Vol. II. Cleveland: Chemical Rubber Co, 1976, p 669.
15. Credo RB, Stenberg P, Tong YS, Lorand L: Fed Proc 35:1631, 1976 (Abstract No. 1390).
15. Lorand L, Chenoweth D, Gray A: Ann NY Acad Sci 202:155, 1972.
16. Credo RB, Stenberg P, Tong YS, Lorand L: Fed Proc 35:1631, 1976 (Abstract No. 1390.
17. Cooke RD, Pestell TC, Holbrook JJ: Biochem J 141:675, 1974.
18. Lorand L, Nilsson JLG: In Ariens EJ (ed): "Drug Design." New York: Academic, 1972, vol 3, p 415.
19. Lorand L, Downey J, Gotoh T, Jacobsen A, Tokura S: Biochem Biophys Res Commun 31:222, 1968.
20. Roberts WW, Lorand L, Mockros LF: Biorheology 10:29, 1973.
21. Mockros LF, Roberts WW, Lorand L: Biophys Chem 2:164, 1974.
22. Lorand L, Campbell-Wilkes LK, Cooperstein L: Anal Biochem 50:623, 1972.
23. Curtis CG, Lorand L: Methods Enzymol 45:177, 1976.
24. LaCelle PL, Kirkpatrick FH, Udkow MP, Arkin B: In Bessin M, Weed RI, Leblond PF (eds): "Red Cell Shape." New York: Springer Verlag, 1973, p 69.
25. Eaton JW, Shelton TD, Swofford HL, Kolpin CE, Jacob HS:Nature 246:105, 1973.
26. Palek J: Blood 42:988, 1973 (abstract).
27. LaCelle PL: In Weed RI, Jaffe ER, Miescher PA (eds): "The Red Cell Membrane." New York: Grune and Stratton, 1971, p 107.
28. Smith B, Siefring G, Parameswaran K, LaCelle P, Lorand L: Blood 50:87, 1977 (Abstract).
29. Siefring GE Jr, Lowe-Krentz L, Parameswaran KN, Lorand L, Smith B, LaCelle P: Biophys J 21:119a, 1978 (Abstract No. TU-PM-G5.
30. Sarkadi B, Szasz I, Gardos G: J Membrane Biol 26:357, 1976.
31. Bessis M: In Bessis M, Weed RI, Leblond PF (eds): "Red Cell Shape." New York: Springer Verlag, 1973, p 1.
32. Beutler E: In "Red Cell Metabolism, A Manual of Biochemistry Methods." 2d ed. New York: Grune and Stratton, 1975, p 104.

Journal of Supramolecular Structure 9:441–452 (1978)
Normal and Abnormal Red Cell Membranes 293–304

Redistribution of Intramembrane Particles of Human Erythrocytes Induced by HVJ (Sendai Virus): A Prerequisite for the Virus-Induced Cell Fusion

Akira Asano and Kiyotoshi Sekiguchi

Institute for Protein Research, Osaka University, Osaka 565, Japan

Aggregation of intramembrane particles of human erythrocytes was found to be induced by HVJ (Sendai virus) under conditions which lead to cell fusion. Degree of polyerythrocyte formation was compared under a variety of conditions with extent of cluster formation observed with the same preparations. Both structural changes of the membranes, ie, fusion and clustering of the particles, behaved very similarly under widely different virus-to-cell ratios and over the time course of cell fusion. Furthermore, by inclusion of high concentrations of antispectrin antibodies within the ghosts, inhibition of clustering of intramembrane particles and hindrance of virus-induced cell fusion were found to occur simultaneously. Antibodies by themselves did not induce aggregation of particles under isotonic conditions, whereas particle clustering could be induced under hypotonic conditions at antibody concentrations causing partial cross-linking of spectrin molecules.

In conclusion, clustering of intramembrane particles seems to be required for virus-induced fusion of human erythrocytes.

Key words: **cell fusion, human erythrocytes, Sendai virus, clustering of intramembrane particles, antispectrin antibody**

Intramembrane particles (IMP) observed by freeze-fracture electron microscopy in human erythrocyte membranes have been identified as cell surface glycoproteins [1, 2]. In reconstitution experiments [3] similar particles have been observed with liposomes containing purified band 3* dimers, and a possible association of glycophorin or other surface proteins with IMP has also been suggested [1, 2, 4]. By freeze-fracture studies of Sendai virus-induced fusion of human erythrocytes, Bächi and co-workers [5, 6] discovered that aggregated distribution of IMP was observed with extensively fused cells in contrast to

*The major polypeptides of the erythrocyte membrane are designated by Steck's nomenclature [39].

Abbreviations: HVJ, hemagglutinating virus of Japan (Sendai virus); HAU, hemagglutinating unit; TBS, tricine-buffered saline (140 mM NaCl, 5.4 mM KCl, 40 mM tricine-NaOH, pH 7.6); BSA, bovine serum albumin; IMP, intramembrane particles; PF and EF, protoplasmic fracture face and extracellular fracture face, respectively. Nomenclature of Branton et al. [25]

Received May 4, 1978; accepted August 7, 1978.

0091-7419/78/0903-0441$02.30

their random distribution in untreated erythrocytes. Because this clustering of IMP was induced by action of the virus, and this change seems to expose protein-free areas on the cell surface which may be sites of fusion of lipid bilayers, this process was thought to be a prerequisite of virus-induced cell fusion [6, 7].

On the other hand, the virus has been known to induce several changes on human erythrocytes; since only some of them may be actually related to cell fusion, critical studies will be required to draw final conclusions about involvement of these phenomena in virus-induced fusion of erythrocyte membranes. Hemagglutination [8, 9] and probably fusion of the viral envelope to the cell membrane (envelope fusion) [10–12] seem to be required for formation of polyerythrocytes, whereas hemolysis, which is induced by fusion of some but not all types of viral envelope to erythrocytes [13, 14], and virus-induced fluidity changes of lipid bilayers [15, 16] may not be required for cell fusion, although these are also induced by the virus.

Therefore, we started a closer examination of the relationship between cluster formation of IMP and fusion of adjacent cell membranes to find out whether the former is required for the latter or not. To this end, the following experiments were undertaken: 1) comparison of the virus-to-cell ratio required for cell fusion and that needed for aggregation of IMP; 2) comparison of the time course of the fusion of erythrocyte ghosts and that of clustering of IMP; 3) inhibition of clustering of IMP by antispectrin antibodies and its relationship to the inhibition of the virus-induced fusion of erythrocyte ghosts. The results of these experiments will be reported together with the effect of salt concentrations on mobility of the IMP-spectrin complex.

MATERIALS AND METHODS

Cells and Virus

Human erythrocytes were obtained from a blood bank (Midori Jugi) and used within four weeks after they had been drawn. Hemagglutinating virus of Japan (HVJ, Sendai virus), kindly propagated in Dr. Y. Okada's laboratory, was grown in the allantoic sac of chick embryos and purified as elsewhere described [17, 18]. Hemagglutination titer was determined by Salk's pattern method [19].

Preparation of Ghosts and Fusion Experiments

Ghosts were prepared according to Dodge et al [20] with 5 mM sodium phosphate (pH 8.0) as hemolyzing buffer. Packed ghosts were washed once with the lysing buffer, incubated with four volumes of tricine-buffered saline (TBS; 140 mM NaCl, 5.4 mM KCl, 40 mM tricine-NaOH, pH 7.6) containing 5% bovine serum albumin (BSA) and other proteins when indicated at 0° for 10 min, and then resealed by incubation at 37° for 60 min as described previously [21]. Albumin-loaded ghosts and intact erythrocytes were washed twice with TBS and suspended in TBS. Fusion experiments were carried out as follows: Cells or ghosts were mixed, to give a final concentration of 2%, with indicated amounts of the virus at 0° for 15 min to allow agglutination; then the aggregates were incubated at 37° for 30 min unless stated otherwise. Degree of fusion was observed by a Nikon-phase contrast microscope.

Electron Microscopy

The samples were fixed by the addition of an equal volume of 4% glutaraldehyde prepared with the same medium and warmed to reaction temperature. This process was performed for 40 min at 37° or for 2 h at 4°. After three washes with the incubation medium, the fixed samples were suspended in 20% (v/v) glycerol in physiologic saline at 4° over night. Then freeze-fracture was performed under standard conditions with a Hitachi freeze-fracture apparatus. Electron micrographs were taken with a Hitachi HU-12 electron microscope.

Preparation and Purification of Antispectrin Antibodies

Spectrin was extracted from ghosts by dialysis against 1 mM ethylenediamine-tetracetic acid (EDTA), pH 10, at 4° for 18–20 h and further purified by gel filtration on Sepharose 4B. Antibodies against spectrin were produced in rabbits. The antisera were first fractionated by ammonium sulfate precipitation and then purified by a spectrin-Sepharose column (2–3 mg spectrin per milliliter of packed gel) prepared by the method of Cuatrecasas [22]. Antispectrin antibody thus purified was 63% precipitable with purified spectrin and formed a single precipitin band on immunodiffusion against solubilized erythrocyte membrane and purified spectrin. Antispectrin F_{ab} fragments were made and purified by the procedure of Porter [23]. Antigen-binding activity of the F_{ab} fragments was checked by ability to prevent precipitation of spectrin-[^{125}I] antibody complex near the equivalence point. Control immunoglobulin (IgG fraction) was prepared form non-immunized sera by ammonium sulfate precipitation and DEAE-cellulose column chromatography.

Reagents

Bovine serum albumin (fraction V) and N-[tris(hydroxymethyl)methyl] glycine (tricine) were purchased from Sigma Chemical Co. Sodium iodide I^{125} was obtained from Dai-ichi Chemical Co. Iodinated bovine serum albumin was prepared by a chloramine-T method [24].

RESULTS

Aggregation of IMP and Polyerythrocyte Formation Induced by Different Amounts of HVJ

As shown in Fig. 1(A–D), fusion frequency of human erythrocytes observed after incubation for 30 min is dependent on the amounts (in hemagglutinating units – HAU) of the virus added A, 50 HAU; B, 100 HAU; C, 400 HAU; D, 800 HAU); further incubation up to 2 h has not appreciably changed the fusion profile. Freeze-fracture observation of the protoplasmic fracture face (PF) [25] of the membrane revealed that the degree of aggregation of the particles roughly paralleled that of polyerythrocyte formation, as shown in Fig. 1 (E, 50 HAU; F, 400 HAU; G, 800 HAU). Incubation at low temperature neither induced cell fusion nor stimulated redistribution of IMP (Fig. 1 H), although a ragged region was sometimes observed on fracture faces of the virus-agglutinated cells. At very low virus doses, such as 50 HAU/ml, when fused samples still contained many unfused single cells, some difference in degree of clustering was evident from fracture face to fracture face. An area showing average clustering is shown in Fig. 1 E as typical of the effect of virus treatment at 50 HAU/ml.

Time Course of Erythrocyte Ghost Fusion and Cluster Formation of IMP

As reported previously [21], erythrocyte ghosts loaded with bovine serum albumin could be fused by virus treatment, although larger amounts of virus were needed to attain the same level of fusion as for intact erythrocytes. The rate of the fusion process was similar to that of erythrocyte fusion. As shown in Fig. 2 (A–D), degree of fusion reached

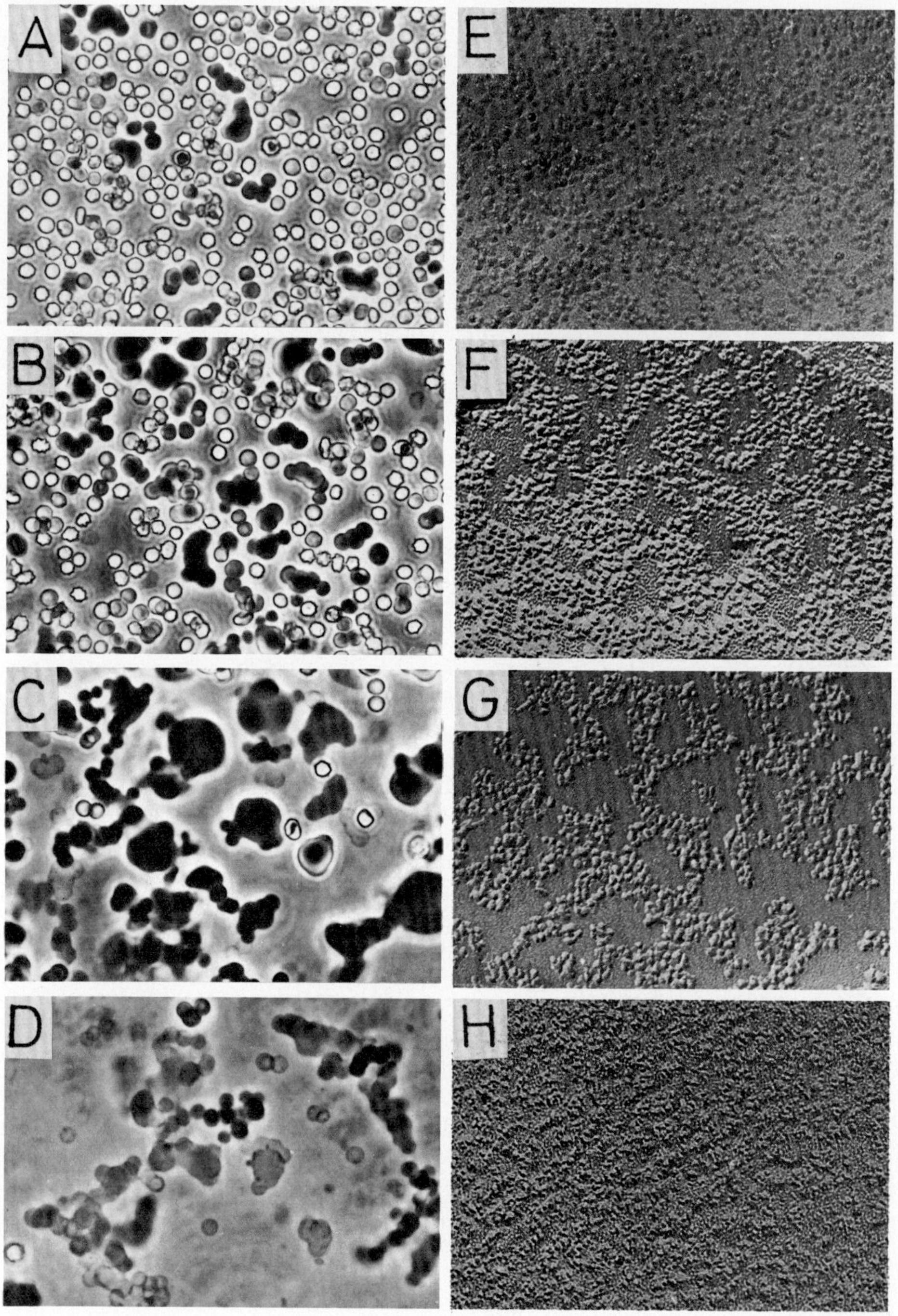

Fig. 1. Comparison of degree of cell fusion with that of cluster formation of intramembrane particles of different virus-to-cell ratios. Intact cells were agglutinated by different concentrations of HVJ for 15 min in an ice bath and subsequently incubated at 37° for 30 min except for H. A, E) 50 HAU/ml; B) 100 HAU/ml; C, F) 400 HAU/ml; D, G, H) 800 HAU/ml; H) no incubation at 37°. A–D) Phase microscopy, × 350; E–H) PF of freeze-fractured sample, × 100,000.

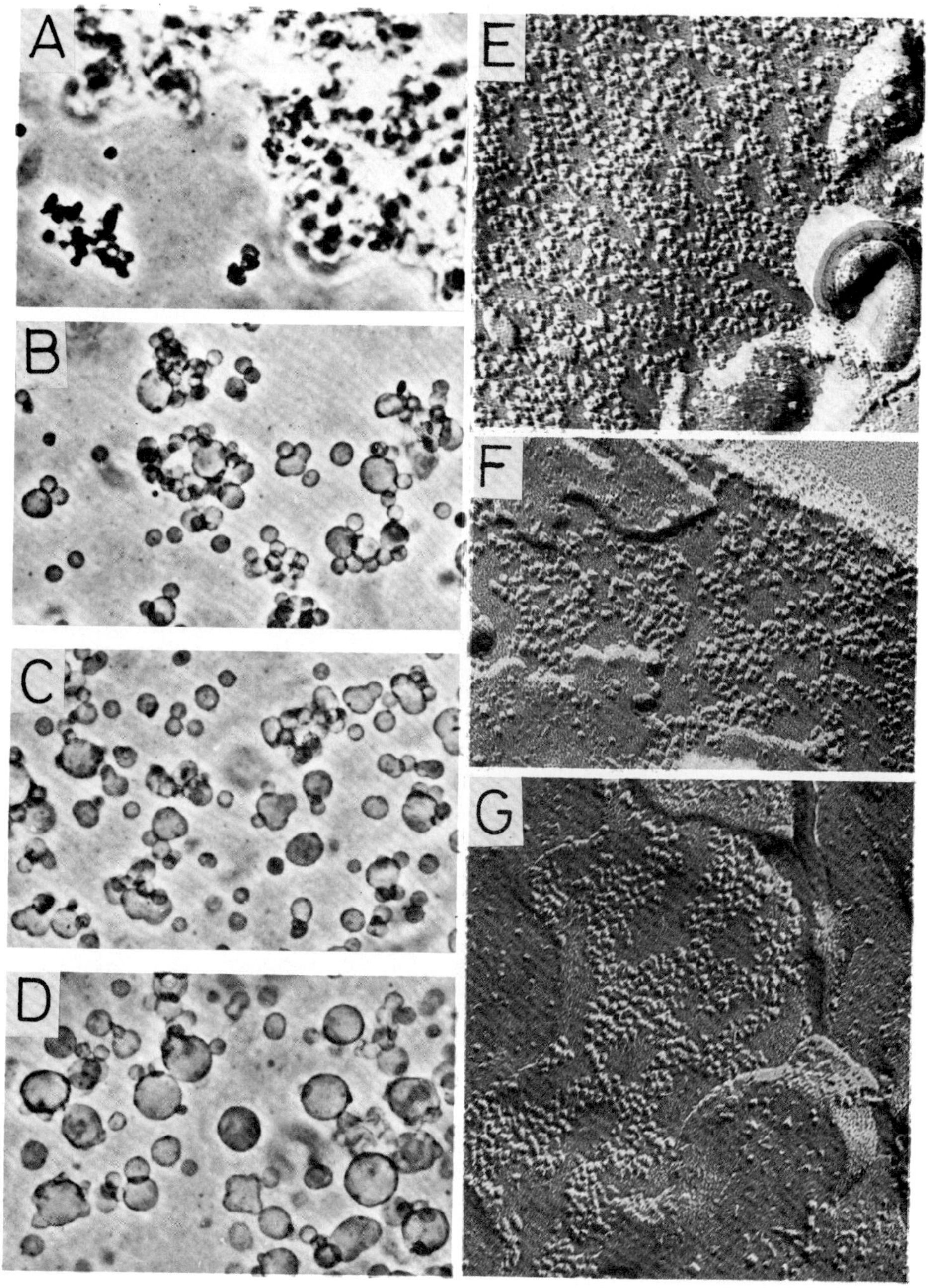

Fig. 2. Time course of the fusion reaction of BSA-loaded ghosts. The ghosts were agglutinated by HVJ (6,000 HAU/ml) for 15 min in an ice bath, then incubated at 37° for A) 0 min; E) 3 min; B) 5 min; C) 10 min; D, F, G) 30 min. A–D) Phase microscopy, × 350; (E–G) PF of freeze-fractured sample, × 100,000; E, F) samples were fixed with 2% glutaraldehyde at 37° for 40 min; G) reaction was stopped by cooling in an ice bath for 30 min, and then fixing with 2% glutaraldehyde was performed for 2 h at 4°.

maximum after 30–60 min incubation at 37°. When the virus-cell aggregate was incubated at 37° for 3 min (Fig. 2E), some redistribution of IMP on the PF could already be detected. Longer incubation (30 min) at 37° resulted in more extensive clustering of IMP (Fig. 2F). Cooling of the fused ghosts to 4° before fixing seems to enhance clustering (Fig. 2G), as recently reported in the case of Ca^{2+}-induced membrane changes of chicken erythrocytes [26], but similar cold treatment of unfused cells showed no appreciable clustering (Fig. 1H).

Inhibition of Virus-Induced Fusion and Clustering of IMP by Antispectrin Antibody Included Within Ghosts

As reported preliminarily [21], antispectrin antibody sequestered in ghosts at a concentration of 1 mg/ml (Fig. 3B) and 4 mg/ml (Fig. 3C) greatly inhibits virus-induced fusion. Figure 3A represents a typical fusion profile of ghosts loaded with bovine serum albumin. Inclusion of IgG fraction prepared from control rabbit sera has no inhibitory effect, as is shown in Fig. 3D. The requirement of relatively high concentrations of antibody (1–4 mg/ml) for inhibition suggests that extensive cross-linking of spectrin by the anti-

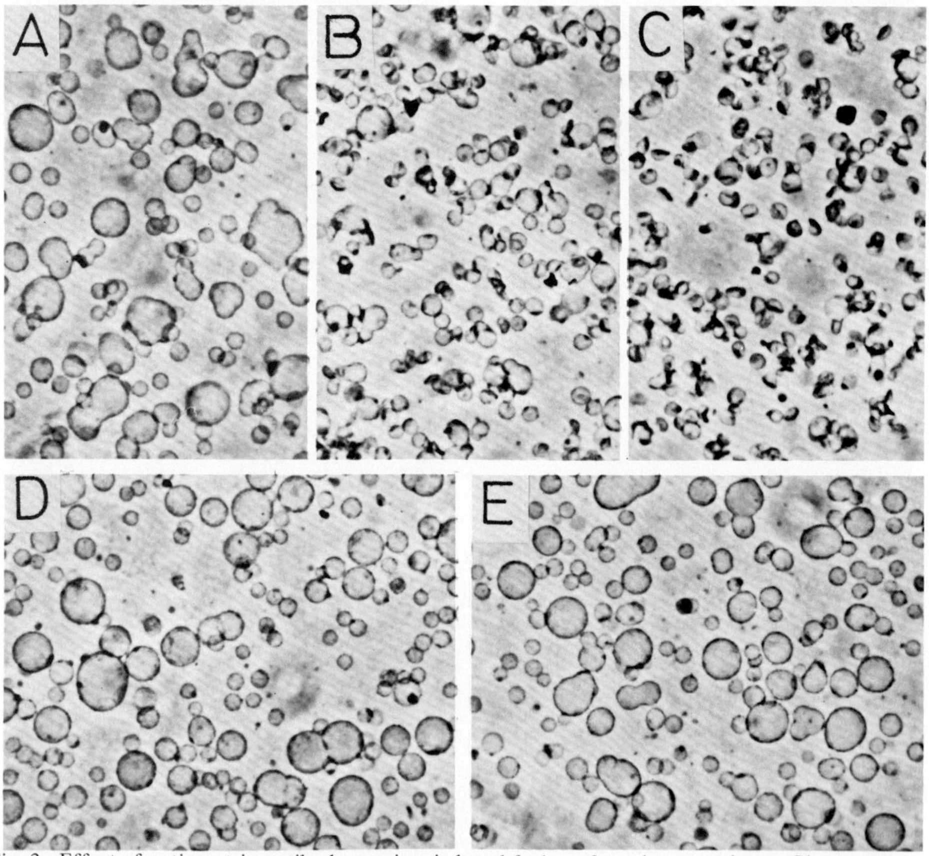

Fig. 3. Effect of antispectrin antibody on virus-induced fusion of erythrocyte ghosts. Ghosts were loaded with 5% BSA containing the following proteins at indicated concentrations by the method described in Materials and Methods. A) No further addition; B) antispectrin antibody, 1 mg/ml; C) antispectrin antibody, 4 mg/ml; D) control immunoglobulin, 4 mg/ml; E) Fab fragments prepared from the antibody, 4 mg/ml. These ghosts were agglutinated by HVJ (10,000 HAU/ml) for 15 min in an ice bath and then incubated at 37° for 30 min. Phase microscopy, × 350.

body might be necessary for inhibition. This assumption was further substantiated by the fact that monovalent F_{ab} fragments loaded at 4 mg/ml did not affect the fusion reaction (Fig. 3E).

Distribution of IMP was studied in inhibited and control samples. As shown in Fig. 4A, fused ghosts containing IgG fractions from control sera exhibited nonrandom distribution of IMP, whereas no such clustering was observed in ghosts loaded with antispectrin antibody at 5 mg/ml (Fig. 4B). Therefore, cross-linking of spectrin with high concentrations of the antibody under the conditions employed seems to restrict the movement of IMP, and this immobilization in turn may lead to the inhibition of virus-induced cell fusion.

Changes Induced by the Virus on External Fracture Face

The extracellular fracture face (EF) of human erythrocyte membranes has fewer IMP than the PF; therefore, it is rather difficult to detect such redistribution as might be induced by the virus. But upon closer examination, pits or depressions corresponding to the places where particles might have been pulled out would be detectable on the EF. As shown in Fig. 5A, the distribution of such pits on EF of fused preparations was nonrandom. In contrast, nonfused preparations had randomly distributed pits and IMP on their EF (Fig. 5B).

Effect of Antispectrin Antibody by Itself on Distribution of IMP:

Several years ago Nicolson and Painter [27] reported that antispectrin by itself induced clustering of cell surface anionic sites (sialic acid residues) in hypotonic conditions. Since we postulated that inhibition rather than induction of cluster formation is responsible for inhibition of virus-induced fusion, the effects of the antibody by itself on distribution of IMP were studied under several conditions. Treatment of ghosts by antibody under the hypotonic shock conditions employed by Nicolson and Painter (Fig. 6, A and B), and simple addition of the antibody to Dodge-type leaky ghosts [20] in the hemolyzing buffer (Fig. 6, C and D). both resulted in cluster formation of IMP at the antibody concentrations optimal for clustering (0.2–1.0 mg/ml). Thus, previous experiments [27] were substantiated by the freeze-fracture method.

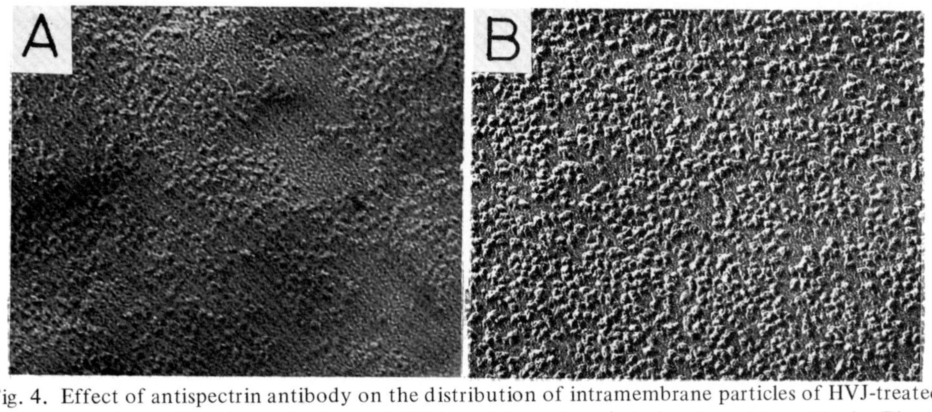

Fig. 4. Effect of antispectrin antibody on the distribution of intramembrane particles of HVJ-treated erythrocyte ghosts. The ghosts, loaded with BSA containing 5 mg/ml of antispectrin antibody (B), were agglutinated with HVJ (8,000 HAU/ml) and then incubated at 37° for 40 min with 2% glutaraldehyde, samples were freeze-fractured as described in Materials and Methods. PF at a magnification of 100,000.

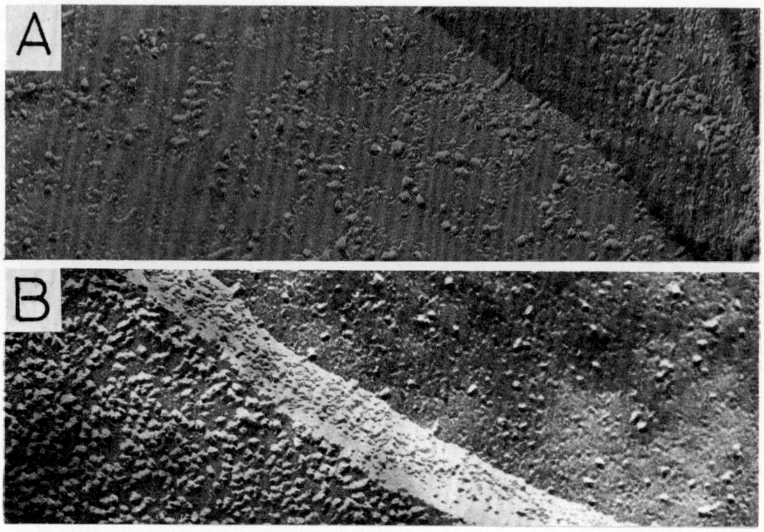

Fig. 5. EF of fused and unfused erythrocyte membranes. A) Fusion conditions were as described in legend of Fig. 1G. A piece of PF can be seen at upper right corner. B) Fusion was inhibited by anti-spectrin antibody as described in Fig. 4B. Random distribution of IMP on PF can be seen at lower left side, and EF is shown at upper right side.

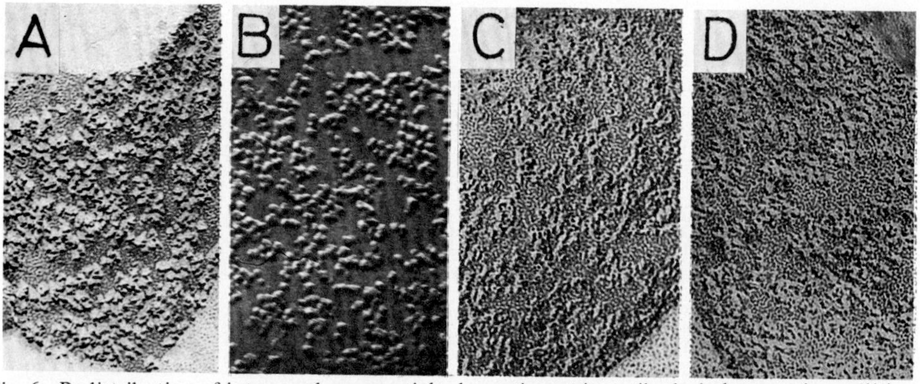

Fig. 6. Redistribution of intramembrane particles by antispectrin antibody in hypotonic conditions. A, B) Ghosts were prepared and processed as described by Nicolson and Painter [27] with slight modification. To pelleted ghosts which were incubated in an isotonic medium (300 PB: 0.05 M sodium phosphate–0.6% sodium chloride buffer, pH 7.5, 300 mOsm) over night at 4°, 10 volumes of 15 PB (300 PB diluted 1:20, pH 7.5) containing antispectrin antibody was added and incubated at 37° for 30 min. After cooling to 4°, the ghosts were washed twice in 15 PB and fixed in 2% glutaraldehyde for 40 min at 37°. Concentrations of the antibody used were 0.2 mg/ml (A) and 1.0 mg/ml (B). C, D) To ghosts prepared by the method of Dodge et al [20], antispectrin antibody in 5 mM sodium phosphate (pH 7.5) was added to give a final concentration of 1.0 mg/ml. After indubation at 37° for 30 min, the samples were fixed by the addition of equal volumes of 4% glutaraldehyde for 40 min at 37°. Freeze-fracturing was performed as described in Materials and Methods. PF was shown at × 100,000.

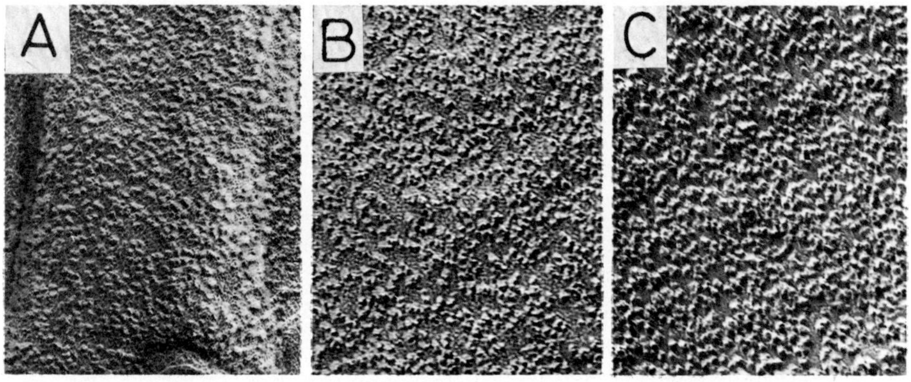

Fig. 7. Distribution of intramembrane particles of ghosts loaded with antispectrin antibody. The ghosts were loaded with 5% BSA containing the indicated concentrations of antispectrin antibody as described in Materials and Methods. Incubation conditions and freeze-fracturing were as described for fusion experiments except that no virus was added. The antibody concentrations employed were (A) 0.2 mg/ml, (B) 1 mg/ml, (C) 5 mg/ml. PF was shown at × 100,000. A ragged appearance was sometimes observed on fracture faces.

However, similar treatment of ghosts with antibody in isotonic salts containing BSA used for the fusion experiments had no effect on redistribution of IMP (Fig. 7, A–C). Therefore, stability of spectrin meshwork on the internal surface of erythrocyte membranes [3, 27–31] may be influenced by the medium composition, and in isotonic conditions partial cross-linking of spectrin by the antibody may not affect distribution of spectrin.

DISCUSSION

Addition of HVJ to erythrocyte suspensions induced several changes in erythrocytes. Amont them, cell agglutination, hemolysis, and redistribution of IMP have been related so far to fusion reaction. Agglutination of cells seems to be a prerequisite for cell fusion, since specific inhibition of hemagglutinating activity of the virus resulted in loss of cell fusion and hemolysis [8, 9]. Furthermore, release of sialic acid by neuraminidase treatment from the cell surface also inhibited both the hemagglutination and fusion reactions [32].

The relationship between hemolysis and cell fusion is more complex. There are several lines of evidence which indicate that fusion of the viral envelope to the cell membrane (envelope fusion) is directly or indirectly responsible for hemolysis [13, 14, 21]. Envelope fusion seems to be required for cell fusion as well as hemolysis, since virus preparations incapable of fusing with the cell membrane either by specific removal of F-glycoprotein through trypsin treatment [33] or by propagation of the virus in cells lacking processing activity (limited proteolysis of F-glycoprotein to an active form) [10] also lose the capacity of cell fusion, hemolysis, and infectious activities.

But envelope fusion does not always induce hemolysis, especially in the case of virus preparations harvested at an early stage of propagation in fertilized eggs. Freeze-thaw or hypotonic treatment of the virus preparations extensively enhanced hemolysis without affecting fusion activity. Furthermore, several other processes, such as sonication [34], heating at 45° [35], and incubation with very low concentrations of glutaraldehyde [36] were found to inhibit cell fusion without affecting hemolysis.

Similar analysis of the relationship between cluster formation of IMP and cell fusion may be required to decide whether IMP aggregation is a prerequisite to cell fusion. Sendai virus-induced redistribution of IMP was first discovered by Bächi and co-workers [5, 6]; however, use of too high concentrations of virus (10–20 times our virus-to-cell ratios as shown in Fig. 1D and G) has been criticized [37]. But, as detected in this study, the appreciable redistribution of IMP with virus levels as low as 50 HAU/ml and the roughly parallel increase of clustering and cell fusion with increase of virus-to-cell ratio seem to substantiate Bächi and Howe's findings.

On the basis of extensive morphologic studies on fusion of the viral envelope to human erythrocytes, Knutton [37] claimed that he did not always observe redistribution of IMP in his preparations, although he noticed clustering of IMP after longer incubation At present we do not know the exact reason for this apparent discrepancy, but one possibility is that his virus strain has rather low frequency and slow rate of cell-to-cell fuision under the conditions employed, although hemolytic activity may be high with his virus preparations. If so, it is possible that freeze-fracture of a mixture of polyerythrocytes and unfused cells would reveal a spectrum of PF of different degrees of IMP aggregation, as described above. Selection of fracture face at an early stage of virus-cell interaction ie, invagination of the viral envelope (a step before occurrence of the virus-cell fusion) might be possible only under these conditions.

In our hands, the initial, rapid phase of hemolysis, which may represent fusion of the viral envelope to the cell membrane, is almost complete within 3 min after onset of incubation at 37° [18]. Invagination of the viral envelope could not be observed in so short a time as the 3 min incubation set by this rapid reaction. Furthermore, some redistribution of IMP seems to occur within this time, as shown in Fig. 2E. Therefore, the rate of the reaction of the virus with the cell membrane seems to be much faster with our virus preparations and under the conditions of our study.

As also shown in a preliminary communication [21], agglutination of cells by the virus and lysis of resealed ghosts (equivalent to fusion of the viral envelope to the cell membrane) were not affected by the inhibition of cluster formation of IMP by anti-spectrin antibodies; thus redistribution of IMP seems to participate at the latter stage of cell fusion, ie, fusion of adjacent cell membranes. In support for this assumption, measurement of envelope fusion by a spin-labeling technique [11, 12] also confirmed the absence of inhibition of this reaction by antispectrin antibody sequestered within ghosts (K. Sekiguchi and K. Kuroda, unpublished observations). As discussed previously [21], induction of redistribution of IMP has also been reported in many cases of membrane fusion phenomena.

As discussed above, clustering of IMP seems to be a necessary step for virus-induced cell fusion; however, it has also been reported that similar aggregation of IMP can be induced by anti-spectrin antibody at low concentrations which might cross-link spectrin only partially when added to erythrocyte ghosts under hypotonic conditions [27]. Because the viral induction of IMP clustering was performed in isotonic salts containing bovine serum albumin, control experiments without addition of the virus were done in the isotonic fusion medium. No such redistribution of IMP was observed by the antibodies by themselves at any concentrations tested. Thus, lateral mobility of spectrin-IMP complex seems to be influenced by the medium employed. Enhanced mobility of spectrin in hypotonic conditions is consistent with higher extractability of spectrin at hypotonic conditions [38, 39]. Clustering of both surface anionic sites (sialic acid residues) [27], and IMP (this report) by antispectrin antibodies further substantiated the well-documented assumption that IMP correspond to a complex of band 3 dimer and glycophorin [1–4].

The questions that need to be addressed next would seem to be the following: 1) What component of the virus is responsible for the redistribution of IMP; 2) what component of erythrocyte membranes is first affected by virus treatment and then brings about the clustered configuration of IMP in the membrane; 3) what and how many components of erythrocytes participate in this reaction; 4) is aggregation of IMP for induction of cell-to-cell fusion or is some change in lipid bilayers also required for fusion of adjacent cell membranes?

ACKNOWLEDGMENTS

We are indebted to Professor Ryo Sato of our institute and to Professor Yoshio Okada of the Research Institute for Microbial Diseases for valuable discussions. Electron microscopy was done in Professor Y. Tashiro's laboratory at Kansai Medical University. We are grateful to him and to Dr. Shiro Matsuura of Kansai Medical University for kindly allowing us to use their equipment and for their help in electron microscopy.

REFERENCES

1. Tillack TW, Scott RE, Marchesi VT: J Exp Med 135:1209, 1972.
2. Pinto da Silva P, Nicolson GL: Biochim Biophys Acta 363:311, 1974.
3. Yu J, Branton D: Proc Natl Acad Sci USA 73:3891, 1976.
4. Shotton D, Thompson K, Wofsy L, Branton D: J Cell Biol 76:512, 1978.
5. Bächi T, Howe C: Proc Soc Exp Biol Med 141:141, 1972.
6. Bächi T, Aguet M, Howe C: J Virol 11:1004, 1973.
7. Ahkong QF, Fisher D, Tampion W, Lucy JA: Nature 253:194, 1975.
8. Portner A, Scroggs RA: Virology 67:179, 1975.
9. Ozawa M, Asano A, Okada Y: FEBS Lett 70:145, 1976.
10. Homma M, Ohuchi M: J Virol 12:1457, 1973.
11. Maeda T, Asano A, Ohki K, Okada Y, Ohnishi S: Biochemistry 14:3736, 1975.
12. Maeda T, Asano A, Okada Y, Ohnishi S: J Virol 21:232, 1976.
13. Apostolov K, Damjanovic V: Microbios 8:257, 1973.
14. Homma M, Shimizu K, Shimizu Y-K, Ishida N: Virology 71:41, 1976.
15. Tanaka K, Ohnishi S: Biochim Biophys Acta 426:218, 1976.
16. Lyles DS, Landsberger FR: Proc Natl Acad Sci USA 74:1918, 1977.
17. Okada Y: Biken's J 1:103, 1958.
18. Sekiguchi K, Asano A: Life Sci 18:1383, 1976.
19. Salk JE: J Immunol 49:87, 1944.
20. Dodge JT, Mitchell CD, Hanahan DJ: Arch Biochem Biophys 100:119, 1963.
21. Sekiguchi K, Asano A: Proc Natl Acad Sci USA 75:1740, 1978.
22. Cuatrecasas P: Biochem Biophys Res Commun 35:531, 1969.
23. Porter RR: Biochem J 73:119, 1959.
24. Hunter WH: In Weir DM (ed): "Handbook of Experimental Immunology." Oxford: Blackwell Scientific Publications, 1973, p 17.3.
25. Branton D, Bullivant S, Gilula NB, Karnovsky MJ, Moor H, Mühlethaler K, Northcote DH, Packer L, Satir B, Satir P, Speth V, Staehlin LA, Steere RL, Weinstein RS: Science 190:54, 1975.
26. Volsky D, Loyter A: Biochim Biophys Acta 471:243, 1977.
27. Nicolson GL, Painter PG: J Cell Biol 59:395, 1973.
28. Nicolson GL, Marchesi VT, Singer SJ: J Cell Biol 51:265, 1971.
29. Elgsaeter A, Branton D: J Cell Biol 63:1018, 1974.

30. Steck TL, Yu J: J Supramol Struct 1:220, 1973.
31. Ji TH, Nicolson GL: Proc Natl Acad Sci USA 71:2212, 1974.
32. Howe C, Lee LT: Adv Virus Res 17:1, 1972.
33. Shimizu K, Ishida N: Virology 67:427, 1975.
34. Hosaka Y: J Gen Virol 8:43, 1970.
35. Okada Y, Tadokoro J: Exp Cell Res 26:108, 1962.
36. Toister Z, Loyter A: J Biol Chem 248:422, 1973.
37. Knutton S: J Cell Sci 28:189, 1977.
38. Marchesi VT, Steer E: Science 159:203, 1968.
39. Steck TL: J Cell Biol 62:1, 1974.

Journal of Supramolecular Structure 9:453–458 (1978)
Normal and Abnormal Red Cell Membranes 305–310

Bilayer Balance and Regulation of Red Cell Shape Changes

Narla Mohandas, Alfred C. Greenquist, and Stephen B. Shohet

Departments of Laboratory Medicine and Medicine, the Division of Hematology (N.M., A.C.G., S.B.S.); and the Cancer Research Institute, University of California at San Francisco (N.M., S.B.S.), San Francisco, California 94143

Discocytic human red cells undergo discocyte-echinocyte and discocyte-stomatocyte transformations under the action of a wide variety of lipid-soluble anionic and cationic agents respectively. These shape transformations are explained by the bilayer couple hypothesis of Sheetz and Singer to be the result of preferential distribution of the anionic agents in the outer half of the bilayer and the cationic agents in the inner half of the bilayer. We demonstrate that echinocytogenic effects indeed occur when the naturally occurring phospholipid lysophosphatidylcholine (LPC) is localized in the outer half of the bilayer, and stomatocytogenic effects occur when LPC is in the inner half. However, in contrast to the bilayer couple hypothesis, our results show that simple equivalent membrane surface area expansion on each layer is insufficient to maintain the discocytic shape and there exists a differential concentration effect of LPC on the two halves of the bilayer.

Key words: **red cell, membranes, bilayer, morphology, echinocyte, stomatocyte, phospholipid, lysolecithin**

Excellent evidence now exists that the protein and lipid components of the biologic membrane are asymmetrically distributed within the two monolayers [1, 2]. In human red cells phosphatidylcholine (PC) and sphingomyelin lie mainly in the external monolayer, while the aminophosphatides (phosphatidylethanolamine and phosphatidylserine) are for the most part in the internal or cytoplasmic monolayer [2–4]. Sheetz and Singer have made the attractive suggestion that this asymmetrical distribution of phospholipids produces the separation of electrostatic charge, leading to differences in the transmembrane localization of compounds that induce shape changes in red cells [5, 6]. They proposed that, at equilibrium, anionic and cationic drugs are preferentially distributed in the outer and inner half of the lipid bilayer respectively. According to this hypothesis, anionic drugs

Received March 23, 1978; accepted August 8, 1978.

would expand the area of the outer surface of the membrane relative to the inner surface and cause the cells to become echinocytic (crenated), and cationic compounds would expand the inner surface area relative to the outer and cause the cells to become stomatacytic (cup shaped) [7].

In this paper we show that varying the leaflet location of the natural membrane phospholipid lysophosphatidylcholine (LPC) indeed induces different red cell shape changes. However, the changes occur with differing sensitivity to LPC in the inner and outer halves of the bilayer, and indicate that simple membrane leaflet expansion cannot explain the shape change effects of LPC.

MATERIALS AND METHODS

Blood was drawn from healthy human volunteers into heparinized vacutainers, and the red cells were washed twice in saline. Washed red cells were incubated at a 5% hematocrit in phosphate-buffered saline (PBS) (pH 7.4, 290 mOsm) with glucose, 0.5% human se serum albumin, and 70 μmoles/liter of the echinocytic agent, LPC. Lysopalmitoyl phosphatidylcholine (Palmityl-^{14}C) was used as a tracer to determine membrane concentration of LPC by radioactive counting.

The incubations were carried out at 37°C. Five min after the start of incubation and at 2.5-h subsequent intervals, two 0.25-ml aliquots of the red cell suspension were taken, one washed four times (15 ml wash solution) with PBS and the other four times with 1% bovine serum albumin in PBS. After the final wash the red cells were dissolved in 0.75 ml Protosol (New England Nuclear), decolorized with H_2O_2, and subsequently counted in a liquid scintillation counter using Aquasol as counting fluid.

To determine the extent of acylation of LPC into phosphatidylcholine, aliquots of the incubating red cell suspension were also taken at the same time intervals to determine the percentage of total radioactivity in the LPC and PC fractions after albumin and saline washings by thin-layer chromatography [8]. Red cell morphology was monitored by phase contrast microscopy and scanning electron microscopy [9].

RESULTS

LPC Content

Red cell membrane localization of ^{14}C-LPC at regular incubation intervals is shown in Figure 1. LPC was incorporated into the red cell membrane as evidenced in 5 min by the rapid rise of ^{14}C counts in saline-washed red cells. Subsequently, LPC content of the red cells increased linearly with time in both the saline- and albumin-washed cells (Fig. 1). Because of the high affinity of albumin for LPC and the large amounts of albumin used in washing, it is reasonable to assume that the LPC of red cells after saline washing represented the total LPC in both halves of the bilayer, while the LPC after albumin washing represented the inaccessible LPC present in only the inner half of the bilayer. The outer leaflet LPC was calculated by subtracting the inner leaflet content from the total.

This proposed localization of residual LPC in the inner monolayer of albumin-washed cells was confirmed by our experiments with resealed and unsealed ghosts made from red cells after 7.5 hours of incubation and subsequent albumin washing. None of the residual LPC could be removed from the resealed ghosts by further albumin washes, whereas 95% of the LPC was removed by albumin washing of the unsealed ghosts. An increase in the ^{14}C-labeled phosphatidylcholine content of the red cell also occurred as a result of

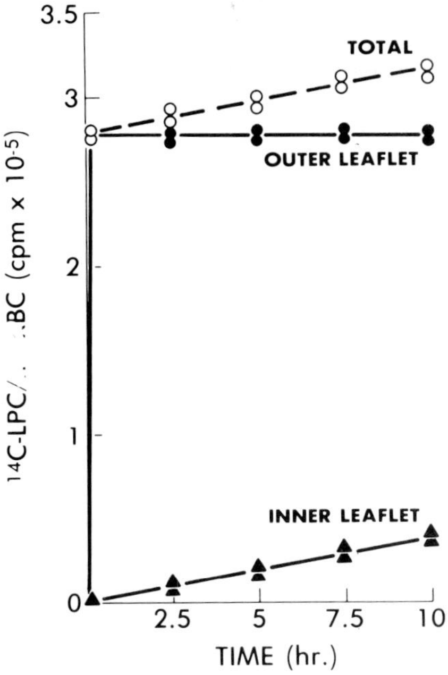

Fig. 1. Radioactive LPC content of red blood cell membranes as a function of incubation time. The total LPC content of the red cells (○) was obtained after four saline washes and the inner leaflet LPC (▲) after four albumin washes. The outer leaflet LPC (●) is calculated by subtracting the residual counts after albumin washes from those after saline washes. Data from two separate experiments using red cells from two different donors are presented and are indicated by the separate characters.

acylation of the incorporated LPC. Since PC does not induce either echinocytic or stomatocytic shape changes and the PC synthesized by acylation accounts for less than 4% of the naturally occurring PC in red cell membrane, its role in red cell shape changes was not considered significant.

Shape Changes

Red cell morphologic changes at various stages of incubation are shown in Figure 2. Five minutes after the start of incubation the red cells were transformed into echinocytes (spherical cells with uniformly distributed spicules [7]); they retained this shape when washed with saline, but resumed their discocytic shape when washed with albumin. In contrast, the morphology of the red cells at 7.5 h was discocytic and remained so after saline washing, but after albumin washing the shape became stomatocytic (stomatocyte III: deeply cup-shaped cells with membrane invagination [7]). Between 5 min and 7.5 h there was a gradual reversal of the morphology of red cells from echinocytic (echinocyte III) to discocytic in spite of the progressive increase in total LPC content. At the same time

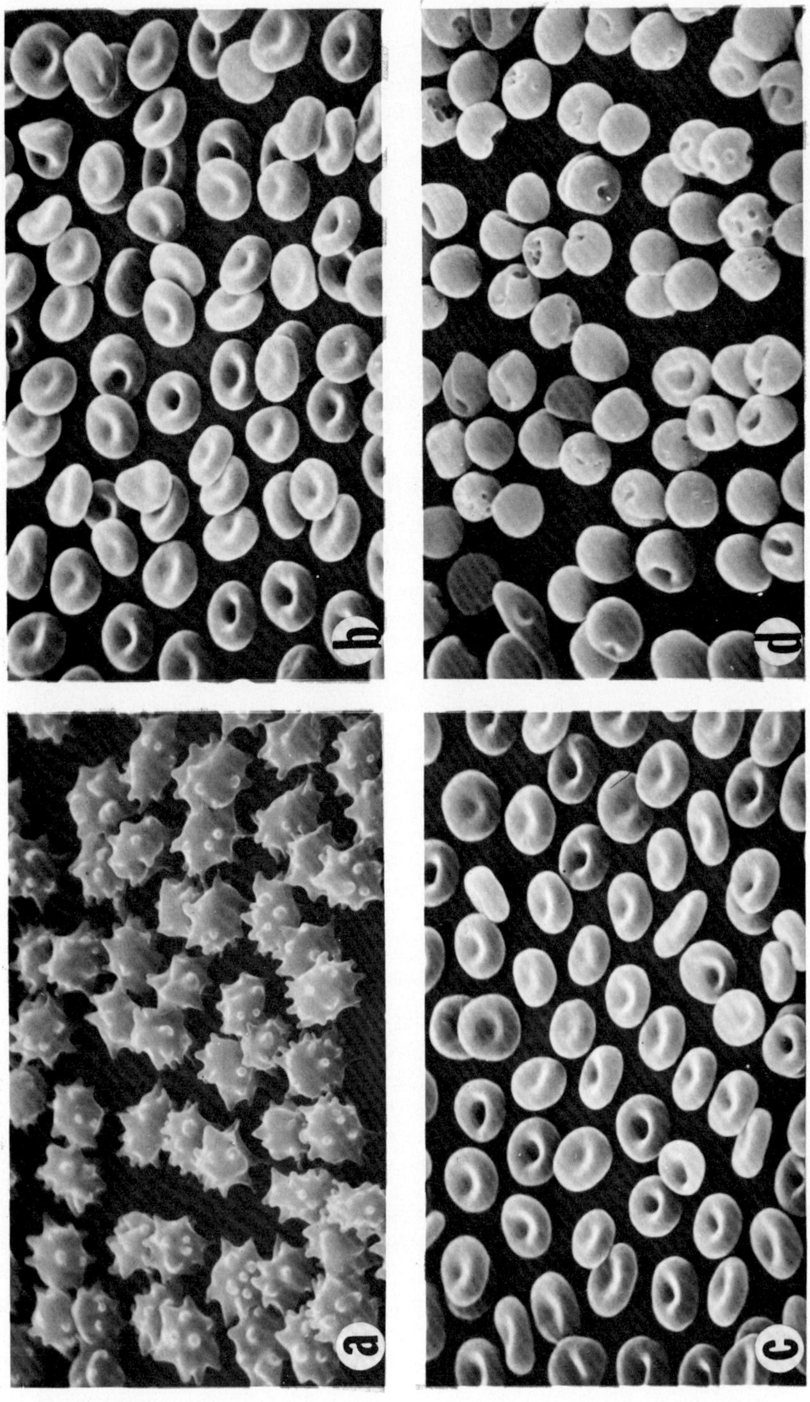
b
d
a
c

intervals after albumin washing, the morphology changed from discocytic to stomatocytic, with progressive accumulation of albumin-inaccessible LPC.

In summary, these results demonstrate that five minutes after the start of incubation, the discocytes were transformed into echinocytes with 160 nmoles LPC/ml RBC found in the outer half of the bilayer, and no LPC in the inner half. At 7.5 h 160 nmoles LPC/ml RBC was still present in the outer half as consequence of the equilibrium partition of LPC between the suspending medium and the outer half; however, 20 nmoles LPC/ml RBC was now present in the inner half and the red cells were transformed back into discocytes. This indicates that the echinocytic effect of the LPC in the outer monolayer had been nullified or counterbalanced by the much lower concentration of LPC which had now entered the inner monolayer. Albumin washing of these discocytes produced stomatocytes with 20 nmoles LPC/ml RBC remaining in the inner monolayer and none in the outer monolayer, showing the morphologic effect of unbalanced LPC in the inner leaflet.

DISCUSSION

These results demonstrate the different echinocytogenic (with LPC outside) and stomatocytogenic (with LPC inside) effects that occur when this naturally occurring agent is localized in different areas of the bilayer. They further emphasize the importance of the balance between the inner and outer leaflet concentrations of this agent in determining cell shape. The increasing concentration of LPC in the inner monolayer over the period of observation appears to have been due to its translocation from the outer to the inner leaflet as suggested by previous studies [8].

The kinetics observed for LPC translocation during this study agree well with those obtained for PC translocation using other techniques [10, 11]. The translocation of other echinocytic agents from the outer half of the bilayer to the inner half could also explain the spontaneous reversal of spheroechinocytes into discocytes, as reported by Hoffman [12].

Our observation that shape changes produced by a higher concentration of LPC in the outer monolayer can be balanced by a much lower concentration of LPC in the inner monolayer indicates a differential concentration effect of LPC on cell shape in the inner and outer halves of the bilayer. It has also been reported [9] that a ten-fold increase in cellular concentration of anionic phenothiazines was needed to produce sphero-echinocytes, compared with the concentration of cationic phenothiazines needed to produce spherostomatocytes. Data from both these studies show that an equivalent concentration level of these compounds in the inner and outer monolayers, and the consequent simple equivalent area expansion of each monolayer as previously proposed [5], is insufficient to wholly explain these morphologic changes. The differential concentration

Fig. 2. Red blood cell morphology as a function of incubation time. a) Scanning electron micrograph of echinocytes after 5 min incubation in the medium containing LPC; b) discocytes obtained by washing these echinocytes with 1% albumin solution; c) discocytes which reformed after 7.5 h incubation in the medium containing LPC; d) stomatocytes obtained by washing these discocytes at 7.5 h with 1% albumin solution.

dependence also suggests that either differential charge effects, or surface tension effects of the shape-active agents in the two halves of the bilayer, may mediate these changes.

ACKNOWLEDGMENTS

The work was supported in part by US Public Health Service grants AM 16095 and HL 07100 and by career development award AM 37237 to S.B.S.

REFERENCES

1. Rothman ME, Lenard J: Science 195:743, 1977.
2. Bretscher MS: Nature (New Biol) 236:11, 1972.
3. Gordesky SE, Marinetti GV: Biochem Biophys Res Commun 50:1027, 1973.
4. Verkleij AJ, Zwaal RFA, Roelofson B, Comfurius P, Kastalijn D, Van Deenen LLM: Biochim Biophys Acta 323:178, 1973.
5. Sheetz MP, Singer SJ: Proc Natl Acad Sci USA 71:4457, 1974.
6. Sheetz MP, Singer SJ: J Cell Biol 70:247, 1976.
7. Bessis M: In Bessis M, Weed RI, Leblond PF (eds): "Red Cell Shape." New York: Springer-Verlag, 1973, pp 1–25.
8. Shohet SB: J Clin Invest 49:1668, 1970.
9. Mohandas N, Feo C: Blood Cells 1:375, 1975.
10. Rousselet A, Guthmann C, Matrican J, Bienvenue A, Devaux P: Biochim Biophys Acta 426:357, 1976.
11. Renooij W, Van Golde LMG, Zwaal RFA, Van Deenen LLM: Eur J Biochem 61:53, 1976.
12. Hoffman JF: In Bessis M, Weed RI, Leblond PF (eds): "Red Cell Shape." New York: Springer-Verlag, 1973, pp 51–54.

Journal of Supramolecular Structure 9:537–554 (1978)
Normal and Abnormal Red Cell Membranes 311–328

Membrane Alterations in Irreversibly Sickled Cells: Hemoglobin–Membrane Interaction

Lawrence S. Lessin, Joseph Kurantsin-Mills, Charles Wallas, and Henri Weems

Division of Hematology and Oncology, Department of Medicine (L.S.L., C.W., H.W.); and Department of Physiology (J.K.-M.); George Washington University Medical Center, Washington, DC 20037

Irreversibly sickled cells (ISCs) are sickle erythrocytes which retain bipolar enlongated shapes despite reoxygenation and owe their biophysical abnormalities to acquired membrane alterations. Freeze-etched membranes both of ISCs produced in vitro and ISCs isolated in vivo reveal microbodies fixed to the internal (PS) surface which obscure spectrin filaments. Intramembranous particles (IMPs) on the intramembrane (PF) surface aggregate over regions of subsurface microbodies. Electron microscopy of diaminobenzidine-treated ISC ghosts show the microbodies to contain hemoglobin and/or hemoglobin derivatives. Scanning electron microscopy and freeze-etching demonstrate that membrane–hemoglobin S interaction in ISCs enhances the membrane loss by microspherulation. Membrane-bound hemoglobin is five times greater in in vivo ISCs than non-ISCs, and increases during ISC production, paralleling depletion of adenosine triphosphate. Polyacrylamide gel electrophoresis of ISC membranes shows the presence of high-molecular-weight heteropolymers in the pre–band 1 region, a decrease in band 4.1 and an increase in bands 7, 8, and globin. The role of cross-linked membrane protein polymers in the generation of ISCs is discussed and is synthesized in terms of a unified concept for the determinants of the genesis of ISCs.

Key words: **irreversibly sickled cells, freeze-etching, scanning electron micrography, membrane-bound hemoglobin, membrane proteins and glycoproteins**

The irreversibly sickled cell (ISC), a dense, rigid bipolar cell which can be isolated from the blood of sickle cell patients has been shown to contribute to the abnormal rheologic properties of oxygenated sickle cell blood. Visualization of sickle cells through the microvasculature of animal models suggests that ISCs may initiate microvascular occlusion and thus play an important pathophysiologic role in the generation of the vasooclusive crises [1]. Although the rheologic abnormality of the ISC has been attributed to alterations

Received May 4, 1978; accepted August 4, 1978.

0091-7419/78/0904-0537$03.20

of its membrane, the precise nature of the biochemical lesion in terms of rearrangement of macromolecular architecture has not been elucidated. A minor controversy has arisen regarding the origin of the ISCs. Some studies suggest that ISCs emerge from the bone marrow of sickle cell patients with low hemoglobin F and thus are predestined to undergo rapid membrane alteration and shortened circulatory survival [2, 3]. Studies of in vitro production of ISCs from our laboratory and others indicate that the membrane alteration in the ISC is a cumulative, progressive change [4–7]. We have previously shown that when sickle cells are incubated under anoxic conditions, there is progressive accumulation of membrane-bound hemoglobin [4]. Padilla et al [6] demonstrated that ISCs may be generated by repetitive sickling and unsickling of individual sickle cells with progressive membrane loss by microspherulation. In a preliminary study we have shown that with repetitive sickling and unsickling, there is selective loss of hemoglobin F from sickle cells by microspherulation [8]. This may occur because hemoglobin F does not copolymerize with hemoglobin S in the deoxygenated state [9] and thus is rapidly lost from the cell surface within vesicles which fragment during unsickling. Eaton et al [10] and Palek [11] have shown that sickle cells manifest accumulation of calcium within the cell, with a significant fraction bound to the membrane. Lux and co-workers [12], utilizing Triton-extracted membrane residues of ISCs have demonstrated that the shape alteration of the ISC is conferred by irreversible changes within the "spectrin-actin lattice." It is our contention that these events work together to bring about a progressive and cumulative alteration in the membrane of sickle cells as their shape and deformability become irreversibly altered in the generation of the ISC.

In the present study, ISCs were obtained from two sources: 1) in vivo ISCs were derived from centrifugal separation of whole blood of sickle cell anemia patients in which greater than 90% of the total ISC content is localized in the 15% bottom fraction, and 2) ISCs were produced in vitro by incubation under anoxic conditions for up to 24 h, with and without adenosine triphosphatase (ATP) depletion. These studies have been designed to permit concomitant observation of ISC membrane changes, both morphologically and biochemically. They employed scanning electron microscopy, freeze-etching with transmission electron microscopy, and histochemical staining of membranes for hemoglobin. Cells obtained from the same experiments are subjected to concomitant analyses for membrane associated hemoglobin, ATP, 2,3-diphosphoglycerate (2,3-DPG), age-dependent enzymes, and sodium dodecyl sulphate (SDS) polyacrylamide gel electrophoresis of their membrane proteins and glycoproteins.

METHODS

Preparation of Red Cells and Membranes

Fresh blood was obtained by venipuncture from normal control (AA) subjects and individuals with sickle cell anemia (SS). The blood was anticoagulated with sodium heparin (14 units/ml). Hemoglobin genotypes of the patients were verified by cellulose acetate (pH 8.4) and citrate agar (pH 6.4) electrophoresis. Hemoglobin F levels were determined by the alkaline denaturation technique [13]. Blood specimens were drawn from the patients during clinical steady states, and hematocrit values ranged from 25% to 40%.

Hemoglobin-free red cell membranes were prepared by the method of Dodge et al [14] using 20 mOsm Tris-HCl buffer, pH 7.6. Membranes were used in various analyses, including residual hemoglobin [15], as soon as possible. Membranes not immediately used for assays were stored at −70°C.

Electron Microscopy

Cells or membrane preparations for electron microscopy were fixed in 1% glutaraldehyde in phosphate buffer (pH 7.4) and processed by the method of Bessis and Weed [16] for scanning electron microscopy (SEM). Samples for transmission electron microscopy (TEM) were fixed in 1% glutaraldehyde, washed twice with buffer, postfixed in 1% osmium tetroxide in phosphate buffer (pH 7.4), dehydrated in graded ethanol, and embedded in Epon 812. Thin sections were stained with uranyl acetate and lead citrate [17] and examined in an AEI EM 801 transmission electron microscope.

Freeze-Etching

Freeze-etching was carried out in a Balzers 360M ultra-high-vacuum device by the method previously described [18]. After the initial red cell or membrane preparation procedures, cells or membranes were cryoprotected in serial glycerol solutions to final concentrations from 25 to 40% in phosphate-buffered saline (pH 7.4). Droplets of cell suspension were then frozen on gold disks in liquid Freon 22 (−160°C) and stored in liquid nitrogen. Specimens were placed on the freeze-etching microtome stage and the chamber was evacuated to 10^{-6} torr. The specimen was then fractured by a single stroke or multiple chips using the cold (−100°C) microtome blade and sublimated (etched) for periods of time varying from one to ten minutes. The replica was produced by evaporation of platinum and carbon onto the fractured surface. The replica was removed from the freeze-etching device, cleaned of cellular debris by flotation in distilled water, 70% sulfuric acid, and dilute sodium hypochlorite, and rinsed in distilled water. Replicas thus obtained were studied and photographed in an AEI EM 801 electron microscope at 10,000–40,000 times magnification.

Incubation of Sickle Cells and the Determination of ISCs

Normal and sickle cells were incubated for 24 h in isoosmotic Krebs-Henseleit buffer of the following composition in mM: NaCl 110, KCl 5.9, $CaCl_2$ 2.0, $MgSO_4 \cdot 7H_2O$ 1.2, $NaH_2PO_4 \cdot H_2O$ 2.4, $NaHCO_3$ 25.0, glucose 30.0, bovine serum albumin 0.51% (pH 7.4, 290 mOsm) under 95% O_2 or 95% N_2 with 5% CO_2. Cells were sampled at intervals for determination of %ISCs, ATP, membrane-bound hemoglobin, Na^+, and K^+, and for freeze-etch and transmission EM of whole cells and membrane preparations.

Differential Centrifugation of Sickle Cells

In vivo ISCs were isolated from freshly packed sickle cell blood by ultracentrifugation for 1 h at 100,000g and fractionated into bottom 15%, middle 70%, and top 15% of the densely packed cells. Various analytical procedures and chemical determinations were performed on these cell fractions.

Morphologic Characterization of Irreversibly Sickled Cells

ISCs were defined as Hb-SS cells with one or more pointed extremities under oxygenated conditions, as defined by Jensen et al [19].

Analytical Procedures

ATP content of cell preparations were determined by the method of Kornberg [20] as modified by Lamprecht and Trautschold [21] by enzymatic determination of neutralized perchloric acid extracts. 2,3-DPG was determined by the method of Rose and Liebowitz [22]. Intracellular sodium and pottassium were analyzed as described elsewhere [23]. Membrane-bound hemoglobin was analyzed histochemically by the method of Breton-Gorius using diaminobenzidine [24]. Membrane-bound hemoglobin was determined for 20-μl aliquots of membrane preparation employing the benzidine reaction method of Crosby and Furth [15].

Electrophoresis of membrane proteins and glycoproteins in 5.6% polyacrylamide gels with 0.2% bis-acrylamide as cross-linker in 1% sodium dodecyl sulfate was executed as described by Fairbanks et al [25]. Each gel was loaded with 30 μg protein. Membrane proteins were determined by the method of Lowry et al using bovine serum albumin as a standard [26]. After electrophoresis, gels were stained for protein with Coomassie Blue R-250 and for protein-bound carbohydrate with periodic acid-Schiff (PAS) reagent and were photographed through a medium red filter (Kodak #25). Densitometry was performed at 560 nm using a Beckman ACTA CIII spectrophotometer.

RESULTS

Ultrastructural Studies

Scanning electron microscope observations. ISCs obtained from whole blood of SS patients by ultracentrifugation have a characteristic shape (Fig. 1A–C). They are fusiform cells in the shape of crescents with two pointed extremities. The membrane surface of the ISC in the oxygenated state is often irregular but without visible organization. In the deoxygenated state the surface of the ISC tends to reflect polymerization of submembrane deoxyhemoglobin S with the presence of subsurface fibers and irregular indentation of the membrane (Fig. 1D). ISCs produced in vitro by an anoxic incubation show a different shape abnormality from those isolated from blood of SS patients. In vitro ISCs show a much greater degree of spiculation and membrane distortion, often displaying multiple spicules and holly-leaf (drepanoechinocyte) configurations. These cells appear to have arisen from echinocytic forms. Both in vitro and in vivo ISCs show evidence of membrane loss by fragmentation.

Freeze-etching and transmission electron microscopy. Freeze-etch electron micrographs of ISCs and their membranes isolated by hypotonic lysis and centrifugation show the accumulation of microbodies on the internal membrane (PS) surface (Fig. 2A,B). These microbodies measure ca. 50 × 10 nm and show a random distribution over what appears to be the internal membrane (PS) surface. The microbodies obscure filamentous structures usually visible on the PS surface. In some preparations, the microbodies appear to be associated with a rearrangement of membrane-associated particles on the intramembrane (PF) surface. In vivo ISCs isolated from whole blood of SS patients show similar microaggregates on the internal (PS) aspect of the ISC membrane. In some cases, aggregates of this material seen in cross-section in the submembrane region resemble small Heinz bodies (Fig. 3A). The degree of microaggregate formation is less prominent within in vivo than in vitro ISCs. When ISCs are generated by repetitive sickling and unsickling, the

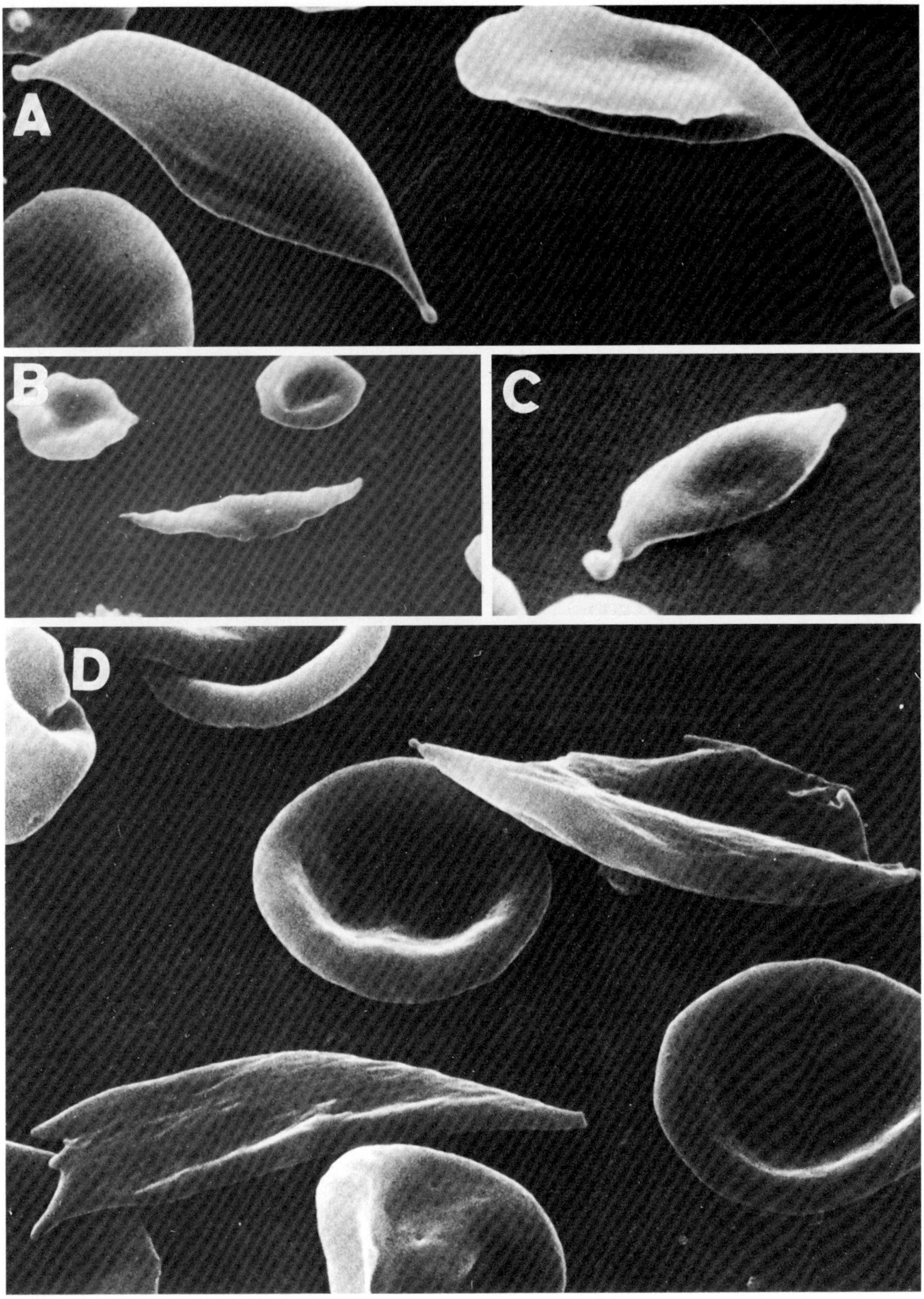

Fig. 1. Scanning electron micrographs of ISCs isolated from whole SS blood by ultracentrifugation. Cells were prepared as described in Methods [16]. Final magnification A ≃ 10,000 × B, C ≃ 4,000 ×, D ≃ 10,000 ×.

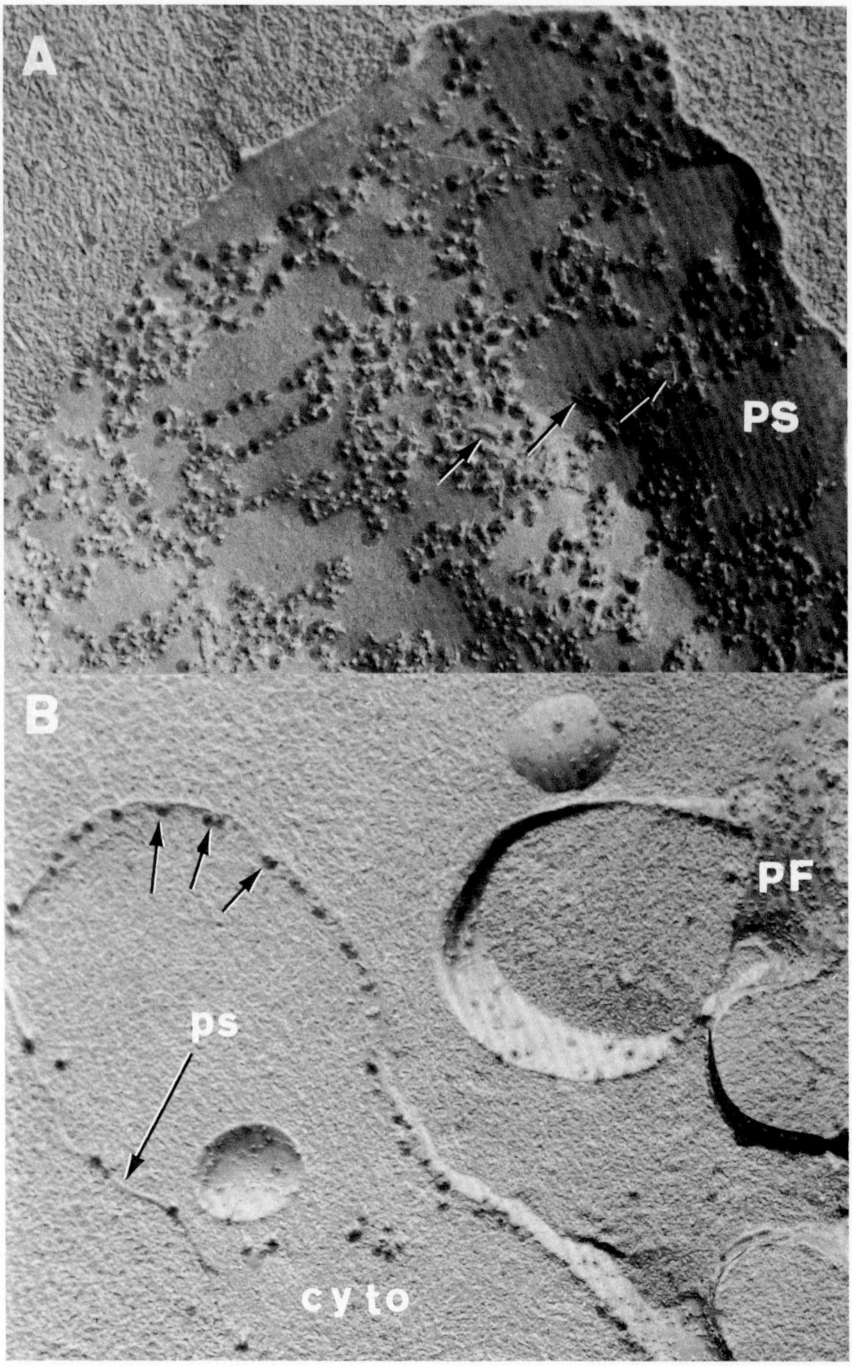

Fig. 2. Freeze-etch electron micrographs of ISCs showing microbodies on the internal (PS) surface of the membrane and the aggregation of intermembranous particles on the PF surface. Note the marked distortion of the PS surface by large numbers of adherent microbidies. Filamentous structures can also be seen (A, arrows). Alignment of microbodies along the PS surface is also clear in the cross section (B). Cyto = cytoplasm. Final magnification: A = 100,000 ×, B = 100,000 ×.

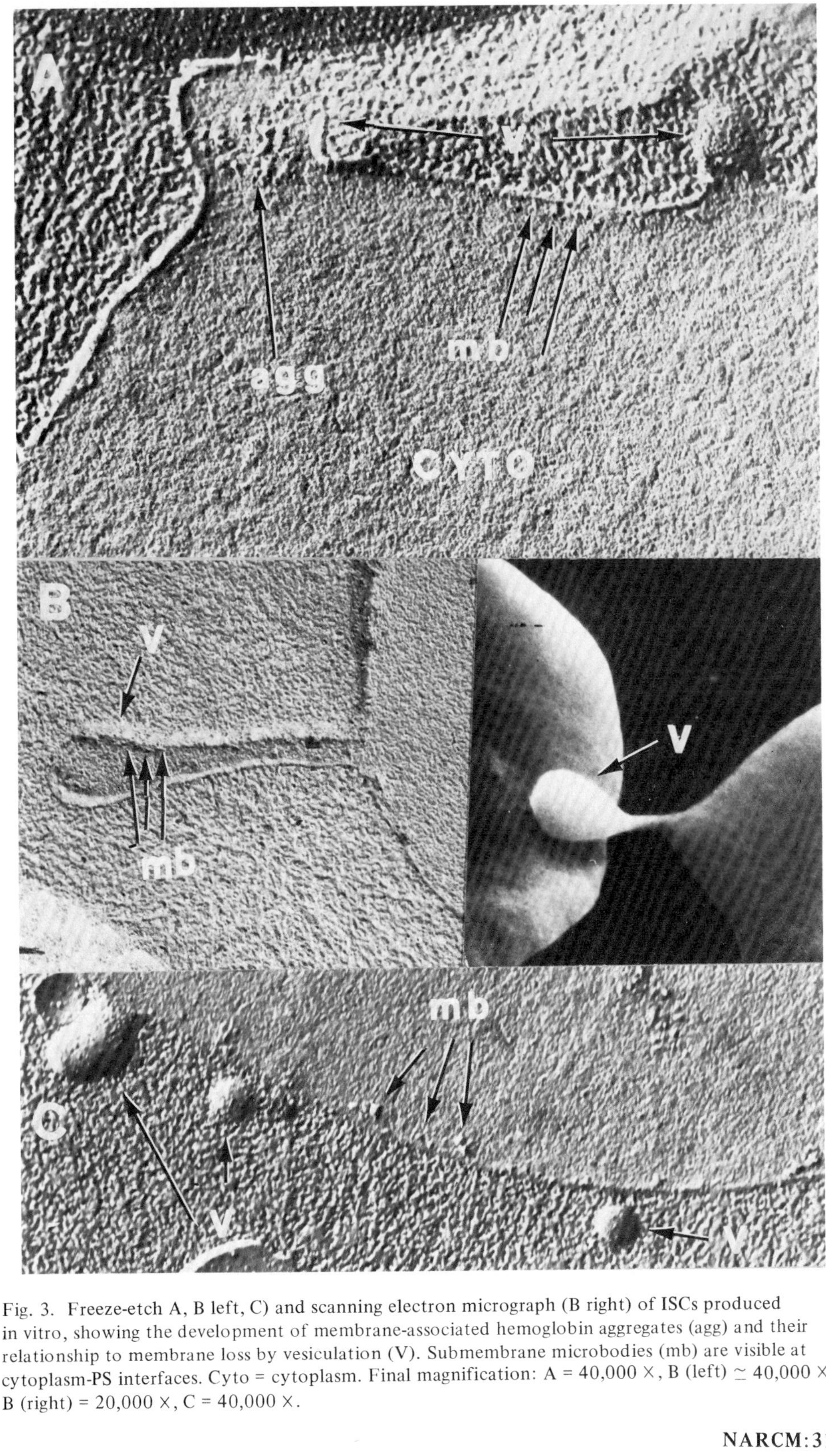

Fig. 3. Freeze-etch A, B left, C) and scanning electron micrograph (B right) of ISCs produced in vitro, showing the development of membrane-associated hemoglobin aggregates (agg) and their relationship to membrane loss by vesiculation (V). Submembrane microbodies (mb) are visible at cytoplasm-PS interfaces. Cyto = cytoplasm. Final magnification: A = 40,000 ×, B (left) ≃ 40,000 ×, B (right) = 20,000 ×, C = 40,000 ×.

development of submembrane microaggregates is shown to accompany the fragmentation process (Fig. 3A–C). Aggregates occur initially in the region of the retracting spicules during the unsickling process and appear to play a role in fragmentation and microvesiculation, perhaps by annealing apposing internal membrane (PS) surfaces, thus fostering disjunction of the vesicle from the main body of the cell (Fig. 3B,C).

In order to determine the nature of the submembrane aggregates, ISCs produced in vitro by anoxic incubation (with increased membrane-associated hemoglobin and decline of ATP levels) were subjected to hypotonic lysis and stained histochemically for hemoglobin with diaminobenzidine (DAB). Figure 4A shows control membranes in which no membrane-bound hemoglobin is visible. Figure 4B represents DAB-stained membranes of in vitro ISCs and shows numerous aggregates of submembrane DAB-positive material. This suggests that the submembrane aggregates seen in such preparations are hemoglobin or derivatives of hemoglobin.

In Vitro Production of ISCs and Binding of Hemoglobin to ISC Membranes

ISCs were produced by incubation for 24 h in isotonic Krebs-Henseleit buffer under 95% N_2 with 5% CO_2, with continuous shaking in an oscillating waterbath at 37°C. Control sickle cells were incubated with 95% O_2/5% CO_2 and control normal cells were incubated under identical oxygenated and anoxic conditions. Cells incubated 0–24 h were sampled at intervals for determination of percentage of ISCs, ATP, and membrane-bound hemoglobin, as well as freeze-etch and transmission electron microscopy. As indicated in Figure 5A, ISC generation from SS cells during the 24-h incubation showed a sigmoid curve with gradual increment in the initial 8 h, a sharp rise during the second 8-h period, and plateauing in the final 4 h. ATP levels were maintained in oxygenated SS and control cells for the entire incubation, but fell slightly in SS cells after 16 h under deoxygenated conditions (Fig. 5B). Membrane-bound hemoglobin showed a 100-fold increase during the 24-h incubation, rising from 2 mg% to 250 mg%, as indicated in Fig. 6. Incubated control AA cells and oxygenated SS cells showed no appreciable accumulation of hemoglobin with the membrane fraction.

In the ATP maintenance experiments, shown in Fig. 7, membrane-bound hemoglobin rose from 40 mg% to 90 mg%, whereas no significant rise was seen in SS cells incubated under oxygen, or in control cells. In both experiments, whether ATP was allowed to fall or was maintained, a significant fall in cellular potassium and a concomitant rise in cellular sodium occurred in the SS cells incubated under N_2, whereas control sickle and normal cells under O_2 showed only minor alterations in intracellular potassium and sodium.

Chemical Characterization of ISCs Isolated From Blood of SS Patients

Whole blood from sickle cell patients was fractionated by ultracentrifugation at 100,000g for 1 h and cells were separated into the upper 15% "reticulocyte-rich" fraction, a middle 70% non-ISC fraction, and a bottom 15% "ISC-rich" fraction. Table I shows data from a representative separation, with determinations of ATP, 2,3-DPG, pyruvate kinase (an age-dependent enzyme) activity, cellular sodium, and membrane-associated hemoglobin. Values for normal control AA erythrocytes subjected to similar analysis are also shown. The ISC fraction shows membrane-associated hemoglobin to be three times greater than the middle (non-ISC) fraction. The reduction in ATP level seen in the ISCs is significant but does not represent total depletion and should not substantially impair cellular functions dependent upon the availability of high-energy phosphate. The high level of membrane-associated hemoglobin seen in reticulocytes is an expected finding because of continued hemoglobin synthesis in polyribosomes associated with the reticulocyte membrane [27].

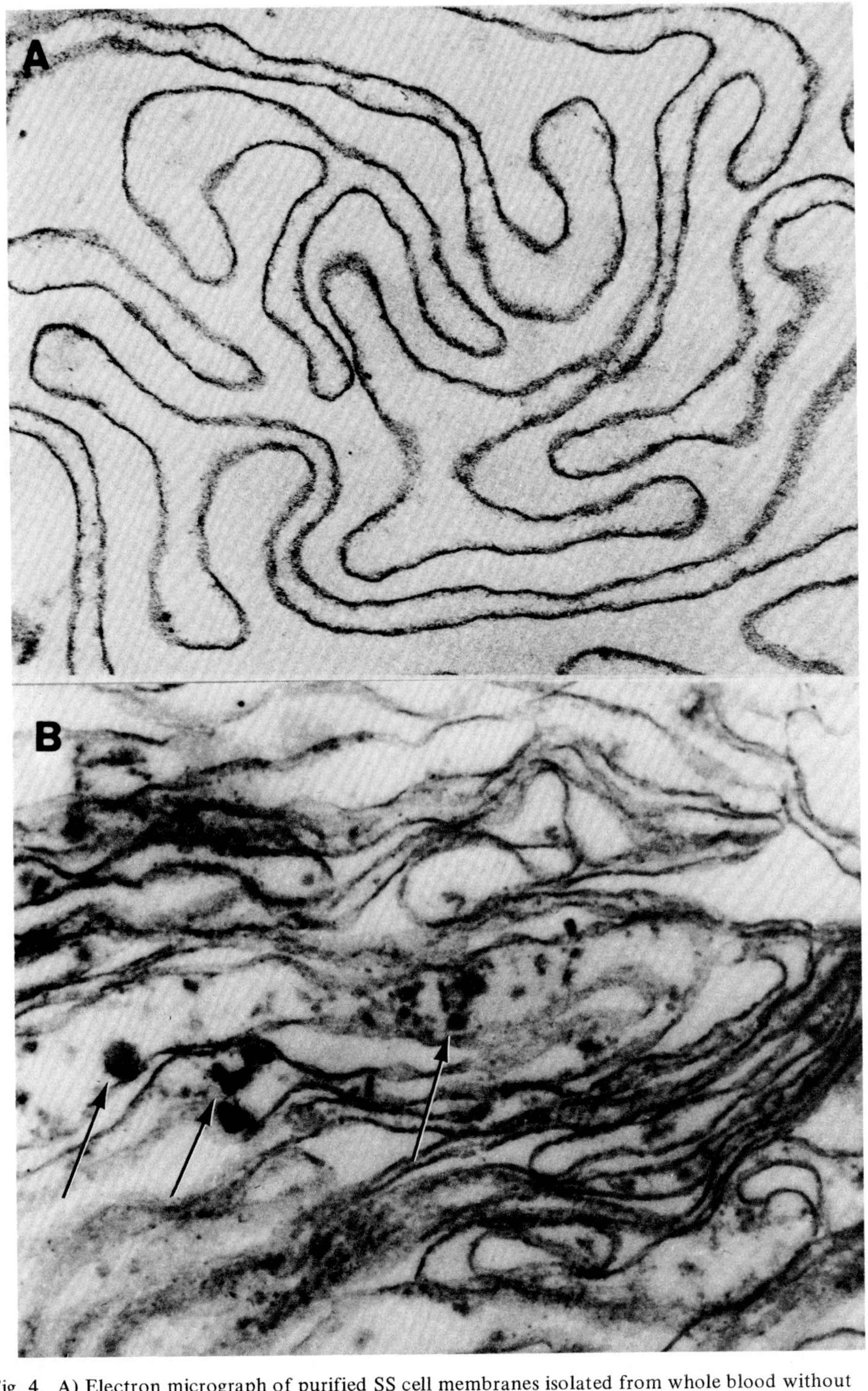

Fig. 4. A) Electron micrograph of purified SS cell membranes isolated from whole blood without anaerobic incubation of cells. The micrograph shows the richness of the preparation, and the minimal residual heme compounds associated with the membranes. B) SS cell membranes isolated from cells incubated under anaerobic conditions (95% N_2, 5% CO_2, 37°C, 12–18 h). Membranes were stained with diaminobenzidine [24]. Dark membrane-associated clumps represent hemoglobin and/or its derivatives. Final magnification = 25,000 ×.

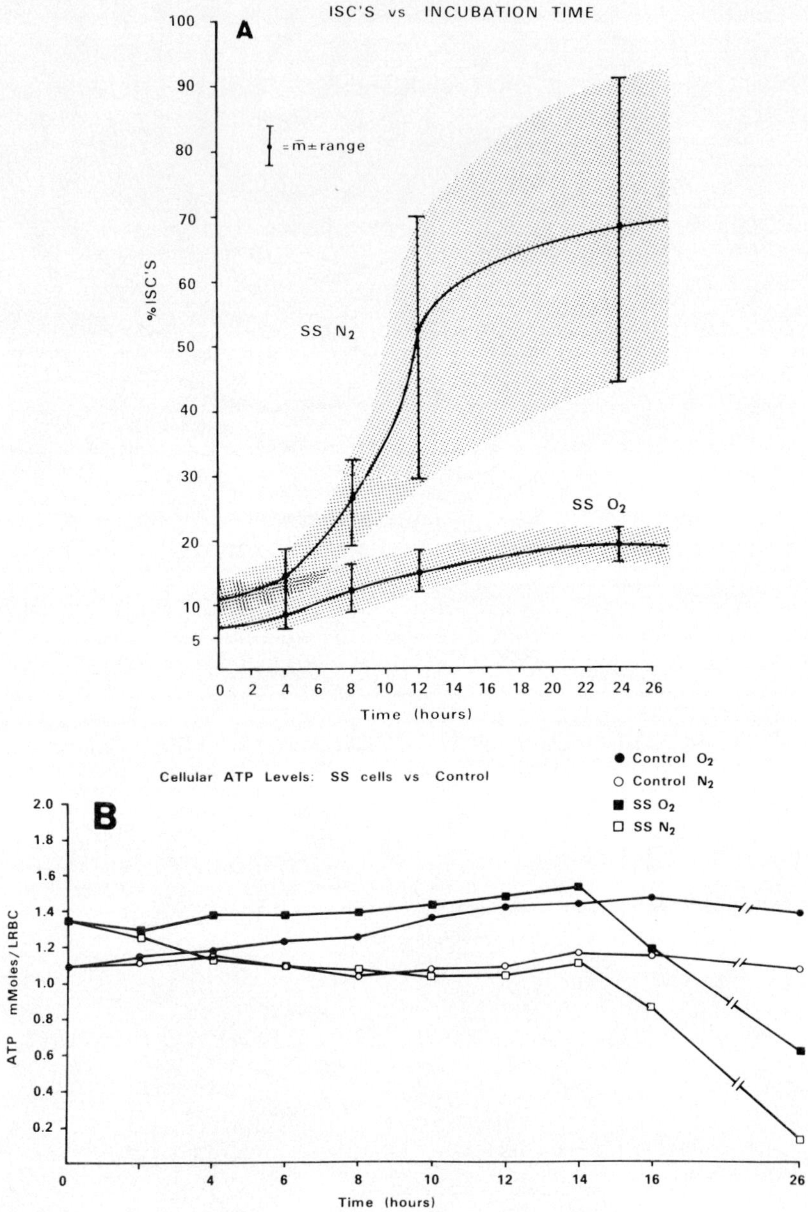

Fig. 5. A) Production of ISCs in vitro as a function of time, under oxygenated (95% O_2 and 5% CO_2) and deoxygenated (95% N_2 and 5% CO_2) conditions. Incubation conditions are described in Methods. B) Intracellular ATP concentration of AA and SS erythrocytes during in vitro production of ISCs. Graph represents mean of three determinations. For details see Methods. Note the early decline of ATP concentrations in the SS cells.

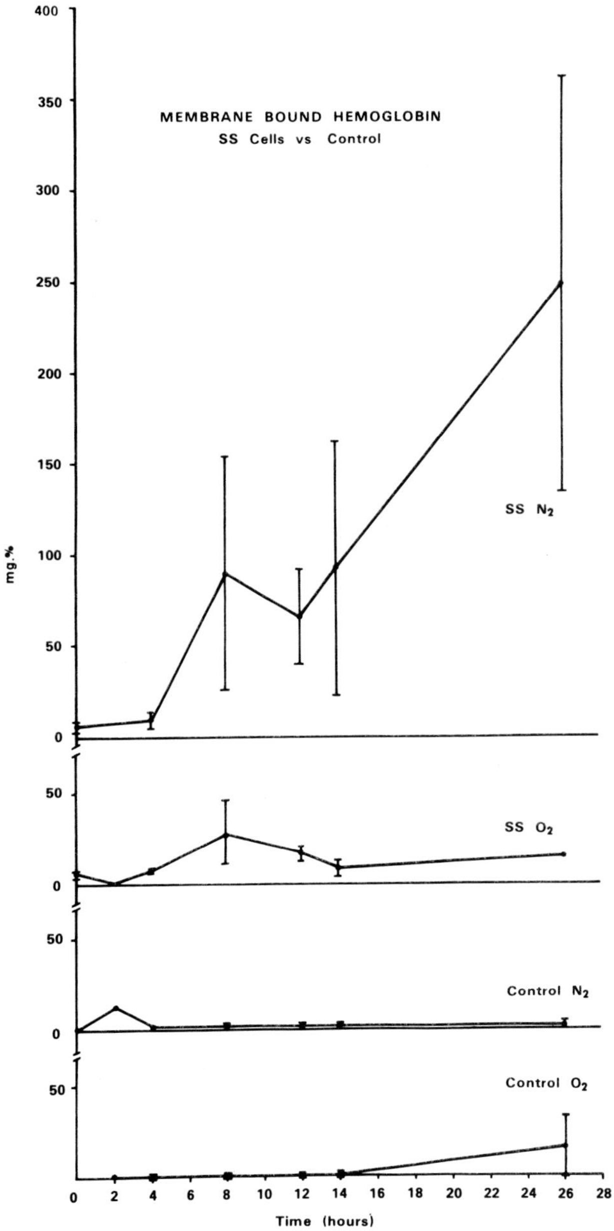

Fig. 6. Membrane-bound hemoglobin of control (AA) and sickle cells (SS) as a function of time during incubation under oxygenated (95% O_2 and 5% CO_2) and deoxygenated (95% N_2 and 5% CO_2) conditions. Ordinate expressed as mg% of hemoglobin from a standard curve; 20 μl of ghost suspension used for assay.

SDS Polyacrylamide Gel Electrophoresis Analysis of ISC Membranes

When cells from top, middle, and bottom fractions are lysed and their membranes are solubilized with sodium dodecyl sulfate and electrophoresed in SDS-polyacrylamide gels after reduction of protein disulfide bonds with dithiothreitol, significant differences are evident between the membranes from non-ISC and ISC fractions, as shown in Fig. 8A. The membrane protein and glycoprotein profile of membranes from the non-ISC fraction does

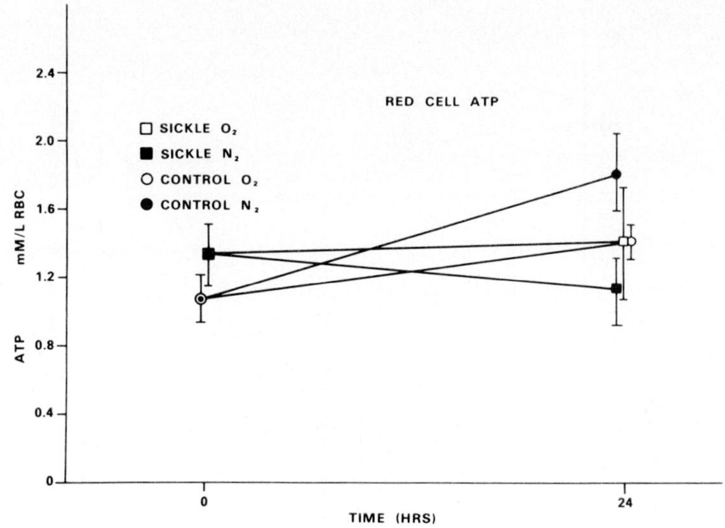

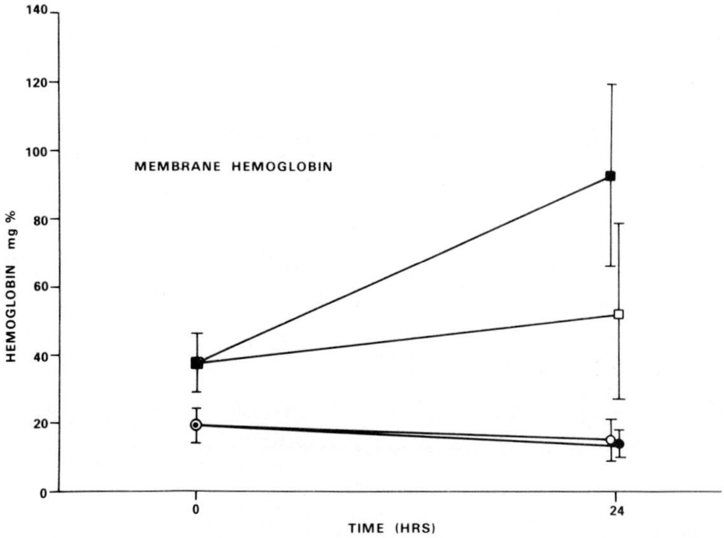

Fig. 7. Above) ATP concentrations of control (AA) and sickle cells (SS) before and after incubation under oxygenated and deoxygenated conditions. Below) Membrane-bound hemoglobin of normal (AA) cells and sickle cells (SS) before and after incubation under oxygenated and deoxygenated conditions. Ordinate expressed as mg% of hemoglobin from a standard curve. A 1-ml aliquot of ghost suspension was used for assay; final data are expressed as mg% Hb for a liter of ghosts, taking into account the packed cell volume used.

TABLE I. Separation of Sickle Cell Fractions by Ultracentrifugation Comparison With Control AA Red Cells

	Hct %	ATP (mmoles/ liter RBC)	2,3-DPG (mmoles/ liter RBC)	Pyruvate kinase (EU/gmHb)	Na (mmoles/ liter RBC)	Membrane Hb (mg%)	Retics (%)	ISC (%)
Sickle								
Top	0.4195	1.93	5.67	15.32	7.3	74.5	97.5	6.3
Middle	0.4288	1.48	7.92	4.14	8.2	18.5	—	6.4
Bottom	0.3927	1.17	5.51	3.13	33.3	49.9	3.6	62.0
Control								
Top	0.4781	1.24	4.75	3.49	9.4	70.5	3.2	0
Middle	0.3683	1.24	4.88	1.75	11.1	26.6	—	0
Bottom	0.1908	1.23	3.70	1.46	14.1	26.0	0	0

Packed red cells from fresh sickle cell blood was fractionated, by ultracentrifugation at 100,000g for 1 h, into reticulocyte-rich (top 15%), non-ISC (middle 70%), and ISC fractions (bottom 15%). The table shows a 62% ISC yield in the bottom fraction and characterizes the in vivo ISC as a cell with low ATP and pyruvate kinase, increased sodium, and high membrane-bound hemoglobin.

EU, Enzyme Units = Activity of enzyme as μmole substrate transformed per minute per gm Hb.

not differ significantly from the SDS polyacrylamide gel electrophoresis (PAGE) pattern seen in normal erythrocytes. In the ISCs, however, several important differences can be seen. There is a marked increased in the globin band, presumably derived from the membrane-associated hemoglobin of the ISCs. Band 4.1 has decreased staining intensity, whereas bands 7 and 8 were increased. At the pre–band 1 region of the gel were high-molecular-weight complexes (greater than 270,000–280,000 daltons) which may be heteropolymers of certain low-molecular-weight proteins. The exact nature of these heteropolymers was not determined in the present study. No differences were observed in the glycoprotein (PAS) bands (Fig. 8, right panel). Figure 9 illustrates representative densitometric scans of the stained polyacrylamide gels. Reticulocytes also show an increase in membrane-associated globin by this method, as well as high-molecular-weight complexes which may represent membrane-associated ribosomal material. There is no decrease, however, in band 4.1 in the reticulocyte membrane fraction.

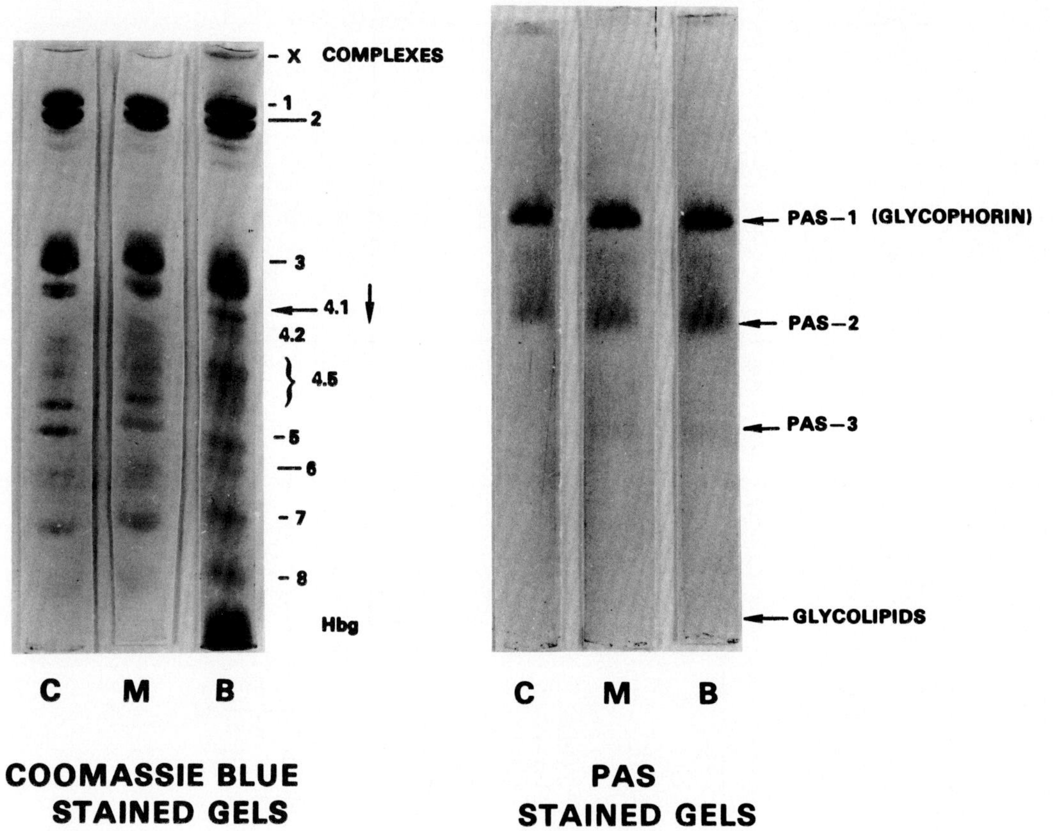

Fig. 8. Sodium dodecyl sulfate and polyacrylamide gel electrophoretograms of red cell ghost proteins from normal controls (C), middle fraction of packed sickle cells (M), and bottom fraction of packed sickle cells (B). Ghosts [14] were dissolved in 1% SDS, 0.1% dithiothreitol, and buffer, incubated at 37°C for 30 min, and electrophoresed as described in Methods [25]; 30 μg protein was loaded on each gel. Gels were stained with Coomassie Blue for the proteins (left); and periodic acid-Schiff reagent (PAS) for the glycoproteins (right). The top fraction of packed sickle cells is not included because of the high proportion of reticulocytes.

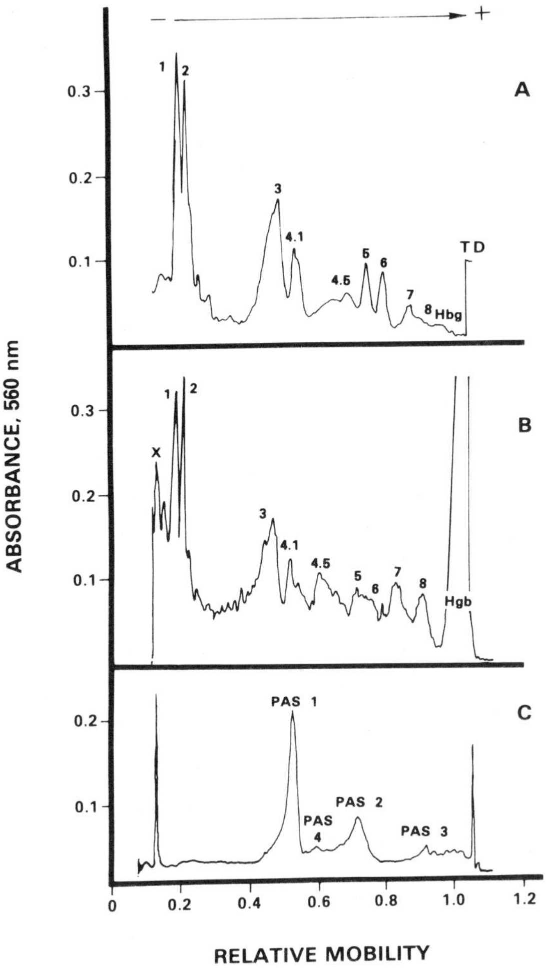

Fig. 9. Densitometric scans of Coomassie Blue-stained proteins of control cell membranes (A), and bottom fraction of packed sickle cell membranes (ISC-rich) (B). The scan of the PAS-stained gel (C) represents the common profile observed in both control cells and fractionated sickle cell membranes. Note the presence of all four bands, PAS 1, 2, 3, and 4, as previously described [25].

DISCUSSION

Using concomitant ultrastructural and biochemical methods, we have assessed the membrane alteration both in ISCs isolated in vivo and in ISCs generated in vitro. Morphologically, the ISC is a bipolar fusiform cell with two or more pointed excrescences, often showing microspherulation from the extremities of the cell. When deoxygenated, the ISC does not undergo a basic shape change, but shows membrane surface (ES) alterations which reflect the polymerized state of submembrane deoxyhemoglobin S. ISCs produced in vitro show shape and membrane alterations similar to those found in in vivo ISCs; however, distortions are much more marked and the cells appear to have arisen from echinocytic forms, thus assuming drepanoechinocyte shapes. Cell membrane loss by vesiculation is a common finding in both in vitro and in vivo ISCs. Vesiculation of sickle cells during unsickling [6] and upon agitation in the deoxygenated state [28] leads to net membrane loss which further contributes to ISC generation.

We have previously reported that freeze-etching and TEM of ATP-depleted ISCs revealed microbodies on the internal membrane (PS) surface [4, 18]. These microbodies distort intramembrane PF and EF surfaces at sites containing intramembranous particles (IMPs). Submembrane microbodies are accompanied by aggregation of IMPs on the overlying PF surface, which suggests binding of microbodies to intrinsic membrane proteins. When in vivo ISCs are examined as whole cells or ghosts, microbodies similar to those seen in the in vitro ISCs can be readily identified. However, they appear less numerous, and appear to be present at the membrane-cytoplasm interface (PS), where they are associated with aggregated IMPs on the PF surface. When the in vivo ISC is subjected to a single cycle of deoxygenation-reoxygenation, submembrane microbodies appear in the region of the spicules, from which segments of the membrane are lost by vesiculation [18]. The association of microbody formation with membrane loss by vesiculation is morphologically evident. Most vesicles that are seen in cross-section contain microaggregates which in some way foster the loss of vesicles from the cell. We therefore postulate that the interaction of deoxyhemoglobin S with membrane proteins may serve to anneal apposing internal membrane (PS) surfaces and thus lead to formation of vesicles from the cell.

EM histochemistry of ISC membranes has demonstrated that submembrane aggregates found only in the ISC fraction were diaminobenzidine-positive, indicating the presence of hemoglobin and/or hemoglobin derivatives. Increased content of methemoglobin has been demonstrated in sickle cells, and recently Asakura et al [29] have shown spectrophotometrically that the heme compounds associated with membranes of sickle cells are predominately methemoglobin [29]. Fischer et al [30] have found increased "retention" of hemoglobin in membranes of ISCs compared to normal cells.

ISCs produced in vitro by anoxic incubation [31] acquired increasing amounts of membrane-associated hemoglobin. This membrane hemoglobin was not observed in AA and SS control cells and occurred prior to substantial ATP depletion. Similar experiments with an ATP-maintenance medium demonstrated that membrane-associated hemoglobin in ISCs increased irrespective of intracellular ATP levels and that simultaneously intracellular sodium and potassium concentrations were altered. Other studies have demonstrated that during anoxic incubation of sickle cells, calcium accumulation occurs largely in the membrane fraction, and correlates directly with ISC content [11].

Our results, and current studies of the ISC membrane, suggest that the acquired defect of the ISC membrane lies in the protein components [4, 12, 34–36]. Durocher and Conrad [32] reported that the SDS PAGE protein profiles from AA and SS membranes are similar, and others have made similar observation [33]. By contrast, Riggs and Ingram [34] found decreases in bands 1, 2, 2.2, 2.3, and 3, and increases in bands 4.5, 6, 7, and globin, as well as a marked decrease in sialic acid content of SS cell membranes. Lux et al [12], studying Triton X-100-extracted ghosts of ISCs, found that the membrane residues retained the shape of the original ISC and suggested that the defective morphology of the ISC probably lies in the "spectrin-actin lattice." In our studies of ISCs isolated in vivo, SDS PAGE revealed significant differences between ISCs and non-ISC fractions. The marked increase in the globin band in the Coomassie Blue-stained gels is consistent with the increase in membrane-associated hemoglobin shown by the other methods. The decrease in band 4.1 may be due to the involvement of these proteins in the formation of the pre–band 1 heteropolymer. Although the components of this high-molecular-weight complex have not been determined in the present study, cross-linking studies of AA cell membranes using diamine (diazine dicarboxylic acid bisdimethylamide) [39] suggest that proteins such as bands 1, 2, 3, and 4.1 may be components of the pre–band 1 heteropolymer. Palek et al [35], employing catalytic oxidation of protein SH groups, found that ISC membrane proteins formed a 450,000-dalton complex of spectrin 1 + 2, a 260,000-dalton complex of bands 2 + 4.9, and a small amount of bands 3 and actin dimers. Lorand and co-workers [36] have attributed the formation of high-molecular-weight complexes within normal (AA) membranes in the presence of calcium [37, 38] to protein cross-linking mediated by a transglutaminase. Lorand et al [36] suggest that calcium influx into the red cell activates this enzyme, which would conceivably induce the cross-linking of membrane proteins by means of γ-glutamyl–ϵ-lysine bridges. Formation of these cross-linked polymers is generally accompanied by reduction in band 4.1 [36, 38, 39], suggesting the involvement of this band in the polymerization. The relation of these membrane protein heteropolymers to the microbodies observed in ISC membranes is at present unknown. However, variations in experimental conditions such as electrophoresis, staining, and destaining procedures may influence the resultant gel pattern and explain the divergent findings from several laboratories.

The ISC has a markedly decreased cellular deformability as demonstrated by micropipette elastimetry [5], cell filtration [40, 41], and viscometric studies [42]. This alteration in deformability is due to increased membrane rigidity [5, 43]. The chemical basis for this alteration in the biophysical characteristics of the ISC membrane may be considered in terms of alteration of molecular organization of the ISC. It has been our contention that the membrane defect of the ISC is an acquired cumulative or progressive lesion in which several factors can be identified and synthesized into a unified concept: 1) Deoxyhemoglobin S or denatured hemoglobin S binds to the membrane of the ISC. 2) This deoxyhemoglobin S–membrane interaction is associated with an apparent increase in membrane and cellular calcium in the ISC, and may occur independently of alteration in cellular ATP level. 3) The association of deoxyhemoglobin S and calcium with the membrane may be indicators of alterations in the macromolecular (protein) organization of the membrane, rather than principal events in the generation of the ISC membrane lesion. 4) The irreversible shape alteration in the ISC and perhaps its membrane rigidity can be attributed to irreversible cross-linking or protein components, perhaps through disulfide bridges, of the spectrin-actin lattice of the cell membrane. 5) This cross-linking may be mediated by a calcium-dependent transglutaminase enzyme and explain the presence of high-molecular-weight complexes found in polyacrylamide gel electrophoresis patterns of ISC membranes.

ACKNOWLEDGMENTS

This study was supported in part by contract No. N01-HL-2-2946B from the National Heart and Lung Institute, and a World Health Organization Fellowship to J. Kurantsin-Mills.

The authors thank Mr Frank Stewart, departmental secretary, for his assistance in typing the manuscript and the Audio-Visual Division of the George Washington University Medical Center for processing illustrations.

REFERENCES

1. Klug PP, Lessin LS, Radice P: Arch Intern Med 133:577, 1974.
2. Bertles JF, Milner PFA: J Clin Invest 47:1731, 1968.

3. Sergeant GR, Sergeant BE, Milner PFA, Br J Haematol 17:527, 1969.
4. Lessin LS, Wallas C: Blood 42:978, 1973.
5. Havell T, Hillman D, Lessin LS: Am J. Hematol 4:9, 1978.
6. Padilla F, Bromberg PA, Jensen WN: Blood 41:653, 1973.
7. Palek J: Blood 42:988, 1973.
8. Yoo D, Lessin LS, Jensen WN: Clin Res 23:285, 1975.
9. Bookchin RM, Nagel RL: Sem Hematol 11:577, 1974.
10. Eaton J, Skelton T, Swofford H, Kolpin C, Jacob H: Nature 246:105, 1973.
11. Palek J: J Lab Clin Med 89:1365, 1977.
12. Lux SE, John KM, Karnovsky MJ: J Clin Invest 58:955, 1976.
13. Singer K, Chernoff AI, Singer L: Blood 6:413, 1951.
14. Dodge JT, Mitchell C, Hanahan DJ: Arch Biochem Biophys 100:119, 1963.
15. Crosby WH, Furth FW: Blood 11:380, 1956.
16. Bessis M, Weed RI: In Johari O, Corvin I (eds): "Scanning Electron Microscopy, Part II." Chicago: Illinois Institute of Technology Research Institute, 1972, p 289.
17. Reynolds ES: J Cell Biol 17:208, 1963.
18. Lessin LS: Nouv Rev Franc Hematol 12:151, 1972.
19. Jensen WN, Ruchnagel DL, Taylor WJ: J Lab Clin Med 56:854, 1960.
20. Kornberg A: J Biol 182:779, 1950.
21. Lamprecht W, Trautschold I: In Bergmeyer HU (ed): "Methods in Enzymatic Analysis." New York: Academic, 1974, p 2101.
22. Rose ZB, Liebowitz J: Anal Biochem 35:177, 1970.
23. Kurantsin-Mills J, Kudo M, Addae SK: Clin Sci Mol Med 46:679, 1974.
24. Breton-Gorius J: Nouv Rev Franc Hematol 10:243, 1970.
25. Fairbanks G, Steck TL, Wallach DFH: Biochemistry 10:2606, 1971.
26. Lowry OH, Rosebrough NJ, Farr AL, Randall RJ: J Biol Chem 193:265, 1951.
27. Bessis M: "Living Blood Cells and Their Ultrastructure." New York: Springer-Verlag, 1973, p 134.
28. Bessis M, Bricka M: Rev Hematol 7:407, 1952.
29. Asakura T, Minakata K, Adachi K, Russel MO, Schwartz E: J Clin Invest 59:633, 1977.
30. Fischer S, Nagel RL, Bookchin RM, Roth EF, Tellez-Nagel I: Biochem Biophys Acta 375:422, 1975.
31. Shen SC, Fleming EM, Castle WB: Blood 4:498, 1949.
32. Durocher JR, Conrad ME: Proc Soc Exp Biol Med 146:373, 1974.
33. Dzandu J, Johnson RM: J Supramol Struct (Suppl) 2:209, 1978.
34. Riggs MG, Ingram VM: Biochem Biophys Res Commun 74:191, 1977.
35. Palek J, Liu SC, Liu A: In Kruckeberg WC, Eaton JW, Brewer GJ (eds): "Progress in Clinical and Biological Research." New York: Alan R Liss, 1978, vol 20.
36. Lorand L, Weissman LB, Epel DL, Bruner-Lorand J: Proc Nat Acad Sci USA 73:4479, 1976.
37. Carraway KL, Triplett RB, Anderson DR: Biochim Biophys Acta 379:571, 1975.
38. King LE, Morrison M: Biochim Biophys Acta 471:162, 1977.
39. Kurantsin-Mills J, Lessin LS: Biophys J 21:119a, 1978.
40. Lessin LS, Kurantsin-Mills J, Weems HB: Blood Cells 3:241, 1977.
41. Lessin LS, Kurantsin-Mills J, Klug PP, Weems HB: In Kruckeberg WC, Eaton JW, Brewer GJ (eds): "Progress in Clinical and Biological Research." New York: Alan R Liss, 1978, vol 20.
42. Chien S, Usami S, Bertles J: J Clin Invest 49:623, 1970.
43. LaCelle PL: Blood Cells 1:269, 1975.

Journal of Supramolecular Structure 9:555–567 (1978)
Normal and Abnormal Red Cell Membranes 329–341

Role of Physiologic Autoantibody in the Removal of Senescent Human Red Cells

Marguerite M. B. Kay

Molecular and Clinical Immunology Laboratory, Geriatric Research, Education and Clinical Center (GRECC), VA Wadsworth Hospital Center, Los Angeles, California 90073, and The Department of Medicine, University of California at Los Angeles, Los Angeles, California 90024

The mechanism by which mononuclear phagocytes distinguish mature "self" from senescent "self" was investigated. Evidence is presented indicating that human mononuclear phagocytes distinguish senescent RBC from mature RBC on the basis of selective Ig attachment to the membranes of senescent cells. This Ig, eluted from senescent human RBC, was shown to be IgG and free of other Igs by immunodiffusion, immunoelectrophoresis, and polyacrylamide gel electrophoresis. The IgG was polyclonal with respect to light chains. The eluted IgG reattaches to homologous stored RBC, but not to mature autologous or allogeneic RBC, via the Fab region. It then initiates phagocytosis of these stored RBC by mononuclear phagocytes. Evidence suggests that the IgG is directed against altered membrane receptors. Thus, this IgG may be a "physiologic" autoantibody and contribute to the maintenance of homeostasis by performing regulatory functions.

Key words: scanning electron microscopy, cellular aging, autoantibodies, red blood cells

Mononuclear phagocytes* can distinguish mature "self" from senescent "self" cells. This is reflected by their ability to phagocytize cells that have reached the end of their functional life-span, while sparing the mature cells. For example, mononuclear phagocytes

*A select WHO committee [1] has recommended that actively phagocytic mononuclear cells of any system, including those of the reticuloendothelial system, be reclassified as the mononuclear phagocyte system (MPS) on the basis of common functional properties (ie, phagocytosis) and of their common origin from the blood monocyte which is itself derived from a bone marrow precursor cell. In accordance with this recommedation, the terminology, "mononuclear phagocyte," will be used throughout this manuscript.

Abbreviations: ID, immunodiffusion; IEP, Immunoelectrophoresis; Ig, Immunoglobulin; PAGE, polyacrylamide gel electrophoresis; RBC, red blood cells.

Publication No. 020 from GRECC, VA Wadsworth Hospital Center, Los Angeles, CA 90073.

Received April 8, 1978; revision accepted September 20, 1978.

0091-7419/78/0904-0555$02.60

of the liver and spleen remove syngeneic lymphocytes as well as antibody-coated red blood cells (RBC) [2–4]. Studies on the fate of aged RBC indicate that they are eliminated intracellularly by mononuclear phagocytes rather than by osmotic lysis both in vitro and in situ [2–9]. In this way, mononuclear phagocytes may perform an essential homeostatic role by permitting the more efficient mature cells to carry out their vital functions without hindrance from the less efficient senescent cells, or by pathological reactions that could arise as a consequence of senescent cells dying and decaying within the organism.

Previous experiments performed in this laboratory suggest that mononuclear phagocytes can distinguish senescent from mature self RBC on the basis of selective attachment of autologous immunoglobulin (Ig)G to the membrane of senescent RBC [10]. The presence of IgG on senescent cells is presumptive evidence that an immunological receptor-IgG binding has occurred. However, such evidence by itself does not establish that the Ig is a homeostatic autoantibody directed against normal constituents of the cell membrane. Definitive evidence for the role autoantibodies play in the selective removal of senescent cells can be obtained by first dissociating the antibodies from senescent cells and by then demonstrating their specific immunologic reattachment to homologous senescent but not to mature cells, leading to destruction of only the senescent cells by mononuclear phagocytes. This report presents evidence that IgG binds to the surface of senescent cells via the Fab region and initiates their phagocytosis by macrophages. The evidence suggests that the IgG may be an autoantibody directed against altered cell membrane molecules.

Human RBC were utilized as a model system because mononuclear phagocytes routinely phagocytize RBC at the end of their 120 day life-span, and they are an ideal experimental system in many respects. Large numbers of RBC are readily available, and senescent cells can be easily be separated from mature cells. RBC membranes have been extensively characterized biochemically, and they have a smooth regular surface that does not "cap" or ingest labels. Two biological assays are available: a phagocytosis assay, which assesses recognition of senescent cells by mononuclear phagocytes [2, 10], and a scanning immunoelectron microscopy labeling technique, which enables detection of as few as 2 IgG molecules per cell and assesses density and distribution of receptor sites [10–13].

MATERIALS AND METHODS

Isolation of Ig From Old RBC

Blood was obtained from 18 healthy individuals 19 to 34 years of age and one who was 50 years old. Young RBC were removed, and the remaining RBC were washed 3 times with 50 volumes of phosphate buffered saline (PBS), pH 7.4. Ig was eluted from 50–250 ml of packed RBC by the method of Kochwa and Rosenfield [14], because methods of elution which did not result in dissociation of antigen-antibody bonds (eg, temperature and glycine-NaOH buffer, pH 8), did not result in Ig elution in our hands. Preliminary experiments indicated that Ig could be eluted from old, but not young, RBC. The RBC eluate from nine individuals was assessed without further purification. Antibody from the RBC eluates of each of 10 individuals was isolated with an anti-Fab immuno-absorbent column. Fab was obtained from normal human IgG by papain digestion and column chromatography [15, 16]. Purity was determined by immunodiffusion (ID), immunoelectrophoresis (IEP), and polyacrylamide gel electrophoresis (PAGE). Antisera to Fab was obtained by immunizing a goat with 8 weekly injections of 1 mg of Fab that was pure as determined by ID and IEP. After 10 weeks, the goat was bled and the immune serum was incubated with an immunoabsorbent that was made by binding Fab covalently to Sepharose 4B through a 13 atom spacer (aminohexyl derivative of Sepharose 4B, [17]). After thorough washing, the beads were poured into a 7.5 ml glass column (Bio Rad), and the antibodies specific for Fab were eluted with 0.1 M glycine-HCl, pH 2.3. The eluted antibody, determined with a recording spectrophotometer, was neutralized with 1 N NaOH, concentrated, and dialysed against PBS, pH 7.4. The anti-Fab antibodies obtained by this procedure were specific for Fab and reacted with pure IgA and IgM as well as IgG, as determined by ID and IEP. Conversely, specific anti-IgA, IgG, and IgM reagents reacted only with the specific Ig class. Anti-Fab specific antibodies were coupled to aminohexyl Sepharose 4B and used to isolate Ig from RBC eluates. The Ig was eluted from the anti-Fab column in the same manner as described for anti-Fab antibodies, then concentrated with an Amicon Diaflow with PM 10 filter. The quantity of IgG eluted per 100 ml of packed RBC was 10.27 ± 3.03 μg (mean ± SE), as determined by radial immunodiffusion with Ultra Low Level Diffu-gen plates, lot #55822 (Oxford Laboratories, Foster City, CA).

Mononuclear Phagocytes

Mononuclear cells from human peripheral blood were isolated on "Lymphoprep" and washed three times with Medium 199. The percentage of mononuclear phagocytes was determined by spreading an aliquot of mononuclear cells on a slide, or by making a cytocentrifuge preparation of mononuclear cells, staining with May-Gruenwald-Giemsa or with peroxidase [18], and performing differential cell counts with a 100X oil-immersion objective (Zeiss). The number of mononuclear phagocytes was calculated by multiplying the total number of mononuclear cells times the percentage of mononuclear phagocytes. Polymorphonuclear leukocyte contamination was less than 1%. Mononuclear cells were diluted with bicarbonate buffered Medium 199 with Methicillin/Gentamycin (100 μg/ml) and glutamine so that the concentration of mononuclear phagocytes was $6–10 \times 10^5$/ml, and 1 ml was pipetted into each tube. After a 1 h incubation at 37° in an atmosphere of humidified air containing 5% CO_2, nonadherent cells were removed by vigorous washing.

Phagocytosis Assay

The phagocytosis assay utilized for these studies measured phagocytosis rather than attachment, osmotic lysis, or adhesion of RBC to glass tubes. Light microscopy and transmission electron microscopy of cultures after 30 min and 3 h demonstrated that RBC in various stages of degradation were present inside mononuclear phagocytes, with some phagocytes having as many as 20 RBC inside them [2, 19]. Scanning electron microscopy of the cultures after 3 h demonstrated that only RBC that were partially engulfed were visible on the surface [2]. When young RBC were added to 20 tubes containing mononuclear phagocytes, 100% of the RBC were recovered 3 h later. When RBC stored without Ig were added to 16 tubes containing mononuclear phagocytes, 98–100% of the RBC were recovered 3 h later. Negative controls were utilized throughout the study. These included young RBC, RBC aged in vitro and incubated in medium without serum or in Ig-depleted serum, neuraminidase-treated RBC incubated in culture medium, and young RBC incubated in allogeneic Ig eluted from senescent cells. These cells were not phagocytized, as indicated by the recovery rates noted above. Mononuclear phagocyte viability at the end of culture was 98–100%, as determined by trypan blue dye exclusion.

Young and Senescent RBC

RBC from freshly drawn blood were depleted of white cells and reticulocytes, then separated into young, middle-aged, and old (senescent) populations by their difference in density [20, 21]. At the end of the density separation, young RBC are at the top of the gradient, and old RBC are at the bottom, as determined by the distribution of recently synthesized ^{59}Fe-labeled RBC [20, 21].

Stored RBC

Freshly isolated young RBC were washed 3 times with 50 volumes of Medium 199, resuspended at a concentration of 10% in Medium 199 without serum to avoid IgG binding, and transferred to tissue culture flasks. RBC were stored for 2–4 wk at 4°.

Not all of the RBC populations were needed for the purpose of these experiments. Those in excess of the required numbers remained in storage for a total of five months. When these cells were subsequently examined, it was found that all old RBC and approximately half of the middle-aged RBC had lysed. The young RBC populations, however, were essentially free of lysed cells. This reaffirms that the method of cell separation employed in the present experiment is successful and that different cell populations have different membrane properties. It suggests that storage of RBC in vitro may be a reasonable parallel model for aging in vivo because young RBC survive at least 150 days, and that old RBC have the potential for lysis if stored, without macrophages, for an extended period of time. It is possible that the mechanism by which membrane lesions are generated during storage in vitro may not be the same as that by which lesions are generated in vivo as cells age. It is possible, however, that the lesions themselves are identical.

Incubation of RBC With Ig Eluted From Senescent Cells

Stored RBC were washed and resuspended to a concentration of $1.5–2.0 \times 10^9$ RBC per ml. Twenty micrograms of Ig were added to 1 ml of the cell suspension which was incubated at 37° for 30–60 min in a shaking water bath. The RBC were then washed 3 times with medium and incubated with mononuclear phagocytes. Approximately 15–20 RBC were added per phagocyte, and the volume was adjusted to 0.24–0.40 ml per tube. Following incubation for 3 h at 37°, the percentage of phagocytized RBC was calculated as described previously [10]. This culture method supports a maximum of $\approx$ 50% phagocytosis.

The maximum percentage of phagocytosis obtainable appears to be limited by depletion of nutrients in the media. Addition of new medium at the end of 3 h results in additional phagocytosis of RBC: 46 ± 11% of the RBC were phagocytized during 6 h when new medium was not added, whereas 61 ± 2% were phagocytized when new medium was added after the first 3 h incubation. If old RBC are added to cultures that have been incubated without RBC for the first 3 h, without changing medium, there is no significant phagocytosis (only 8 ± 7% of the RBC were phagocytized). Finally, an additional 40 ± 3% of the old RBC, harvested from cultures after a 3 h incubation, are phagocytized when added to new cultures with fresh medium.

Neuraminidase-Treated RBC

Freshly isolated young RBC were washed 3 times with 50 volumes of Medium 199; incubated with 3.35 units of Vibrio Cholerae neuraminidase (Behring Diagnostics, which was tested and found to be lipase and protease free) per 10^{10} RBC at 37° in PBS, pH 6.8,

TABLE I. Characterization of Antibody Eluted From Senescent RBC*

Individ-	IgA			IgG			IgM			Albumin			Kappa		Lambda	
uals	ID	IEP	PAGE	ID	IEP	PAGE	ID	IEP	PAGE	ID	IEP	PAGE	ID	IEP	ID	IEP
1	–	–	–	+	+	+	–	–	–	–	+	+	+	–	+	+
2[a]	–	–	–	+	+	+	–	–	–	–	–	–	+	+	+	+
3[b]	–	–	–	+	+	+	–	–	–	–	–	–	+	+	+	+
4[b]	–	–	–	+	+	+	–	–	–	–	+	+	+	–	+	+
5	–	–	–	+	+	+	–	–	–	–	–	–	ND	ND	ND	ND
6	–	–	–	+	+	+	–	–	–	–	–	+	ND	ND	ND	ND
7	–	–	–	+	+	+	–	–	–	–	–	–	ND	ND	ND	ND
8	–	–	–	+	+	+	–	–	–	–	–	–	ND	ND	ND	ND
9[b]	–	–	–	+	+	+	–	–	–	–	–	–	+	–	+	+

*The results of the first 9 out of 15 individuals are presented here, for the latter 6 individuals gave similar results; ND, not done. Eluted antibody was identified by ID, IEP, and PAGE. For PAGE, 50 and 100 μg of protein were loaded on the gels. A "plus" indicates that the component was present; a "minus" indicates that it was not detected. ID was performed with Hyland ID plates (pattern C). IEPs were performed with barbital-barbital sodium buffer, pH 8.2 ($\Gamma = 0.05$), at a constant current of 34 mamp (approximately 51 volts) for 3 h at room temperature using IEP plates from Meloy. PAGE was performed by the method of Laemmli (22). The following anti-sera were used anti-human: whole serum and anti-human albumin (Meloy, Springfield, VA), anti-kappa, anti-lambda, anti-IgA, anti-IgG, anti-IgM, and anti-$F(ab)_2$ (Tago Immunodiagnostics, Burlingame, CA), and anti-Fc (Miles Labs., Kankakee, IL).

[a] Sodium dodecyl sulfate polyacrylamide gel electrophoresis was also performed and the results revealed only one Ig.

[b] Antibody eluted but not purified with anti-Fab immunoabsorbent.

TABLE II. IgG Binding and Specificity

	RBC group	Macrophage source	IgG source[a]	% Phagocytosis ± SEM[b]
Control groups				
Positive	Senescent, freshly isolated	Autologous	none added	50 ± 4
Negative	Young, freshly isolated	Autologous	none added	0
	Young, freshly isolated	Autologous	Allogeneic	5 ± 3
	Young, stored	Autologous	none added	0
	Young, stored	Allogeneic	none added	0
Experimental groups				
	Young, stored	Autologous	Autologous	46 ± 0
	Young, stored	Autologous	Allogeneic	27 ± 0
	Young, stored	Allogeneic	Autologous	56 ± 4

[a] Twenty μg of IgG eluted from senescent cells was added to 1 ml of RBC suspension containing $1.5-2.0 \times 10^9$ cells. In contrast, when stored RBC were incubated in either 0.6 mg or 6 mg of pooled, normal human IgG, the percentage of phagocytosis was 13 ± 2 and 35 ± 9, respectively. This confirmed the specificity of the binding of IgG eluted from senescent cells, since even a 300-fold greater concentration of pooled, normal human IgG was not as efficient as the eluted IgG in initiating phagocytosis.

[b] SEM, standard error of the mean from three triplicate cultures from each of three experiments.

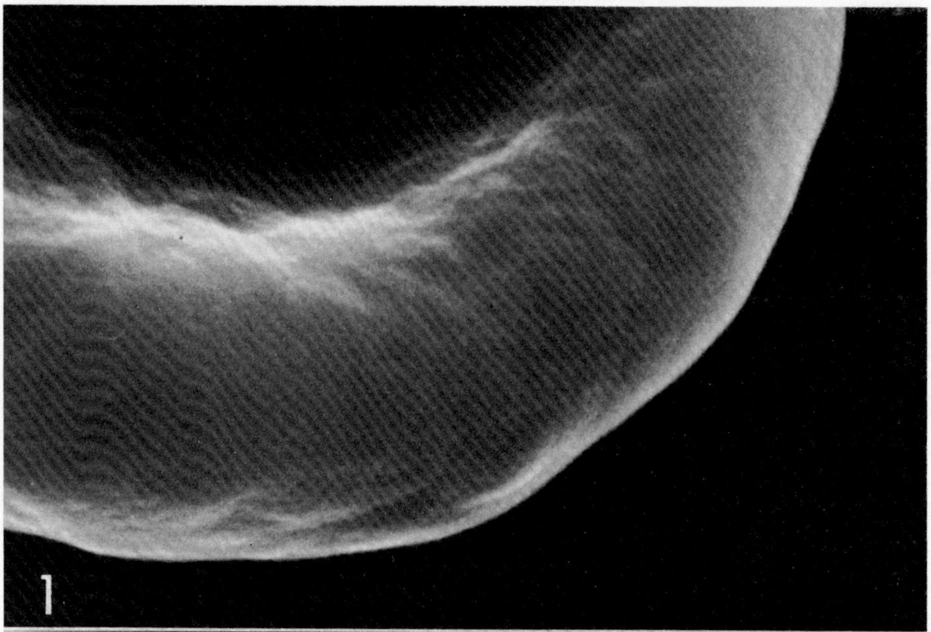

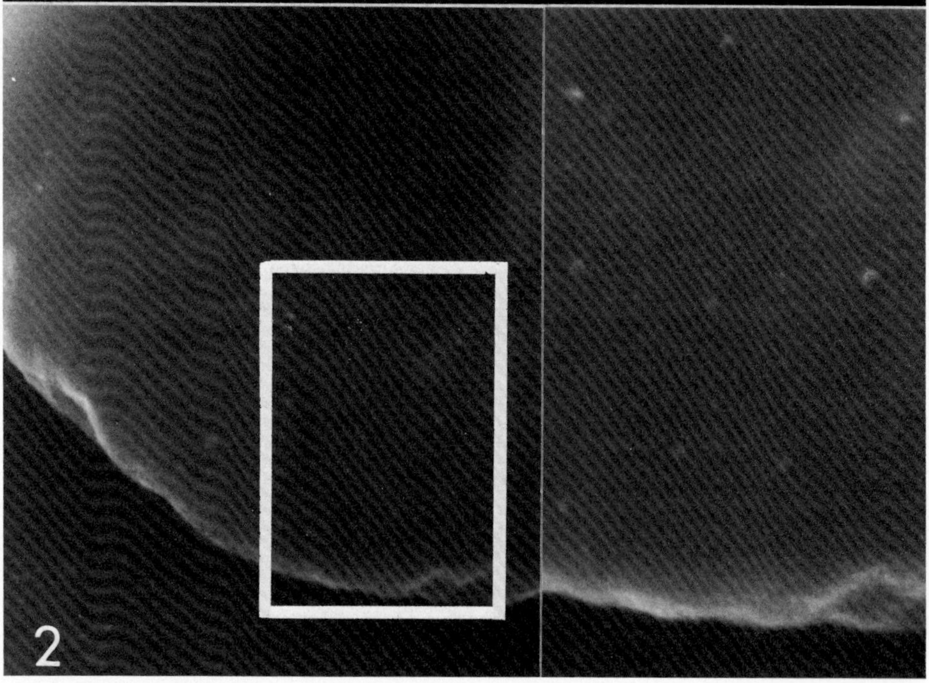

Fig. 1. Scanning electron micrograph of a typical stored RBC, incubated with goat antihuman IgG, and then rabbit antigoat conjugated to ferritin as a control for the antibody binding and specificity experiments. No ferritin is visible (× 31,250).

Fig. 2. Scanning electron micrograph of stored RBC, incubated with autologous IgG eluted from senescent cells, and then goat antihuman IgG followed by rabbit antigoat conjugated to ferritin. Ferritin is visible on the cell surface, even at low magnification. All RBC in these preparations were labeled with the ferritin. × 22,857. The inset on the right shows a higher magnification of the area within the white square (× 56,500).

for 30–60 min; and washed again. They were incubated in Medium 199 containing 20 μg of either autologous or allogeneic Ig eluted from senescent cells, washed 3 times, and incubated with autologous mononuclear phagocytes.

Scanning Immunoelectron Microscopy

Aliquots of the RBC used in phagocytosis experiments were incubated in the IgG fraction of goat antihuman IgG for 30 min at 37°, washed, incubated in rabbit antigoat IgG conjugated to ferritin for 30 min at 4°, washed again, and prepared for scanning electron microscopy [10–13]. Preparations were viewed with an Hitachi HFS-2 field emission, scanning electron microscope with 3 nm resolution. Between 220 and 300 cells were viewed in each preparation at magnifications from 20,000 to 100,000. Scanning time per preparation was 18–36 h.

RESULTS

Identification and Characterization of Old RBC Ig

The Ig eluted from RBC aged in situ was shown to be an IgG containing kappa and lambda light chains by immunodiffusion and immunoelectrophoresis (Table I). Other Igs were not detected by immunodiffusion, immunoelectrophoresis, or polyacrylamide gel electrophoresis.

IgG Binding and Specificity Experiments

In order to determine whether the IgG eluted from old RBC aged in situ would reattach to homologous cells, the IgG was incubated with autologous or allogeneic young stored RBC. These RBC were then washed and incubated with autologous mononuclear phagocytes. The results of these experiments are summarized in Table II. The percentage of phagocytosis of stored RBC incubated with autologous IgG and then with autologous mononuclear phagocytes is essentially the same as that of RBC aged in situ. Mononuclear phagocytes phagocytized autologous stored RBC incubated with autologous IgG, as well as allogeneic stored RBC incubated with autologous IgG. However, they did not phagocytize allogeneic cells that had not been incubated with IgG, nor did they phagocytize young allogeneic cells that were incubated with allogeneic IgG. IgG was demonstrated on the surface of stored RBC incubated with IgG eluted from autologous or allogeneic cells with scanning immunoelectron microscopy (Figs. 1 and 2).

TABLE III. Phagocytosis of Stored RBC ("0" RBC) Incubated With IgG Eluted From Senescent Cells Before and After Absorption With Stored RBC or Freshly Isolated Young RBC (YRBC)

Experiment	Quantity[a] (μg)	Phagocytosis (%) ± SEM[b] Before absorption	After absorption with YRBC	After absorption with "0" RBC
1	3	49 ± 2	43 ± 9	0
2	3	35 ± 1	34 ± 7	0
3	3	43 ± 11	46 ± 16	0

[a]Quantity (μg) of IgG added to 1.5×10^8 RBC in 1 ml of Medium 199.
[b]SEM, standard error of the mean of triplicate or quadruplicate cultures.

TABLE IV. Phagocytosis of Stored RBC Incubated With Pooled Human IgG Before or After Absorption of the IgG With Stored RBC*

Experiment	Quantity of IgG (μg)[a]	Phagocytosis (%) Before absorption (Mean ± SEM)[b]	Phagocytosis (%) After absorption
1	30	42 ± 17	0
2	30	32 ± 4	0
3	300	52 ± 2	0
4	300	28 ± 6	0

*IgG was absorbed overnight at 4° with RBC aged in vitro.
[a]The quantity of IgG (μg) was added to 2×10^8 RBC which were incubated for 30 min at 24° and then for 30 min at 4°, washed, and incubated with autologous mononuclear phagocytes. The quantity of IgG (μg) was adjusted so that it was the same both for absorbed and unabsorbed IgG, as determined by radial immunodiffusion.
[b]Mean ± the standard error of the mean of quadruplicate cultures.

TABLE V. Phagocytosis of Neuraminidase-Treated Young RBC Incubated With IgG Eluted From RBC Aged In Situ

IgG source	% Phagocytosis ± SEM
None	0
Autologous	35 ± 2
Allogeneic	46 ± 6

Absorption of the eluted IgG with stored RBC, but not with freshly isolated young RBC, abolished its phagocytosis-inducing ability (Table III). Likewise, absorption of pooled normal human IgG with stored RBC abolished its phagocytosis-inducing ability (Table IV).

To confirm these findings and to determine the nature of the membrane molecules that are altered during RBC aging in situ, young RBC were treated with neuraminidase, a microbial enzyme that cleaves sialic acid groups from glycoprotein molecules. Neuraminidase was selected for this purpose because it is known that: 1) approximately 10% of the RBC membrane is composed of glycoproteins, 2) removal of sialic acid from circulating glycoproteins can result in their removal, 3) transient autoimmune hemolytic anemias sometimes follow respiratory infection with viruses such as influenza which contain neuraminidase, and 4) IgG will bind to neuraminidase-treated RBC [10]. Neuraminidase-treated RBC incubated in medium alone were not phagocytized, whereas those incubated in autologous and allogeneic IgG eluted from old RBC aged in situ were phagocytized (Table V). IgG was observed with scanning immunoelectron microscopy on the surface of neuraminidase-IgG-treated RBC, but not on RBC treated with neuraminidase alone.

The following experiments were performed in order to determine whether the Fab region of IgG binds to old RBC, thus indicating an immunological receptor binding, or whether old RBC simply develop Fc receptors. One group of stored RBC was incubated first with human Fab, then with goat antihuman Fab, and finally with rabbit antigoat IgG conjugated to ferritin. An identical group of stored RBC were incubated with human Fc,

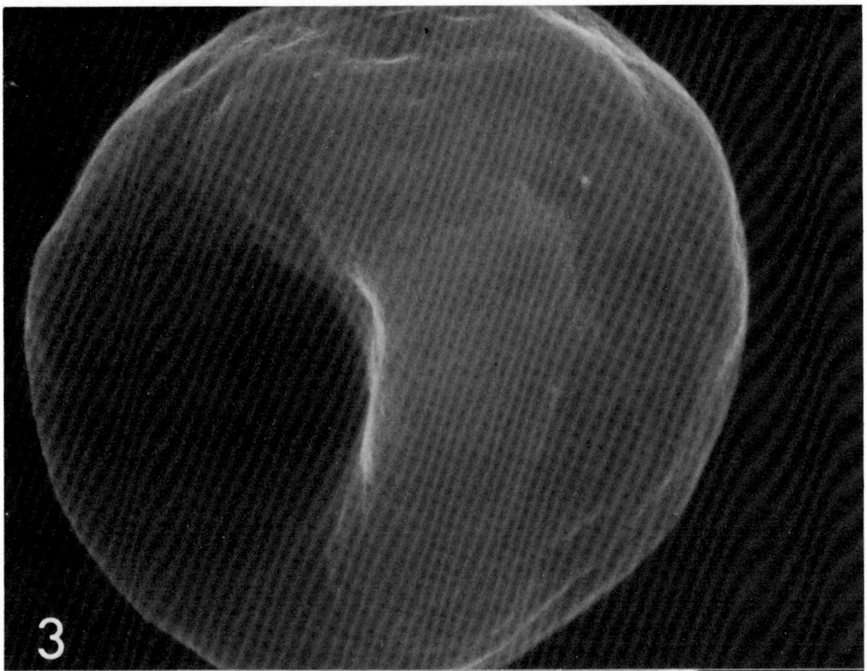

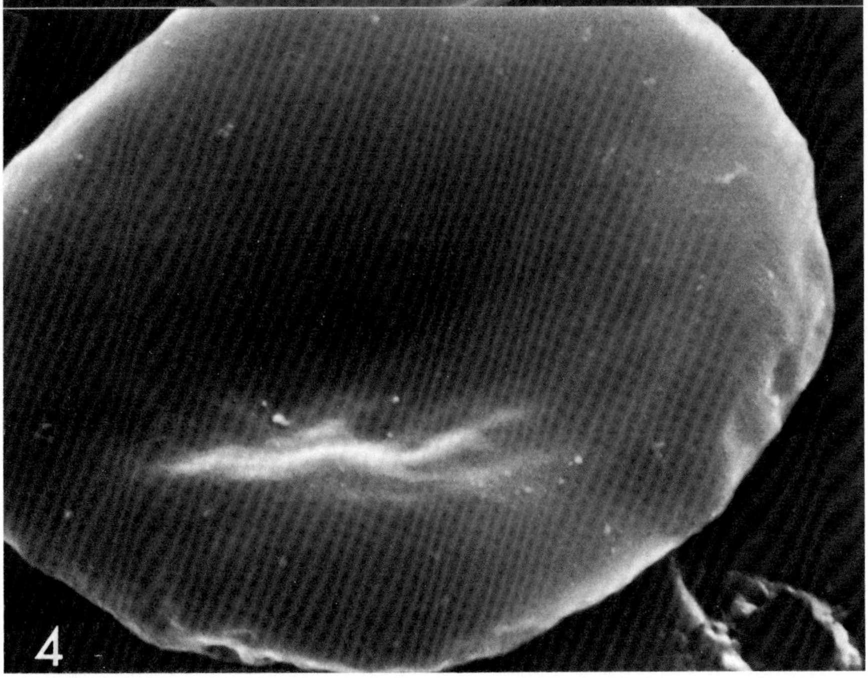

Fig. 3. Scanning electron micrograph of a typical stored RBC, incubated with human Fc, then goat anti-human Fc followed by rabbit antigoat conjugated to ferritin. RBC is essentially unlabeled (× 23,500).

Fig. 4. Scanning electron micrograph of a typical stored RBC, incubated with human Fab, then goat anti-human Fab followed by rabbit antigoat conjugated to ferritin. RBC is labeled with ferritin (× 22,979).

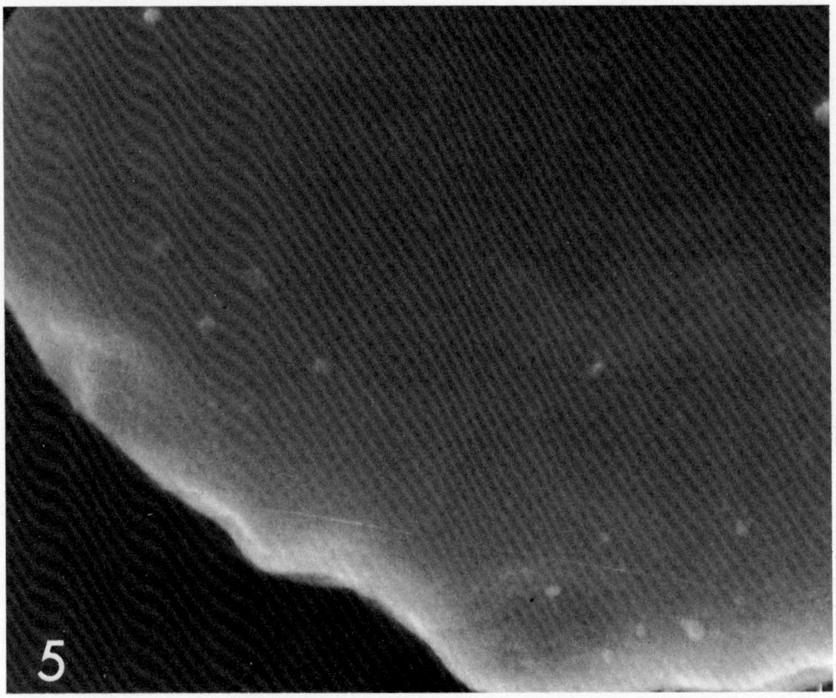

Fig. 5. Higher magnification of RBC from same preparation as that shown in Figure 4. Ferritin label indicating Fab is easily visible (× 57,065).

then with goat antihuman Fc, and finally with rabbit antigoat IgG conjugated to ferritin. Controls consisted of untreated RBC incubated with either goat antihuman Fab or anti-Fc, and then with rabbit anti-goat IgG conjugated to ferritin. As an additional control, stored RBC were incubated with either Fab and goat antihuman Fc, or Fc and goat antihuman Fab, followed in both cases by incubation with rabbit antigoat IgG conjugated to ferritin. Cells were then viewed with scanning electron microscopy. The results of these scanning experiments showed that the Fab but not the Fc region of IgG binds to stored RBC (Figs. 3–5).

To determine whether the Fab or Fc portion of IgG attaches to RBC, by a method independent of scanning immunoelectron microscopy, receptor blockade studies were performed. The results are summarized in Figure 6. Stored RBC were incubated for 30 min with either pooled normal human IgG, its Fab fragment, or its Fc fragment. The RBC were washed, and all three groups were incubated with IgG for another 30 min. RBC were washed again and incubated with autologous mononuclear phagocytes (Fig. 6A). For the control cultures, stored RBC were treated with IgG, Fab, or Fc before they were exposed to mononuclear phagocytes (Fig. 6B). Control results show that phagocytosis was achieved by exposing the RBC to IgG. Treatment with Fab or Fc did not promote phagocytosis. Experimental results show that treatment of RBC with Fab prior to incubation with IgG reduced the phagocotyosis to essentially 0, whereas pretreatment with Fc did not inhibit phagocytosis (Fig. 6A). Thus, these blockade studies also demonstrate that IgG binds old RBC via its Fab region.

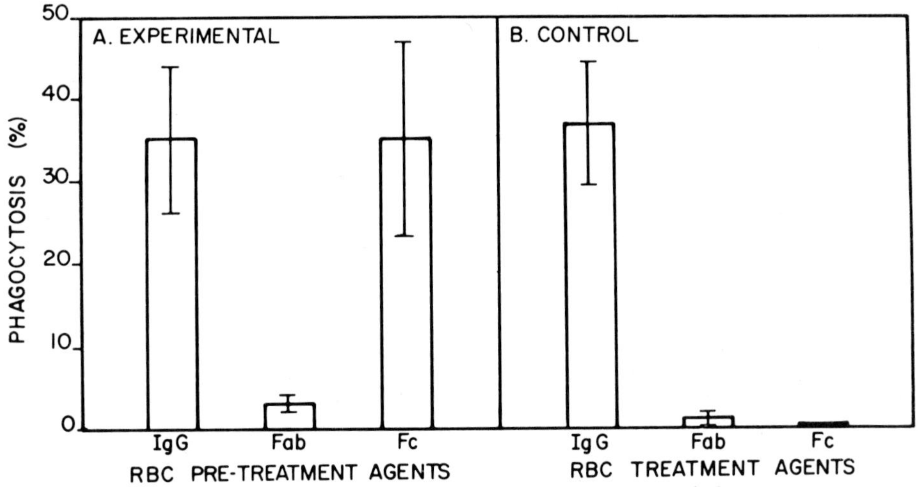

Fig. 6. A. Susceptibility to phagocytosis of aged RBC as influenced by their pretreatment with either IgG, Fab, or Fc before exposure to IgG. Stored RBC were incubated with either IgG, Fab, or Fc for 30 min, washed, and incubated with IgG for 30 min. The RBC were washed and incubated with mononuclear phagocytes for 3 h. B. Susceptibility to phagocytosis of aged RBC as influenced by their exposure to either IgG, Fab, or Fc. Stored RBC were incubated with either IgG, Fab, or Fc for 30 min, washed and then incubated with mononuclear phagocytes for 3 h. Bars indicate standard error of the mean; sample size was 6.

DISCUSSION

An earlier study from this laboratory [10] revealed that stored RBC were phagocytized by mononuclear phagocytes only after they had been exposed to IgG. The same study demonstrated that freshly isolated RBC aged in situ had IgG, but not IgA or IgM, on their surface. These RBC were phagocytized by mononuclear phagocytes, whereas young RBC were not. The experiments reported here confirm and extend this earlier study by showing that the Ig isolated from senescent cells is an IgG that is polyclonal with respect to light chains.

The binding and specificity experiments indicate that 1) IgG is required for the phagocytosis of stored autologous and allogeneic RBC; 2) nonspecific binding of IgG does not play a major role in these experiments because absorption of both pooled normal human IgG and IgG eluted from senescent cells with stored RBC abolishes its phagocytosis-inducing activity; 3) IgG eluted from senescent RBC is reactive against stored, but not young, cells; and 4) IgG eluted from senescent RBC cannot discriminate between autologous and allogeneic cells. The last two findings suggest that the receptor site appearing on the surface of cells aged in situ and that appearing on stored cells is the same, or closely related, for all individuals. This was confirmed by binding experiments utilizing neuraminidase-treated RBC, which showed that the IgG eluted from RBC aged in situ binds to neuraminidase-treated young autologous or allogeneic RBC, initiating their phagocytosis by mononuclear phagocytes. The observation that the IgG eluted from RBC aged in situ recognizes the receptor exposed by removal of sialic acid groups suggests that the receptor exposed as cells age naturally in situ may be the same as, or analogous to, that exposed by the removal of sialic acid in vitro. This would suggest that membrane glycoproteins may be losing sialic acid as cells age, thus exposing the molecular determinants to which IgG binds. Another possibility is that the structural association between glycophorin and integral membrane proteins may be disrupted during aging, leading to exposure of cryptic antigens [23]. In such a case, one could speculate that neuraminidase acts, not by exposing new sugars, but by changing glycophorin–protein interactions through removal of sialic acid.

Although the antibody eluted from senescent cells has been found to bind only to senescent RBC aged in situ and to stored RBC, it is possible that it also binds and initiates the removal of damaged cells. Thus, this antibody could be participating in a generalized mechanism by which altered cells are removed from the circulation.

The evidence that indicates that the Fab region of the IgG molecule binds to aged RBC is consistent with an immunological binding of IgG with a surface receptor. Preliminary experiments suggest that the IgG eluted from senescent RBC belongs to the IgG_1 and IgG_3 subclasses. It is interesting that reports in the literature show that macrophages have receptors for the Fc region of complement-binding IgG_1 and IgG_3 subclasses [24].

The IgG eluted from senescent RBC may be considered an autoantibody, as it specifically reattaches to homologous RBC and initiates their selective destruction by mononuclear phagocytes. Indeed, this IgG may be a "physiologic" autoantibody. It appears to contribute to the maintenance of homeostasis by collaborating with macrophages in the removal of sensecent and damaged cells. This collaboration may permit the more efficient mature cells to carry out their vital functions without hindrance from less efficient cells, or by pathological reactions that could arise as a consequence of cells dying or decaying within the organism. Since the IgG autoantibodies may be part of the normal immune mechanism for removing cells, the data allow for the suggestion that the B cell clones producing these antibodies are not "forbidden" [25]. Further, the presence of these autoantibodies need not be attributed to an age-related decrease in suppressor cell function [26, 27].

Greater than 90% of the Ig molecules in human serum are of the IgG class, which supports the concept that IgG may perform homeostatic functions. Human serum contains an average of 12.1 mg/ml of IgG, 2.5 mg/ml of IgA, 0.93 mg/ml of IgM, 0.023 mg/ml of IgD, and 0.0003 mg/ml of IgE [28]. The total mass of IgG in the extravascular fluids is about the same as that in blood [28]. Thus, if one uses the averages figure for the plasma volume of a 70 kg male (ie, 3.5 liters) and the average figure for the extracellular fluid of a 70 kg male (ie, 10.5 liters), one arrives at the startling amount of 42.35 g of IgG in the plasma and 127.06 gm in the extracellular fluid, for a total of 169.40 gm or 1.13×10^{-3} moles of IgG in the average adult male. By comparison, the plasma mass of IgM is approximately 3.26 gm, or 3.6×10^{-6} moles. This can be considered the total body mass of IgM, as there is no evidence that IgM enters the extravascular fluids under normal conditions.

In view of these considerations, it may be appropriate to speculate that a collaboration between "humoral factors" and phagocytes may have evolved as a "safeguard" to ensure the specificity of surveillance mechanisms.

ACKNOWLEDGMENTS

I am grateful to Sam Wong and Ernest Yamamoto for their technical assistance; to Doctors Robert C. Johnson, Takashi Makinodan, Gerald Price, Jacinto Vasquez, An-Chuan Wang, and Fred Wilt for reviewing the manuscript, and to An-Chuan Wang for providing anti-human IgG subclass reagents. This work was carried out, in part, at the Gerontology

Research Center, National Institute of Aging, National Institutes of Health, Baltimore and Bethesda, Maryland, and was supported, in part, by USPHS grant HL 22671.

REFERENCES

1. Furth R, Van A, Cohn AA, Hirsch JG, Humphrey JH, Spector WG, Lungwoort HL: Bull Wld Hlth Org 6:845, 1972.
2. Key MMB: "Lifer and Aging." ed Platt D, Springer-Verlag, Berlin (in press).
3. Klausner MA, Hirsch LI, Leblond PF, Chamberlain JF, Klempeser MR, Segel GB: Blood 46:695, 1975.
4. Silobrčicć V, Vitale B, Sušnjić M, Tomazic V, Basić: I Exp Hematol 4:103, 1976.
5. Gemsa D, Woo CH, Fudenberg HH, Schmid RJ: Clin Lab Invest 52:812, 1973.
6. Jenkin CR, Karthigasu K: Compt Rend Soc Biol 161:1006, 1962.
7. Morita T, Perkins EH: J Reticuloendothel Soc 2:406, 1965.
8. Nelson DS: "Macrophages and Immunity." American Elsevier Publishing Co, New York: 247, 1969.
9. Stuart AE, Cumming RA: Vox Sang 13:270, 1967.
10. Kay MMB: Proc Natl Acad Sci USA 72:3521, 1975.
11. Kay MMB: Nature 254:424, 1975.
12. Kay MMB: "Principles and Techniques of Scanning Electron Microscopy. " (ed) Hayat MA, Van Nostrand and Reinhold Co, New York (in press).
13. Kay MMB: "Immunology and Aging." (eds) Makinodan T, Yunis E, Plenum Press, New York: 135, 1977.
14. Kochwa S, Rosenfield R: J Immunol 92:682, 1964.
15. Cebra JJ, Givol D, Silman HI, Katchalski EJ: Biol Chem 236:1720, 1961.
16. Nisonoff A, Wissler FC, Lipman LN, Woernley DL: Arch Biochem Biophys 89:230, 1960.
17. Cambiasco CL, Goffinet A, Vaerman J-P, Feremans JF: Immunochemistry 12:272, 1975.
18. Kaplow LS: Blood 26:215, 1965.
19. Kay MMB: Recent Results Cancer Res 56:111, 1976.
20. Borun ER, Figueroa WG, Perry SM: J Clin Invest 36:676, 1957.
21. Murphy JR: J Lab Clin Med 82:334, 1973.
22. Laemmli UK: Nature 227:680, 1970.
23. Evolved from discussions with Dr. Hans Lutz.
24. Berken A, Benacerraf B: J Exp Med 123:119, 1966.
25. Burnet FM: "Immunological Surveillance." Pergamon Press, Oxford, England, 1970.
26. Fudenberg HH: Amer J Med 51:295, 1971.
27. Gershwin MD, Steinberg AD: Clin Immunol Immunopathol 4:38, 1975.
28. Eisen HN: "Immunology." Harper and Row, Inc, Hagerstown, Md, 1974.

Journal of Supramolecular Structure 10:79–96
Normal and Abnormal Red Cell Membranes 343–360

Membrane Protein Organization in ATP-Depleted and Irreversibly Sickled Red Cells

J. Palek and S.C. Liu

Department of Research, St Elizabeth's Hospital of Boston, and Tufts University School of Medicine, Boston, Massachusetts

It has been proposed that the spectrin-actin submembrane network participates in control of red cell shape and deformability. We have examined ATP- and calcium-dependent changes in organization of spectrin in the membrane employing cross-linking of the nearest membrane protein neighbors by spontaneous or catalyzed ($CuSO_4$, O-phenanthroline) intermolecular disulfide couplings and two-dimensional sodium dodecyl sulfate polyacrylamide gel electrophoresis.

Cross-linking of fresh red cells resulted in the formation of spectrin and actin dimers and tetramers. ATP-depleted red cells differed from fresh cells in the presence of an additional reducible polymer of $MW > 1 \times 10^6$ selectively enriched in spectrin. This polymer formed spontaneously when red cells were depleted of ATP under aerobic conditions. After anaerobic ATP depletion, the polymer formed in ghosts after cross-linking by catalytic oxidation. Polymerization was prevented by maintenance of ATP and coincided with an ATP-dependent discocyte-echinocyte transformation. This suggests that, in ATP-depleted red cells, spectrin is rearranged to establish closer contacts, and that this may contribute to the discocyte-echinocyte transformation.

The introduction of greater than 0.5 mM Ca^{++} into ghosts by inclusion in hemolysis buffer or into fresh red cells (but not ATP-depleted red cells) by treatment with ionophore A23187 spontaneously produced a nonreducible polymer which others have attributed to transamidative cross-linking of spectrin, band 3, and other proteins. Spontaneous formation of both polymer types (reducible in aerobically ATP-depleted red cells and nonreducible in fresh, Ca^{++} enriched red cells) resulted in stabilization ("autocatalytic fixation") of spheroechinocytic shape.

Irreversibly sickled cells, which have increased calcium and decreased ATP, and exhibit a permanent membrane deformation, failed to form any of the above polymers. This suggests that in contrast to normal cells depleted of ATP

Abbreviations: ATP – adenosine triphosphate, ISCs – irreversibly sickled cells, HEPES – N_2 hydroxyethyl piperazine N'2-ethane sulphonic acid, SDS – sodium dodecylsulphate, PAGE – polyacrylamide gel electrophoresis, DTT – dithiothreitol, SEM – scanning electron microscopy, G6PD – glucose 6-phosphate dehydrogenase, EDTA – ethylenediaminotetracetic acid, A23187 – calcimycin, HbSS – sickle cell anemia.

Received May 4, 1978; accepted September, 11, 1978.

0091-7419/79/1001-0079$03.20

in vitro, fixation of ISC shape in vivo is not related to Ca- and ATP-dependent membrane protein polymerization. However, ISCs had an increased propensity to form the reducible, spectrin-rich polymer during a subsequent metabolic depletion in vitro. This was associated with transformation of ISCs into spheroechinocytes. Similar echinocytic ISCs were found to constitute 5–10% of the densest fractions of freshly separated ISCs. ISCs then exhibit sphero-echniocyte transformation, both in vitro and in vivo. We propose that this is due to spectrin reorganization that presumably results from the progressively increasing calcium and decreasing ATP of ISCs.

These data provide evidence of altered spectrin organization in membranes of ATP-depleted, calcium-enriched red cells in vitro and in vivo.

Key words: **red cell membrane proteins, spectrin, red cell shape, deformability, membrane protein cross-linking, membrane protein disulfide coupling, red cell adenosine triphosphate, calcium, membrane protein polymerization, discocyte–echinocyte transformation, irreversibly sickled cells, sickle cell anemia**

Viscoelastic properties of erythrocyte membranes are principally determined by the two-dimensional network of peripheral membrane proteins spectrin and actin, laminating the internal side of the membrane [1–4]. Changes in physical properties and molecular organization of these proteins in red cells undergoing decrease in intracellular ATP and accumulation of calcium have been implicated in alterations of cell shape, deformability, and membrane stability [5–8].

In this review, we examine the organization of spectrin and other membrane proteins in red cell membranes as a function of intracellular ATP and calcium concentrations in vitro, and we discuss their possible significance for the control of cell shape and deformability. We further report our studies on membrane protein organization of irreversibly sickled cells, which exhibit increased calcium [9–10], and a decreased ATP content [11, 12]. Their stabilization in an irreversibly sickled shape has been related to a permanent deformation of their membranes [13]. We employed cross-linking of nearest membrane protein neighbors by intermolecular disulfide couplings produced by catalytic oxidation of red cell ghosts or by spontaneous oxidation during aerobic incubation of intact red cells.

MATERIALS AND METHODS

Venous blood was collected into heparin Vacutainers, red cells were separated by centrifugation and washed, and white cells and platelets were removed by aspiration of the buffy coat after each washing. Red cells were suspended at 20% hematocrit in an isotonic solution containing 50 mM glycylglycine (pH 7.4 at 37°C), 5 mM KCl, 2 mM $CaCl_2$, 2 mM $MgCl_2$, and NaCl to 290 mOsm and were incubated under air or nitrogen with gentle mixing [14]. At specified times, red cells were separated from supernatants and white ghosts were prepared by hemolysis in 30 volumes of 10 mM Tris-HCl buffer (pH 7.4) followed by two washings [14]. Part of the ghost pellet was subjected to oxidative cross-linking by reacting the ghosts with 30 volumes of $CuSO_4$ (10 μM), O-phenanthroline (50 μM), at 25°C for 10 min. Selected samples were also cross-linked with 2 mM glutaraldehyde in 10 mM HEPES (pH 7.4) at 25°C for 30 min. The details have been described previously [15, 16].

Ghosts were solubilized in SDS solution and subjected to two-dimensional PAGE [17]. In analyzing cleavable (oxidative) cross-linkings, membrane proteins were first separated in cylindrical gels without DTT reduction. The composition of the cross-linked complexes was identified by placing the first-dimension gels horizontally on the top of the second-dimension slab gel. After passage through a DTT zone to cleave the intermolecular disulfide crosslinks, membrane proteins were separated in the second dimension on the slab gels and identified according to their relative mobilities as compared to a standard membrane sample. In some examples, the proteins of the cross-linked complexes were quantified by densitometric scanning of Coomassie blue-stained gels [14].

Venous blood of patients with the homozygous form of sickle cell anemia was fractionated on discontinuous stractan gradients [18] to yield ISC-rich fractions. ISCs were identified according to criteria described by Bertles and Milner [19] by phase contrast microscopy and SEM [20]. ATP and GSH were measured as detailed by Beutler [21].

RESULTS

Oxidation-Induced Membrane Protein Cross-linkings

The two-dimensional electrophoresis of membrane proteins from fresh red cells not exposed to cross-linking is illustrated in Figure 1A. The stained replica of the first-dimension cylindrical gel is positioned horizontally on top of the slab gel. After electrophoresis in the second dimension, membrane proteins separated, forming a skewed line. The individual spots were identified from their relative mobilities as compared to a reference membrane sample in an identical gel system and denoted by arabic numerals according to Fairbanks et al [22]. The dotted circles represent glycoproteins [14]. No off-diagonal spots are noted in the second dimension, indicating the absence of spontaneous oxidative cross-links in fresh red cell membranes immediately subjected to SDS PAGE.

Two-dimensional separation of membrane proteins from fresh ghosts subjected to mild catalytic oxidation (20 mM $CuSO_4$, 50 mM O-phenanthroline, 25°C, 10 min) is illustrated in Figure 1B. On the replica of the first-dimension gel, a band corresponding to MW 450,000 can be seen (first vertical arrow). After DTT cleavage and subsequent separation in the second dimension, this band can be identified as the spectrin 1 + 2 heterodimer, as indicated by the presence of these polypeptides as off-diagonal spots positioned in the same vertical line as the original complex. Additional complexes include spectrin tetramers; complexes of spectrin polypeptide 2 and band 4.9; dimers, trimers, and tetramers of band 3; and dimers of band 4.1, 4.5, and 5.

The two-dimensional separation of ATP-depleted red cell membrane proteins cross-linked by catalytic oxidation is illustrated in Figure 1C. ATP depletion was achieved by 22 h incubation (37°C) in a buffered solution without glucose. Anaerobic conditions were used to avoid spontaneous membrane protein oxidation. The cross-linking pattern of membrane proteins from ATP-depleted cells differed from that of fresh red cells in that a polymer of very high mw ($> 1 \times 10^6$) was present at the origin of the first dimension gel (note asterisk, Fig 1C). This complex was completely dissociated by DTT reduction and separated into multiple components, which include spectrin polypeptides 1 and 2; polypeptides 3, 4.5, 5; and other less easily identified components. A similar complex was formed spontaneously when red cells were incubated to deplete their ATP under aerobic conditions, and their ghosts were subsequently solubilized without cross-linking (Fig. 2). We concluded that under the latter conditions, the intermolecular disulfide couplings producing the high-molecular-weight membrane protein polymer took place spontaneously during aerobic incubation.

Densitometric scan of the large complex of cross-linked ghosts from ATP-depleted red cells is illustrated in Figure 3 and compared to a reference sample of normal mem-

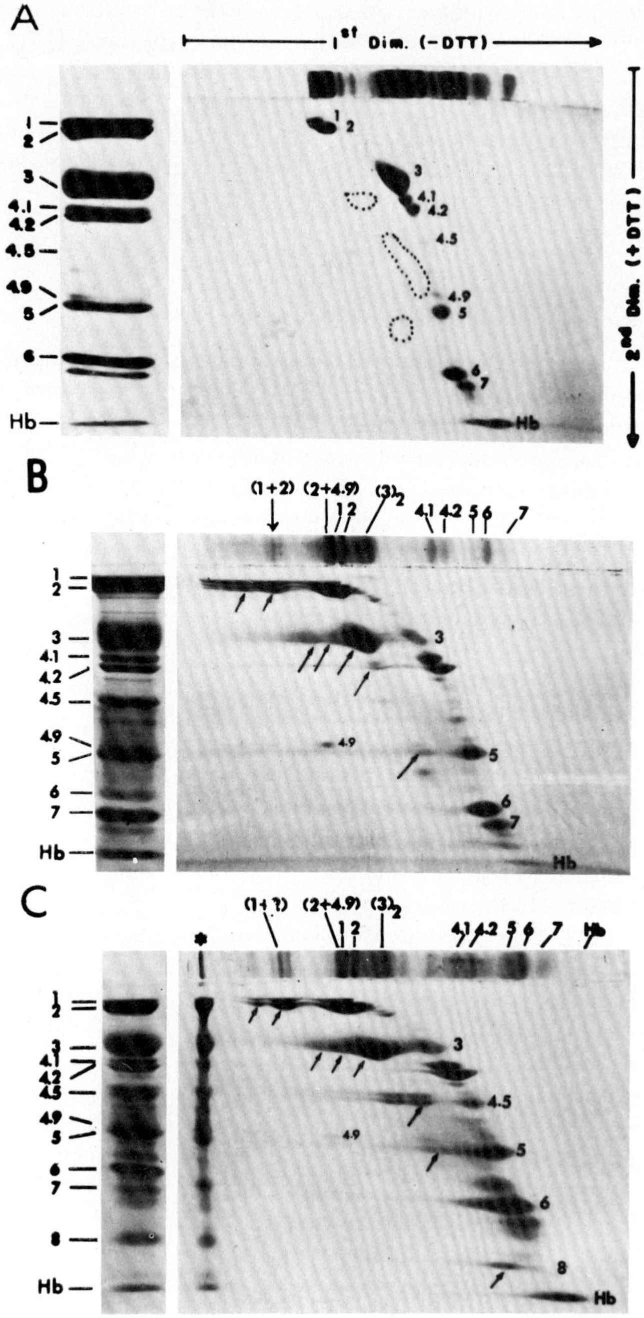
A
1st Dim. (-DTT)
2nd Dim. (+DTT)
1
2
3
4.1
4.2
4.5
4.9
5
6
7
Hb
B
(1+2)
(2+4.9)
1 2
(3)2
4.1 4.2 5 6 7
C
(1+?)
(2+4.9)
1 2
(3)2
4.1 4.2 5 6 7 Hb
8

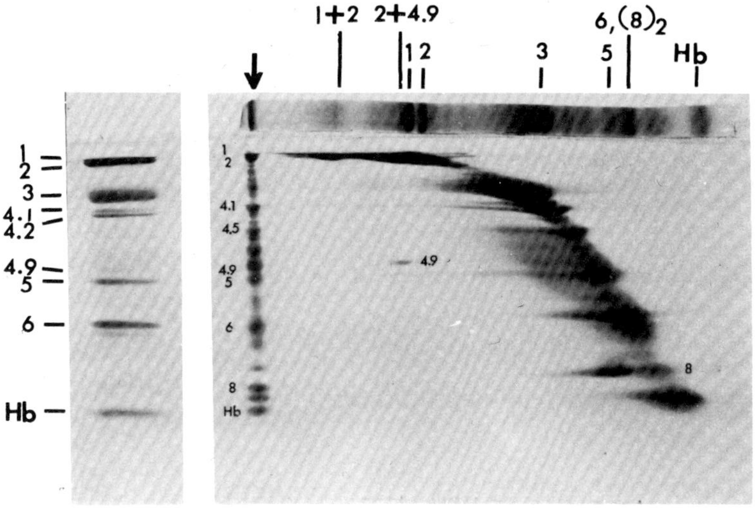

Fig. 2. Two-dimensional PAGE of membrane proteins (250 μg) from red cells depleted in ATP by incubation under air for 24 hours. These were not subjected to catalytic oxidation. Arrow indicates a spontaneously formed large molecular weight polymer (> 10^6 daltons) in the first dimension and the cleaved components in the second dimension. (Reprinted from Ref 14 with permission of publishers.)

Fig. 1. Two-dimensional PAGE of cross-linked proteins ($CuSO_4$/O-phenanthroline) in isolated membranes from fresh and ATP-depleted erythrocytes.
A) Fresh ghosts (100 μg protein) that were not subjected to cross-linking were fractionated in the first dimension by electrophoresis in SDS agarose (0.3%)-polyacrylamide (2.5%) composite gels without DTT reduction. Electrophoresis in the second dimension was performed in a slab, incorporating a DTT zone to cleave the possible disulfide bonds. The pattern of membrane sample applied directly is shown at the left for reference. The pattern obtained by electrophoresis in the first dimension is shown in a stained replicate gel placed on top of the slab. Off-diagonal elements indicated by a dotted curve probably represents glycoproteins. The indiviudal polypeptides are numbered according to Fairbanks et al [22].
B) Ghosts from fresh erythrocytes were cross-linked by catalytic oxidation with $CuSO_4$ (10 μM) + O-phenanthroline (50 μM) at 25°C for 10 min. Membrane proteins were electrophoresed in the first dimension without a prior DTT reduction. Second dimension was run as described in Figure 1A. Arrows indicate polymers of spectrin – ie, (1 + 2), $(1 + 2)_2$ – band 3 – ie, $(3)_2$, $(3)_3$, $(3)_4$ – and dimers of 4.1, 4.5, and 5.
C) Ghosts from ATP-depleted erythrocytes (37°C, under nitrogen, 24 hours) were analyzed as in Figure 1B. The asterisk at the origin represents the large molecular weight polymer (>1 × 10^6 daltons). Note also a dimer of band 8. (Reprinted from Ref 23 with permission of publishers.)

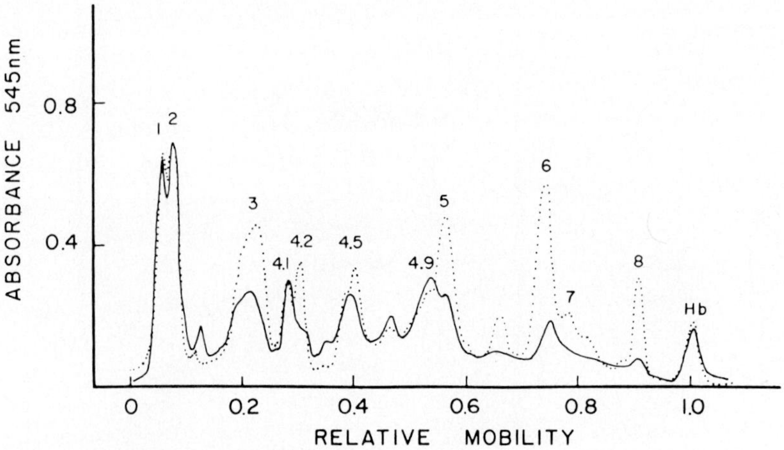

Fig. 3. Densitometric scans of Coomassie blue-stained proteins released from the > 1 × 10^6 daltons polymer after DTT reduction. (This polymer is depicted in Figure 1C.) Dotted line shows a reference membrane sample separated in an identical gel system. (Reprinted from Ref 23 with permission of publishers.)

brane proteins separated in an identical gel system. It can be seen that this high-molecular-weight complex was selectively enriched in spectrin, whereas the ratio of band 3 to spectrin (0.45) was considerably less than in normal red cell membranes (1.0). In the following text, this large complex of mw > 1 × 10^6 is referred to as spectrin-rich polymer.

Glutaraldehyde Cross-Linking

We investigated whether the spectrin-rich polymer of ATP-depleted red cells reflected an altered spectrin organization in the membrane in which spectrin neighbors came into closer contact. For this we employed another cross-linking agent, glutaraldehyde, which produces irreversible cross-links between the adjacent amino groups in the red cell membrane.

Glutaraldehyde cross-linking of red cells depleted of ATP under anaerobic conditions produced a polymer resembling that produced by catalytic oxidation in failing to enter the gel. In contrast, such polymers were not formed by glutaraldehyde cross-linking of ghosts from fresh cells (not shown). Reproducible demonstration of differences in membrane protein cross-linking between fresh and ATP-depleted red cells required careful maintenance of temperature, time, and concentration of the reactants. Increased temperature, cross-linking times or concentrations of these reagents produced high-molecular-weight complexes both in membranes of depleted and fresh cells, presumably due to membrane perturbation resulting from a more extensive cross-linking.

ATP Dependence on the Spectrin-Rich Polymer

Spontaneous formation of the spectrin-rich polymer is markedly dependent on red cell ATP content, as illustrated in Fig. 4. The amount of spectrin-rich polymer increases progressively as red cells undergo ATP depletion under aerobic conditions. The formation of this complex was completely inhibited by maintenance of red cell ATP level (Fig. 4B, 1st gel). In addition, aerobically ATP-depleted erythrocytes exhibited a spontaneous formation of two additional complexes of mw, 450,000 and 260,000. These represented complexes 1 + 2 and 2 + 4.9, respectively, as documented by analysis in the second dimension after DTT reduction, shown in Fig. 2.

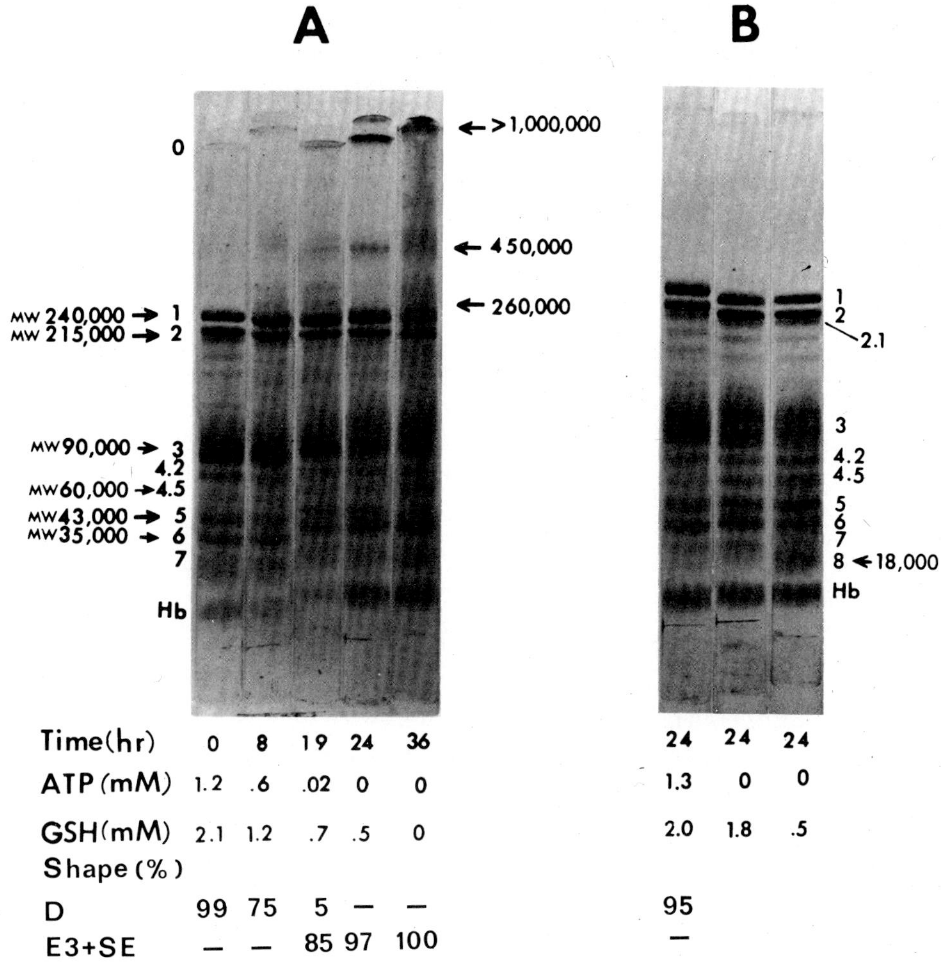

Fig. 4. Formation of large molecular weight complexes of membrane proteins during red cell ATP depletion in vitro.
A) Relationships between changes in red cell ATP, GSH, shape, and membrane protein composition during aerobic incubation of red cells at 37°C without glucose. Membrane proteins were separated by electrophoresis in SDS agarose (0.3%)-acrylamide (2.5%) composite gels without DTT reduction.
B) Inhibition of the formation of large molecular weight complexes by a maintenance of red cell ATP with adenine (0.5 mM), inosine (12.7 mM), glucose (2 gm/liter, 1st gel), anaerobic incubation (N_2, 2nd gel), or DTT (25 mM) reduction before electrophoresis (3rd gel). D, E3, and SE depict the percent of discocytes, echinocytes 3, and spheroechinocytes classified according to Ref 24. (Reprinted from Ref 14 with permission of publishers.)

The bottom part of Fig. 4 indicates a relationship of the spectrin-rich complex to cellular shape. It can be seen that appreciable amounts of the spectrin-rich polymer were noted in cell populations showing 80% conversion to echinocytes 3 or spheroechinocytes (classified according to Bessis [247]). ATP repletion was associated with a partial recovery of biconcave shape and a decrease (40–60%) in the staining intensity of the high-molecular-weight complex (not shown). The spectrin-rich polymer was absent in cross-linked ghosts from red cells in which echinocytic shape was produced by lysolecithin (0.1 mM). On the other hand, a spectrin-rich complex was noted in aerobically ATP-depleted erythrocytes in which biconcave shape was maintained by the addition of cationic anesthetic (such as 40 mM procaine HCl) to the incubation medium (not shown). These data indicate direct relationships of the spectrin-rich polymer to cellular ATP content; on the other hand, ATP-independent shape changes appeared to be without effect on the formation of this polymer.

Since aerobic ATP depletion or ghost exposure to catalytic oxidation is associated with a marked decrease in GSH, we investigated the relative contributions of GSH and ATP in the formation of the spectrin-rich polymer and the complexes of 1 + 2 and 2 + 4.9. We have incubated G6PD-deficient red cells aerobically with adenine, inosine, and glucose and an oxidant, acetylphenylhydrazine (4 mM). These cells maintained normal ATP levels (70% of preincubation value) while they exhibited a marked GSH depletion (10% of pre-incubation value). The oxidative injury to these cells was manifested morphologically by the formation of five or more Heinz bodies per cell in more than 90% of these cells (not shown). As shown in Figure 5, such cells exhibited spontaneous formation of spectrin heterodimer 1 + 2 and a complex of 2 + 4.9. They further contained a high-molecular-weight protein complex at the start of the first-dimension gel (arrow of Fig. 5); however, after dissociation by DTT and subsequent separation in the second dimension, this polymer was found to consist almost exclusively of globin subunits. Thus, oxidative damage to cells containing normal ATP content resulted in an extensive disulfide coupling of globin and a formation of complexes 1 + 2 and 2 + 4.9. However, it failed to produce the large spectrin-rich polymer.

The above data suggest that the spontaneous formation of the high-molecular-weight spectrin-rich polymer of ATP-depleted red cells is a consequence of two processes. First, spectrin and other membrane proteins rearrange to close contact with each other, presumably because of protein aggregation. Second, these aggregated proteins are subsequently coupled by disulfide cross-links. These take place spontaneously when ATP depletion is performed under aerobic conditions. We have shown that i) the first process, that is, the "rearrangement" of spectrin, is prevented by a maintenance of ATP content, and ii) the

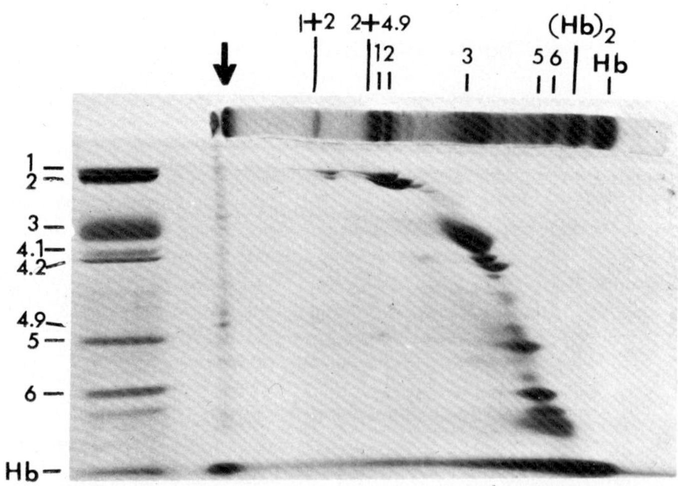

Fig. 5. Two-dimensional PAGE of membrane proteins of acetylphenylhydrazine-treated G6PD-deficient erythrocytes. Red cells were incubated under air with 4 mM acetylphenylhydrazine for 3 hours. Arrows indicate the large aggregate at the origin of the first dimension. (Reprinted from Ref 14 with permission of publishers.)

second process can be reversed by reducing agents which dissociate the above disulfide cross-links. We further explored whether the first process, ie, the spectrin "rearrangement," is reversible with ATP repletion. We have depleted red cells in ATP under anaerobic conditions (to prevent a spontaneous protein disulfide coupling) and subsequently restored ATP content with adenine and inosine. Ghosts from both ATP-depleted and -repleted cells were subsequently subjected to cross-linking with catalytic oxidation and examined for the presence of spectrin-rich polymer. Maintenance of ATP content completely suppressed the propensity of the cells to form the spectrin-rich complex after catalytic oxidation. In contrast, ATP-depleted red cells in which the ATP content was subsequently restored to 40–60% of the original level (90% of which recovered their discoidal shape) continued to form this polymer after a subsequent catalytic oxidation (not shown). This suggests that the rearrangement of spectrin to closer contacts, as reflected by the formation of this complex, is ATP-dependent. However, once this rearrangement occurs, it cannot be reversed by a subsequent ATP repletion, and it does not appear to relate directly to changes in cell shape.

Role of Calcium

Since shape and deformability alterations of red cells undergoing ATP depletion can be mimicked by introduction of calcium into red cells or ghosts [5, 8, 25, 26], we tested the role of Ca^{++} in the formation of the spectrin-rich polymer The following three approaches were used. First, exclusion of calcium from the incubation medium failed to prevent the formation of this complex during aerobic incubation without metabolizable substrates (not shown).

Second, we tested the effect of chelating agents on ghosts of ATP-depleted red cells. We have previously observed that the calcium accumulating in red cell membranes during ATP depletion was nearly completely extracted by washing ghosts with EDTA [27]. However, EDTA washing did not prevent the formation of spectrin-rich polymer after catalytic oxidation of ghosts from ATP-depleted red cells (not shown).

The third approach consisted in loading fresh red cells or their ghosts with increasing calcium concentration. When red cells were exposed to the calcium ionophore A23137 and 0.1 mM Ca^{++} (60 min, 37°C) and their ghosts were subsequently subjected to oxidative cross-linking, a high-molecular-weight complex was again found, provided that the same concentration of external calcium was maintained during ghost preparation prior to cross-linking (not shown). However, such cells also exhibited a decrease in ATP (to 40% of preincubation values), as also shown by others [28].

Exposure of washed, white ghosts to Ca^{++} followed by oxidative cross-linking failed to produce a reducible high-molecular-weight polymer unless the Ca^{++} concentration exceeded 2 mM. The introduction of 10^{-6} to 10^{-4}M Ca^{++} into ghosts during hemolysis, followed by oxidative cross-linking, produced an extensive background smearing which did not permit examination of the above high-molecular-weight protein complexes (not shown). Hemolysis in Ca^{++} at 0.5 mM followed by incubation at 37°C yielded spontaneous formation of a protein polymer at the start of the gel (Fig. 6) which differed from the spectrin-rich polymer of ATP-depleted red cells by its complete resistance to DTT cleavage. This polymer could not be reproduced when ghosts were washed prior to the exposure to calcium. However, a subsequent addition of a ghost-free hemolysate restored the spontaneous formation of this complex (not shown). In contrast to fresh red cells, ATP-depleted erythrocytes (both under O_2 or N_2) exposed to similar calcium concentrations during hemolysis failed to produce such a complex. Subsequent exposure of

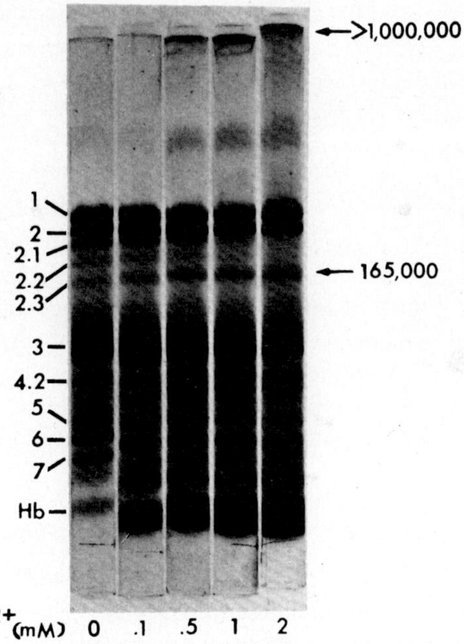

Fig. 6. Ca^{2+}-induced membrane protein polymerization. Fresh washed erythrocytes were lysed with 10 mM Tris buffer, pH 7.4, containing various Ca^{2+} concentrations and incubated at 37°C for 30 min. Ghosts were subsequently washed twice with 10 mM Tris, pH 7.4, and then subjected to PAGE in the presence of DTT. (Reprinted from Ref 23 with permission of the publishers.)

washed ghosts from ATP-depleted red cells to a ghost-free hemolysate from fresh red cells restored their propensity to form the high-molecular-weight nonreducible polymer. These data suggest i) requirement of a cytoplasmic constituent for polymer formation and ii) its dependence on intracellular ATP levels (eg, inhibition by ATP depletion). Others have shown that the formation of this polymer is related to calcium activation of cytoplasmic transglutaminase, which forms covalent cross-links among δ-glutamyl—ϵ-lysine residues of spectrin, band 3, and presumably other membrane and cytoplasmic proteins [29, 30]. The enzyme is dependent on ATP level [31].

Stabilization of Red Cell Shape by Membrane Protein Polymerization

Since some cross-linking agents are used as biologic fixatives, we investigated whether the above-mentioned membrane protein polymers contributed to irreversibility of spheroechinocytic shape. Table I depicts the propensity of ATP-depleted echinocytes to resume biconcave shape after a subsequent ATP repletion. The restoration of ATP levels in red cells previously depleted of ATP under aerobic conditions (producing the spectrin-rich polymer in the membrane) was associated with a considerably slower and incomplete restoration of biconcave shape when compared to anaerobically ATP-depleted red cells which did not form the complex spontaneously [14]. The exposure of the cross-linked cells to DTT reduction (which completely dissociates the polymer) markedly improved their ability to resume biconcave shape. No major differences were noted in the kinetics of restoration of ATP levels under both conditions (Table I). These data suggest that the delayed and incomplete reversal of aerobically ATP-depleted echinocytes to discocytes

TABLE I. Restoration of Biconcave Shape and ATP and GSH Levels of ATP-Depleted Red Cells During Subsequent Incubation (37°C) With Glucose, Adenine, and Inosine*

	Time (hours)			
	0	1	2	4
Discocytes (%)				
N_2	0	92	98	98
O_2	0	31	48	68
O_2 & DTT	0	86	88	89
ATP (%)				
N_2	10	32	38	37
O_2	10	30	32	33
Air & DTT	10	31	30	32
GSH (%)				
N_2	90	80	90	100
O_2	0	35	65	75

*Red cells were depleted in ATP by 18 hours (37°C) of incubation without glucose under 100% nitrogen or oxygen. DTT was added at a final concentration of 4 mM. Mean values of three experiments. ATP and GSH are expressed as % of preincubation levels.

TABLE II. Dependence of the Formation of the Nonreducible Membrane Protein Polymer and the Percentage of Irreversible Spheroechinocytes on Ca^{2+} Concentration

External Ca^{2+} concentration (mM)[a]	0.1	0.5	1.0	2.0	2.0 + histamine
Nonreducible[b] polymer (%)	0	7	25	100	8
Irreversible spheroechinocytes (%)[c]	7	12	36	100	11

[a]Fresh red cells were exposed to A23187 and Ca^{2+} (1 hour, 37°C). Histamine concentration (last column) was 40 mM.
[b]The polymer is expressed as percent of the amounts produced by 2 mM Ca^{2+}, as measured planimetrically after densitometric scanning of Coomassie blue-stained gels.
[c]Counted after 16 hours of incubation with glucose, adenine, and inosine. ATP was repleted to 80–120% of preincubation values and > 95% of ^{45}Ca was extruded from the cells after incubation. Mean values of four experiments.

during ATP repletion was related to oxidative cross-linking of membrane proteins which stabilized the altered spectrin arrangement in such cells.

The nonreducible polymer produced by 0.5 mM Ca^{++} + A23187 had a similar stabilizing effect on cell shape. Table II illustrates that a progressively increased formation of this complex, produced by exposure of cells to increasing external concentrations of Ca^{++} (in the presence of A23187) coincided with increased percentage of cells which retained spheroechinocytic shape after a subsequent ATP repletion and extrusion of calcium from the cells. Transglutaminase inhibition by histamine prevented the formation of the nonreducible polymer and nearly completely restored the propensity of such cells to transform into biconcave and stomatocytic shapes (Fig. 7).

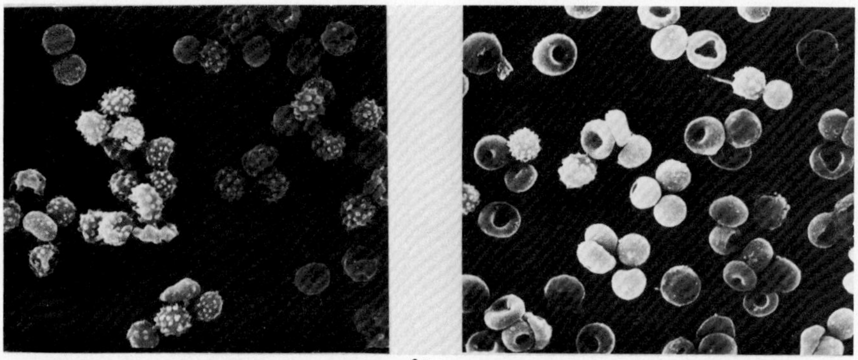

Fig. 7. 1. SEM of red cells treated with 2 mM Ca^{2+} and A23187 for 1 hour, followed by 17 hours of incubation with glucose, adenine, and inosine (left). 2. The SEM on the right depicts the same conditions, except that 40 mM histamine was present at the time of exposure of cells to Ca^{2+}.

Irreversibly Sickled Cells

The calcium content of ISC-enriched (54 ± 8%) HbSS red cells is higher than that of non-ISC HbSS cells (ISCs: 66 ± 12 μmoles/liter cells; unseparated HbSS red cells: 50 ± 21 μmoles/liter cells). It is almost four times higher than that of normal erythrocytes (18 ± 6 μmoles/liter of cells [9]. Furthermore, ISCs exhibit a decrease in ATP content [11, 12]. We have examined ISC membrane protein composition in order to evaluate a possible role of the membrane protein polymerization in irreversibly sickled shape.

ISCs were separated from blood of individuals with the homozygous form of sickle cell anemia (HbSS) using a five-step discontinuous stractan gradient. HbSS red cells were separated thereby into five fractions (Fig. 8). Fraction 1 (top) contained no ISCs; fractions 3, 4, and 5 all contained > 80% ISCs. Fractions 1–5 also exhibited progressively increasing mean corpuscular hemoglobin concentrations (MCHC) from 34 to 41% and decreasing mean volumes (MCV) from 96 to 61. ISCs from the two densest fractions were subsequently washed and subjected to analysis of membrane protein composition before and after cross-linking with catalytic oxidation or glutaraldehyde.

Figure 9A illustrates protein composition of ISC-free HbSS red cell ghosts (fraction 1), HbSS cells containing 90% ISCs (fraction 4 + 5), and ghosts, from aerobically ATP-depleted red cells. It is apparent that both ISC-free and ISC-rich HbSS red cells failed to exhibit large complexes of proteins in untreated membranes. However, both ISCs and to a lesser extent non-ISC HbSS cells shared with ATP-depleted red cells an increased retention of band 4.5 (membrane-attached catalase [33, 34]) and globin. Likewise, ISC membrane protein cross-linking with both catalytic oxidation (Fig. 9B) and glutaraldehyde (not shown) failed to produce high-molecular-weight protein complexes in these membranes under conditions that readily induce cross-linking in membranes from ATP-depleted cells. Thus, the ISC lesion does not appear to result from a stabilization of ISC shape by membrane protein cross-linking; presumably the degree of ATP depletion and calcium accumulation in ISCs is not sufficiently high to produce these changes.

ISC-Spheroechinocyte Transformation

Figure 10 depicts scanning electron micrographs of ISCs from fractions 3 and 5. It is apparent that ISCs exhibited a considerable morphologic heterogeneity: ISCs of relatively low densities (fraction 3) had an elongated shape with a central concavity, while 5–10%

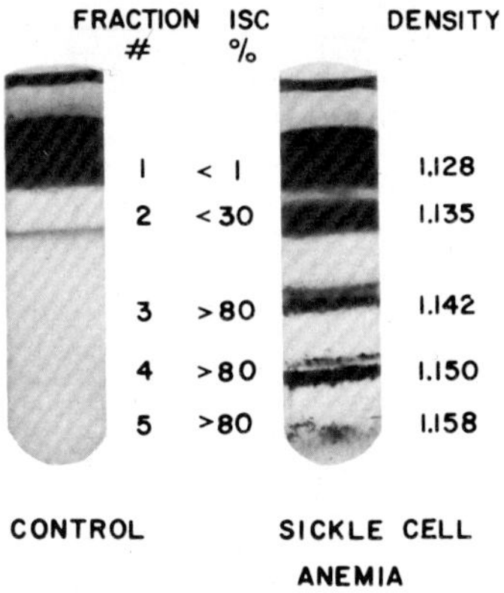

Fig. 8. ISC separation on a discontinuous stractan gradient. (Reprinted from Ref 32 with permission of publishers.)

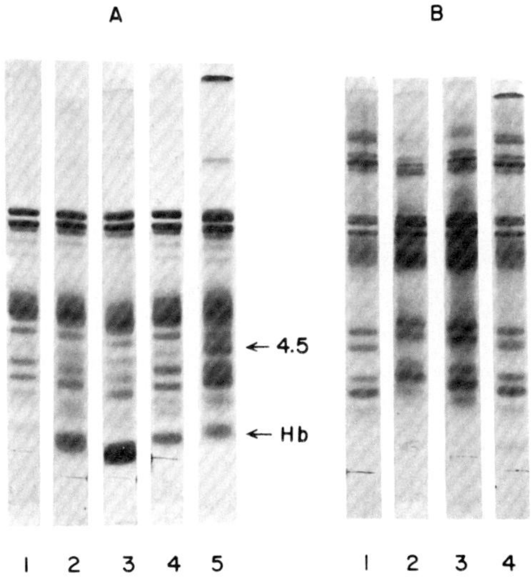

Fig. 9. PAGE of ISC ghost proteins before (A) and after (B) cross-linking by catalytic oxidation, as described in Figure 1. All samples were prepared in the absence of DTT. Otherwise, the gel system was the same as that described in Figure 3. 1) Fresh normal red cells; 2) Top HbSS fraction 1 containing no ISCs; 3) Bottom ISC-rich fractions 4 + 5 (combined); 4) ATP-depleted red cells (22 hours, 37°C) under anaerobic conditions; 5) ATP-depleted red cells under aerobic conditions. (Reprinted from Ref 23 with permission of publishers.)

of the densest cells (fraction 5) had an elliptical shape and an extensive surface speculation. These shape changes were not artifacts of stractan separation, as pooling of all the cells followed by differencial counting yielded a percentage of echinocytic ISCs (1%) similar to the fresh, unseparated HbSS blood. These data suggest that ISCs undergo a discocyte-to-echinocyte transformation in vivo, presumably as a result of progressively increasing calcium accumulation and ATP depletion.

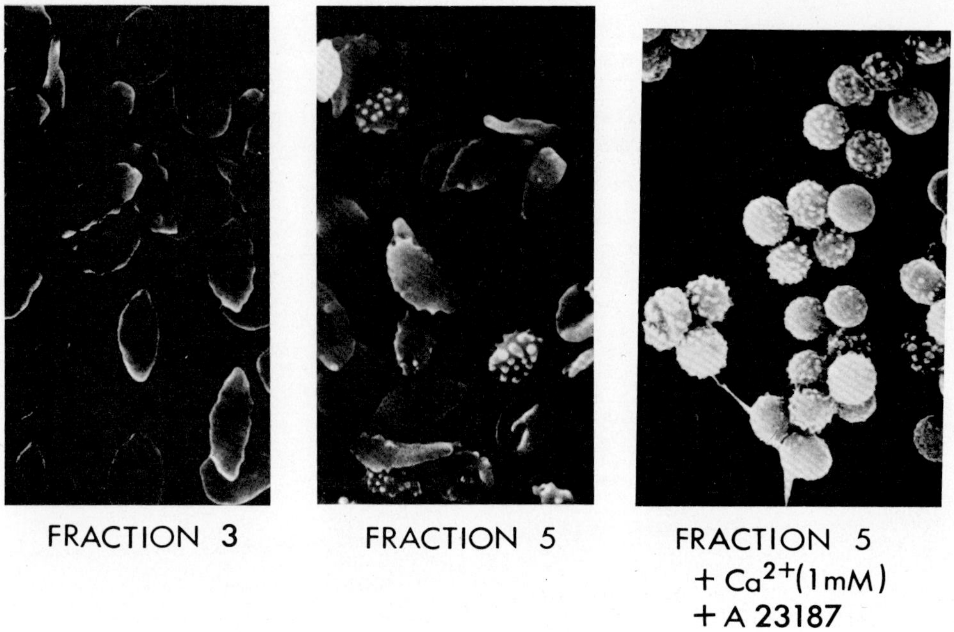

Fig. 10. SEM of ISCs from fraction 3, fraction 5, and combined fractions 4 + 5 exposed to Ca^{2+} (1 mM) and calcium ionophore A23187 (10 μM) for 60 min at 37°C. (Adapted from Refs 23 and 32 with permission of publishers.)

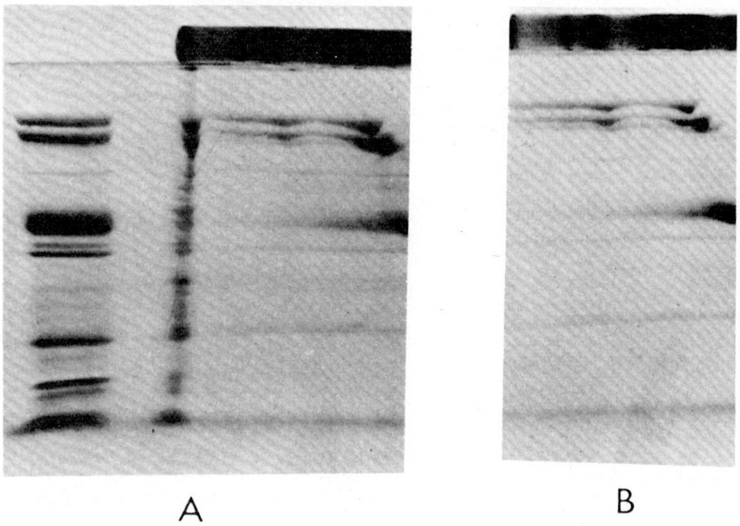

Fig. 11. Accelerated formation of the spectrin-rich complex during incubation (6 hours, 37°C) of ISCs without glucose. A) ISC-rich fractions 4 + 5 (combined); B) HbSS cells from fraction 1, containing no ISCs. Cross-linking of ghosts from incubated ISCs and PAGE was done as described in Figure 1. (Reprinted from Ref 32 with permission of publishers.)

The above hypothesis is supported by the data shown in Fig. 10, which illustrates that ISCs (fraction 5, 90% ISCs) can be efficiently (90%) converted into spheroechinocytes after exposure to 2 mM Ca^{++} + A23187. Furthermore, ISCs exhibited an increased propensity to form the spectrin-rich reducible polymer during aerobic incubation without glucose. Figure 11 illustrates that after 6 h of incubation, the top, ISC-free HbSS red cells did not form any spectrin-rich polymer, while the dense ISC-rich fraction 4 + 5 produced considerable amounts of this complex. More than 80% of these incubated ISCs were converted to type 3 echinocytes or spheroechinocytes (not shown). The increased propensity of ISCs to form the spectrin-rich reducible complex and transform into echinocytic shapes during a subsequent incubation without glucose is presumably related to their decreased ATP and increased calcium content in vivo.

DISCUSSION

ATP-Calcium Dependence of Membrane Protein Organization

Our cross-linking studies revealed major differences between the nearest membrane protein neighbors of fresh and ATP-depleted red cell membranes. Oxidation of the intermolecular SH groups of fresh red cell ghosts resulted in formation of dimers and tetramers of spectrin, dimers of band 3 and actin, and a 2 + 4.9 complex. In contrast, disulfide coupling of ATP-depleted erythrocyte ghosts produced an additional protein complex of mw $> 1 \times 10^6$ (Table III).

This polymer was produced by three different types of cross-linking: a) $CuSO_4$, O-phenanthroline-catalyzed intermolecular disulfide coupling, b) spontaneous disulfide couplings in intact red cells during their aerobic ATP depletion, and c) glutaraldehyde cross-linking. The reducible polymer of ATP-depleted red cells was selectively enriched in spectrin, while the relative amounts of actin and band 3, the major transmembrane polypeptide, were lower than in normal red cell membranes. We conclude that red cell ATP depletion alters spectrin organization within the membrane to produce more intimate contacts, which in turn allow an easier cross-linking of the individual spectrin subunits into the large polymer. It is not likely that the increased propensity of spectrin to cross-linking relates to 1) a conformational change exposing a previously masked SH group, or 2) a dissociation from the membrane binding site that increases its lateral mobility and hence increases the chance of collisions. The first possibility is unlikely because other agents, such as glutaraldehyde, which cross-links protein amino groups, produced a similar polymer. Likewise, we exclude the second possibility, as the cross-linking could also be produced at temperatures close to 0°C, when membrane proteins exhibit only a limited lateral mobility.

The dependence of the formation of spectrin-rich polymer on red cell ATP depletion is suggested by an absence of this polymer in cells in which ATP has been maintained during incubation. These ATP-maintained cells failed to exhibit this polymer after cross-linking with both catalytic oxidation and glutaraldehyde. In contrast, this polymer was produced by the above-mentioned cross-linkings in cells which were first depleted in ATP and subsequently ATP-repleted by incubation with adenine-inosine, which suggests an irreversibility of the ATP-dependent reorganization of spectrin to closer contacts. It should be pointed out that the partial disappearance of this complex during ATP repletion of cells previously depleted in ATP under aerobic conditions should not be interpreted as indicating the reversibility of this process. Under the latter circumstances, cells apparently generate a reducing power which cleaves the disulfide cross-linkages but spectrin remains rearranged into closer contacts.

TABLE III. Oxidative Membrane Protein Cross-Linkings of Fresh and ATP-Depleted Red Cells

	Fresh	ATP-depleted
$(1 + 2)_2$	+	+
(2 + 4.9)	+	+
$(3)_2$	+	+
$(5)_2$	+	+
Spectrin-rich (10^3K) complex	−	+

Polymer formation is apparently not controlled by intracellular Ca^{++}, but our data on this point are not conclusive. First, the formation of the spectrin-rich polymer during aerobic ATP depletion was not influenced by exclusion of calcium from the incubation medium. However, normal red cells contain 3.5 μM of exchangeable calcium per liter of cells (presumably as a calcium ATP complex [27]), which after depletion of intracellular ATP may interact with the membrane, thereby producing the spectrin-rich polymer even in the absence of a net calcium accumulation. Second, Ca^{++} treatment of washed, white ghosts from fresh red cells, followed by oxidative cross-linking, failed to produce the polymer unless the Ca^{++} concentrations exceeded 2 mM. In contrast, treatment of fresh red cells with 0.1 mM Ca^{++} + A23187 virtually duplicated the effects of ATP depletion. However, these cells also exhibited a marked decrease in intracellular ATP. Third, the exposure of ghosts from anaerobically ATP-depleted cells to EDTA, which extracts calcium accumulating in membranes of ATP-depleted red cells [27], failed to prevent the formation of this polymer after subsequent ghost cross-linking with catalytic oxidation. The latter data suggest, but do not prove, that ATP depletion alone rather than a concomitant calcium-membrane interaction is responsible for changes in spectrin organization of ATP-depleted erythrocytes.

In contrast to the formation of a reducible spectrin-rich polymer in ATP-depleted erythrocytes, red cells exposed to 0.5 mM Ca^{++} + A23187 spontaneously produced a high-molecular-weight polymer which resisted cleavage by DTT. This complex was recently shown to result from covalent cross-links between δ-glutamyl—ε-lysine residues of the nearest spectrin, band 3, and other membrane protein neighbors catalyzed by a Ca^{++}-activated cytoplasmic transglutaminase [29, 30]. This polymer could not be reproduced in ATP-depleted red cells, presumably because the enzyme is inhibited by ATP depletion [31].

Role of Spectrin-Rich Polymer in Discocyte-Echinocyte Equilibrium

Several laboratories [35–38] provided indirect support for the hypothesis that the stomatocyte-discocyte-echinocyte equilibrium depends on the relationships between the surface areas of the inner and outer halves of the membrane lipid bilayer. We speculate that the echinocyte transformation of ATP-depleted red cells is related to a reorganization of spectrin to establish closer contacts. Assuming that spectrin and actin form a two-dimensional network [4], this rearrangement could produce a decrease in surface area both of the spectrin-actin network and the closely associated inner half of the membrane lipid bilayer. The resulting bilayer asymmetry would then be reflected in an echinocytic shape change. However, this model cannot account for the observation that during ATP repletion cells restore their biconcave shape despite the fact that spectrin remains reorganized into closer contacts.

Although no direct comparisons between the formation of the reducible spectrin-rich polymer and changes in membrane deformability are to be found in the literature, it is likely that altered spectrin interactions in ATP-depleted red cells may result in changes of membrane deformability. This possibility is suggested by recent observations of decreased membrane deformability of cells exposed to cross-linking agents such as glutaraldehyde [39] and kinetic similarities in the formation of spectrin-rich polymer and changes in red cell deformability [5, 14].

Irreversibly Sickled Cells

ISCs which maintain their characteristic elongated shape even after prolonged oxygenation are rigid, dehydrated cells with a markedly shortened survival in the circulation (for references see Palek [13]). ISC shape deformation has also been found in ghosts and in spectrin-actin residues prepared by extraction of lipids and integral membrane proteins from red cell membranes [40].

Since both the reducible spectrin-rich polymer of aerobically ATP-depleted red cells and the nonreducible polymer of calcium-enriched fresh erythrocytes contributed to a stabilization of red cells in the spheroechinocytic configuration, and since ISCs exhibit increased calcium and decreased ATP content, we evaluated the role of membrane protein polymerization in the stabilization of ISC shape.

Although HbSS red cell separation on the discontinuous stractan gradient allowed us to isolate HbSS red cell populations containing > 90% USCs (Fig. 8), we were unable to find either of the two polymers in freshly isolated ISCs, including the densest ISC-rich fraction 5 (Fig. 9). Likewise, no high-molecular-weight polymer was seen after a subsequent exposure of ISC ghosts to cross-linking by catalytic oxidation or glutaraldehyde. Thus, it is unlikely that spectrin rearrangement and polymerization contributed to a permanent shape fixation of these cells, presumably because the calcium gain and ATP depletion in ISCs did not reach the levels required for spectrin rearrangement and polymerization.

The shape heterogeneity of ISCs separated on a discontinuous stractan gradient suggested that ISCs undergo an ISC discocyte-to-echinocyte transformation in vivo which may be related to a progressive calcium accumulation and ATP depletion in these cells. This possibility is supported by the following findings. First, ISC exposure to Ca^{++} + A23187 resulted in their transformation to spheroechinocytes. Second, during incubation without glucose, ISCs formed a spectrin-rich polymer considerably earlier than the non-ISC HbSS red cells; at the same time, the incubated ISCs assumed an echinocytic shape. Third, when ISCs were formed in vitro during incubation of deoxygenated HbSS red cells under conditions leading to progressive ATP depletion and calcium accumulation, the resulting ISC-shaped cells exhibited an extensive surface spiculation [27]. In contrast, when deoxygenated HbSS red cells were incubated in the absence of the external calcium and under conditions maintaining intracellular ATP levels, the resulting in vitro ISCs lacked a surface spiculation and occasionally exhibited a central concavity.

On the basis of these observations, we conclude that the permanent stabilization of ISC shape does not require ATP depletion and calcium accumulation. In contrast, the additional physical alterations of ISCs, namely, their dehydration [41], decreased deformability, and ultimately echinocyte transformation, may be related to a progressive calcium accumulation and ATP depletion of these cells. The preferential calcium accumulation in ISCs may be related to their high concentration of hemoglobin S relative to hemoglobin F [19] and a known dependence of calcium influx on the concentration of hemoglobin S in the cells [9]. Thus, the progressive calcium accumulation and ATP depletion in ISCs may result in their progressive dehydration, decrease deformability, and ultimately a transformation into spheroechinocytic ISCs. Presumably, the latter ISCs represent an end-stage lesion, resulting in a removal of these cells from circulation.

ACKNOWLEDGMENTS

This study was supported by National Institutes of Health grant HL15157. We appreciate the skilled technical help of Maureen Monroe, Brian Timura, and Robert Lundin.

REFERENCES

1. Evans EA, Hochmuth RM: J Membrane Biol 30:351, 1977.
2. Evans EA, LaCelle PL: Blood 45:29, 1975.
3. LaCelle PL, Kirkpatrick FH: Erythrocyte Structure and Function (Proc 3rd Int Conf Red Cell Metabolism and Function) 535, 1974.
4. Steck TL: J Cell Biol 62:1, 1974.
5. Weed RI, LaCelle PL, Merrill EW: J Clin Invest 48:795, 1969.
6. Lux SE, John KM: In Revel JP, Henning U, Fox CF (eds): "Cell Shape and Surface Architecture." New York: Alan R Liss, 1977.
7. Lutz HU, Liu SC, Palek J: J Cell Biol 73:548, 1977.
8. Palek J, Stewart G, Lionetti FJ, Blood 44:583, 1974.
9. Palek J: J Lab Clin Med 89:1365, 1977.
10. Eaton JW, Skelton TD, Swofford HS, et al: Nature 246:105, 1973.
11. Weed RI, Bessis M: Clin Res 23:442A, 1975.
12. Glader BE, Lux SE, Muller A, et al: Clin Res 24:309A, 1976.
13. Palek J: Br J Haematol 35:1, 1977.
14. Palek J, Liu SC, Snyder LM: Blood 51:385, 1978.
15. Steck TL: J Mol Biol 66:295, 1974.
16. Wang K, Richards FM: J Biol Chem 249:8005, 1974.
17. Liu SC, Fairbanks G, Palek J: Biochemistry 16:4066, 1977.
18. Corash LM, Piomelli S, Chen AC, et al: J Lab Clin Med 84:147, 1974.
19. Bertles JF, Milner P: J Clin Invest 47:1731, 1968.
20. Palek J, Liu A, Liu D, et al: Blood 50:1955, 1977.
21. Beutler E: "Red cell metabolism – A Manual of Biochemical Methods," ed 2. New York: Grune & Stratton, 1975.
22. Fairbanks G, Steck TL, Wallach DFH: Biochemistry 10:2606, 1971.
23. Palek J, Liu SC, Liu A: In Kruckenberg WC, Eaton JW, Brewer GJ (eds): "Erythrocyte Membranes: Recent Clinical and Experimental Advances." New York: Alan R Liss, 1978.
24. Bessis M: Nouv Rev Fr Hematol 12:1, 1972.
25. Kirkpatrick FH, Hillman DG, LaCelle PL: Experientia 31:653, 1975.
26. White JG: Am J Pathol 77:507, 1974.
27. Palek J, Church A, Fairbanks G: In Leaf A, Hoffman JF, Bolis L (eds): "Membranes and Diseases." New York: Raven Press, 1976.
28. Taylor D, Baker R, Hochstein P: Biochem Biophys Res Commun 76:205, 1977.
29. Lorand L, Weissman LB, Epel DL, et al: Proc Natl Acad Sci USA 73:4479, 1976.
30. Anderson DR, Davis JL, Carraway KL: J Biol Chem 252:6617, 1977.
31. Brenner SC, Wold F: Biochim Biophys Acta 522:74, 1978.
32. Palek J, Liu SC, Liu PA: In Caughey WS (ed): "Clinical and Biochemical Aspects of Hemoglobin Abnormalities." New York: Academic Press, 1978.
33. Allen DW, Cadman S, McCann SR, et al: Blood 49:113, 1977.
34. Snyder LM, Liu SC, Palek J, et al: Biochim Biophys Acta 470:290, 1977.
35. Sheetz MP, Singer SJ: Proc Natl Acad Sci USA 71:4457, 1974.
36. Sheetz MP, Painter RG, Singer SJ: J Cell Biol 70:193, 1976.
37. Palek J, Njoku G, Liu A, et al: Blood 50:155, 1977.
38. Evans EA: Biophys J 14:923, 1974.
39. Heusinkveld RS, Goldstein DA, Weed RI, et al: Blood Cells 3:175, 1977.
40. Lux SE, John KM, Karnovsky MJ: J Clin Invest 58:955, 1976.
41. Glader BF, Miller A: Pediatr Res 9:321, 1975.

Journal of Supramolecular Structure 10:97–109 (1979)
Normal and Abnormal Red Cell Membranes 361–373

Cross-Linkings Between Spectrin and Band 3 in Human Erythrocyte Membranes

Shih-Chun Liu and Jiri Palek

Department of Research, St Elizabeth's Hospital, Boston, and Tufts University School of Medicine, Boston, Massachusetts 02135

A specific structural association between spectrin component 1 and band 3 in human erythrocyte membrane has been demonstrated by covalent cross-linkings, specific labeling, and the technique of two-dimensional gel electrophoresis. A complex of 330,000 daltons, representing 1 + 3, was produced in mildly oxidized membranes at physiologic pH and isotonic conditions but not at hypotonic conditions (< 10 mM KCl or NaCl). The yield of this complex decreased dramatically as the monovalent cation concentration decreased from 90 mM to 30 mM. The presence of Mg^{++} or Ca^{++} (2 mM) at low ionic strength promoted 1 + 3 cross-linking in an amount similar to that produced at isotonic conditions. The specific segment of band 3 involved in the cross-linking was also investigated by means of chymotrypsin digestion of band 3 in the intact red cells. The results showed the cross-links between spectrin component 1 and the 55,000-dalton fragment of band 3 at physiologic pH and isotonic conditions. This is consistent with the idea that band 3 is anchored on or contacted with the submembrane meshwork at the cytoplasmic membrane surface.

Key words: **spectrin, band 3, covalent cross-linking, two-dimensional gel electrophoresis, ^{125}I-labeling, chymotrypsin digestion**

Spectrin, the major "peripheral" protein located at the cytoplasmic surface of erythrocyte membrane [1–3], is thought to form a submembrane meshwork with actin, which influences cell shape, viscoelastic properties, and transmembrane communications [4–15]. This submembrane meshwork may also provide anchoring sites at the inner membrane surface for transmembrane proteins, thereby affecting their surface topography and lateral mobility. However, detailed interactions between spectrin and transmembrane proteins at molecular level are not clear.

Abbreviations: SDS) sodium dodecyl sulfate, PAGE) polyacrylamide gel electrophoresis, ATP) adenosine triphosphate, PAS) periodic acid Schiff (stain), Tris) tris-(hydroxymethyl)-aminomethane, HEPES) N-2-hydroxy-ethyl piperazine-N-2-ethanesulfonic acid, DTT) dithiothreitol, CuP) $CuSO_4$/o-phenanthroline mixture.

Received March 5, 1978; accepted September 27, 1978.

0091-7419/79/1001-0097$02.60

Recently, the techniques of covalent cross-linking and two-dimensional sodium dodecyl sulfate polyacrylamide gel electrophoresis have been employed to identify the nearest neighbors among membrane proteins of red cells [16–21]. The data suggest that the proteins in the red cell membrane are organized into stable homooligomers and, less commonly, into heterocomplexes derived from different proteins. The spontaneous cross-linkings among spectrin, actin, and band 3 (the major integral membrane protein) were first observed in ghosts incubated at acid pH (4.0–5.5) [20]. These cross-linkings were disulfides and were related to the isoelectric precipitation of spectrin (and probably band 3) at this pH.

In this investigation, we studied further the protein cross-linkings at physiologic pH and isotonic conditions. The data indicate structural contacts between spectrin component 1 (240,000 daltons) and band 3 (90,000 daltons) at physiologic conditions, the amount of which was affected by the concentration of mono- and divalent cations present. In addition, the segment of band 3 that was cross-linked with spectrin was also investigated by pretreating the intact cells with a proteolytic enzyme, chymotrypsin. The enzyme cleaved band 3 at the outer surface into two fragments of 55,000 daltons and 38,000 daltons [22]. We now demonstrate that the 55,000-dalton fragment of band 3 can be cross-linked to spectrin component 1 at the cytoplasmic surface.

MATERIALS AND METHODS

Lactoperoxidase, glucose oxidase, chymotrypsin, and o-phenanthroline were purchased from Sigma Chemical Co. Sodium iodide I^{125} was obtained from New England Nuclear Co. Erythrocyte membranes were prepared from freshly drawn blood by the hypotonic lysis method of Fairbanks et al [23] except the buffer, which was adjusted to pH 7.4. All membrane preparations were carried out as described at 0–4°C. Catalytic oxidation of ghosts with $CuSO_4$/o-phenanthroline mixture was performed as described by Steck [16] except that some ghosts were suspended in isotonic buffer (5 mM Na phosphate, 150 mM KCl or NaCl, pH 7.4) and the reaction temperature was 0°C. The two-dimensional SDS-PAGE and the designation of the major membrane polypeptides in both first and second dimensions were the same as described previously [20]. The 2.5% polyacrylamide/0.3% agarose composite gels were used in the first dimension. The discontinuous gel system described by Laemmli [42] was employed in the second dimension. Radioactive iodination of surface proteins with lactoperoxidase, glucose oxidase and sodium iodide I^{125} in intact cells was done according to Reichstein and Blostein's procedures [24]. Chymotrypsin treatment of red cells (10% suspension) was carried out in the ATP-maintaining buffer which contains 50 mM glycylglycine, 5 mM KCl, 2 mM $MgCl_2$ 200 mg% glucose, 0.54 mM adenine, 12.7 mM inosine, 2 mM phosphate, and NaCl to obtain 290–300 mOsm, pH 7.4. Chymotrypsin (0.2 mg/ml) was added to initiate the digestion. After 22 h incubation at 37°C under nitrogen, digestion was terminated with diisopropyl phosphofluoridate (final concentration 0.05 mM [22]).

RESULTS

Mild Oxidation and Two-Dimensional SDS PAGE

Disulfide couplings of proteins in isolated erythrocyte membranes were produced by catalytic oxidation with $CuSO_4$/o-phenanthroline mixture (CuP) [16, 17]. The results depended on the tonicity of the suspending solution (Fig. 1A). Under hypotonic condition (5 mM Na phosphate, pH 7.4), the complexes of 450,000, 260,000, and 175,000 daltons were observed (gel II) as previously described by others [16, 17]. Under isotonic conditions (5 mM Na phosphate, pH 7.4, 150 mM KCl or NaCl) (gels III–V), an additional complex of 330,000 daltons were found. More extensive oxidation did not increase the yield of 330,000-dalton complex (gels III–V). Instead, it produced additional large aggregates retained at the origin of the gel, (gel V). The disulfide couplings were reversible by reduction (gel VI), and were utilized subsequently to identify the participating components.

The cross-linked products in the first dimension were reversed by DTT reduction, and reelectrophoresed into the second dimension, in which the released constituents appeared as "off-diagonal" spots (Fig. 1B–E). We have identified the constituents of the complexes from membrane samples oxidized under isotonic conditions. Several off-diagonal spots appear to represent dimers (ie, 1 + 2, 3_2, 4.1_2 and 5_2) and trimers (ie, 3_3) of membrane proteins. Heterocomplexes of 1 + 3 and 2 + 4.9 are also evident on the slabs of higher resolution (Fig. 1C and 1D). The very high-molecular-weight material at the origin of the gel produced by more extensive oxidation contained essentially all of the membrane protein components (Fig. 1E) and is enriched with spectrin. The data are summarized in Table I.

Cross-Linkings of ^{125}I-Labeled Band 3 With Spectrin

To further substantiate that the above 330,000-dalton complex was in fact 1 + 3, we labeled band 3 with ^{125}I and studied the incorporation of the label into the complexes (Fig. 2). With the enzymes lactoperoxidase and glucose oxidase, band 3 and a 150,000-dalton band in intact cells were labeled extracellularly (Fig. 2C) as shown previously by others [24]. The 150,000-dalton band probably represents the major sialoglycoprotein, PAS-1, as judged from the relative mobility of PAS-1 in the gel system of low concentration of polyacrylamide [20, 25]. Catalytic oxidation of isolated ghosts derived from ^{125}I-labeled intact cells under isotonic conditions produced new radioactive peaks corresponding to 330,000, 240,000, and 175,000 daltons (Fig. 2D). The 330,000-dalton peak has the same relative mobility as 1 + 3. The 240,000- and 175,000-dalton peaks probably represent dimers and trimers, respectively, of band 3. The involvement of PAS-1 in the 330,000-dalton peak is unlikely because the size of PAS-1 is too large to be accounted for; the complex of spectrin and PAS-1 would be about 390,000 rather than 330,000 daltons.

Effect of Salt Concentration on Protein Cross-Linkings

It is known that the interaction of spectrin with membrane is influenced by the ionic strength in the medium [26]. We explored the effect of salt on protein cross-linkings and specifically the cross-linkings of spectrin itself and those between spectrin and band 3 (Fig. 3A). The quantitative analysis (Fig. 3B) showed that the decrease of salt gradually diminished the amount of 1 + 3 and 1 + 2. On the other hand, the amount of band 3 dimer did not change significantly. The change of the amount of 1 + 3 was most noticeable in the salt concentration ranging from 30 to 90 mM (Fig. 3B).

A concomitant depletion of monomeric band 6 (glyceraldehyde 3-phosphate dehydrogenase) was also shown in membranes incubated with high concentration of salt. This was due to the release of band 6 from membranes by salt [27–29] rather that its involvement in the cross-linking reactions, because the subsequent DTT reduction did not normalize the amount of band 6 in the gel (Fig. 1A, gel VI). The range of salt concentration

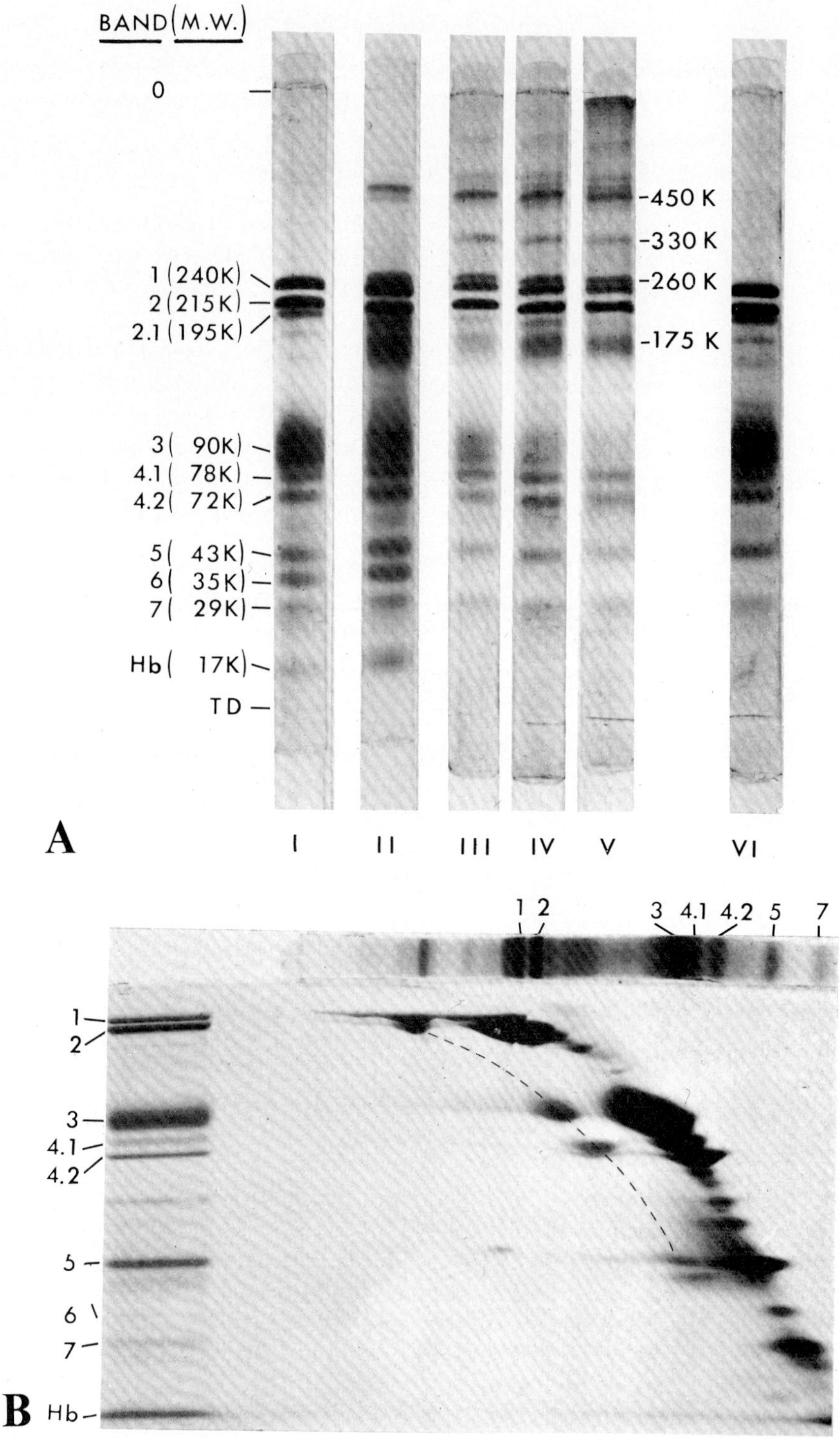

Fig. 1. The cross-linking of proteins in isolated erythrocyte membranes produced by oxidation catalyzed by $CuSO_4$/o-phenanthroline (CuP). A: Cross-linkings under hypotonic and isotonic conditions. Gel I) Untreated ghosts. Packed ghosts (10 μl or 25 μg of protein) dissolved in SDS without reduction were electrophoresed. Gel II) Ghosts in hypotonic buffer (Na phosphate, 5 mM, pH 7.4) were incubated with CuP(5μM/25μM) at 0°C for 20 min. The reaction was quenched by ethylinediaminetetracetic acid (EDTA) (2 mM). Gels III–V) Ghosts in isotonic buffer (Na phosphate 5 mM, KCl 150 mM, pH 7.4) were incubated at 0°C for 20 min with the following concentrations (μM/μM) of

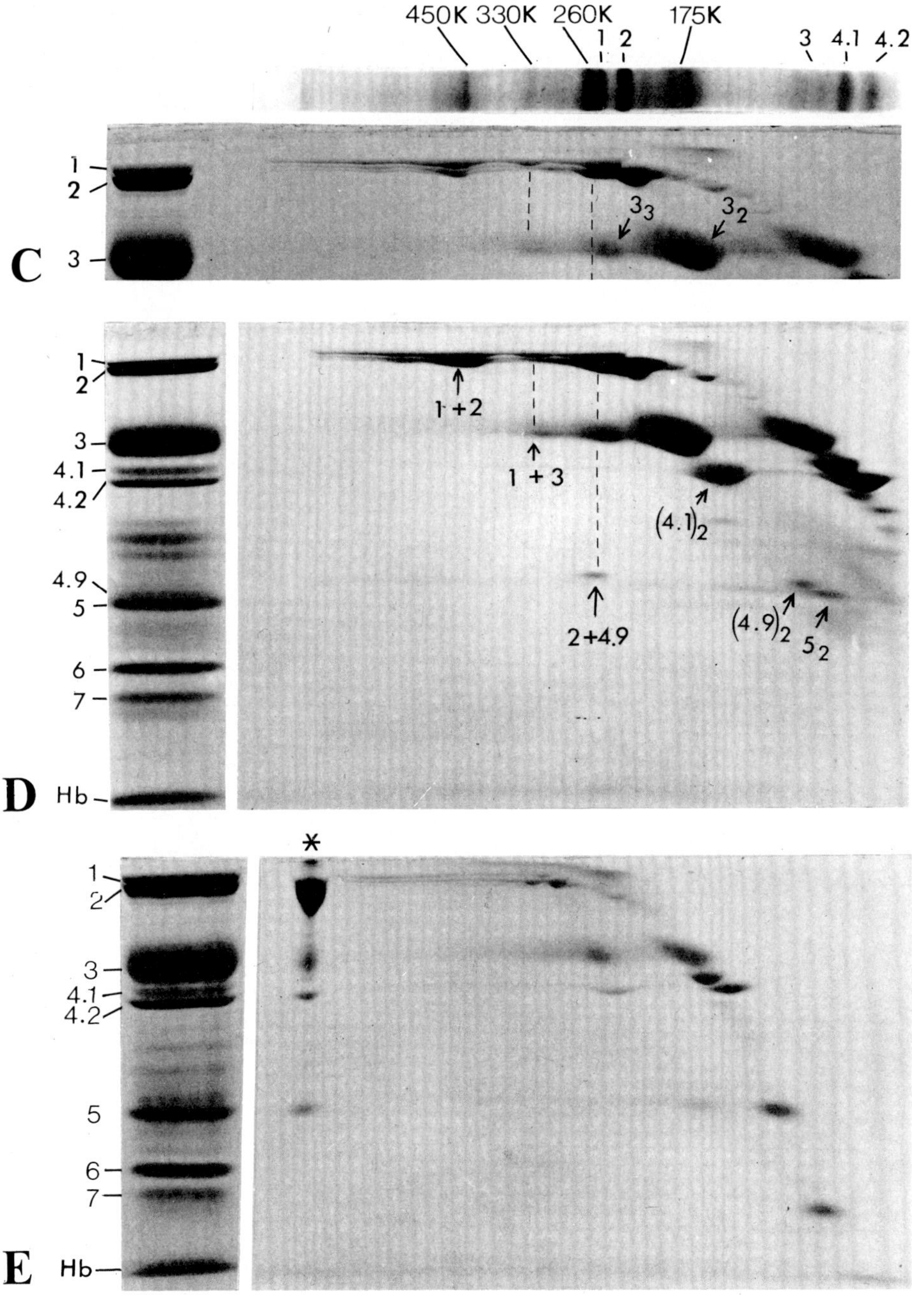

CuP: 1/5, 5/25, 10/50, respectively. Gel VI) Same as in gel IV, except that the sample was reduced with 25 mM DTT prior to electrophoresis. B–E: Two-dimensional analysis of protein cross-linkings under isotonic conditions. B: Ghosts were oxidized the same as in gel III; 150 μg of membrane protein was applied. A replicate gel of the first dimension is placed at the top of the slab. A membrane sample applied directly on the second-dimension slab is shown at the left for reference. Dashed curve indicates alignments of spots corresponding to polypeptides released after cleavage of the dimers of membrane proteins. C: Ghosts were oxidized the same as in gel IV. The cross-linked sample (100 μg of protein) was subjected to prolonged electrophoresis in the first dimension. The spectrin and band 3 zones of the two-dimensional pattern are shown. D: Same as in C, except that 150 μg of protein was applied. Tentative identification of the cross-linked complexes giving rise to off-diagonal spots is indicated. E: Ghosts were reacted with CuP(10 μM/50 μM) at 0°C for 1 h; 75 μg of protein was applied. The asterisk denotes protein components released from the large aggregates at the origin of the first dimension.

TABLE I. Tentative Identification of the Major Cross-Linked Protein Complexes From Human Erythrocyte Ghosts

Approx MW × 10^{-3} [a]	Estimated composition
450	1 + 2
330	1 + 3
260	2 + 4.9
175	3_2

[a] A calibration curve for the estimation of aggregate molecular weights was constructed by extrapolating the curve for the major membrane polypeptides through the point representing 1 + 2 complex, which was readily identified before [20].

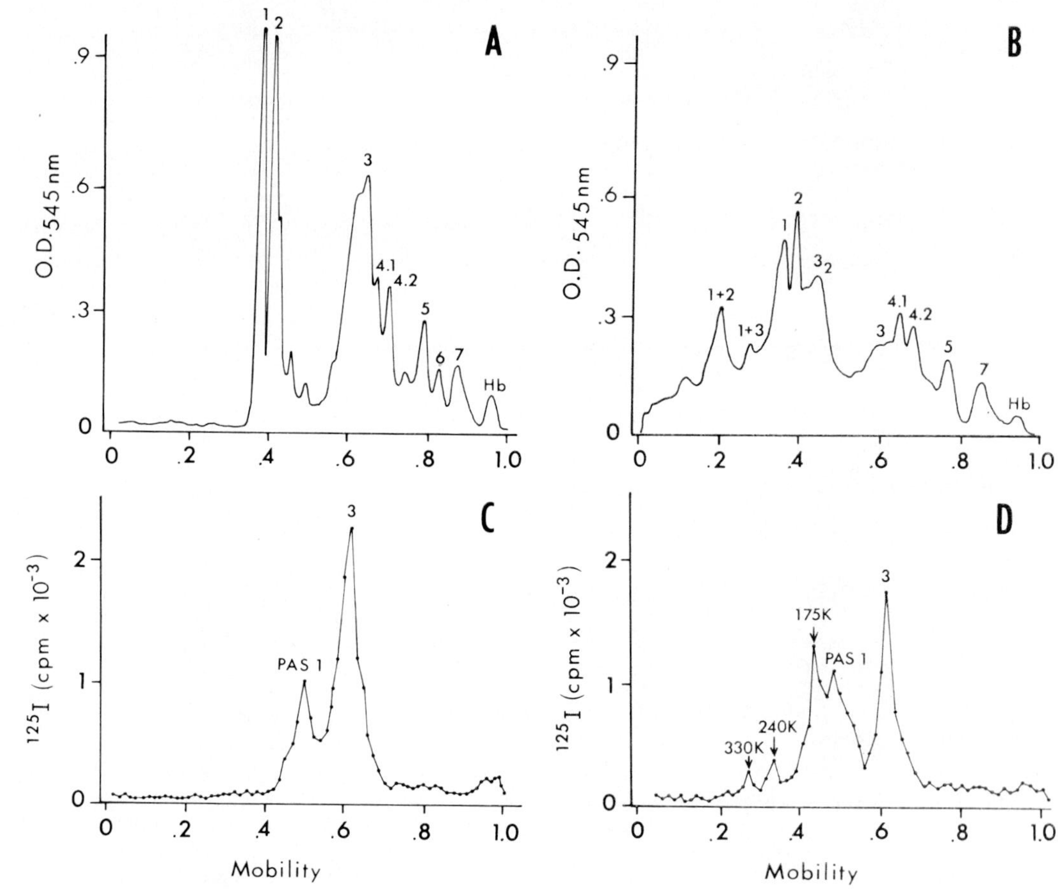

Fig. 2. Cross-linking of ^{125}I-labeled erythrocyte membrane proteins. Intact erythrocytes were labeled with ^{125}I on the outer surface. The isolated ghosts were reacted with CuP(5 μM/25 μM) and electrophoresed as described in the text. Scans of the Coomassie blue-stained gels of the untreated (A) and mildly oxidized (B) ghosts. Radioactive profiles are of the untreated (C) and mildly oxidized (D) ghosts. Radioactivity was determined in 1 mm minced segments of gel.

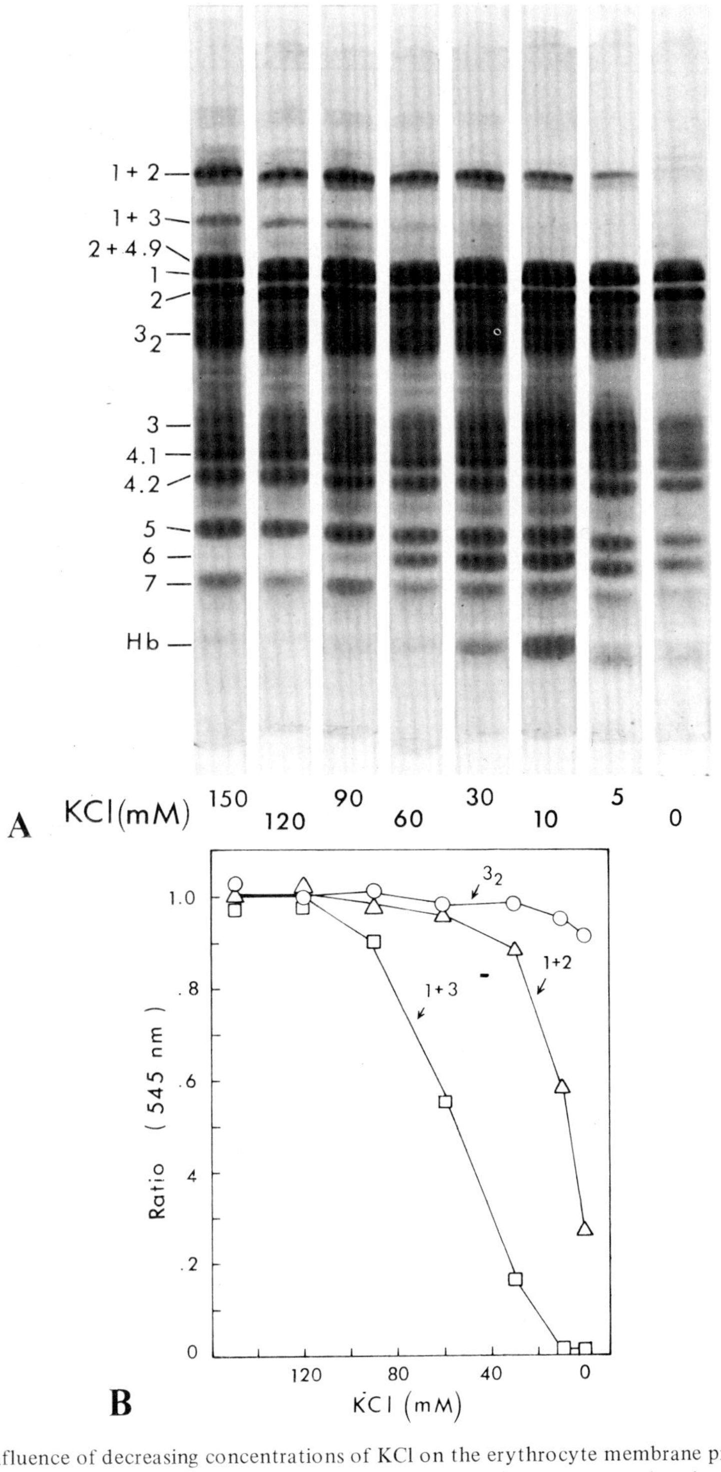

Fig. 3. Influence of decreasing concentrations of KCl on the erythrocyte membrane protein cross-linkings. A: Ghosts were catalytically oxidized with CuP(5 μM/25 μM) in Na phosphate buffer (0.5 mM, pH 7.4) with different concentrations of KCl at 0°C for 20 min. B: Changes in the relative amount of 1 + 3, 1 + 2, and 3_2 as a function of KCl concentration. Depicted are the ratios of the area under each complex (after they were cut out, weighed, and normalized by the total Coomassie stain in the gel) to the area of the same complex produced under isotonic conditions.

(30–90 mM) that influences the retention of band 6 by the membrane has been shown above to affect the amount of 1 + 3. However, a direct correlation between them is not evident (see Discussion).

The effect of Ca^{++} (or Mg^{++}) on membrane protein cross-linking is observed at much lower concentrations than that of KCl (Fig. 4A). Under hypotonic conditions 2 mM Ca^{++} (or Mg^{++}) produced the same effect as that of NaCl (or KCl) at 90 mM or more. In addition, Ca^{++} clearly enhanced the degree of protein cross-linkings when added to the isotonic salt solution (Fig. 4B). A distinct smearing of Coomassie blue stain was shown at the slow-migrating zone of the upper region of the gel.

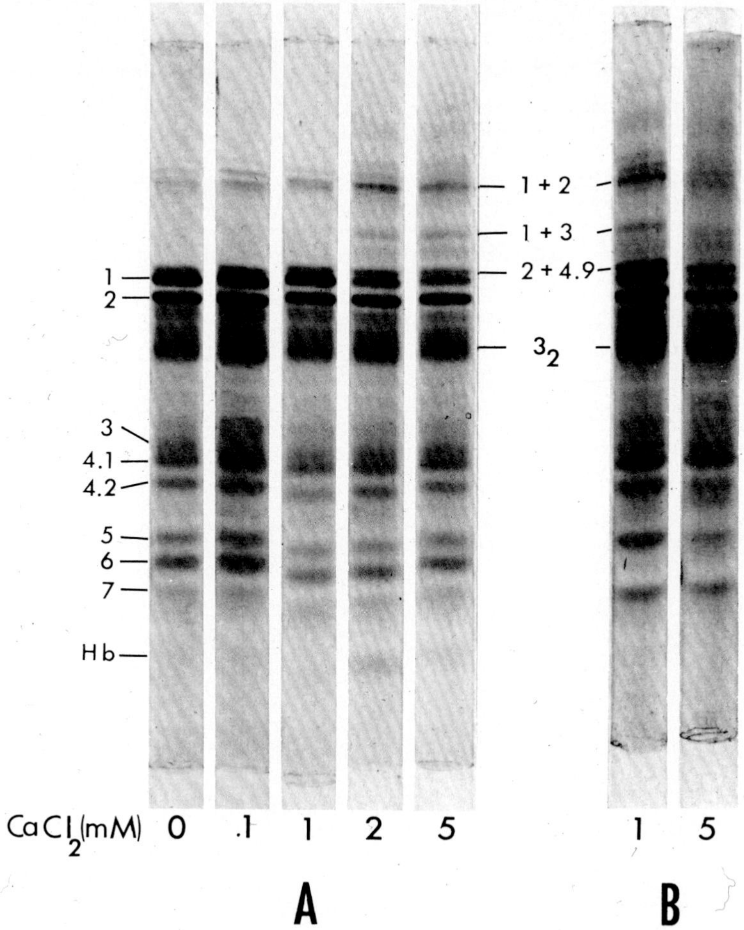

Fig. 4. Influence of $CaCl_2$ on the erythrocyte membrane protein cross-linkings. A: Ghosts were catalytic oxidized with CuP(5 μM/25 μM) in hypotonic buffer (HEPES 2 mM, pH 7.4) with different concentrations of $CaCl_2$ at 0°C for 20 min. B: Ghosts were oxidized in isotonic buffer (HEPES 2 mM, 150 mM KCl, pH 7.4) with 1 or 5 mM $CaCl_2$.

Effect of Chymotrypsin Digestion of Band 3 in Intact Cells on Protein Cross-linking

The mild digestion of intact cells with chymotrypsin cleaved band 3 specifically into two fragments of 55,000 and 38,000 daltons (Fig. 5, gel II; Fig. 6, gel I), which confirmed the previous observation by Steck et al [22]. To examine which fragment was structurally associated with band 1, we oxidized catalytically the ghosts from digested cells with CuP. Three new complexes (110,000, 165,000, and 300,000 daltons) were produced in addition to the 260,000- and 450,000-dalton complexes which were observed previously in undigested cells (Fig. 5, gels III and IV). The two-dimensional analysis revealed that these new complexes were 1 + 55k (300,000 daltons) as well as dimers (110,000 daltons) and trimers (165,000 daltons) of 55k fragments. Two other familiar complexes 2 + 4.9 (260,000) and 1 + 2 (450,000 daltons) were also seen. The 38k fragment of band 3 appeared on the slab as a monomeric spot, involving neither self-polymerization (ie, dimer, trimer) nor coupling with band 1. Compared with the amount of band 3 trimer in undigested sample, the yield of 55k trimer is markedly enhanced (Fig. 1C and Fig. 6C).

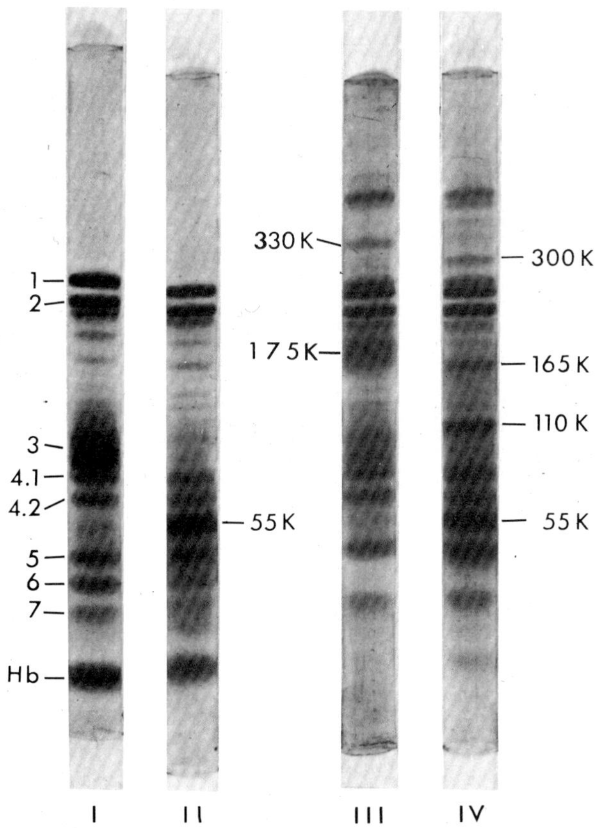

Fig. 5. Protein cross-linkings in isolated ghosts from chymotrypsin-digested erythrocytes. Ghosts were prepared from red cells which had been incubated for 22 h in an ATP maintaining buffer at 37°C lacking (gel I) or containing 0.2 mg/ml of chymotrypsin (gel II). Subsequent oxidation of undigested (gel III) and digested (gel IV) samples were carried out in isotonic buffer (Na phosphate 5 mM, KCl 150 mM) with CuP(5 μM/25 μM) at 0°C for 20 min.

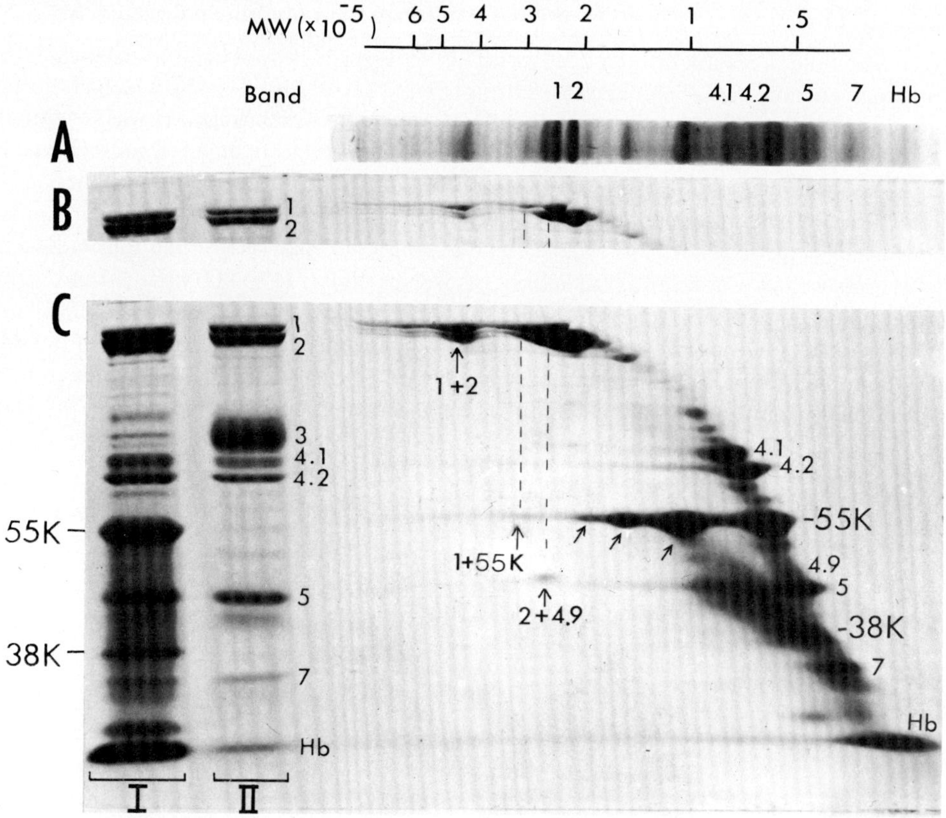

Fig. 6. Two-dimensional analysis of protein cross-linkings in ghosts from chymotrypsin-treated erythrocytes. A. Replicate gel identical to gel IV in Fig. 5. B: Spectrin zone of the two-dimensional pattern with low loading (75 μg of protein). C: Same as (B) with 150 μg of protein applied. Constituents of some complexes are labeled. Arrows indicate the trimers, dimers, and tetramers of 55,000-dalton fragment. Column I) pattern of a membrane sample from chymotrypsin-treated erythrocyte applied directly on the slab, column II) untreated ghost sample in which band 6 has been eluted by salt.

DISCUSSION

The 330,000-dalton complex is one of the major cross-linked products produced by the mild oxidation of ghosts at physiologic pH and isotonic conditions. The complex was identified as 1 + 3 from both the analysis of two-dimensional gel electrophoresis and the specific ^{125}I-labeling of band 3. In addition, prior chymotrypsin digestion of band 3 in intact cells led to the subsequent formation of a smaller complex of 300,000 daltons between spectrin 1 and the 55,000-dalton fragment of band 3.

Previous studies by others [16, 17] using CuP in protein cross-linking of isolated ghosts did not detect the 330,000-dalton complex. This is apparently due to the low tonicity employed in these experiments. The amount of 1 + 3 and 1 + 2 complexes depended on the concentration of mono- and divalent cations in the reaction mixture (Figs. 3 and 4). This is not unexpected, since both the spectrin and band 3 segments exposed at the cytoplasmic surface are known to contain a large amount of glutamic and aspartic acid residues [22, 30, 31]. In the absence of salt, the charge repulsion arising from these residues at neutral pH is likely to be enormous; and they may limit the physical contacts of protein chains that are necessary for intermolecular disulfide couplings to occur. In fact, at low ionic strengths and alkaline conditions, spectrin is known to detach from the membrane [1, 2, 23] and dissociate primarily into noncovalent dimers or tetramers (ie, $(1 + 2)_{1,\,2}$) in the solution [2, 32, 33]. In contrast to the 1 + 3 or 1 + 2 complexes, the yield of band 3 dimers in membranes was essentially unchanged at various ionic strengths (Fig. 3B). Whether this is due to the close proximity of hydrophobic segments of these transmembrane polypeptides in the membrane is not known. Recently, the band 3 proteolysis in membrane was also found to be affected by salt [34]; band 3 became more resistant to trypsin digestion under isotonic conditions. This phenomenon is consistent with the interpretation of our cross-linking data; the closer contacts of spectrin to band 3 under isotonic conditions decrease the accessibility of the proteolytic enzyme to band 3. The amount of spectrin-band 3 cross-linkings gradually diminished as the salt concentration (NaCl or KCl) decreased from 90 mM to 30 mM. This range of concentration is higher than that detected by Bennett and Branton in the study of spectrin-membrane interactions [26]. They reported the saturation of spectrin binding by inside-out vesicles at 10 mM KCl. Recent data of Litman et al [35] suggest that band 2, rather than band 1, binds to the inside-out vesicles. The discrepancies probably represent the measurement of two different parameters in these experiments: i) the molecular interactions and ii) the degree of physical contacts. It is recognized that cross-linked products may not necessarily represent the stable protein complexes in the membrane. Random collisional interferences may be introduced from either the lateral mobility or the concentration of protein constituents in the membrane [21, 36]. However, recent studies using fluorescein isothiocyanate labeling show that integral proteins (mainly band 3 and the major sialoglycoprotein) have a diffusion coefficient of the order of 10^{-11} $cm^2 \cdot s^{-1}$ at 37°C, or 10^{-12} $cm^2 \cdot s^{-1}$ at 23°C in the erythrocyte membrane [37, 38]. These diffusion coefficients are about two orders below that of rhodopsin in the photoreceptor membranes [39], or of surface antigens in the membranes of cultured muscle fibers [40]. The mobility of these integral proteins is curtailed dramatically at cold temperatures. Following the fusion of labeled and unlabeled cells, incubation at 0°C for up to 20 h failed to produce any fluorescent label redistribution [37]. Since we have oxidized the ghost proteins at 0°C (Fig. 1), and the complexes of 1 + 3 appeared within a minute of oxidation (Liu and Palek, unpublished observations), the interference from the lateral mobility of band 3 in the membrane is probably not significant. Furthermore, the fact that the yield of 1 + 3 complex is dependent on the tonicity (Fig. 3) or pH [20] of the reaction mixture suggests that the cross-linking is governed by the electrostatic interaction rather than by the concentration or lateral mobility of protein constituents in the membrane. However, the exact relationship between the implicated contacts and the molecular interactions is not clear. Recent studies of direct molecular bindings suggest that another protein component may be involved as an intermediate between spectrin and band 3 [26, 35]. Therefore, the sulfhydryl groups involved in the couplings between spectrin and band 3 may not reside directly in the molecular binding site. On the other hand, our cross-linking data suggest a gradual change of structural proximity, which is not detected in binding studies, between spectrin and band 3 in the salt concentration (KCl or NaCl) ranging from 30 to 90 mM. It should be pointed out here that spectrin-band 3 cross-linkings have not yet been detected in intact red cells. Therefore, the conclusive association between these two proteins in situ requires further elucidation. The possibility of subtle rearrangements of membrane proteins during the ghost preparation cannot be excluded at the present time.

A concomitant increase of band 6 (G3PD) retention by the membrane was observed as the NaCl concentration decreased from 90 mM to 30 mM in the incubation mixture (Fig. 3A). Although it has previously been shown by Yu and Steck [41] that G3PD interacts with band 3 in the membrane, the elution of G3PD from membrane (eg, with NaCl (150 mM) or NADH (2 mM)) prior to cross-linking did not affect the amount of 1 + 3 complex subsequently produced (data not shown). Therefore, the binding of G3PD to band 3 seems to have no direct effect on 1 + 3 formation.

The chymotrypsin-produced 55,000-dalton fragment of band 3 that could cross-link with spectrin (Fig. 5) is probably the same segment as that shown by Steck et al [22] to extend from the extracellular space to the cytoplasmic surface. This segment of band 3 appears to contain the reactive SH groups which could form dimers and trimers as the intact band 3 does in the membrane (Fig. 1). The yield of 55k trimers appears markedly enhanced compared to band 3 trimer in intact ghosts (Fig. 1C and Fig. 6). The reason for this is not yet known. Some subtle rearrangement of 55k fragments may occur as a consequence of chymotrypsin treatment. On the other hand, the 38,000-dalton fragment of band 3 did not polymerized into homopolymers or cross-link with spectrin 1. The data are consistent with the idea that the 38,000-dalton fragment resides mainly on the outer surface and within the lipid bilayer core but does not extend to the cytoplasmic side and hence is not in contact with spectrin. However, a definite conclusion of the lack of physical contacts between spectrin and the 38,000-dalton fragment of band 3 awaits further investigation by some other means, because the absence of their cross-linkings may be due to the lack of adequate sulfhydryl groups of two adjacent polypeptide chains [36].

Our cross-linking data reveal a major difference in the behavior of the two spectrin chains at physiologic pH and isotonic conditions (ie, the preferential cross-linking of chain 1 relative to 2 with band 3). While 1 + 3 is one of the major complexes promoted by the presence of salt, the 2 + 3 apparently is not (Fig. 1). The low yield of 2 + 3 does not appear to be due to the lack of -SH groups of chain 2, since the two spectrin chains have virtually identical amino acid composition [31] and they have previously been shown to produce about the same amount of disulfide couplings with band 3 under acidic conditions (pH 4.0–5.5) [20]. Presumably, these results reflect differences in detailed structure or localization of the two chains in the membrane. Other observations of preferential depletion of monomeric chain 1 relative to chain 2 in ghosts incubated at acid pH (4.0–5.5), and the differential cross-linking in complexes (eg, 2 + 4.9, 1 + 5), are added evidence for this suggestion. However, the physiologic implication of the difference of these two chains is not yet evident. One potentially significant difference is that only spectrin 2 is phosphorylated [43–45] by a cAMP-independent protein kinase. The degree of spectrin 2 phosphorylation has recently been shown to correlate with the shape changes of isolated ghosts [46]. The observation that both 1 + 3 cross-linkings and spectrin 2 phosphorylation are affected significantly by mono- and divalent cations is of particular interest and certainly merits further investigation.

ACKNOWLEDGMENTS

This work was supported by National Institutes of Health grant HL-15157 and by the Boston Sickle Cell Center. We appreciate the skilled technical help of Mr. Robert Lundin and Mr. Jim Monroe.

REFERENCES

1. Marchesi VT, Steers E Jr: Science 159:203, 1968.
2. Clarke M: Biochem Biophys Res Commun 45:1063, 1971.
3. Nicolson GL, Marchesi VT, Singer SJ: J Cell Biol 51:265, 1971.
4. Steck TL: J Cell Biol 62:1, 1974.
5. Lux SE, John KM, Karnovsky MJ: J Clin Invest 58:955, 1976.
6. Palek J, Stewart G, Lionetti FJ: Blood 44:583, 1974.
7. Tilney LG, Detmers P: J Cell Biol 66:508, 1975.
8. Pinder JC, Bray D, Gratzer WB: Nature 258:765, 1975.
9. Nicolson GL, Painter RG: J Cell Biol 59:395, 1973.
10. Ji TH, Nicolson GL: Proc Natl Acad Sci USA 71:2212, 1974.
11. Elgsaeter A, Branton D: J Cell Biol 63:1018, 1974.
12. Elgsaeter A, Shotton DM, Branton D: Biochim Biophys Acta 426:101, 1976.
13. Yu J, Branton D: Proc Natl Acad Sci USA 73:3891, 1976.
14. Sheetz MP, Painter RG, Singer SJ: Cold Spring Harbor Conference on Cell Proliferation 3:651, 1977.
15. Kirkpatrick FH: Life Sci 19:1, 1976.
16. Steck TL: J Mol Biol 66:295, 1972.
17. Wang K, Richards FM: J Biol Chem 249:8005, 1974.
18. Huang CK, Richards FM: J Biol Chem 252:5514, 1977.
19. Mikkelsen RB, Wallach DFH: J Biol Chem 251:7413, 1976.
20. Liu SC, Fairbank G, Palek J: Biochemistry 16:4066, 1977.
21. Kiehm DJ, Ji TH: J Biol Chem 252:8524, 1977.
22. Steck TL, Ramos B, Strapazon E: Biochemistry 15:1154, 1976.
23. Fairbanks G, Steck TL, Wallach DFH: Biochemistry 10:2606, 1971.
24. Reichstein E, Blostein R: J Biol Chem 250:6256, 1975.
25. Silverberg M, Marchesi VT: J Biol Chem 253:95, 1978.
26. Bennett V, Branton D: J Biol Chem 252:2753, 1977.
27. Tanner MJA, Gray WR: Biochem J 125:1109, 1971.
28. Kant JA, Steck TL: J Biol Chem 248:8457, 1973.
29. Shin BC, Carraway KL: J Biol Chem 248:1436, 1973.
30. Marchesi SL, Steer E, Marchesi VT, Tillack TW: Biochemistry 9:50, 1970.
31. Fuller GM, Boughter JM, Morazzani M: Biochemistry 13:3036, 1974.
32. Ralston GB: Aust J Biol Sci 28:259, 1975.
33. Ralston GB, Dunbar J, White M: Biochim Biophys Acta 491:345, 1977.
34. Jenkons R, Tanner MJA: Biochem J 161:131, 1977.
35. Litman D, Chen JW, Marchesi VT: J Supramol Struct Suppl 2, 209, 1978.
36. Peters K, Richards FM: Ann Rev Biochem 46:523, 1977.
37. Fowler L, Branton D: Nature 268:23, 1977.
38. Peters R, Peters J, Tews KH, Bahr W: Biochim Biophys Acta 367:282, 1974.
39. Poo M, Core RA: Nature 247:438, 1974.
40. Edidin M, Fambrough D: J Cell Biol 57:27, 1973.
41. Yu J, Steck UL: J Biol Chem 250:9176, 1975.
42. Laemmli UK: Nature 227:680, 1970.
43. Gurthrow CE, Allen JE, Rasmussen H: J Biol Chem 247:8154, 1972.
44. Rubin C, Rosen O: Biochem Biophys Res Commun 50:421, 1973.
45. Avruch J, Fairbanks G: Biochemistry 13:5507, 1974.
46. Birchmeier W, Singer SJ: J Cell Biol 73:647, 1977.

Journal of Supramolecular Structure 10:215–225 (1979)
Normal and Abnormal Red Cell Membranes 375–385

Properties of (Mg^{2+} + Ca^{2+})-ATPase of Erythrocyte Membranes Prepared by Different Procedures: Influence of Mg^{2+}, Ca^{2+}, ATP, and Protein Activator

Sidney Katz, Basil D. Roufogalis, Amiram D. Landman, and Larry Ho

Faculty of Pharmaceutical Sciences, University of British Columbia, Vancouver, British Columbia, Canada V6T 1W5

Erythrocyte membranes prepared by three different procedures showed (Mg^{2+} + Ca^{2+})-ATPase activities differing in specific activity and in affinity for Ca^{2+}. The (Mg^{2+} + Ca^{2+})-ATPase activity of the three preparations was stimulated to different extents by a Ca^{2+}-dependent protein activator isolated from hemolysates. The Ca^{2+} affinity of the two most active preparations was decreased as the ATP concentration in the assay medium was increased. Lowering the ATP concentration from 2 mM to 2-200 μM or lowering the Mg:ATP ratio to less than one shifted the (Mg^{2+} + Ca^{2+})-ATPase activity in stepwise hemolysis membranes from mixed "high" and "low" affinity to a single high Ca^{2+} affinity. Membranes from which soluble proteins were extracted by EDTA (0.1 mM) in low ionic strength, or membranes prepared by the EDTA (1–10 mM) procedure, did not undergo the shift in the Ca^{2+} affinity with changes in ATP and $MgCl_2$ concentrations. The EDTA-wash membranes were only weakly activated by the protein activator. It is suggested that the differences in properties of the (Mg^{2+} + Ca^{2+})-ATPase prepared by these three procedures reflect differences determined in part by the degree of association of the membrane with a soluble protein activator and changes in the state of the enzyme to a less activatable form.

Key words: **(Mg^{2+} + Ca^{2+})-ATPase, erythrocyte membranes, endogenous protein activator**

Controversy exists as to the properties, number and function of (Mg^{2+} + Ca^{2+})-ATPase(s) present in erythrocyte membranes. Quist and Roufogalis [1, 2], employing a stepwise hemolysis procedure for preparation of erythrocyte membranes, identified mixed "high" and "low" Ca^{2+} affinity (Mg^{2+} + Ca^{2+})-ATPase activity. A correlation of ATPase

Received March 5, 1978; accepted August 29, 1978.

0091-7419/79/1002-0215$02.30

activity in the low Ca^{2+}-affinity range and calcium transport has been found in intact erythrocytes as well as in preparations of resealed "ghosts" and vesicles [1, 3, 4]. Katz and Blostein [5] employing an EDTA-wash procedure for preparation of erythrocyte membranes and low ATP concentrations (2 μM) observed an association of (Mg^{2+} + Ca^{2+})-ATPase activity and related Ca^{2+}-dependent phosphoprotein formation in the high Ca^{2+} affinity range. The recent discovery of a soluble protein activator [6–8] of (Mg^{2+} + Ca^{2+})-ATPase further increases the difficulty in determining whether there are two distinct ATPases or two states of a single (Mg^{2+} + Ca^{2+})-ATPase regulated by other proteins in the membrane. In the present study, we have utilized three different erythrocyte membrane preparations, all of which are currently being used to study the properties of the (Mg^{2+} + Ca^{2+})-ATPase activity, to investigate a number of factors that affect the Ca^{2+} affinity and activity of this enzyme complex.

MATERIALS AND METHODS

Human erythrocyte membranes were prepared by three different procedures Essentially they were the following: i) a 1:10 hemolysis of packed cells in distilled water followed by washing in EDTA (1–10 mM), then further washes and storage in Tris-HCl, pH 7.4 [9, 10]; ii) a stepwise 1:10 hemolysis in decreasing concentrations of NaCl (0.08–0.015 M) followed by washing and storage in 0.015 M NaCl and 0.005 M Tris-maleate, pH 7.2 [2]; and, iii) a 1:14 hemolysis in 20 imOsm imidazole, pH 7.4, followed by washing and storage in imidazole medium [11]. Complete details of these procedures are given in the references cited.

Extracted erythrocyte membranes containing low affinity (Mg^{2+} + Ca^{2+})-ATPase activity were prepared by the procedure of Fairbanks et al [12] as previously described [2]. Essentially, membranes prepared by the stepwise hemolysis procedure were incubated in 5 vol of 1 mM Tris- 0.1 mM EDTA, pH 8, and agitated at 37° for 30–45 minutes. Membranes separated by centrifugation at 20,000 × g for 10 minutes were resuspended in 5 mM Tris-15 mM NaCl, pH 7.2, to the original volume of packed cells from which the membranes were derived. Since this procedure removes up to 25% of membrane protein [12, 13], activities of membranes and extracted membranes were compared per ml of packed cells.

The preparations of (γ-^{32}P)ATP and the procedures for measuring ATPase activity as $^{32}P_i$ released from (γ-^{32}P)ATP have been described previously [9, 10] and are summarized in the legend to Fig. 1. Incubation times at the various ATP concentrations were chosen so that the assays were linear with respect to time and membrane concentration. Free Ca^{2+} was buffered in the incubation medium, with ethyleneglycolbis (β-aminoethyl)-N,N-tetraacetate (EGTA) in a final concentration of 0.1 mM. The free Ca^{2+} concentration was determined by the association constants for the interaction of EGTA and ATP with Ca^{2+} for the pH and ATP concentrations at which the experiment was conducted [14].

Protein activator was prepared from erythrocyte hemolysates by the method of Luthra et al [6] using a carboxy methyl Sephadex column (CM 50, Pharmacia) and concentrating the desired fraction by ultrafiltration. An endogenous soluble activator was also isolated from erythrocyte membranes: 12 ml of membranes prepared by the stepwise hemolysis procedure were incubated in 5 vol of 1 mM Tris-HCl-0.1 mM EDTA, pH 6.5 for 35 minutes at 37°. The 100,000 × g supernatant was concentrated 20-fold by ultrafiltration (Amicon XM-100 A filter), layered on a 5–20% isokinetic sucrose gradient and centrifuged at 38,000 × g for 16–18 h. Activator was assayed by incubating 300 μl of various fractions with extracted membranes under standard conditions (see Fig. 3) at 300 μM Ca^{2+}.

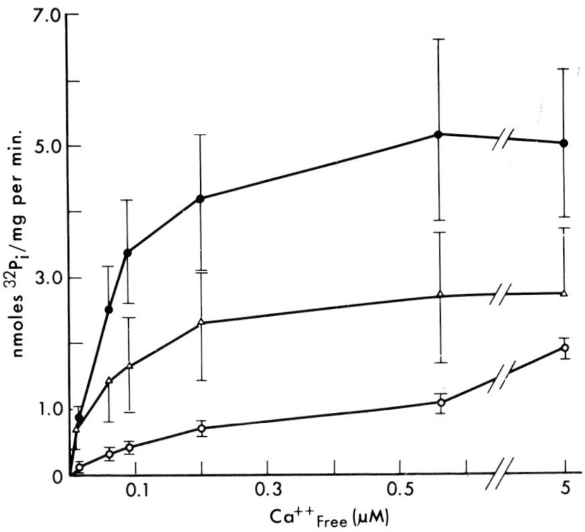

Fig. 1. $(Mg^{2+} + Ca^{2+})$-ATPase activity of erythrocyte membranes prepared by different procedures. Erythrocyte membranes prepared by stepwise hemolysis (●——●), imidazole-wash (△——△) or EDTA-wash (○——○) procedures were first incubated at 37° for 10 min in the presence of 0.1 mM Tris-EGTA, pH 7.4. The membranes were assayed at 37° for 10 min in a final volume of 0.125 ml containing 0.075 ml membranes (2–3 mg protein/ml), 40 mM Tris-HCl, pH 7.4, 0.2 mM [γ-^{32}P] ATP (50×10^3 cpm per 0.125 ml final volume), 1.0 mM $MgCl_2$ in the presence of various amounts of added $CaCl_2$ (0.02–5.0 μM Ca^{2+} free). The reaction was terminated by the addition of 0.75 ml cold trichloroacetic acid (5%) containing 5 mM Na_2ATP and 2 mM KH_2PO_4. 0.45 ml of charcoal (0.15 g/ml in 5% trichloroacetic acid) was added and following centrifugation for 2 min (Eppendorf microcentrifuge) aliquots (0.4 ml) were counted in 10 ml Aquasol scintillation fluid. The results shown are the mean ± SE of at least 3 different membrane preparations in each case. The ATPase activity refers to Ca^{2+}-stimulated components after subtraction of values measured without Ca^{2+} added.

Materials: All chemicals were purchased from Sigma Chemical. $^{32}P_i$ (carrier free) and Aquasol were purchased from New England Nuclear. All inorganic chemicals used were Reagent grade. Charcoal (Norit A) was purchased from Fisher Scientific.

RESULTS

$(Mg^{2+} + Ca^{2+})$-ATPase Activities of Different Erythrocyte Membrane Preparations

The $(Mg^{2+} + Ca^{2+})$-ATPase activities of the three erythrocyte membrane preparations in the presence of various free Ca^{2+} concentrations (0.02–5 μM) is illustrated in Fig. 1. The ATP concentration in these experiments was 200 μM. The imidazole-wash preparation and the stepwise hemolysis preparation produced $(Mg^{2+} + Ca^{2+})$-ATPase activity curves of a similar shape, although in our hands, the $(Mg^{2+} + Ca^{2+})$-ATPase activity was higher in membranes prepared by the stepwise hemolysis procedure. The EDTA-wash preparation produced a $(Mg^{2+} + Ca^{2+})$-ATPase activity curve of low activity, particularly at low free Ca^{2+} concentrations. Figure 2 is a reciprocal plot of the same data illustrating the K_{diss} for Ca^{2+} and the maximum velocity at saturating Ca^{2+} concentrations ($V_{Ca^{2+}}$) of the $(Mg^{2+} + Ca^{2+})$-ATPase of the three erythrocyte membrane preparations. The plots were constructed using the weighted statistical analysis of Wilkinson [15]. At this ATP concentration, membranes prepared by the step-wise hemolysis procedure and the imidazole-wash

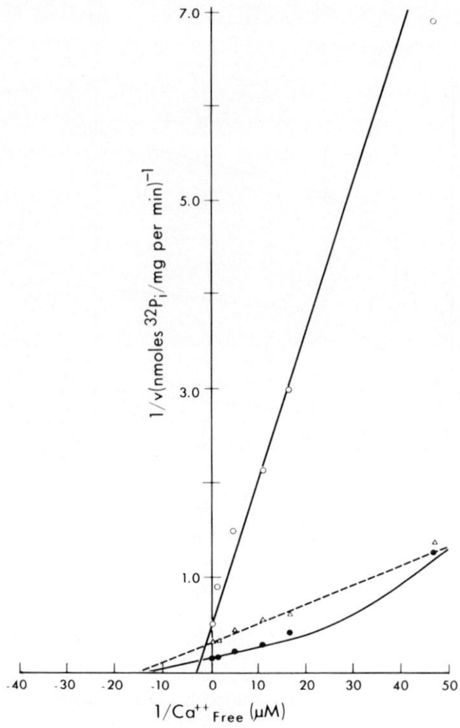

Fig. 2. K_{diss} and $V_{Ca^{2+}}$ of the (Mg^{2+} + Ca^{2+})-ATPase activity of erythrocyte membranes prepared by different procedures. Reciprocal plots of data illustrated in Fig. 1 at 200 μM ATP in the (●——●) stepwise hemolysis preparation, (△– – –△) imidazole-wash preparation and (○——○) EDTA-wash preparation. Plots were constructed according to the weighted statistical analysis of Wilkinson [15].

procedure have a similar K_{diss} for Ca^{2+}, but the EDTA-wash preparation has a significantly lower Ca^{2+} affinity than either of the other two preparations ($P < 0.001$, student t-test). The EDTA-wash preparation also has a significantly lower $V_{Ca^{2+}}$ than either of the other two preparations ($P < 0.001$).

The effect of ATP concentration on the K_{diss} for Ca^{2+} and the $V_{Ca^{2+}}$ for the (Mg^{2+} + Ca^{2+})-ATPase activities of the three erythrocyte membrane preparations is illustrated in Table I. The K_{diss} and the $V_{Ca^{2+}}$ values were determined by the statistical analysis of Wilkinson [15]. At ATP concentrations of 2-200 μM the K_{diss} for Ca^{2+} increased as the ATP concentration was increased. The K_{diss} values were not statistically different between the stepwise and imidazole-wash preparations. The EDTA-wash preparation, on the other hand, showed a significantly higher K_{diss} for Ca^{2+} at all three ATP concentrations ($P < 0.001$). At 2,000 μM ATP the differences among the three preparations in K_{diss} for Ca^{2+} were eliminated. As expected, $V_{Ca^{2+}}$ values in the three preparations increased progressively as the ATP concentration increased. At ATP concentrations of 20–2,000 μM the $V_{Ca^{2+}}$ of the stepwise preparation was significantly higher than that of the EDTA-wash preparation ($P < 0.001$) and the imidazole-wash preparation ($P < 0.01$ at 20 μM ATP and $P < 0.001$ at 200 and 2,000 μM ATP).

Effect of ATP Concentration on Ca^{2+} Affinity

Since ATP affected the affinity of the (Mg^{2+} + Ca^{2+})-ATPase in the membrane preparations, the effect of ATP on the shape of the Ca^{2+}-activation curve was examined in detail in membranes prepared by the stepwise hemolysis procedure (Fig. 3). In these experiments, $MgCl_2$ was kept constant (6.4 mM). At 2 mM ATP (Fig. 3A) Ca^{2+} activation of the (Mg^{2+} + Ca^{2+})-ATPase activity occurred over a wide range of Ca^{2+} concentrations (0.3–300 μM), demonstrating mixed high and low Ca^{2+}-affinities [2, 16]. By contrast, at 2 or 20 μM ATP, (Mg^{2+} + Ca^{2+})-ATPase activity was saturated at around 10 μM Ca^{2+}, the ATPase activity reaching a plateau at higher Ca^{2+} concentrations (Fig. 3A). At 200 μM ATP the Ca^{2+}-activation curve was intermediate but tended to exhibit mainly high Ca^{2+}-affinity ATPase activity (Fig. 3A). To determine whether these ATP-dependent changes in the shape of the Ca^{2+}-activation curve were associated with soluble proteins in the erythrocyte membrane, the effect of ATP on the shape of the Ca^{2+}-activation curve was again examined following extraction of soluble proteins in 1.0 mM Tris-0.1 mM EDTA, pH 8 for 35 min at 37°. As shown previously [2], loss of soluble proteins resulted in (Mg^{2+} + Ca^{2+})-ATPase activity of predominantly low Ca^{2+}-affinity. The ATP dependence of the

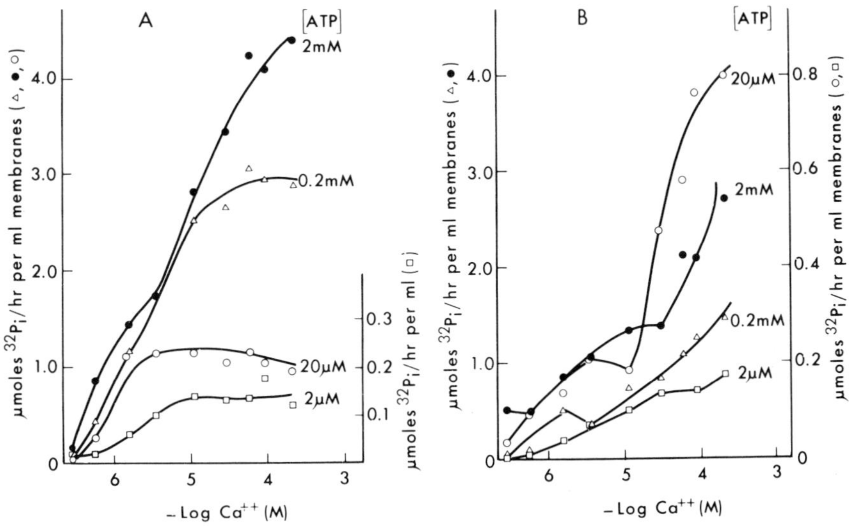

Fig. 3. Effect of ATP on the Ca^{2+} affinity of (Mg^{2+} + Ca^{2+}) -ATPase in erythrocyte membranes (A) and pH 8-extracted membranes (B). Erythrocyte membranes were prepared by the stepwise hemolysis procedure. Extracted membranes were obtained as described in Methods. (Mg^{2+} + Ca^{2+})-ATPase activity was assayed in a final volume of 0.6 ml containing 0.05 ml of membranes or 0.10 ml of extracted membranes (approximately 4 and 3 mg protein/ml), 55 mM Tris-maleate, pH 7.2, 6.4 mM $MgCl_2$, 66 mM NaCl, 0.1 mM EGTA, 0.1 mM ouabain, 0.002-2.0 mM Na_2ATP containing [γ-^{32}P]ATP (15–30 × 10^3 cpm) and $CaCl_2$ (0.3-300 μM Ca^{2+} free). Membranes were incubated at 37° for 2 min (2–20 μM ATP), 20 min (200 μM ATP) and 60 min (2000 μM ATP). The reaction was terminated with 0.2 ml of 5% cold trichloroacetic acid. 0.4 ml of charcoal (0.15 g/ml in 5% trichloroacetic acid) was added and following centrifugation for 2 min (Eppendorf microcentrifuge) aliquots (0.4 ml) were counted in 10 ml Aquasol scintillation fluid. The influence of 2–2,000 μM ATP on free Ca^{2+} was calculated (14) and found to be negligible. The curves shown represent a typical experiment from the same batch of erythrocyte membranes.

TABLE I. K_{diss} for Ca^{2+} and $V_{Ca^{2+}}$ of $(Mg^{2+} + Ca^{2+})$-ATPase of Erythrocyte Membranes Prepared by Different Procedures: Effect of ATP Concentration.

	ATP (μM)	Preparations Stepwise	EDTA-wash	Imidazole-wash
K_{diss} (μM)	2	0.018 ± 0.006	0.185 ± 0.021[a]	0.018 ± 0.004
	20	0.020 ± 0.005	0.192 ± 0.031[a]	0.030 ± 0.007
	200	0.062 ± 0.012	0.398 ± 0.039[a]	0.060 ± 0.006
	2000	0.118 ± 0.013	0.149 ± 0.012[f]	0.165 ± 0.023
$V_{Ca^{2+}}$ (nmoles $mg^{-1} min^{-1}$)	2	0.398 ± 0.026	0.303 ± 0.011[f]	0.322 ± 0.013[c]
	20	1.781 ± 0.080	1.155 ± 0.061[b]	1.036 ± 0.049[d]
	200	5.419 ± 0.235	2.042 ± 0.078[a]	2.896 ± 0.077[e]
	2000	11.340 ± 0.377	4.250 ± 0.104[b]	7.474 ± 0.331[e]

Erythrocyte membranes prepared by different procedures were assayed for $(Mg^{2+} + Ca^{2+})$-ATPase activity as described in Fig. 1, in the presence of the following ATP and $MgCl_2$ concentrations: i) 2 μM ATP (5×10^3 cpm [γ-^{32}P]ATP per 0.125 ml final volume) and 25 μM $MgCl_2$, ii) 20 μM ATP (5×10^3 cpm [γ-^{32}P]ATP per 0.125 ml final volume) and 100 μM $MgCl_2$, iii) 200 μM ATP (50×10^3 cpm [γ-^{32}P]ATP per 0.125 ml final volume) and 1,000 μM $MgCl_2$ and, iv) 2,000 μM ATP (500×10^3 cpm [γ-^{32}P] ATP per 0.125 ml final volume) and 6,000 μM $MgCl_2$. Membranes were incubated at 37° for 2 min (2 μM ATP), 3.5 min (20 μM ATP), 10 min (200 μM ATP) and 25 min (2,000 μM ATP). The results are expressed as the K_{diss} ± SE and $V_{Ca^{2+}}$ ± SE of 3 pooled experiments in each case.

[a] Indicates a significant difference between the EDTA-wash preparation and the other two preparations ($P < 0.001$).

[b] Indicates a significant difference between the EDTA-wash preparation and the stepwise hemolysis preparation ($P < 0.001$).

[c] Indicates a significant difference between the stepwise hemolysis preparation and the imidazole-wash preparation ($P < 0.05$).

[d] Indicates a significant difference between the stepwise hemolysis preparation and the imidazole-wash preparation ($P < 0.01$).

[e] Indicates a significant difference between the stepwise hemolysis preparation and the imidazole-wash preparation ($P < 0.001$).

[f] Not significantly different.

Ca^{2+}-affinities seen in the erythrocyte membranes (Fig. 3), the prominantly low Ca^{2+}-affinity of the $(Mg^{2+} + Ca^{2+})$-ATPase activity was maintained at all ATP concentrations examined (2–2,000 μM).

Effect of $MgCl_2$ Concentration on Ca^{2+}-Affinity

The relationship of Mg:ATP ratio to the Ca^{2+}-affinity of the $(Mg^{2+} + Ca^{2+})$-ATPase was examined in both erythrocyte membranes and extracted membranes prepared by the stepwise hemolysis procedure. In these experiments, ATP was kept constant at 2 mM. In the erythrocyte membranes, lowering the $MgCl_2$ concentration from 6.4 mM (Mg:ATP = 3.2:1) to 1.0 mM (Mg:ATP = 0.5:1) resulted in a change in the Ca^{2+} activation curve from a mixed high and low affinity to predominantly high Ca^{2+}-affinity activity saturating at 10 μM free Ca^{2+} or less (Fig. 4). Lowering the Mg:ATP ratio from 1 to 0.5 resulted in an abrupt decrease in maximal velocity. The extent to which these effects were related to soluble membrane proteins were examined in the extracted membranes. In contrast to the erythrocyte membranes, lowering the $MgCl_2$ from 6.4 mM to 1 mM progressively reduced the activity of the $(Mg^{2+} + Ca^{2+})$-ATPase without any apparent effect on Ca^{2+}-affinity, the enzyme requiring higher than 10 μM Ca^{2+} for saturation throughout (Fig. 5).

Characterization of Soluble Protein Activator

We confirmed a previous finding [2] that addition of the soluble fraction (extracted from membranes with 1 mM Tris-0.1 mM EDTA, pH 8) to the extracted membranes restored the original high Ca^{2+}-affinity and velocity of $(Mg^{2+} + Ca^{2+})$-ATPase activity (not shown). A similar result was obtained with soluble fraction extracted under the same conditions at pH 6.5 for 35 min at 37° (not shown). When the soluble protein fraction was layered on a 5–20% isokinetic sucrose gradient, an activator of the $(Mg^{2+} + Ca^{2+})$-ATPase activity of the extracted membranes wàs found in the fraction above the hemoglobin band. The failure of the activator protein to penetrate the sucrose gradient suggests that it may be similar to the low molecular weight $(Mg^{2+} + Ca^{2+})$-ATPase activator isolated from hemolysates of erythrocytes [6–8]. Work is in progress to further investigate this aspect.

Endogenous protein activator isolated from hemolysates by the method of Luthra et al [6] stimulated the $(Mg^{2+} + Ca^{2+})$-ATPase activity of all three preparations studied but to varying degrees (Table II); erythrocyte membranes prepared by the imidazole-wash procedure were stimulated to a greater degree than membranes prepared by the two other procedures.

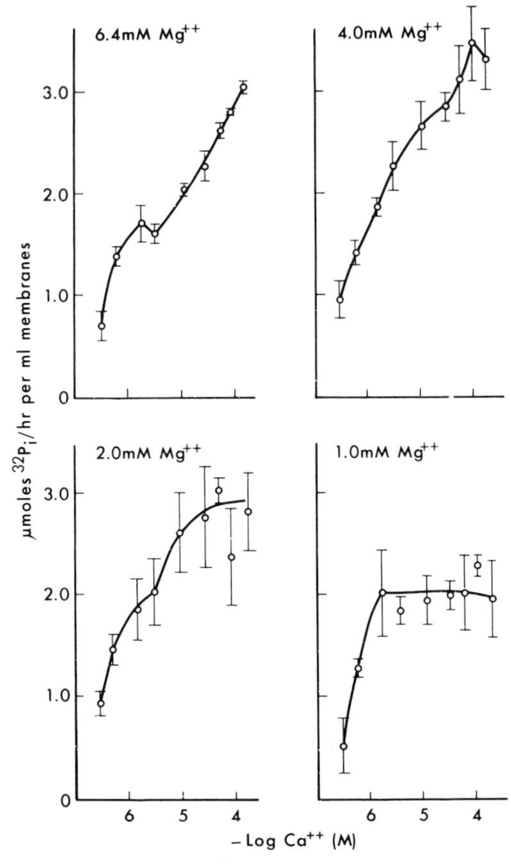

Fig. 4. Effect of $MgCl_2$ on the Ca^{2+} affinity of $(Mg^{2+} + Ca^{2+})$-ATPase in erythrocyte membranes. Erythrocyte membranes were prepared by the stepwise hemolysis procedure. $(Mg^{2+} + Ca^{2+})$-ATPase was assayed as described in Fig. 3, in the presence of 2 mM ATP and various $MgCl_2$ concentrations (1–6.4 mM). The results are the mean ± SE of three membrane preparations.

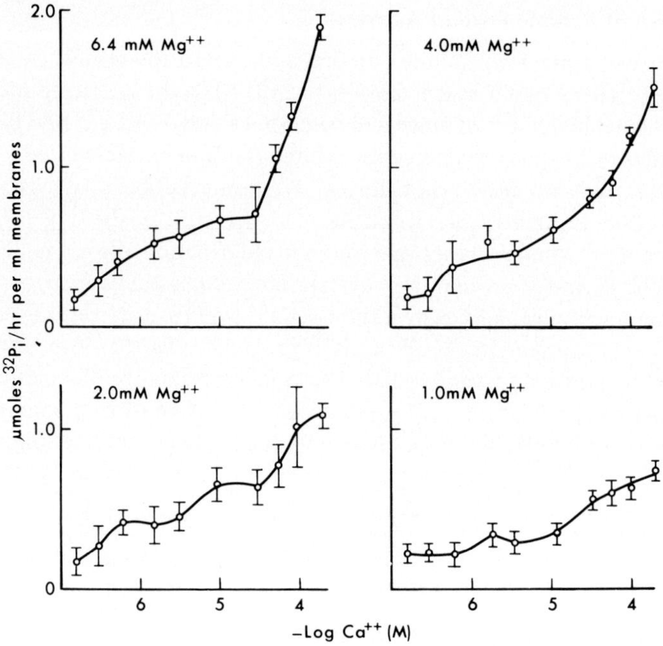

Fig. 5. Effect of $MgCl_2$ on the Ca^{2+} affinity of (Mg^{2+} + Ca^{2+})-ATPase in extracted membranes. Extracted membranes were obtained from erythrocyte membranes prepared by stepwise hemolysis, as described in Methods, and assayed as described in Fig. 3 for 60 min at 2 mM ATP. Results are the mean ± SE of three extracted membrane preparations.

TABLE II. Effect of Endogenous Protein Activator on (Mg^{2+} + Ca^{2+})-ATPase Activity of Erythrocyte Membranes Prepared by Different Procedures.

Preparation		% Stimulation
Stepwise	[3][a]	48.0 ± 13.6
EDTA-wash	[7]	111.1 ± 17.4
Imidazole-wash	[3]	311.0 ± 104.1[b]

Erythrocyte membranes prepared by three different procedures were assayed for (Mg^{2+} + Ca^{2+})-ATPase activity as described in Fig. 1 (200 μM ATP, 1,000 μM $MgCl_2$, and 0.1 μM free Ca^{2+}) in the presence and absence of protein activator (35 μg/0.25 ml final incubation volume) prepared by the method of Luthra et al [6]. Results are expressed as the mean % increase ± SE over activity observed in the absence of activator in at least three preparations in each case.

[a]indicates number of preparations in each group.

[b]indicates a significant difference between the imidazole-wash preparation and the EDTA-wash preparation ($P < 0.02$).

DISCUSSION

In this study we examined the factors responsible for differences in (Mg^{2+} + Ca^{2+})-ATPase activity and Ca^{2+}-affinity of three different erythrocyte membrane preparations commonly used to investigate the properties of this enzyme. The differences in K_{diss} for Ca^{2+} activation of (Mg^{2+} + Ca^{2+})-ATPase in the three preparations were dependent on the

ATP concentration. Membranes prepared by the stepwise and imidazole-wash procedure had a significantly higher Ca^{2+}-affinity than the EDTA-wash preparation at low ATP concentrations (2–200 μM). However, the Ca^{2+}-affinity of the former preparations progressively decreased as the ATP concentration in the assay medium was increased; at 2 mM ATP the K_{diss} of the three preparations was not significantly different. The EDTA-wash preparation exhibited a low Ca^{2+}-affinity at all of the ATP concentrations investigated. The EDTA-wash preparation also had the least active $(Mg^{2+} + Ca^{2+})$-ATPase activity. It is possible that the differences in Ca^{2+}-affinity and $V_{Ca^{2+}}$ noted in the three preparations were due to the different extent of association of the protein activator of $(Mg^{2+} + Ca^{2+})$-ATPase [11, 17] with the membranes. The protein activator has been shown to affect both these parameters [7] and is removed from membranes by EGTA [17, 18] or EDTA. However, the loss of activator from the EDTA-wash preparation may not be the only factor accounting for the low $(Mg^{2+} + Ca^{2+})$-ATPase activity and Ca^{2+}-affinity in these membranes, since this preparation was less activated by the addition of purified protein activator than the imidazole-wash membranes, a preparation with significantly higher $(Mg^{2+} + Ca^{2+})$-ATPase activity.

The influence of soluble membrane proteins on the properties of $(Mg^{2+} + Ca^{2+})$-ATPase was examined further in membranes prepared by the step-wise hemolysis procedure. This preparation, like the imidazole-wash preparation [11] contained a low molecular weight activator of $(Mg^{2+} + Ca^{2+})$-ATPase, extractable from the membranes by incubation in low ionic strength medium (1mM Tris) containing 0.1 mM EDTA. Whereas mixed high (saturation at 10 μM Ca^{2+}) and low Ca^{2+} affinity (not saturated up to 300 μM Ca^{2+}), $(Mg^{2+} + Ca^{2+})$-ATPase activities were apparent at 2 mM ATP, only high Ca^{2+} affinity activity was expressed at low ATP concentrations (2–20 μM). A similar shift to higher Ca^{2+} affinity activity was obtained when the $MgCl_2$ concentration was decreased, an abrupt change occurring when the Mg/ATP ratio was decreased below one. This shift in Ca^{2+}-affinity was also noted in the imidazole-wash preparation but not in the EDTA-wash preparation (Table I). Thus ATP and $MgCl_2$, or possibly Mg-ATP, appear to regulate the Ca^{2+}-affinity of the more active membranes.

Changes in Ca^{2+}-affinity of $(Mg^{2+} + Ca^{2+})$-ATPase with variation in ATP and $MgCl_2$ were not observed following extraction of soluble proteins from the membranes. Extraction resulted in the loss of approximately 25% of the membrane protein, including spectrin and actin (band 5) [13] and protein activator, producing a preparation of predominantly low Ca^{2+}-affinity $(Mg^{2+} + Ca^{2+})$-ATPase activity. Whether the change in Ca^{2+}-affinity in the extracted membranes resulted from the loss of a high affinity $(Mg^{2+} + Ca^{2+})$-ATPase from the membranes [2, 17], loss of a protein activator [18] or a change in state of the enzyme protein [20] is unclear. The addition of soluble protein extracts [2, 17], or purified $(Mg^{2+} + Ca^{2+})$-ATPase activator [7, Roufogalis and Mauldin, unpublished observations] to the extracted membranes restored their original high Ca^{2+}-affinity. The failure of ATP and Mg^{2+} to modulate the Ca^{2+}-affinity in extracted membranes suggests that their modulation is mediated through the soluble protein(s). Failure of ATP to alter the Ca^{2+}-affinity of the EDTA-wash preparation (Table I) suggests that this preparation was deficient in soluble proteins and perhaps protein activator compared to the other two preparations.*

*Predominantly high Ca^{2+}-affinity $(Mg^{2+} + Ca^{2+})$-ATPase has been reported in some membrane preparations at a Mg:ATP ratio equal to or less than one [21–23] indicating that other factors, such as membrane Ca^{2+} content [23–25] or the abundance of protein activator [18] can counteract the influence of these modulators.

However, failure of the partially purified activator to restore the activity of the EDTA-wash preparation to that of the other preparations (Table II) suggests that additional changes in membrane-bound (Mg^{2+} + Ca^{2+})-ATPase can occur as a result of the preparation conditions. This could result from the loss of other soluble proteins (spectrin and actin) from the membranes, a mechanism for which there is no direct experimental evidence at present, or an irreversible change in the state of the (Mg^{2+} + Ca^{2+})-ATPase [20] to a non-activatable form. An irreversible change in state does not appear to occur following the limited treatment of membranes with 1 mM Tris- 0.1 mM EDTA at 37° [2], but may have occurred on prolonged washing in EDTA (1-10 mM) during the preparation of the EDTA-wash membranes.

This work suggests that the differences in properties of the (Mg^{2+} + Ca^{2+})-ATPase prepared by different procedures may be due to the state of the enzyme determined at least in part by the degree of association of a protein activator and the Mg^{2+} and ATP concentrations used. This work also emphasizes that for the study and the comparison of (Mg^{2+} + Ca^{2+})-ATPase a careful definition be made of the method of erythrocyte membrane preparation, the subsequent treatment of the membranes at various ionic strengths and the conditions for assay with respect to Mg^{2+}, Ca^{2+} and ATP.

ACKNOWLEDGMENTS

This work was supported by the Medical Research Council of Canada, the British Columbia Heart Foundation and the Canadian Cystic Fibrosis Foundation.

REFERENCES

1. Quist EE, Roufogalis BD: Proc Can Fed Biol Soc 16:13, 1973.
2. Quist EE, Roufogalis BD: Arch Biochem Biophys 168:240, 1975.
3. Quist EE, Roufogalis BD: J Supramol Struct 6:375, 1977.
4. Sarkadi B, Szasz I, Gerloczy A, Gardos G: Biochim Biophys Acta 464:93, 1977.
5. Katz S, Blostein R: Biochim Biophys Acta 389:314, 1975.
6. Luthra MG, Hildenbrandt GR, Hanahan DJ: Biochim Biophys Acta 419:164, 1976.
7. Gopinath RM, Vincenzi FF: Biochem Biophys Res Commun 77:1203, 1977.
8. Jarrett HW, Penniston JT: Biochem Biophys Res Commun 77:1210, 1977.
9. Blostein R: J Biol Chem 243:1957, 1968.
10. Blostein R: J Biol Chem 245:270, 1970.
11. Farrance ML, Vincenzi FF: Biochem Biophys Acta 471:49, 1977.
12. Fairbanks G, Steck TL, Wallach DF: Biochemistry 10:2606, 1971.
13. Marchesi VT, Steers Jr E: Science 159:203, 1968.
14. Katz AM, Repke DI, Upshaw JE, Polascik MA: Biochim Biophys Acta 205:473, 1970.

15. Wilkinson GN: Biochem J 80:324, 1961.
16. Schatzmann HJ, Rossi GL: Biochim Biophys Acta 241:379, 1971.
17. Scharff O: Biochim Biophys Acta 509:67, 1978.
18. Farrance ML, Vincenzi FF: Biochim Biophys Acta 471:59, 1977.
19. Weidekamm E, Brdiczka D: Biochim Biophys Acta 401:51, 1975.
20. Wolf HU: Biochem J 130:311, 1972.
21. Wolf HU, Schoffeniels E: Biochim Biophys Acta 219:521, 1970.
22. Ronner P, Gazzotti P, Carafoli E: Arch Biochem Biophys 179:578, 1977.
23. Scharff O: Biochim Biophys Acta 443:206, 1976.
24. Carraway KL, Triplett RB, Anderson DR: Biochim Biophys Acta 379:571, 1975.
25. Porzig H: J Memb Biol 31:317, 1977.

Journal of Supramolecular Structure 10:227–239 (1979)
Normal and Abnormal Red Cell Membranes 387–399

Substructure of Human Erythrocyte Spectrin

C. J. Hsu, A. Lemay, Y. Eshdat, and V. T. Marchesi

Department of Pathology, Yale University School of Medicine, 310 Cedar Street, New Haven, CT 06510

The human erythrocyte structural protein spectrin and its subunits I, II were isolated in the presence of Na-dodecyl-sulfate by gel filtration and preparative gel electrophoresis. After removal of the detergent, spectrin alpha-helical content is comparable to spectrin isolated without detergent. Subunits I and II formed single bands in isoelectric focusing (pI = 5.6) and in Ornstein-Davis disc gel electrophoresis systems, indicating the individual subunits are homogenous in nature. The molecular weights of the subunits I and II, determined by Ferguson plot, are 237,500 and 238,600, respectively, which is in good agreement with values obtained by the standard SDS gel relative mobility method. Limited tryptic digestion of spectrin and two-dimensional peptide maps of the individual subunits cleaved by S-cyanylation reaction showed dissimilar patterns, suggesting differences in primary structure between the two subunits.

Key words: spectrin, actin, red cell membranes

Many current models of membrane organization favor the idea that transmembrane glycoproteins play a pivotal role in determining binding sites on the cell surface and in regulating interactions between other membrane proteins. Such transmembrane glycoproteins, which have polypeptide segments facing both sides of the lipid bilayer, are uniquely placed to sample the external environment of the cell and at the same time have portions of their polypeptide chains in close proximity to the protein components which are arranged along the inner surface of the membrane. In the case of the human red blood cell membrane, the two major glycoproteins, glycophorin A [1] and the so-called band 3 polypeptide [2] both have the molecular features to accommodate these dual functions.

Abbreviations: PMSF – phenylmethane sulfonyl fluoride, EDTA – ethylenediaminetetracetic acid, β-Me – β-mercaptoethanol, SDS – sodium dodecyl sulfate, MW – molecular weight, Bis – N,N'-methylene bisacrylamide, R_m – relative mobility, K_R – retardation coefficient, CBB – Coomassie Brilliant Blue, NTCB – 2-nitro-5-thiocyanobenzoic acid, DTT – dithiothreitol, RBC – red blood cell, TPCK – L-1-Tosylamide-2-phenylethylchloro-methyl ketone

C. J. Hsu is now at Syva Research Institute, 3181 Porter Drive, Palo Alto, CA 94303.

A. Lemay is now at the Laboratoire D'Endocrinologie Moleculaire CHUL, Ste-Foy, P. Québec, Canada.

Y. Eshdat is now at the Department of Biophysics, The Weizmann Institute of Science, Rehovot, Israel.

Received June 22, 1978; accepted July 31, 1978.

0091-7419/79/1002-0227$02.60

The evidence in support of the idea that the cytoplasmic segments of these transmembrane glycoproteins interact directly with a submembranous cytoskeletal network is largely indirect and can be summarized as follows. Incubating leaky red cell ghost membranes with multivalent antispectrin antibodies causes a significant shift in the topography of the sialoglycopeptide components [3]. This is most easily explained by assuming that shifts in the distribution of the spectrin network caused by the antispectrin antibodies result in a corresponding shift in the overlying (and associated) transmembrane glycoproteins. The same results can also be obtained more indirectly by incubating partially spectrin-depleted red cell ghosts in media buffered at pH 5.5, which is close to the isoelectric point of spectrin. This treatment causes the intramembranous particles to form irregular clumps [4, 5]. Since the latter are assumed to contain most, if not all, of the major transmembrane glycoproteins [6, 7] it is again reasoned that perturbation of the spectrin network causes corresponding perturbations in the distribution of the transmembrane glycoproteins, the simplest interpretation being that there are direct noncovalent connections between the cytoplasmic domains of the transmembrane proteins and the underlying spectrin network.

A recent and more direct attempt to demonstrate associations between the transmembrane glycoproteins and spectrin has been reported by Yu and Branton, who have shown that reconstituted liposomes containing the band 3 polypeptide are able to bind significant amounts of spectrin and band 5 (actin) [8], and these spectrin-actin-band 3 complexes also seem to respond to pH manipulations.

If we accept these data at face value, they provide provocative evidence that spectrin and the cytoplasmic segments of the major glycoproteins do indeed reside close together when all are organized as components in the membrane. The data fall short of providing us with any clear idea as to how spectrin attaches to the inner surface of the red cell membrane and what segments of the transmembrane glycoproteins it actually binds to.

It is obvious that further insight into this complex multiprotein system depends upon our knowing more about the chemical and molecular properties of the spectrin molecules. The purpose of this report is to summarize what is now known (or assumed) about spectrin and then to present some recent data on the substructure of human erythrocyte spectrin.

When spectrin was first described almost a decade ago [9], it was assumed on the basis of preliminary findings that the principal components were composed of two homogeneous high-molecular-weight polypeptide chains. Although the available evidence favored a two-chain model, it was certainly not compelling, and in fact when additional studies were carried out in different laboratories just the opposite interpretation was proposed. Three different groups of investigators reported that their purified spectrin preparations contained multiple N-terminal amino acid residues [10–12], and two laboratories reported that purified spectrin preparations were distinctly heterogeneous when analyzed by isoelectric focusing [13, 14]. Both sets of observations strongly favored the idea that spectrin prepared by essentially similar techniques was composed of distinctly different polypeptide chains all of which seemed to have roughly equivalent polypeptide chain length. Further studies on the properties of the spectrin preparations analyzed in nonionic detergents provided a somewhat paradoxical result in that each of the apparently heterogeneous bands of spectrin seemed to react with the same antispectrin antisera, suggesting that each of the heterogeneous forms of spectrin shared common antigenic determinants [14].

METHODS

Spectrin and actin were extracted from human erythrocyte membranes by incubating ghost membranes in 5 volumes of 0.1 mM EDTA (pH 9.5), 0.5 mM β-Me, 0.03 mM PMSF, at 37°C for 30 min. The membranes were removed by centrifugation at 30,000g for 45 min, and the supernatant was concentrated by isoelectric precipitation at pH 5.1 by titrating with 1 N HCl. After incubating on ice for 1 h, the precipitated spectrin were pelleted at 1,400g for 5 min. The precipitate was redissolved in small volumes of column buffer (0.1% SDS, 10 mM Tris-HCl (pH 9.0), 0.5 mM β-Me, 0.5 mM EDTA, 0.03 mM PMSF, 0.02% NaN_3) and applied on a Sepharose 4B column (5 × 90 cm) equilibrated in column buffer. The column was eluted at 50 ml/h, and the effluent was monitored by OD_{280} and SDS gel electrophoresis. Pure spectrin fractions were pooled and dialyzed exhaustively against 2 mM Na phosphate (pH 9.0), 0.5 mM β-Me, 0.5 mM EDTA, 0.03 mM PMSF, 0.02%

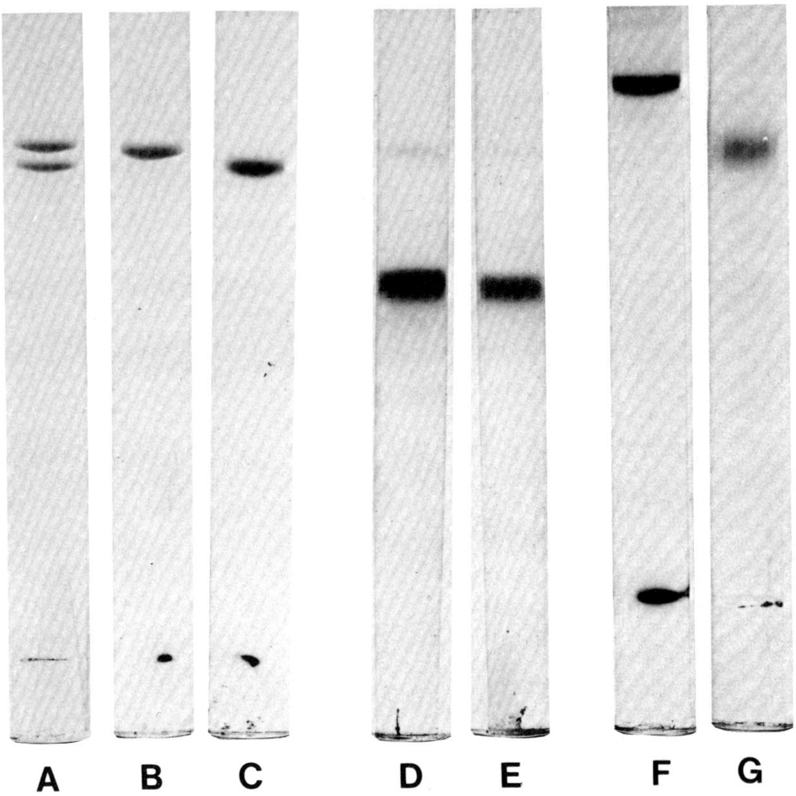

Fig. 1. Electrophoretic and isoelectric focusing analysis of different spectrin preparations. Purified spectrin (A), isolated band 1 (B), and isolated band 2 (C) on 4% SDS gels (Fairbanks); purified spectrin (D) and isolated band 1 (E) analyzed by isoelectric focusing gels containing pH 3–7 ampholytes with 8 M urea (pI of band 1 is 5.5); isolated band 1 (F) and isolated band 2 (G) on 5.5% gels run in Tris-glycine buffer, pH 8.9 (Ornstein and Davis).

NaN_3 at 4°C. After removal of SDS, spectrin solution was concentrated to 1 mg/ml in an Amicon cell with XM-100 membrane and stored at 0°C.

In 0.1% SDS, spectrin was dissociated and fractionated by subunit size. Subunit band 1 can be obtained by rechromatography of the leading edge of the peak. Spectrin subunit band 2 was purified by preparative SDS gel electrophoresis on 4% acrylamide Fairbank's gel (0.6 × 9 × 33 cm). Purified spectrin (2 mg) in 10 mM Na borate (pH 9.0) was reacted with 0.1 mg fluorescamine (Roche) in 2 μl acetone, and 4 mg unlabeled spectrin was added to the labeled spectrin. The mixture (~ 4 ml) was made to 20 mM Tris-HCl (pH 7.5), 3% SDS, 1.5% β-Me, 2 M urea, with a small amount of Bromophenol Blue added. The protein was applied on the slab gel and electrophoresed at 50 mA for 36 h. Band 2 was excised from the gel under a UV lamp and protein was eluted from the pulverized gel in column buffer. SDS was removed by prolonged dialysis against the buffer used for pure spectrin.

Isoelectric Focusing

Isoelectric focusing was done on acrylamide tube gel matrix, according to the method of Bhakdi et al [13]. The gels (0.5 × 10 cm casted in glass tubes) contained 4% acrylamide cross-linked with 2.5% Bis, 10% sucrose, 8 M urea, and 1% ampholines (pH range 3.5–7.0 or 3.5–10.0). The polymerization was catalyzed by the addition of tetramethylethylene-diamine and ammonium persulfate. The anodal buffer (0.03 M NaOH) and cathodal buffer (0.05 M H_2SO_4) were thoroughly degased and the gels were preelectrophoresed at 1 mA/gel for 15 min to remove persulfate. Samples containing 10 μg protein in 8 M urea were applied on top of the gel, protected by a 0.5-cm layer of 0.1% ampholine in 5% sucrose. Current at 0.5 mA/gel was applied during the first 5 h of electrofocusing and then changed to constant voltage of 40 V/cm for another 12 h. The final current had dropped to 0.1 mA/gel. The gels were fixed in 25% 2-propanol after two changes to completely remove ampholine, then stained in 0.05% CBB in 25% 2-propanol for 5 h, then in 0.0025% CBB in 25% 2-propanol for 16 h.

Molecular Weight Determination

The molecular weights of the spectrin bands 1 and 2 were determined by Ferguson plot [19] in the Ornstein [36] and Davis [37] gel system. The gels (0.5 ×11 cm casted in glass tubes) contained 3.0, 3.75, 4.0, 4.5, 5.0, 5.5, 6.0, 6.5, 7.5, and 9.0% acrylamide with constant Bis:acrylamide = 1:30, in 3.75 mM Tris-HCl (pH 8.9). Electrode buffer was Tris-glycine buffer containing 25 mM Tris, 0.2 M glycine (pH 8.9). Samples contained 10–25 μg protein in 50% sucrose Tris-glycine buffer with Bromphenol Blue as tracking dye. Electrophoresis was run at 4 mA/gel for 3 h, and the gels were stained in 0.05% Coomassie Brilliant Blue. The relative mobility R_m was measured in different percentage acrylamide gels and the values of log (R_m × 100) versus percentage acrylamide concentrations T were plotted (Fig. 2). According to the Ferguson equation:

$$\log R_m = -K_R T + \log Y_0$$

The retardation coefficient, K_R, is proportional to molecular weight at constant Bis/acrylamide ratio. The free mobility $Y_0 = R_m$ at $T = 0$. Linear regression analyses were made on all Ferguson plots to determine K_R and Y_0. K_R of molecular weight protein standards were also determined on identical gel systems to construct the molecular weight standard plot (Fig. 3) [ie, plot K_R versus molecular weight]. The molecular weight of spectrin bands 1 and 2 were obtained by interpolation on the molecular weight standard curve.

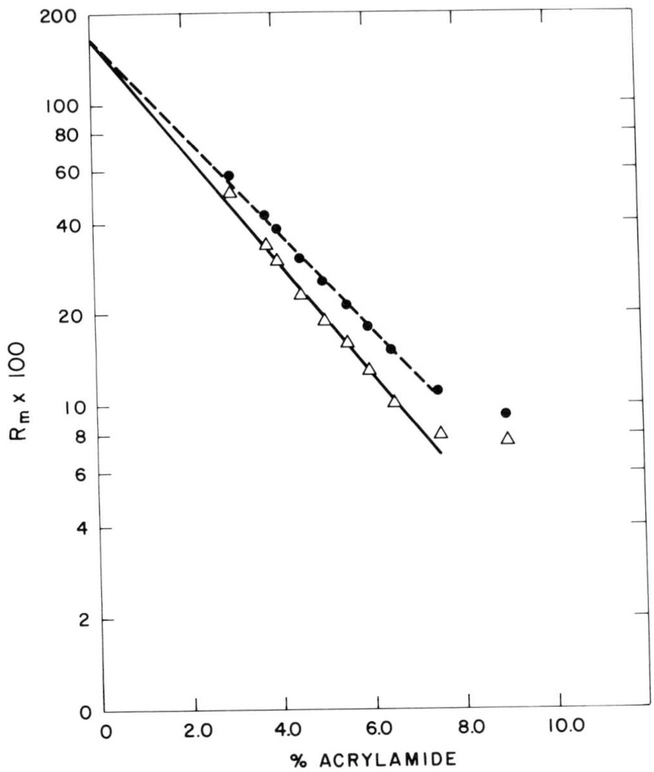

Fig. 2. Ferguson plot of spectrin band I (△——△) and band II (●- - -●). Relative mobilities R_m were measured as described in Methods. The logarithm of $R_m \times 100$ versus the gel acrylamide concentration were plotted. Linear regression analysis results: for band 1 $K_R = -0.157$, for band 2 $K_R = -0.140$.

NTCB Cleavage

Purified spectrin or subunits band 1 or band 2 (1–3 mg) was reduced with 10 mM DTT in 6 M guanidine-HCl (pH 8.0), 1 mM EDTA. After reduction, DTT was removed by dialysis against 100 vol 8 M urea, 1 mM EDTA followed by two more dialyses against the cleavage reaction medium (8 M urea, 0.2 M Tris-HCl (pH 8.0), 1 mM EDTA). Sulfhydryl groups were cyanylated by a two-fold excess of NTCB as described by Jacobson et al [21]. Hydrolysis was achieved by adjusting the pH to 9.0 and incubating over night at 37°C. After cleavage, 10 μl of β-Me per milliliter of reaction mixture was added and incubated for 20–30 min. The reaction mixture was dialyzed twice against 1 mM Tris base, 2 M urea, 0.1 M NaCl, then against 1 mM Tris base. Finally, the reaction mixture was dialyzed against distilled water and lyophilized. The cleavage proteins were analyzed by two-dimensional polyacrylamide gel electrophoresis. The first dimension was run on 5% alkaline urea gel [36, 37] and the second dimension was run on 7.5% acrylamide Fairbank's slab gel.

Amino acid analysis was performed on a Durrum-D500 amino acid autoanalyzer. Determinations on three different preparations of spectrin and subunits gave similar results. Partial tryptic cleavage of spectrin subunits are described in the figure legend of Figure 4.

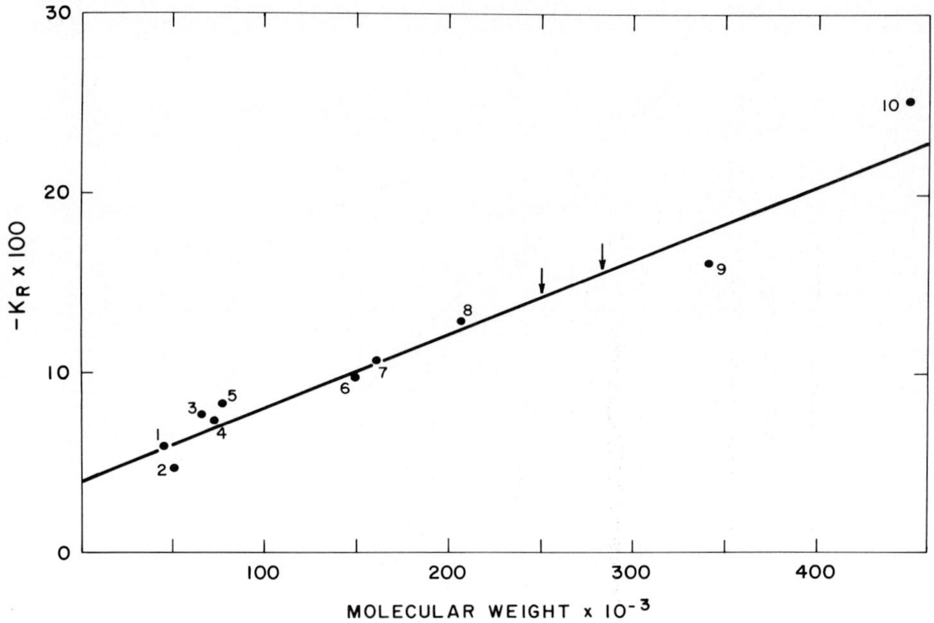

Fig. 3. The retardation coefficient vs molecular weight standard curve. The retardation coefficient K_R was obtained as described in Methods. The proteins used are: 1) Ovalbumin, 45,000; 2) hog pancreas α-amylase, 50,000; 3) bovine albumin, 66,200; 4) lactate dehydrogenase (lactobacillus leichmanni), 72,000 (monomer); 5) human transferrin, 76,500; 6) rabbit muscle aldolase, 149,000; 7) sheep IgG, 160,000; 8) sweet potato β-amylase, 206,000; 9) bovine fibrinogen, 340,000; 10) Apo ferritin, 450,000. Linear regression analysis yielded the following results: slope = −0.0043551, Y intercept = −0.0384, standard deviation of Y = 0.061, correlation coefficient of the regression = −0.9796. K_R of bands I and II were the averages of three determinations as described in Figure 2. The molecular weights obtained by interpolation on the standard curve are band I = 273,500 and band II = 238,600.

RESULTS

We have recently reinvestigated the question of the homogeneity of the spectrin polypeptides by analyzing spectrin purified by both a high-salt gel filtration procedure [15] and by purifying different spectrin polypeptides by gel chromatography and/or preparative gel electrophoresis in the presence of sodium dodecyl sulfate [15]. Purified fractions of spectrin band 1 and spectrin band 2 can be prepared by preparative SDS chromatography, in the case of band 1, or by preparative SDS gel electrophoresis, in the case of band 2 (Fig. 1). In the course of these studies we have never found any indication that the high-molecular-weight polypeptides of spectrin are aggregated forms of low-molecular-weight polypeptides. We also feel that the previous reports which describe low-molecular-weight forms of spectrin polypeptides are undoubtedly due to artifactual proteolytic digestion of the spectrins either from contaminating leukocytes and/or platelets or the action of proteases bound to the red cell membrane itself [16–18]. Spectrin prepared by the high-salt procedure has a tendency to break down slowly during storage at 4°C, while spectrin prepared by SDS chromatography remains stable for long periods of time at 4° and also retains its capacity to bind to inside-out red cell membrane vesicles [15].

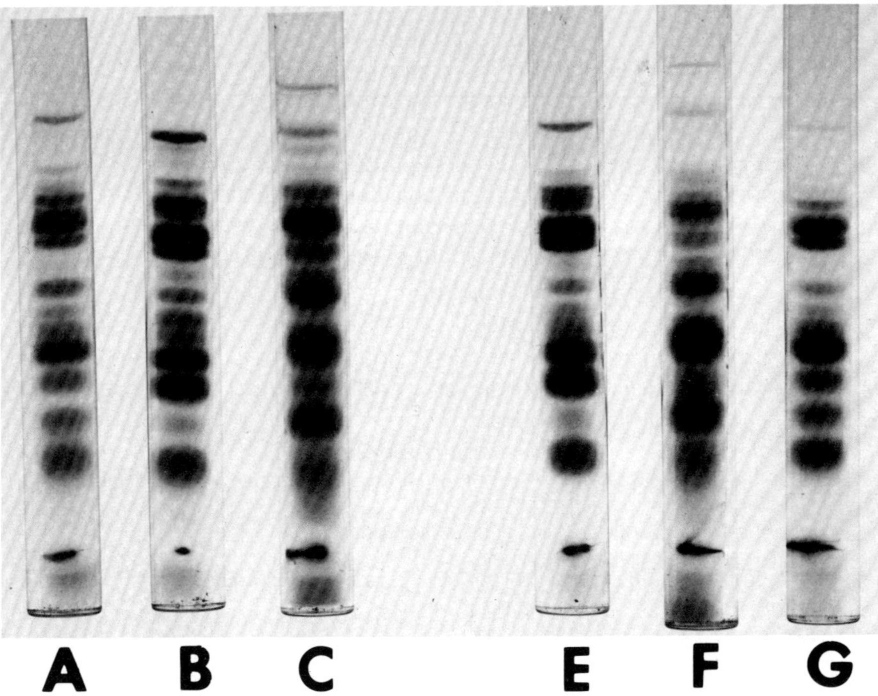

Fig. 4. Partial tryptic digestion of spectrin subunits. The spectrin subunits band I, band II, and unfractionated spectrin (Ca 0.5 mg/ml in 20 mM Tris-HCl, pH = 8.0) were digested with TPCK-trypsin (enzyme:substrate = 1:100) at 0°C, 50 μl aliquots were taken at 15-min intervals, and the digestion was stopped by adding 50 μl boiling SDS solubilizing buffer, following which the mixtures were boiled for 2 min. The samples were analyzed on 5.6% Fairbanks SDS gel system. A) band I, B) band II, C) band I digested for 60 min at 0°C.

Spectrin purified in the presence of SDS also has another interesting property. When spectrin is dissolved in SDS its circular dichroism (CD) spectrum is significantly altered, and a relatively large amount of α-helicity is lost [15]. However, when the SDS is dialyzed away from such preparations the α-helical content of the spectrin molecules is essentially restored, and the CD spectra of SDS-purified spectrin are indistinguishable from the spectra of spectrin purified by conventional high-salt treatment. As mentioned above, SDS-purified spectrin also binds as efficiently to inside-out red cell vesicles as spectrin prepared in the absence of detergents [15].

The ability of spectrin to regain tertiary structure after SDS treatment is surprising, since it is such an enormous polypeptide chain. It is possible that some parts of the molecule, not part of the helical segments or the membrane-binding sites, are irreversibly altered by the SDS treatment. However, the ability to purify spectrin in SDS offers certain operational advantages, in that SDS chromatography is probably the best way to prepare spectrin free of proteases, and is the only way we have been able to purify the individual subunits.

We have also studied the isoelectric focusing properties of spectrin purified in the presence of SDS and have obtained results which differ significantly from previously published reports. SDS-purified band 1 of spectrin forms a reasonably homogeneous band on isoelectric focusing in acrylamide gels (Fig. 1), which is distinctly more focused than bands obtained by previous investigators [13, 14]. SDS-purified band 2 also forms a single band but the latter is more diffuse and less properly focused than the band 1 subunit. In order to explain the discrepancy between our results and those of previous investigators, we have studied the focusing properties of spectrin in some detail and have discovered that the capacity to achieve well-focused bands depends upon the amount of spectrin polypeptide which is applied to the gel. Relatively small amounts of the individual spectrin peptides focus as narrow bands, but if increasing amounts of the same material are applied to different gels, the resulting bands become increasingly broad. Thus we feel that the very broad bands previously achieved by isoelectric focusing may have been due to excessive sample loads and/or secondary aggregation states of the spectrin polymers which take place even in the presence of nonionic detergents.

Further evidence in support of spectrin homogeneity has been obtained by analyzing purified spectrin subunits by standard gel electrophoresis without SDS or other denaturing agents. SDS-purified band 1 forms remarkably sharp bands (Fig. 1); SDS-purified band 2 forms a band which is more diffuse and is reminiscent of the diffuse band achieved when the latter polypeptide is analyzed by isoelectric focusing. It is interesting that the isolated individual bands of spectrin can be analyzed in these gel systems even though the complete spectrin molecule, composed of equal amounts of bands 1 and bands 2, does not migrate into these gels without denaturing agents.

We have taken advantage of this ability to electrophorese the spectrin subunits under these conditions to reinvestigate their molecular weights using the Ferguson method of analysis, which is based on free-mobility calculations [19]. Plots of the mobilities of a set of standard proteins are illustrated in Fig. 3, and the plots obtained when purified band 1 and purified band 2 are analyzed under the same conditions are shown in Fig. 2. Molecular weights of spectrin subunits calculated by this approach give values of 273,500 for band 1 and 238,600 for band 2, which are in remarkably good agreement with the molecular weights calculated using the standard SDS relative mobility method, a result which represents a welcome confirmation of the latter procedure.

The results of analyzing purified spectrin subunits by SDS gel electrophoresis, isoelectric focusing, and standard gel electrophoresis all support the original claims that the spectrin polymers represent homogeneous high-molecular-weight polypeptides. These findings do not support more recent suggestions that spectrin represents a heterogeneous mixture of chemically different proteins. However, it should be realized that the evidence in favor of spectrin being composed of two homogeneous chains is not as rigorous as one would like, and it must be admitted that some heterogeneity in the polypeptide chains could easily pass undetected by these studies. We also have not provided an entirely satisfactory explanation for the multiple N-terminal residues reported by others [10, 12]. It is conceivable that the N-terminal analysis of such mammoth polypeptides could be misleading, particularly since quantitative recoveries of terminal amino acids have not been obtained. It is also conceivable that some of the amino acids detected in these studies represent those exposed by proteolytic cleavage of the spectrin polypeptides. The latter possibility must be considered in the face of clear evidence that spectrin peptides are extremely sensitive to such degradation [20].

Is the smaller subunit of spectrin (band 2) simply a shorter version of band 1?

The amino acid compositions of SDS-purified spectrin band 1 and SDS-purified band 2 are similar (Table I), although there are differences in individual residues. A more revealing attempt to determine the degree of molecular overlap between the two bands has been provided by study of the peptide fragments of the two forms produced by two different methods. Purified band 1 and band 2 have been subjected to tryptic cleavage for different time periods, and the resulting peptide fragments analyzed by SDS gel electrophoresis. Figure 4 shows the electroferograms obtained when both peptides are digested at 30 and 60 min. Although these comparative maps are complex and not easy to interpret, it seems clear that the major Coomassie Blue staining peptides generated by tryptic cleavage from each of the spectrin subunits differ significantly in their SDS mobility. Peptide differences are evident after both 30 and 60 min of cleavage and thus indicate that there are significant differences in the location of lysine and arginine residues in the two polypeptide chains. Comparative studies of peptides generated from both spectrin subunits by S-cyanylation have also been carried out, with comparable results. Figure 5 shows two-dimensional electroferograms of S-cyanylation-induced fragments of both SDS-purified band 1 and SDS-purified band 2. Since S-cyanylation cleaves peptide bonds under relatively mild conditions at sites of cystine linkages [21], the different peptide maps obtained from the two peptides further reinforce the idea that spectrin band 1 and spectrin band 2 represent significantly different primary sequences. The cleavage maps prepared by S-cyanylation of the spectrin subunits were carried out in urea or guanidine; thus this method of generating peptides is not influenced by the conformational states of the different peptides. One drawback of the S-cyanylation procedure evident here and in other studies is the fact that such cleavages are often incomplete. We assume that this explains the presence of a relatively large number of high-molecular-weight peptides present in both maps.

TABLE I. Amino Acid Composition of Human Spectrin Subunits (in mole %)

Amino acid	Band 1	Band 2	Spectrin
Asp	11.4	10.5	10.8
Thr	3.8	3.8	3.9
Ser	5.1	5.1	5.2
Glu	20.8	20.1	20.1
Pro	1.7	2.3	2.1
Gly	4.4	5.0	4.7
Ala	9.2	9.4	9.3
Val	4.8	5.1	4.8
Met	0.9	1.1	1.1
Ile	3.4	3.3	3.5
Leu	14.0	14.5	14.2
Tyr	2.2	1.9	2.1
Phe	3.5	3.5	3.4
His	2.9	3.1	3.0
Lys	7.6	6.6	7.1
Arg	5.8	6.7	6.4

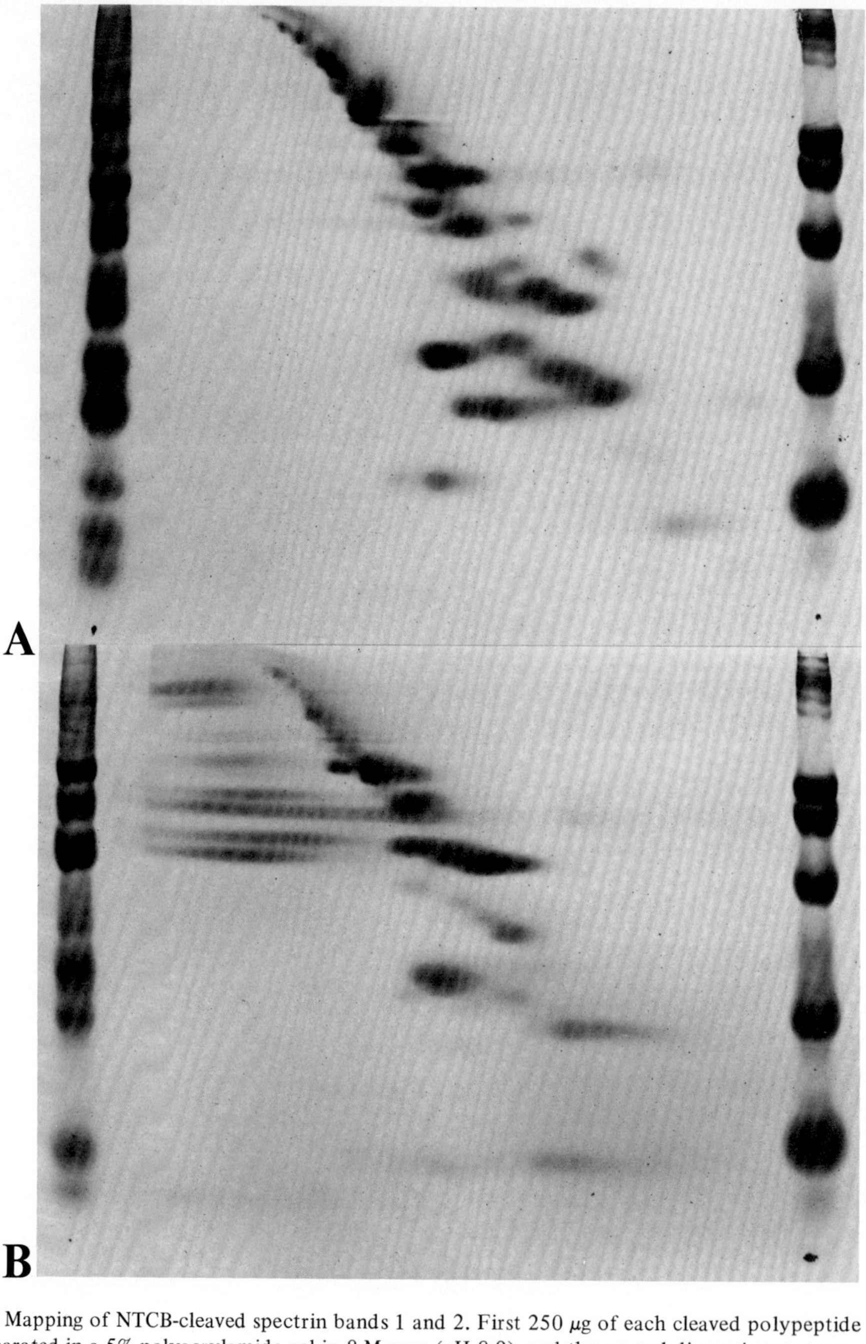

Fig. 5. Mapping of NTCB-cleaved spectrin bands 1 and 2. First 250 μg of each cleaved polypeptide was separated in a 5% polyacrylamide gel in 8 M urea (pH 8.9), and the second dimension was run on a 7.5% acrylamide slab as described under Methods; 150 μg of material and 25 μg of markers were electrophoresed in the lateral slots as controls. Markers used: transferrin (90,000 MW), human albumin (67,000 MW), ovalbumin (45,000 MW), chymotrypsinogen A (23,200 MW), and human hemoglobin (16,000 MW). A) NTCB-cleaved spectrin band 1; B) NTCB-cleaved spectrin band 2.

SUMMARY AND CONCLUSION

Our understanding of the substructure of the spectrin polypeptides is still at a rudimentary stage, but it is possible to draw some tentative conclusions with the evidence at hand. Spectrin bands 1 and 2, which have apparent molecular weights of 250,000 and 225,000 daltons, seem to be composed of single polypeptide chains. The evidence in support of this conclusion is not unequivocal but rests more on the fact that evidence of heterogeneity is less convincing. On the basis of partial enzymatic and chemical cleavage studies, it appears that spectrin band 1, the higher-molecular-weight form, differs significantly in its primary structure from spectrin band 2. Thus spectrin band 2 is not simply a shorter version of the band 1 polypeptide. The evidence suggesting significant differences in amino acid sequence of the two spectrin peptides is amplified by the often repeated observation that only the band 2 of spectrin is phosphorylated [22] and the recent observation that only isolated spectrin band 2 binds to inside-out vesicles [15]. Although the chemical and enzymatic cleavage experiments suggest significant differences in primary structure between the two subunits, it is important to point out that there probably are also large areas of overlap between the two. This conclusion is based on the fact that the isolated components have similar amino acid compositions and closed isoelectric focusing points, and both peptides show significant immunologic cross-reactivity.

Earlier cross-linking studies suggested that the isolated spectrin molecule was made up of heterodimers of bands 1 and 2 [23], and spectrin also appears to be a heterodimer when organized in the intact ghost membrane [24]. Recent immunocytochemical studies indicate that spectrin is localized as a submembranous matrix along the inner surfaces of intact human blood cells [25]. These studies confirm earlier suggestions that the spectrin is located internal to the lipid bilayer of erythrocyte ghosts, as determined both by ferritin-antibody localization [26] and by its inaccessibility to enzymatic digestion or to exogenous chemical labeling [27, 28].

The precise three-dimensional disposition of the spectrin matrix within intact red blood cells is still incompletely understood. Earlier conceptions of the spectrin molecule suggested that it might be myosin-like in form – and idea based on its hydrodynamic properties [29] and by an apparent cross-reactivity between spectrin and muscle myosin [30]. This idea led many to suggest that spectrin might form a submembranous reticulum, perhaps attached to cytoplasmic segments of transmembrane proteins or to other membrane elements. Such a reticulum was thought to confer stability and deformability to the cell membrane. One of the most convincing findings in support of a spectrin network has been provided by analyzing RBC ghost residues prepared by Triton extraction [31]. Triton selectively solubilizes integral membrane proteins and some of the membrane lipids, and it leaves behind a reticular network which still retains the approximate size and shape of the original membrane. Although the exact composition of this network remains undefined, it is reasonable to suppose that its principal components are spectrin and band 5, the putative erythrocyte actin.

These studies illustrate the remarkable stability of spectrin-actin complexes, but leave unanswered how spectrin and actin interact in the intact red cell membrane. Another still unresolved general problem concerns the attachment sites for the submembranous spectrin scaffolding. Earlier studies suggested that spectrin might associate directly with the cytoplasmic segments of at least two transmembrane glycoproteins [3–6], but recent experiments do not support these ideas [15, 32]. The results of binding studies from our laboratory, which are to be reported elsewhere [15], indicate that the spectrin polypeptides bind to specific regions on the inner surface of the red cell membrane which are in close proximity to the cytoplasmic segments of band 3 and to bands 4.1–4.2. We have also shown that spectrin can form specific complexes with isolated bands 4.1–4.2. Although spectrin does not appear to bind directly the cytoplasmic segment of band 3 [32], antibodies to this segment can compete for spectrin binding to inside-out vesicles [15]. Purified spectrin does bind to isolated bands 4.1-4.2 [33] and antibodies to the bands 4.1–4.2 complex also inhibit spectrin binding to the inner surface of the ghost membrane [15]. The close associations between spectrin and band 4.1 suggested by these findings is consistent with earlier cross-linking studies [24] and the recent demonstration that a calcium activated transglutaminase in red cells catalyzes the formation of specific complexes between spectrin and band 4.1 and possibly band 3 as well [34, 35].

The studies to date which have attempted to define the site or sites of spectrin binding to the inner surface of the red cell membrane suggest that spectrin binding sites are concentrated at specific loci which are clustered around or perhaps defined by cytoplasmic segments of the major transmembrane glycoproteins. It is obvious, however, that that available information provides us with only a hazy glimpse of what will undoubtedly prove to be highly complex associations between the spectrin polypeptides and various elements of the red cell membrane.

ACKNOWLEDGMENTS

This study was supported by Membrane Center grant GM 21714 and Patho-Biology Training grant 07562.

We wish to thank Nancy Joyce for her excellent technical assistance.

REFERENCES

1. Tomita M, Marchesi VT: Proc Natl Acad Sci USA 72:2964, 1975.
2. Steck TL, Ramos B, Stapazon E: Biochemistry 15:1154, 1976.
3. Nicolson GL, Painter RG: J Cell Biol 59:395, 1973.
4. Pinto da Silva P: J Cell Biol 53:777, 1972.
5. Elgsaeter A, Branton D: J Cell Biol 63:1018, 1974.
6. Pinto da Silva P, Nicolson GL: Biochim Biophys Acta 363:311, 1974.
7. Shotton D, Thompson K, Wofsy L, Branton D: J Cell Biol 76:512, 1978.
8. Yu J, Branton D: Proc Natl Acad Sci USA 73:3891, 1976.
9. Marchesi VT, Steers EJ: Science 159:203, 1968.
10. Knufermann H, Bhakdi S, Schmidt-Ullrich R, Wallach DFH: Biochim Biophys Acta 330:356, 1973.
11. Fuller GM, Boughter JM, Morazzani M: Biochemistry 13:3036, 1974.
12. Dunn MJ, Maddy AH: FEBS Lett 36:79, 1973.
13. Bhakdi S, Knufermann H, Wallach DFH: Biochim Biophys Acta 345:448, 1974.
14. Green JR, Dunn MF, Spooner RL, Maddy AH: Biochim Biophys Acta 373:51, 1974.
15. Litman D, Hsu CJ, Marchesi VT: Manuscript submitted.
16. Morrison WL, Neurath H: J Biol Chem 200:39, 1953.
17. Bernacki RJ, Bosmann HB: J Membrane Biol 7:1, 1972.
18. Tokes ZA, Chambers SM: Biochim Biophys Acta 389:325, 1975.
19. Ferguson KA: Metabolism 13:985, 1964.
20. Hulla FN: Biochim Biophys Acta 345:430, 1974.
21. Jacobson GR, Schaffer MH, Stark GR, Vanaman TC: J Biol Chem 248:6583, 1973.

22. Birchmeier W, Singer SJ: J Cell Biol 73:647, 1977.
23. Clarke M: Biochem Biophys Res Commun 45:1063, 1971.
24. Wang K, Richards FM: J Biol Chem 249:8005, 1974.
25. Ziparo E, Lemay A, Marchesi VT: Manuscript submitted.
26. Nicolson GL, Marchesi VT, Singer SJ: J Cell Biol 51:265, 1971.
27. Marchesi VT: in Fox CF (ed): "Biochemistry of Cell Walls and Membranes." MTP International Review of Science–Biochemistry Series 1, Volume 2. Baltimore: University Park Press, 1975.
28. Kirkpatrick FH: Life Sci 19:1, 1976.
29. Schechter NM, Sharp M, Reynolds JA, Tanford JA, Tanford C: Biochemistry 15: 1897, 1976.
30. Sheetz MP, Painter RG, Singer SJ: Biochemistry 15:4486, 1976.
31. Hainfeld JF, Steck TL: J Supramol Struct 6:301, 1977.
32. Bennett V, Branton D: J Biol Chem 252:2753, 1977.
33. Hsu CJ, Litman D, Marchesi VT: Manuscript in preparation.
34. Lorand L. Weissmann LB, Epel DL, Bruner-Lorand J: Proc Natl Acad Sci USA 73:4479, 1976.
35. Anderson DR, Davis JL, Carraway KL: J Biol Chem 252:6617, 1977.
36. Ornstein L: Ann NY Acad Sci 121:321, 1964.
37. Davis BJ: Ann NY Acad Sci 121:404, 1964.

Journal of Supramolecular Structure 10:241–251 (1979)
Normal and Abnormal Red Cell Membranes 401–411

Interaction Between Glycophorin and Phospholipids in Recombined Systems

Alice Y. Romans, Philip L. Yeagle, Sally E. O'Connor, and Charles M. Grisham

Department of Pathology, Medical Center of the University of Alabama in Birmingham, Birmingham, AL 35294 (A.Y.R.), Biochemistry Department, Medical School, State University of New York at Buffalo, Buffalo, NY 14214 (P.L.Y.), and Department of Chemistry, University of Virginia, Charlottesville, VA 22901 (S.E.O., C.M.G.)

Both the MN-glycoprotein from human erythrocytes and the hydrophobic fragment from the protein isolated with trypsin treatment, T(is), have been recombined with egg phosphatidylcholine in bilayers at various phospholipid/protein ratios. In order to investigate the effect of the protein on the phospholipid headgroups, ^{31}P nuclear magnetic resonance spectra were obtained with the MN-glycoprotein recombined with egg phosphatidylcholine, which revealed two classes of phospholipid environments, one immobilized and one not immobilized. Electron spin resonance (ESR) of fatty acid methyl ester spin labels provided supporting evidence.

Computer analysis of the ESR spectra indicate that 4–5 moles of phospholipid are immobilized per mole of protein over a wide range of lipid-to-protein ratios. The immobilization of the phospholipids appears mediated by both the polar headgroups and the hydrocarbon tails of the phospholipid.

Key words: **boundary lipid, $^{31}PNMR$, spin labels, glycophorin**

Glycophorin, the major sialoglycoprotein of human erythrocyte membranes, is an integral membrane protein which spans the erythrocyte membrane [1, 2]. The NH_2-terminal region of the glycoprotein contains all the carbohydrate and is exposed to the extracellular milieu [3]. The COOH-terminal region of the molecule is enriched in hydrophilic residues such as aspartic acid, glutamic acid, lysine, and arginine, as compared to the entire molecule [3], and is exposed on the cytoplasmic surface of the membrane [1, 2]. A portion containing 23 amino acid residues connects these two regions and is contained within a tryptic peptide T(is) which is insoluble in aqueous solution [4, 5]. Amino acid

A.Y. Romans is now at Kimberly-Clark Corporation, Neenah, WI 54956.

Received March 5, 1978; accepted September 21, 1978.

0091-7419/79/1002-0241$02.30

analysis and subsequent sequencing showed that this peptide has a high content of nonpolar amino acids [3–5]. The hydrophobicity of this intermediate region of the protein allows it to interact favorably with the hydrocarbon chains of phospholipids as it spans the bilayer.

By the use of electron spin resonance (ESR) spin labels it has been shown that the integral membrane proteins cytochrome b_5 [6], cytochrome oxidase [7], myelin basic protein [8], and the Ca^{++}ATPase [9, 10] immobilize a portion of the lipid in the membrane, called boundary lipid, by contact between the hydrophobic portion of the membrane protein and the hydrocarbon chains of the lipids. Boundary lipid most likely constitutes one or more layers of affected lipid around the protein and may regulate its interaction with the membrane as a whole.

To our knowledge, a detailed structural study of the interactions between phospholipids and protein in a membrane has not been published for any purified membrane protein from the red cell. The purpose of this study is to demonstrate that glycophorin immobilizes lipid when recombined with phospholipid in model membrane systems, and that the immobilization is mediated by the polar headgroups as well as the hydrocarbon chains of the membrane phospholipids.

MATERIALS AND METHODS

Egg phosphatidylcholine was obtained in benzene from Avanti Biochemicals; it exhibited only a single spot on thin layer chromatographic analysis (65:25:4, chloroform, methanol, water) when about 1 mg sample was applied. Phospholipid concentrations were determined using the method of Bartlett [11]. The C-12 spin label, methyl 12-(4′,4′-dimethyloxazolidinyl-N-oxyl) stearate, was synthesized [12].

Glycophorin was isolated from red blood cell ghosts by the Lithium 3,5-diiodosalicylate extraction method of Marchesi and Andrews [13]. T(is) was obtained by trypsin digestion of glycophorin and solubilized in 2,2,2-trifluoroethanol. Its concentration was determined by amino acid analysis on a Beckman 121-M analyzer with computing integration after hydrolysis for 24 h at 110°C in 6 N HCl.

T(is) was associated with egg phosphatidylcholine by first mixing the phospholipid and protein in 2,2,2-trifluoroethanol and, after evaporation of the solvent, hydration with an excess of 100 mM NaCl, 10 mM EDTA, H_2O. For the ESR spin label experiments, the spin label in ethanol was added to the mixture of phospholipid and protein before evaporation of the organic solvent.

Glycophorin was associated with egg phosphatidylcholine by the following procedure. Anhydrous protein and phospholipid were solvated for 3h in 2-chloroethanol and subsequently evaporated under vacuum for three days. The dry mixture was then hydrated in 4 mM histidine, 150 mM NaCl, pH 7.2, overnight. This suspension was used directly for ^{31}P nuclear magnetic resonance (NMR) measurements; for ESR experiments, the spin label in ethanol was dried in a test tube and the aqueous suspension of protein and phospholipid was subsequently incubated in the tube for an hour or more before obtaining ESR spectra. Sucrose density gradient centrifugation indicated that the largest stable protein-to-lipid ratio was 1:20; that ratio was therefore used for both the ESR and NMR experiments with intact glycophorin.

ESR spectra were obtained with a Varian E-109 ESR spectrometer, at 9.07 GHz using a variable temperature controller to maintain the temperature at 23 ± 1°C. Instrument settings were chosen to avoid instrument-induced line broadening or saturation. The ESR spectra for several preparations of the T(is)/egg phosphatidylcholine samples were digitized in a PDP 11/VO3 computer system. Spectral subtraction and numerical integration of spectra were performed using programs developed on the computer (S.E. O'Conner and C.M. Grisham, to be published).

NMR spectra were obtained at 40.48 MHz for ^{31}P on a JEOL PS100/EC100 Fourier transform spectrometer at 23°C, except where noted. ^{31}P NMR spectra were obtained with gated broadband proton decoupling to remove the ^{31}P [^{1}H] nuclear Overhauser effect [14] and to reduce the dipolar contributions to the linewidth [19] so that the magnitude of the effective chemical shift anisotropy could be measured. The decoupler was gated "on" during aquisition to effect proton decoupling and "off" the remainder of the time to prevent buildup of the nuclear Overhauser effect. We used 90° pulses with a repetition rate five times the spin lattice relaxation time of unsonicated egg phosphatidylcholine aqueous dispersions (about 1.5 s [20]). Intensities of spectra were evaluated by cutting and weighing photocopies of the spectra.

RESULTS

T(is)

The hydrophobic peptide obtained from glycophorin by trypsin treatment was associated successfully with egg phosphatidylcholine at initial protein-to-lipid mole ratios of 1:5, 1:10, 1:20, and 1:50. An attempt to associate T(is) with egg phosphatidylcholine at a protein-to-lipid ratio of 1:2.5 left some unassociated protein as a precipitate, so that ratio was not used for the magnetic resonance experiments. Egg phosphatidylcholine was used because it resembles the lipid content of the red cell membrane more closely than a synthetic, saturated phospholipid species, yet can be obtained as a pure phosphatidylcholine.

Methyl esters of fatty acids spin-labeled at various positions produce ESR spectra diagnostic of the motional order of the region of the membrane near their location [15]. The ESR spectra of the C-12 spin label used here, incorporated into the unsonicated bilayers of an egg phosphatidylcholine dispersion at a concentration of 1 mole %, appears in Fig. 1. It is similar to spectra obtained by others [15], reflecting the fluidity of a phospholipid bilayer well above its phase transition temperature. The phospholipid concentration was 5 mg/ml in this and each of the following spin label experiments.

ESR spectra of the 12-doxyl methyl stearate spin label incorporated in T(is)/egg phosphatidylcholine dispersions are shown in Fig. 1. Spectra B–F were taken at the indicated protein-to-lipid mole ratios. Each of the spectra B–E shows that it is composite spectrum consisting of a sum of immobilized and nonimmobilized lipid components. Spectrum B was obtained from the sample containing the largest percentage of immobilized lipid and hence was used to obtain the spectrum of purely immobilized lipid spin label. This spectrum is shown at the top of Fig. 1. Spectrum A′ was synthesized by subtraction of an appropriate amount of the fluid bilayer spectrum (F at the bottom of the fig.) from spectrum B. Spectrum A′ is highly anisotropic and is indicative of lipid spin label in a very immobilized environment. This anisotropic spectrum clearly demonstrates the immobilization of lipids surrounding the protein.

To obtain an estimate of the number of lipids immobilized by the protein in these experiments, the contribution to the total spectral intensity arising from the immobilized lipids was calculated. Spectrum A′ was subtracted from each of spectra B–E until the resulting difference spectrum was indistinguishable from spectrum F. Since spectrum F was taken from a sample containing no protein, it is characteristic of spin labels in fluid bilayers.

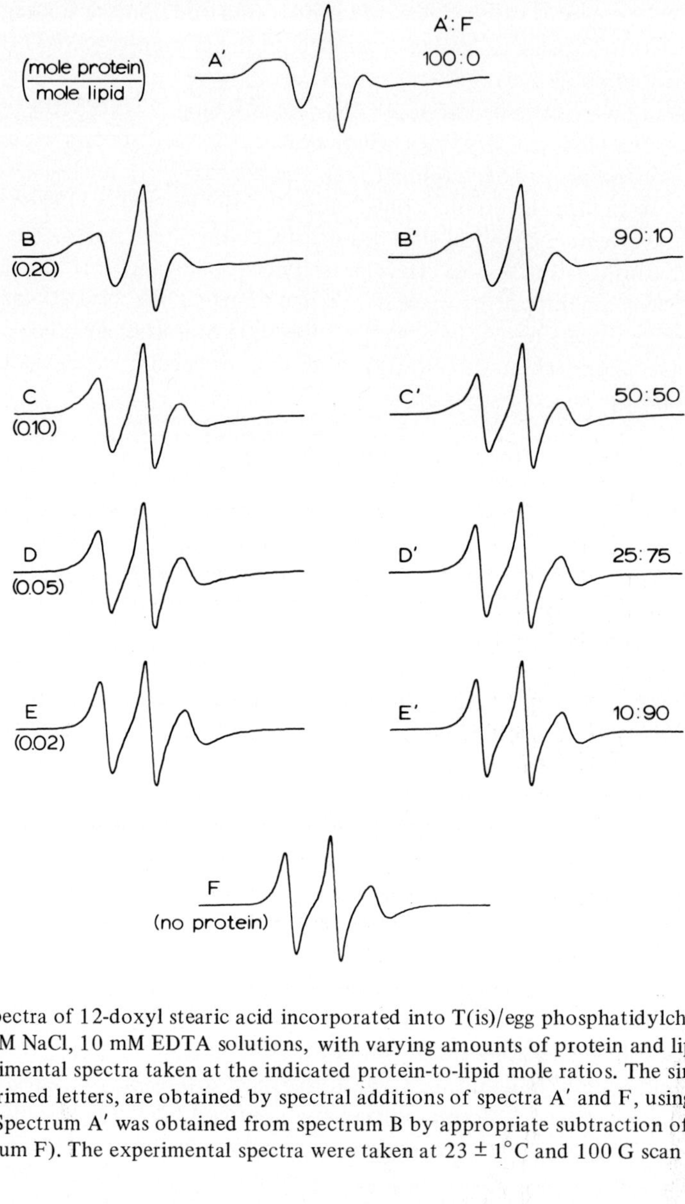

Fig. 1. ESR spectra of 12-doxyl stearic acid incorporated into T(is)/egg phosphatidylcholine dispersions in 100 mM NaCl, 10 mM EDTA solutions, with varying amounts of protein and lipids. Spectra B–F are experimental spectra taken at the indicated protein-to-lipid mole ratios. The simulated spectra, indicated by primed letters, are obtained by spectral additions of spectra A′ and F, using the weighted ratios shown. Spectrum A′ was obtained from spectrum B by appropriate subtraction of the fluid component (spectrum F). The experimental spectra were taken at 23 ± 1°C and 100 G scan range.

Integration of the original spectrum and the difference spectrum gives absorption curves from which the percentage of fluid spin label component can be obtained from the ratios of the areas under the absorption curves. The spectrum of the spin label diffused in T(is) associated with egg phosphatidylcholine at a protein-to-lipid mole ratio of 0.20 shows that 87% of the intensity of its ESR spectrum arises from immobilized spin label. Similar analysis of the other spectra gave percentages of lipid residing in an immobilized environment of 43%, 24%, and 8.1% for the sample containing protein-to-lipid mole ratios of 1:10, 1:20, and 1:50, respectively. As shown in Table I, these results suggest that 4–5 lipids are immobilized by the protein in these experiments.

TABLE I. Quantitative Analysis* of ESR Spectra of 12-Doxyl Methyl Stearate in T(is)-Egg Phosphatidylcholine Dispersions

Sample (lipid/protein mole ratio)	Percentage of total spectral intensity due to bound label	Number of moles of bound lipid per mole of T(is)
5:1	86.9%	4.4
10:1	43.8%	4.4
20:1	23.9%	4.8
50:1	8.1%	4.1

*ESR spectra were resolved into immobilized and nonimmobilized components as shown in Fig. 1 and then integrated to yield absorption and integral mode spectra, which were analyzed as described in the text.

Further support of the values obtained for the number of lipids immobilized by the protein is given by the close correspondence between the experimental spectra and the spectra synthesized by addition of spectrum A and spectrum F. In the right-hand column of Fig. 1 can be seen the spectra obtained by summation of the immobilized and nonimmobilized spectra for varying amounts of each. The weighting factors used in the spectral simulation are shown in the figure. These spectra strongly suggest that the T(is) protein under the conditions of the experiment immobilizes 4–5 lipids per protein monomer. It is also interesting to note that the same number of lipids are immobilized irrespective of the amount of lipid present. The results shown here seem to indicate that there are two environments for the lipids in the presence of the protein. A third spectral component, which was detected in the course of the data analysis, can be seen in the sample containing a protein-to-lipid ratio of 1:10. This third component exhibits an ESR spectrum which is intermediate between the highly immobilized and nonimmobilized lipid spectra, and accounts for less than 10% of the total intensity of spectrum C.

Successful incorporation of T(is) into the bilayers was indicated by the appearance of an immobilized component in the ESR spectrum. Since T(is) is insoluble in water, the perturbation of the bilayer as deep as the location of the C-12 spin label indicates incorporation into the bilayer. Furthermore, density gradient centrifugation at all ratios used in the ESR experiments, with representative material prepared in the identical manner, produced a single band. The density corresponded to the initial ratio of protein to phospholipid recombined, which indicated a stable association of the two components. No significant amount of material appeared at the bottom of the gradient. Freeze-fracture electron microscopy of recombinants revealed bumps on one of the fracture faces.

Glycophorin

The glycophorin/egg phosphatidylcholine complexes were not stable at as high a protein-to-lipid ratio as T(is)/egg phosphatidylcholine complexes. The ESR spectrum of a 1:20 (glycophorin/egg phosphatidylcholine) mixture, the highest ratio obtainable as a stable complex, was essentially the same as for T(is) at the same protein-to-lipid ratio.

It is of interest to know not only whether the hydrocarbon chains of the phospholipids are immobilized by interaction with this integral membrane protein, but also whether the phospholipid headgroups are immobilized by interaction with glycophorin. Recently it was found that the B protein in human low-density lipoprotein immobilized some of the phospholipid of the particle, probably by interaction with the headgroups [16]. This immobilization was detected because it caused, most likely, a large increase in the proton dipolar contributions to the linewidth, leading to phospholipid ^{31}P resonance linewidths so broad that they did not contribute to the high resolution resonance. In an analogous manner, the interactions between phospholipid headgroups and glycophorin was studied.

For these experiments, glycophorin was associated with egg phosphatidylcholine at an initial protein-to-lipid ratio of 1:20. After sucrose density gradient centrifugation of a representative sample prepared in the same fashion as for the magnetic resonance experiments, Lowry and phosphate analyses indicated that a stable lipid/protein complex was formed. A single band was observed at the density expected for a 1:20 mole ratio of glycophorin to phospholipid. No significant amount of material appeared at the bottom of the gradient. Further evidence of the incorporation of glycophorin into bilayers of phosphatidylcholine is seen in the freeze-fracture electron micrograph of Fig. 2, where bumps are seen on one of the fracture faces of the liposomes.

The ^{31}P NMR spectrum of an unsonicated egg phosphatidylcholine dispersion containing glycophorin at a 1:20 initial protein-to-lipid mole ratio appears in Fig. 3. Also in Fig. 3 is the ^{31}P NMR spectrum of an unsonicated egg phosphatidylcholine dispersion, containing the same amount of phospholipid as the glycophorin-phosphatidylcholine sample. These spectra are similar in shape to ^{31}P NMR spectra obtained from the erythrocyte membrane [17], vesicular stomatitus viral coat membrane [18], and unsonicated aqueous dispersions of pure phospholipids [19]. These spectra were obtained with broadband proton decoupling, so the lineshape is dominated by the chemical shift anisotropy of the phosphorus, which can be related to the motional order of the phosphate region of the phospholipid [19]. Furthermore, the proton decoupler was gated to remove the ^{31}P $[^1H]$ nuclear Overhauser effect (about a 40% enhancement of signal intensity in unsonicated egg phosphatidylcholine [20]), and the spectra were obtained with 90° pulses separated by five T_1 of the phosphorus nuclei, so that the intensities would be directly proportional to the amount of phospholipid present. These spectra were obtained twice, from independent samples.

Two important pieces of information are contained in these spectra. First, the intensity of the glycophorin-containing sample is 25–30% less than the sample without the protein. The missing phospholipid must be in an immobilized environment such that the dipolar and/or chemical-shift anisotropy contributions to the lineshape broaden it sufficiently so that it cannot be seen under the conditions of these experiments. This corresponds to five to six phospholipids per glycophorin whose headgroups are immobilized by the protein.

Second, the effective chemical-shift anisotropy is reduced from 45 ± 1 ppm in the pure egg phosphatidylcholine sample to an apparent 36 ± 1 ppm in the glycophorin-containing membrane. The decrease in the apparent chemical-shift anisotropy may indicate a decrease in phospholipid headgroup order (or orientation) and/or a change in organization of those phospholipids not immobilized by the protein.

DISCUSSION

Phospholipids in unsonicated aqueous dispersions produce anisotropic ^{31}P resonances. When the phospholipids are in bilayer form, these ^{31}P resonances generally resemble the spectrum of egg phosphatidylcholine in Fig. 3 (for a review of these phenomena, see Seelig [23]. This spectrum results from partial motional averaging of the ^{31}P chemical-shift tensor by rapid axial motion of the phospholipid perpendicular to the bilayer surface.

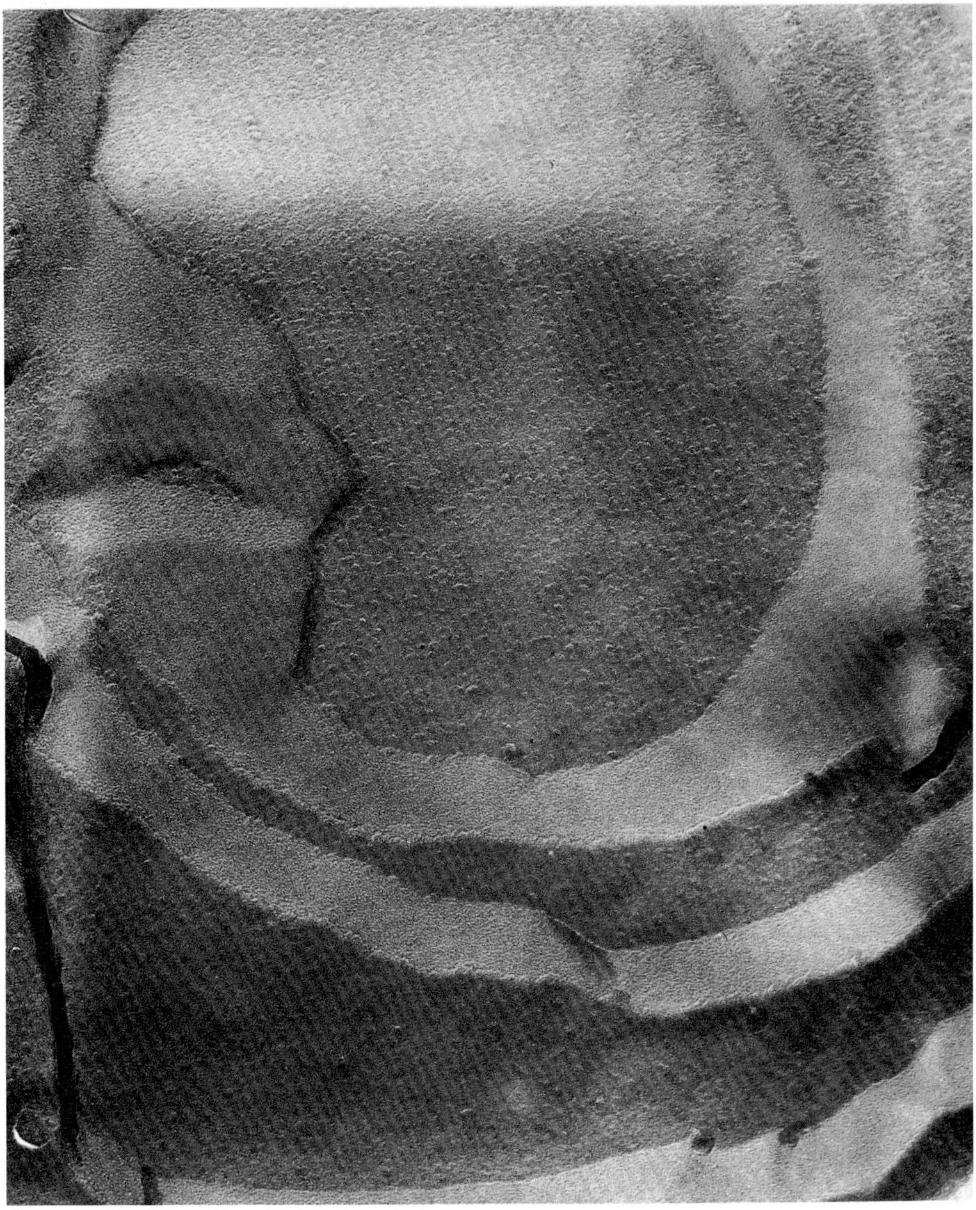

Fig. 2. Freeze-fracture electron micrograph of a 1:50 glycophorin/phosphatidylcholine recombinant at a magnification of 86,000 ×.

The chemical shift tensor describes the three-dimensional behavior of the chemical shift of the phosphate ^{31}P nucleus. The shielding of the nucleus, which determines the chemical shift, is dependent upon the direction from which the nucleus is approached. Because this is a three-dimensional dependence, the chemical shift is described by a tensor, and it is anisotropic because the shielding around the phosphorus is anisotropic. Thus, in a crystal where the molecule containing a phosphorus does not rotate rapidly, the observed chemical shift is a function of the angle of the crystal with the applied magnetic field [22].

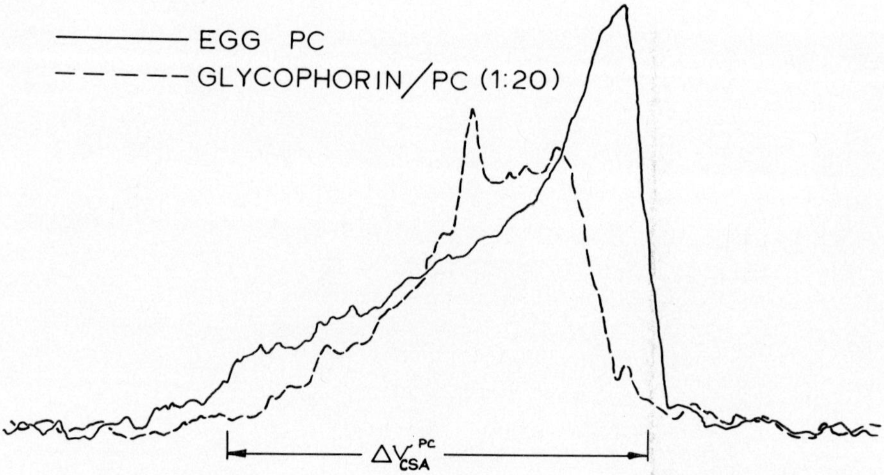

Fig. 3. ^{31}P NMR spectra of unsonicated egg phosphatidylcholine dispersions containing glycophorin. – – –) glycophorin/egg phosphatidylcholine 1:20 (20 mg egg phosphatidylcholine); ——) egg phosphatidylcholine (20 mg). Spectra were obtained with gated broadband proton decoupling. The effective chemical-shift anisotropy for egg phosphatidylcholine is 45 ± 1 ppm (or about 1800 Hz at this field strength) and for the glycophorin-containing sample is 36 ± 1 ppm (or about 1450 Hz at this field strength). Total spectral width is 5,000 Hz; 3,170 scans were obtained with a repetition rate of 7 s; 4,000 data points were collected, with 90° pulses (20 μsec).

When the molecules are randomly oriented, a powder pattern results. For a powder from dry phospholipids the chemical shift is spread over the full range of the chemical-shift tensor with the intensity at any one point proportional to the probability of an orientation in the random powder giving rise to that chemical shift. Discontinuities and shoulders in the spectrum provide the principle values of the chemical-shift tensor.

For phospholipids in randomly oriented bilayers in an aqueous environment rapid axial motion of the phospholipids perpendicular to the bilayer surface (and movement of the motional axis) averages two of the elements of the chemical-shift tensor, producing an apparent axially symmetric spectrum of considerably less breadth than the phospholipid powders. Analysis of ^{31}P NMR spectra of these systems, such as the spectra in Fig. 3, has led to information on motional ordering of the phospholipid head groups [19] and to a description of headgroup orientation in agreement with other, independent approaches [23, 24].

When phospholipids are not in a bilayer, different motional averaging may occur which leads to different spectral shapes. Some phosphatidylethanolamines form a hexagonal phase where additional motional averaging can occur by diffusion of the phospholipids around the cylinders in that phase. The ^{31}P spectra of these hexagonal systems show the opposite sign of the chemical-shift anisotropy and one-half the magnitude of a bilayer system. Similar results have been obtained for some sphingomyelins [25] and for the lipids of the bovine rod outer segment membranes [26].

With this background it is possible to examine the ^{31}P NMR spectra obtained with glycophorin recombined with phosphatidylcholine and obtain some useful information. From the intensity analysis it appears that a portion of the phospholipid is immobilized by the presence of the protein. Approximately five to six lipids appear to be immobilized per glycophorin molecule. This finding is supported by the ESR measurements with the hyrophobic portion of the protein. The identification of immobilized lipid as a separate entity appears justified, because exchange with bulk lipid is slow enough that the spectrum of the bulk lipid is little affected by it. Since these two measurements sense two different portions of the membrane (Fig. 4), apparently the phospholipids interact with the protein through their hydrocarbon tails and their polar headgroups.

These results would be expected to have ramifications for the structure of the erythrocyte cell membrane in which glycophorin is found. Presumably glycophorin would immobilize phospholipid in the erythrocyte membrane just as in the recombined system. Recent work has suggested that there may be preferential interactions between glycophorin and negatively charged phospholipids [21]. Since it appears that glycophorin does bind some phospholipid tightly, and if there is a preferential interaction with negatively charged phospholipids, glycophorin might exert some influence on phospholipid asymmetry of the erythrocyte membrane.

The effects of glycophorin do not appear to be confined to the immediate region of the protein. Figure 3 shows that the ^{31}P resonances of the glycophorin-containing membranes are somewhat less broad than for egg phosphatidylcholine without glycophorin. This result may be interpreted in two different ways. First, the shapes of the two spectra are similar and the lesser breadth of the glycophorin-containing sample may reflect a decrease in the ordering of the headgroups of phospholipids not immobilized by the protein [19]. Alternatively, the spectral difference may reflect a change in organization of the phospholipids not immediately adjacent to the protein. Conversion to a hexagonal phase produces a dramatic change in spectral shape as mentioned earlier [27]. While a hexagonal phase does not appear to dominate here, since the sign of the anisotropy has not changed, a modification of the bilayer structure found in pure phosphatidylcholine systems by the glycophorin might lead to the result observed here. Either interpretation suggests a disorganization of bilayer structure of the phospholipid not immediately adjacent to the protein by the high concentration of glycophorin. Such a result is not altogether surprising, since the protein is no longer in a sea of lipid but rather constitutes a significant portion of the membrane area itself. It is not clear at this point whether glycophorin exhibits long-

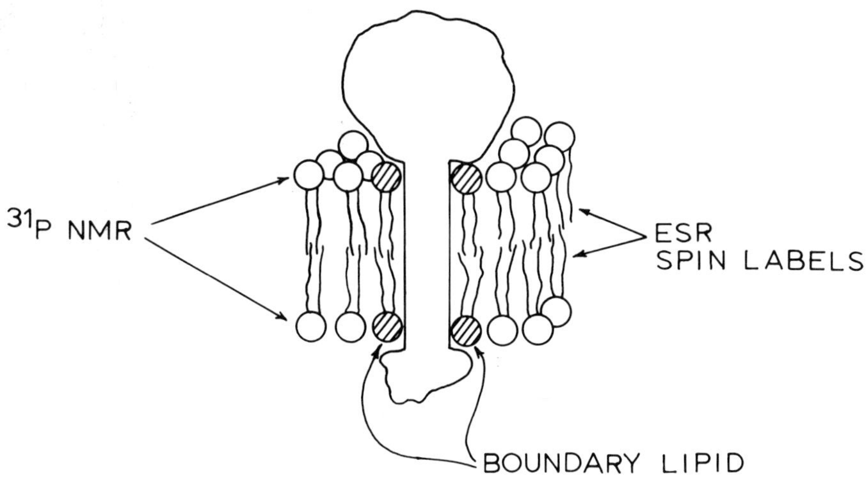

Fig. 4. Schematic of glycophorin in phospholipid bilayer, showing sampling areas of the NMR and ESR measurements.

range effects on the lipids of the erythrocyte membrane of any importance, or whether this effect is merely induced by the close proximity of glycophorin molecules in this recombined preparation. In this regard, it is interesting that rhodopsin at similar protein-to-phospholipid ratios produces no such disordering effect on the phospholipids [26].

ACKNOWLEDGMENTS

PLY thanks Professor R. B. Martin for the opportunity and support for doing this work. We are grateful for the assistance of W.C. Hutton in this project.

This work was also supported by National Institutes of Health grant AM 19419, ACS-PRF grant 87576-4, and grants from the Research Corporation and the Muscular Dystrophy Association of America, as well as grants from the National Science Foundation and the University of Virginia for the ESR spectrometer. We thank Dr. J.P. Segrest for support and David Patton for electron microscopy. We thank Dr. J. Seelig for helpful comments on the manuscript.

REFERENCES

1. Bretscher MS: Nature New Biol 231:229, 1971.
2. Segrest JP, Kahane I, Jackson RL, Marchesi VT: Arch Biochem Biophys 155:167, 1973.
3. Tomita M, Marchesi VT: Proc Natl Acad Sci USA 72:2964, 1975.
4. Segrest JP, Jackson RL, Marchesi VT, Guyer RB, Terry W: Biochem Biophys Res Commun 49:964, 1972.
5. Winsler RJ: In Jamieson GA, Greenwalt TJ (eds): "Red Cell Membrane: Structure and Function." Philadelphia: Lippincott, 1969, p 157.
6. Dehlinger PJ, Jost PC, Griffith OH: Proc Natl Acad Sci USA 71:2280, 1974.
7. Jost PC, Griffith OH, Capaldi RA, Vanderkooi G: Proc Natl Acad Sci USA 70:480, 1973.
8. Boggs JM, Vail WJ, Moscarello MA: Biochim Biophys Acta 448:517, 1974.
9. Hesketh TR, Smith GA, Houslay MD, McGill KA, Birdsall NJM, Metcalf JC, Warren GB: Biochemistry 15:4145, 1976.
10. Nakamura M, Ohnishi S: J Biochem (Tokyo) 78:1039, 1975.
11. Bartlett GR: J Biol Chem 234:466, 1959.
12. Waggoner A, Kingsett T, Roltschaefer S, Griffith OH, Keith A: Chem Phys Lipids 3:245, 1969.
13. Marchesi VT, Andrews EP: Science 174:1247, 1971.
14. Yeagle PL, Hutton WC, Martin RB: J Am Chem Soc 97:7175, 1975.
15. Griffith OH, Jost PC: In Berliner LJ (ed): "Spin Labeling: Theory and Applications." New York: Academic, 1976, p 454.
16. Yeagle PL, Landon RG, Martin RB: Biochemistry 16:3487, 1977.
17. McLaughlin AC, Cullis PR, Hemminga MA, Hoult DI, Radda FK, Ritchie GA, Seeley PJ, Richards RE: FEBS Lett 57:213, 1975.
18. Moore NF, Patzer EJ, Wganer RR, Yeagle PL, Hutton WC, Martin RB: Biochim Biophys Acta 465:173, 1977.
19. Neiderberger W, Seelig J: J Am Chem Soc 98:3704, 1976.
20. Yeagle PL, Hutton WC, Huang C, Martin RB: Biochem 16:4344, 1977.

21. Van Zoelin EJJ, Zwaal RFA, Reuvers FAM, Demel RA, Van Deenen LLM: Biochim Biophys Acta 464:482, 1977.
22. Kohler SJ, Klein MP: Biochemistry 15:967, 1976.
23. Seelig J: Biochim Biophys Acta Biomembr Rev (In press).
24. Yeagle PL: Accounts Chem Res (In press).
25. Yeagle PL, Hutton WC, Martin RB: Manuscript in preparation.
26. Albert AD, Yeagle PL, Litman BJ: Manuscript in preparation.
27. Cullis PR, deKruijff B: Biochim Biophys Acta 507:207, 1978.

Journal of Supramolecular Structure 10:253–263 (1979)
Normal and Abnormal Red Cell Membranes 413–423

Erythrocyte Spectrin Alteration Induced by Low-Density Lipoprotein

David Y. Hui and Judith A. K. Harmony

Chemistry Department, Indiana University, Bloomington, IN 47401

Addition of human plasma low-density lipoproteins (LDL) to intact human erythrocytes induces the erythrocytes to undergo morphologic transition from biconcave disks to echinocytes and spherocytes. The transformation is time-dependent. Two hours are required before echinocytes are detected by scanning electron microscopy. After two hours, LDL also decrease the phosphate content of spectrin by 40% relative to the control, suggesting that these lipoproteins modulate cell shape by influencing phosphorylation-dephosphorylation of a membrane-associated cytoskeletal protein. LDL do not induce depletion of intracellular adenosine triphosphate (ATP), nor do they inhibit cyclic adenosine monophosphate-independent protein kinases which phosphorylate spectrin. LDL stimulate membrane-bound phosphatases by a factor of two, thereby reducing the amount of phosphate covalently bound to membrane proteins. The observed effects are specific for LDL. High-density lipoproteins (HDL) do not stimulate dephosphorylation of spectrin or alter erythrocyte morphology. However, HDL protect the erythrocytes against LDL-induced alterations. These data suggest that the circulating lipoproteins have a role in maintaining erythrocyte morphology by regulating the extent of phosphorylation of spectrin.

Key words: **plasma lipoproteins, erythrocyte morphology, erythrocyte phosphatase, spectrin phosphorylation**

Recent reports [1–3] suggest that the extent of phosphorylation of spectrin determines erythrocyte morphology. According to this concept, spectrin phosphorylation regulates the interaction of actin with spectrin [3, 4], which in turn specifies the structural state of the spectrin-actin complex on the cytoplasmic surface of the membrane [3]. Since patients with certain types of lipoprotein disorders have erythrocytes of altered morphology [5], it is of interest to determine the effects of individual lipoprotein classes on cell morphology and spectrin phosphorylation. In the present communication, we report the influence of human plasma low-density lipoproteins (LDL) and high-density lipoproteins

Received May 1, 1978; accepted November 10, 1978.

(HDL) on erythrocyte morphology and physiology. Results of these studies suggest that LDL but not HDL alter erythrocyte morphology by stimulating dephosphorylation of spectrin.

MATERIALS AND METHODS

Erythrocytes were isolated from normal human plasma by centrifugation. After the plasma and buffy coat were removed by aspiration, the erythrocytes were further fractionated by the method of Poon and Simon [6]. Isolated cells were washed three times in a buffer containing 20 mM Tris-HCl (pH 7.4), 150 mM NaCl, and 20 mM KCl. Human lipoproteins were isolated from the freshly collected plasma of normolipemic fasted donors by sequential ultracentrifugal flotation in KBr [7]. LDL were isolated between densities 1.019 and 1.063 and HDL, between 1.063 and 1.21; densities were measured with a hydrometer. Lipoproteins were dialyzed extensively against 150 mM NaCl (pH 7.4) and used immediately. The isolated LDL did not react at any concentration with antisera prepared against HDL or against the major HDL proteins apoAI and apoAII. However, when high concentrations of HDL were analyzed, a very faint precipitin line was detected between the HDL and antiLDL. The lipid compositions of both LDL and HDL were within the normal range of values [8].

Lipoproteins or albumin were added to erythrocytes which were resuspended to 10–20% hematocrit in a buffer containing 20 mM Tris-HCl (pH 7.4), 150 mM NaCl, 10 mM glucose, 1 μM adenine, and 1 mM $CaCl_2$. LDL were added at a final concentration of 2.5 mg/ml; HDL, at 0.25 mg/ml or 4.5 mg/ml. The concentration of lipoprotein in each case was calculated from the protein concentration assuming that LDL and HDL are 21 wt % and 50 wt % protein, respectively [8]. Bovine serum albumin or defatted human serum albumin was included at a final concentration of 50 mg/ml in the incubation mixture as indicated. In all experiments, the incubation time was 4 h at 37°C.

Protein concentration was determined by a modified method of Lowry et al [9] using 1% sodium dodecylsulfate (SDS); bovine serum albumin was the standard. Cholesterol (free and esterified) was determined by the method of Roeschlau et al [10]. Triglyceride was assayed enzymatically [11]. Phospholipids were separated by thin-layer chromatography on Silica Gel 1B2 (J.T. Baker Chemical Co.) in a solvent system of chloroform:acetone:methanol:acetic acid:water (10:4:2:2:1, v/v). The method of Bartlett [12] was used to quantitate phospholipids; an average molecular weight of 750 was employed to determine phospholipid concentration. Lipids were extracted from erythrocyte ghosts by chloroform-methanol as described by Waku and Lands [13]. The amount of intracellular adenosine triphosphate (ATP) was determined using a phosphoglycerate kinase assay procedure [14]. Phosphatase activity was measured spectrophotometrically employing the exogenous substrate p-nitrophenyl phosphate [15, 16]. Protein kinase activity was determined by measuring the phosphorylation of casein as described by Hosey and Tao [17].

RESULTS

When LDL are added to erythrocytes, cell morphology is significantly altered. As shown in Figure 1, LDL induce a transformation of erythrocytes from normal biconcave disks (Fig. 1A) to echinocytes (Fig. 1B) and cells of poorly defined morphology (Fig. 1C); 2 h at 37° are required to detect the alterations (Table I). A fraction of the poorly defined spherical cells shown in Figure 1C appear to be fused, although microscopic evidence alone

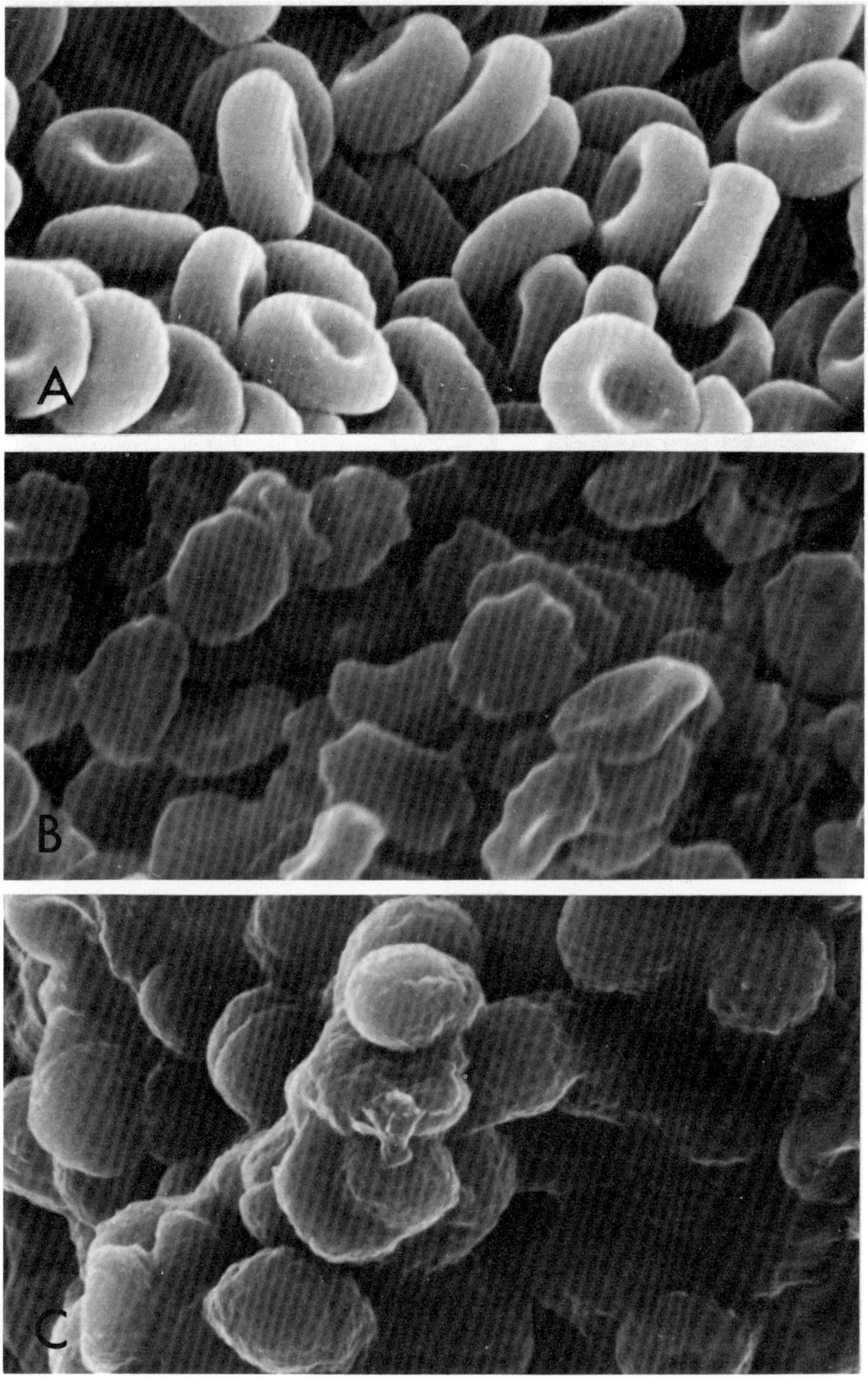

Fig. 1. Effect of LDL on erythrocyte morphology. Erythrocytes were incubated for 4 h at 37°C without LDL (A), and for 3 h (B) and 4 h (C) with LDL (2.5 mg/ml) as described in Materials and Methods. The cells were subsequently fixed at 4° for 1 h by the addition of an equal volume of 1% glutaraldehyde in 150 mM NaCl, 20 mM Tris-HCl (pH 7.4). After extensive washing with distilled water, the packed erythrocytes were dehydrated with acetone and were vacuum-evaporated (1×10^{-5} torr). The specimens were then coated with light carbon and gold-palladium (60:40), and the cells were examined with an ETEC-Autoscann electron microscope.

TABLE I. Erythrocyte Morphology

Experiment	Time (h)	Discocyte	Echinocyte	Spherocyte
Erythrocytes, control	1	++++	–	–
	4	++++	Trace	–
Erythrocytes plus LDL	1	++++	–	–
	2	+++	+	–
	3	+	+++	–
	4	+	++	+
Erythrocytes plus HDL	1	++++	–	–
	4	++++	–	–
Erythrocytes plus LDL and HDL	1	++++	–	–
	4	++++	Trace	–
Erythrocytes plus LDL followed by HDL[a]	4	+	+++	–
Erythrocytes plus LDL followed by heparin[a]	4	$++^{+}/2$	$+^{+}/2$	–
Erythrocytes plus albumin	1	++++	–	–
	4	++++	–	–
Erythrocytes plus albumin and LDL	1	++++	–	–
	4	+	++	+

Erythrocytes were incubated at 37°C and prepared for microscopy as described in Methods and in legend to Fig. 1. Morphology was assessed by scanning electron microscopy and by light microscopy. Morphologic type was scored as follows: ++++) 100%; +++) 75%; ++) 50%; +) 25%; –) 0%.
[a]Erythrocytes were incubated for 3 h with LDL prior to addition of HDL or heparin; incubation was continued for 1 h with HDL or heparin. Concentrations: LDL, 2.5 mg/ml; HDL, 0.25 mg/ml; albumin, 50 mg/ml; heparin, 10 units/ml.

is not conclusive. Once the erythrocytes are transformed to echinocytes by exposure to LDL for 3 h, removal of the LDL with heparin [20] allows the reverse echinocyte-discocyte transformation to occur. The effects of LDL are specific for this class of lipoproteins. HDL do not alter erythrocyte morphology (Table I). However, when added simultaneously with LDL, HDL inhibit the LDL-induced alterations. Inhibition by HDL occurs at a ratio LDL:HDL of 10:1 (wt/wt), a ratio about 10 times normal [8]. HDL are also "protective" when LDL and HDL are added in equal proportions (D.Y. Hui and J.A.K. Harmony, data submitted for publication). If HDL are added to cells which have been exposed to LDL for 3 h (echinocytes), they do not reverse the LDL-induced morphologic alteration; HDL do, however, prevent further alteration which results in formation of spherocytes. Albumin, which is known to reverse lysin-induced sphering [21], does not inhibit the morphologic transformation elicited by LDL (Table I).

To investigate the possible biochemical mechanisms which might account for the morphologic alterations elicited by LDL, we have quantitatively determined intracellular and membrane constituents, the perturbation of which has been associated with changes of erythrocyte morphology. As indicated in Table II, there are no significant differences in the cellular concentration of glucose, inorganic phosphate, or ATP determined for control cells and for cells incubated with LDL, HDL, or LDL plus HDL. Furthermore, no change in the ratios of the major erythrocyte membrane lipids is detected (Table II):

TABLE II. Effect of Lipoproteins on Intracellular and Membrane Constituents of Intact Erythrocytes*

Cell constituent	Erythrocyte control	Erythrocytes plus LDL (2.5 mg/ml)	Erythrocytes plus HDL (0.25 mg/ml)	Erythrocytes plus LDL (2.5 mg/ml) and HDL (0.25 mg/ml)
[^{14}C]-glucose (cpm/mg Hb)	880	880	880	ND
[^{32}P]-phosphate (cpm/mg Hb)	7.0×10^7	6.9×10^7	6.9×10^7	7.1×10^7
ATP (micromoles per liter of packed cells)	400	390	400	395
Membrane lipids[a]				
Phospholipid:cholesterol	3.26 (3.00)	3.28	3.16	3.26
Sphingomyelin: phosphatidylcholine	0.94 (0.84)	0.94	0.89	0.89
Phosphatidylethanolamine: phosphatidylcholine	1.06 (1.00)	1.06	1.00	1.00
Monoacylphosphatidylcholine	Trace	Trace	Trace	Trace

Human erythrocytes were incubated with lipoproteins at the concentration indicated for 4 h at 37°C. At the end of incubation, cells were washed three times with 150 mM NaCl and lysed by the method of Dodge et al [18]. Hemoglobin in the lysate was determined by measuring the absorbance at 576 nm of the supernatant following centrifugation [19]. Erythrocytes were labeled with [^{14}C]-glucose and [^{32}P]-phosphate prior to addition of lipoproteins.
*Abbreviations: Hb) hemoglobin; ND) not determined.
[a]The lipid composition was determined as milligrams lipid per milligram membrane protein; the ratios are subject to an approximate error of 5%. The numbers in parenthesis are from Pennell [39].

cholesterol and the major phospholipids phosphatidylcholine, monoacylphosphatidylcholine, sphingomyelin, and phosphatidylethanolamine are unaltered during incubation of erythrocytes with lipoproteins. Correspondingly, the lipid composition of the lipoproteins is unaltered by interaction with erythrocytes (data not shown).

Subsequently we attempted to determine if the addition of LDL to erythrocytes alters the membrane-associated proteins and, in particular, alters the covalent incorporation of [^{32}P]-phosphate into membrane constituents. Typical polyacrylamide gel electrophoretis patterns of membrane-derived proteins from control cells and from erythrocytes exposed for 4 h to LDL are illustrated in Figure 2. The gel patterns are identical. The amount of protein associated with each stained band as determined spectrophotometrically at 550 nm is not altered by incubation of erythrocytes with LDL, suggesting that membrane proteins are not released. Moreover, exposure of the cells to LDL does not result in the appearance of additional membrane-associated proteins. In agreement with reports of other investigators [22, 23], spectrin band II and band III are the major membrane proteins which are phosphorylated in intact cells in the absence of exogenous cyclic adenosine monophosphate (cAMP) (Fig. 2). When erythrocytes are incubated with LDL there is a 40% (± 5% determined from four separate experiments) reduction of [^{32}P]-phosphate incorporation into spectrin component II; the extent of phosphorylation of band III is not altered by LDL. Furthermore, addition of HDL to erythrocytes does not influence spectrin phosphorylation (data not shown), which is consistent with the fact that HDL do not alter erythrocyte morphology.

Since LDL reduce the level of spectrin phosphate in intact cells, we utilized membrane ghosts and exogenous enzyme substrates to investigate the influence of LDL on phosphorylation and dephosphorylation independently. As is evident in Table III, when ghosts are incubated with [γ-^{32}P]-ATP, membrane-associated protein kinases catalyze the

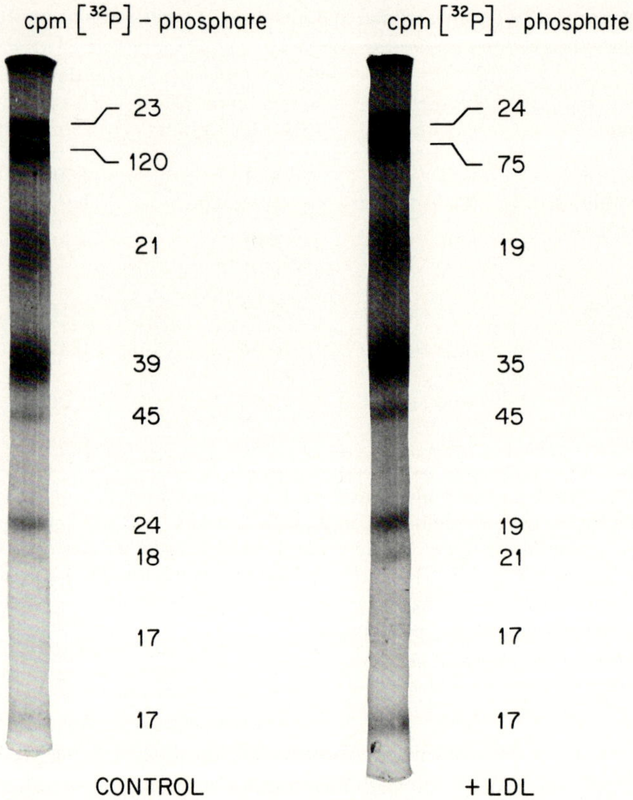

Fig. 2. SDS gel electrophoresis of erythrocyte membrane proteins: A) from control cells; B) from erythrocytes incubated in the presence of LDL (2.5 mg/ml). Human erythrocytes (10% hematocrit) were incubated for 4 h at 37°C. The volume of a typical reaction mixture was 10 ml with final concentrations as follows: 20 mM sodium phosphate (pH 7.4), 150 mM NaCl, 20 mM KCl, 5 mM glucose, 1 μM adenine. The buffer also contained 600 μCi of [^{32}P]-phosphate as $Na_2H^{32}PO_4$. Following incubation, the cells were washed and subsequently lysed according to the method described by Dodge et al [18]. Polyacrylamide gel electrophoresis of membrane ghosts was performed in 6% acrylamide containing 0.16% N,N'-methylene-bis-acrylamide and 0.2% sodium dodecyl sulfate as described by Fairbanks et al [24]. To each gel 50 μg membrane protein was applied. Gels were sliced into 1-mm fractions and each slice was dissolved in 1 ml 30% H_2O_2. The radioactivity of each fraction was determined by liquid scintillation in Aquasol (New England Nuclear).

transfer of [^{32}P]-phosphate to the soluble protein fraction which contains casein. Phosphorylation of casein is diagnostic of the cAMP-independent protein kinase(s) which phosphorylate spectrin [17]. The amount of [^{32}P]-phosphate incorporated into casein is not influenced by preincubating the erythrocyte ghosts for 3 h at 37°C with either LDL or HDL: 1.37×10^4 (± 2%) cpm of [^{32}P]-phosphate are incorporated per milligram casein in the presence or absence of lipoproteins (Table III). Thus, cAMP-independent protein kinase activities are not affected by the LDL-erythrocyte interaction. On the other hand, addition of LDL to the ghost suspension increases twofold the rate of hydrolysis of p-nitrophenyl phosphate catalyzed by membrane-associated phosphatases. Phosphatase activation increases with increasing concentrations of LDL (data not shown): Activation is not maximal at 4 mg/ml LDL. LDL do not catalyze p-nitrophenyl phosphate hydrolysis in the absence of

TABLE III. Effect of Lipoproteins on Phosphorylation-Dephosphorylation

Experiment	Erythrocyte control	Erythrocytes plus LDL (2.5 mg/ml)	Erythrocytes plus HDL (4.5 mg/ml)	Erythrocytes plus LDL (2.5 mg/ml) and HDL (4.5 mg/ml)
Protein kinase activity (^{32}P cpm/mg casein)[a]	1.38×10^4	1.35×10^4	1.34×10^4	1.40×10^4
p-Nitrophenyl phosphatase activity (nmole/mg·h)				
– ATP	162.5	254.2	166.7	165.0
+ ATP	105.0	240.0	101.7	106.3

A volume of freshly prepared membrane ghosts equivalent to 0.8 ml original packed cells was incubated in 20 mM Tris-HCl (pH 7.4) at 37°C. To determine protein kinase activity, erythrocyte ghosts were preincubated for 3 h in the presence and absence of lipoproteins. Lipoproteins suspended in 150 mM NaCl were added to the final concentrations indicated; an equivalent volume of 150 mM NaCl was added to the control experiment. Subsequently, 0.1 ml of the membrane suspension was added to an equal volume of a solution containing 100 μM [γ-^{32}P] ATP and 4 mg/ml casein in 20 mM Tris-HCl (pH 7.4). The final [NaCl] was 50 mM. After incubation for an additional 30 min, the reaction was terminated by the addition of 15 μl of 12 mg/ml bovine serum albumin and 2 ml 33% trichloroacetic acid. The protein precipitate was collected on glass fiber disks (Whatman GF/C, 0.24-mm diameter) and washed exhaustively with 5% trichloroacetic acid; protein-bound ^{32}P was measured by liquid scintillation in Aquasol. To measure phosphatase activity, ghosts were incubated directly with 5 mM p-nitrophenyl phosphate, 0.5 mM $MgCl_2$, and 10 μM ATP, as specified. At the end of incubation, a 1-ml aliquot was removed and the reaction was stopped by the addition of 0.2 ml 33% trichloroacetic acid. Following centrifugation to remove precipitated membranes and lipoproteins, 1 ml of the supernatant was added to 2 ml 0.2 N NaOH and the concentration of p-nitrophenol was determined spectrophotometrically at 418 nm. The maximum hydrolysis of p-nitrophenyl phosphate after a 3-h incubation was less than 20% of the initial amount of substrate present in the assay medium.

[a]Control experiments were performed in the absence of casein; the amount of ^{32}P incorporated into the precipitable fraction was 33% of that in the presence of casein, indicating that the method measures casein phosphorylation and phosphorylation of membrane proteins. The amount of ^{32}P incorporated in the absence of casein was not altered by the addition of LDL or HDL.

erythrocyte ghosts. Although membrane-associated phosphatase activation is inhibited by the addition of ATP, the activity which exists in the presence of LDL is insensitive to ATP. Interestingly, HDL do not enhance phosphatase activity. The lipoproteins of the high-density class do, however, prevent LDL-induced activation of p-nitrophenyl phosphate phosphatase (Table III).

DISCUSSION

Recent reports suggest that a membrane-cytoskeleton complex regulates erythrocyte morphology [1–4]; the cytoskeletal system comprises spectrin, a high-molecular-weight tetrameric protein, and actin – both of which are situated on the cytoplasmic surface of the membrane. One key factor which determines the morphology of the cell is the extent of phosphorylation of spectrin. When spectrin is phosphorylated, erythrocytes are biconcave disks, whereas when spectrin is dephosphorylated by 40–50% [1], the cells are crenated or spherical. Virtually nothing is known concerning the existence of plasma constituents which may modulate erythrocyte morphologic alterations. Since erythrocytes are constantly exposed to the circulating lipoproteins and since the erythrocytes of individuals with abnormal lipoproteins often are spiculated [5], it is of considerable interest to determine if the plasma lipoproteins are the physiologic factors which specify erythrocyte morphology. The results reported herein demonstrate that low-density lipoproteins isolated from normolipemic individuals induce erythrocytes to undergo a transformation from biconcave disks to echinocytes and to poorly defined spherical cells.

The morphologic transformation which occurs when LDL are added to erythrocytes is a time-dependent process requiring at least 2 h at 37°. It is important to note that the ratio of LDL to erythrocytes in the incubation mixture is approximately that found in the blood of normolipemic humans. Two results of the cell morphology studies are significant. First, the morphologic alteration specifically requires LDL; the high-density lipoproteins do not affect cell shape. Second, HDL inhibit the LDL-promoted morphologic transformation. The HDL were present at subphysiologic concentrations; HDL are equally effective when LDL and HDL are present in the physiologic ratio of 1:1 (wt/wt). Thus, normal erythrocyte morphology may depend not only on the concentration of an individual lipoprotein class but also on the ratio of lipoprotein classes in the plasma. It is premature to assess the physiologic significance of these findings, since the structural features of LDL responsible for the LDL-erythrocyte alteration which results in morphologic alteration are unknown. Moreover, our data certainly cannot yet explain why individuals who lack LDL (abetalipoproteinemia) have spiculated erythrocytes and individuals who lack HDL (Tangier disease) have erythrocytes of normal morphology [5]. It is important to note that erythrocyte morphology is altered by numerous chemical agents which act by different mechanisms [21]; thus, a particular morphology is not diagnostic of one specific cellular alteration. Furthermore, the lipoproteins isolated from the plasma of individuals with inherited diseases of lipid metabolism such as Tangier disease [25] frequently have abnormal composition and structure, and these lipoproteins may not behave normally in the lipoprotein-erythrocyte interaction.

The simplest mechanism which would account for the morphologic alteration induced by LDL is a change in the lipid composition of the erythrocyte membrane [21, 26, 27] as a consequence of lipid exchange/transfer between erythrocytes and lipoproteins. While this mechanism may account for results of experiments in which the incubation time is longer than 4 h, no variation in the concentration of membrane cholesterol or phospholipids is detected within the typical four-hour incubation period (Table II). This result rules out the occurrence of net transfer of lipid constituents, although lipid exchange is probable [27].

Since spectrin phosphorylation is critical to erythrocyte morphology, we subsequently investigated the influence of LDL on this cytoskeletal protein. LDL cause a specific reduction of 40% in the amount of exchangeable phosphate associated with spectrin after 4 h incubation (Fig. 2) relative to the control. On the basis of these data alone, it is not evident whether a correlation exists between the extent of spectrin phosphorylation and the morphologic alterations induced by LDL, or whether LDL elicits dephosphorylation of specific spectrin residues. It is of interest that Harris et al [28] reported four phosphorylated sites for spectrin, two of which have significant turnover rates, and it is possible that LDL influence dephosphorylation of the latter two sites. It is of additional interest that our findings are qualitatively similar to those of Loyter et al [29], who reported that Sendai virus which induce cell lysis and fusion also cause dephosphorylation of membrane proteins. In this context, the indication of cell fusion induced by LDL in Figure 1C is particularly intriguing, since it suggests that lipoproteins and certain viruses may interact with erythrocytes by similar mechanisms. The mechanism for lipoprotein-induced dephosphorylation of spectrin differs from that for lipid vesicles, which apparently decrease the phosphate content by increasing the cholesterol:phospholipid ratio of the cell membrane [30].

The phosphate content of spectrin is determined by the intracellular concentration of ATP and by the balance between protein kinase-dependent phosphorylation and phosphatase-catalyzed dephosphorylation. Shore and Shore [31] report that LDL activate a Mg^{+2}-ATPase situated in the erythrocyte membrane, suggesting that LDL may deplete ATP in intact cells. However, the concentration of erythrocyte ATP is not influenced by the presence of the plasma lipoproteins LDL or HDL (Table II); the ATP value 400 μM per liter of packed cells agrees with that reported by Nakao et al [32]. Two possibilities remain to be considered: LDL decrease the amount of phosphate associated with spectrin by 1) inactivating a specific membrane-associated protein kinase and/or 2) stimulating a phosphoprotein phosphatase. As indicated in Table III, cAMP-independent protein kinases are not inhibited by LDL. LDL do, however, stimulate membrane-associated phosphatases twofold. Hydrolysis of p-nitrophenyl phosphate reflects contributions from phosphoprotein phosphatases and from the various ATPases. The fact that LDL also accelerate dephosphorylation of [^{32}P]-phosphorylated erythrocyte membrane proteins (D.Y. Hui and J.A.K. Harmony, data submitted for publication) suggests, not unequivocally, that the target of LDL activation is the phosphoprotein phosphatase. Significantly, HDL do not accelerate dephosphorylation of p-nitrophenyl phosphate (Table III) nor do they induce spectrin dephosphorylation or alteration of erythrocyte morphology (data not shown). HDL prevent both LDL-induced activation of membrane-bound phosphatases and alteration of cell morphology.

The mechanism by which LDL enhance phosphatase activity is not immediately evident. Since erythrocytes do not internalize lipoproteins; regulation of this enzyme does not involve endocytosis and lipoprotein degradation, processes required for LDL to regulate the activity of 3-hydroxy-3-methylglutaryl coenzyme A reductase in nucleated cells [20]. The initial event resulting in phosphatase activation is attachment of LDL to the erythrocyte membrane: About 10^6 [^{125}I]-LDL particles bind to the surface of each erythrocyte, and the binding event requires just 10–15 min at 37° (D.Y. Hui and J.A.K. Harmony, data submitted for publication). Moreover, HDL inhibit the LDL-induced alterations by preventing the attachment of LDL to the cell surface (D.Y. Hui and J.A.K. Harmony, data submitted for publication). There is some evidence to suggest that phosphatase activity may be regulated by a cyclic AMP-dependent conversion of an inactive enzyme-inhibitor complex to an active enzyme [33]. This possibility is particularly attractive, since LDL activate the membrane adenylate cyclase of human adipocytes [34]. However, the mature erythrocyte lacks a functional adenylate cyclase system [35], and analogous activation of the erythrocyte phosphatase must be controlled by other signals. One possible alternative signal is the perturbation by LDL of the concentration of intracellular ions. LDL do not induce a permeability defect for sodium ion in the cell membrane such as that introduced by the addition of sonicated phosphatidycholine vesicles to intact erythrocytes [36]. The concentration of sodium ion in intact cells incubated for 4 h with LDL is identical to the value obtained for cells incubated without lipoproteins (D.Y. Hui and J.A.K. Harmony, data submitted for publication.) Studies are currently under way to determine whether LDL influence the intracellular concentration of other ions, particularly calcium and potassium.

This is the first report that plasma lipoproteins, in particular the LDL, induce dephosphorylation of membrane-associated proteins. The significance of this finding is augmented by the fact that the target for dephosphorylation is spectrin, a cytoskeletal protein which specifies cell morphology [1–4] and the distribution of receptors at the cell surface [37]. Spectrin has so far been identified in the erythrocyte only, although the existence of high-molecular-weight cytoskeletal proteins which interact with actin is postulated in other cell types. [38]. Our observations suggest a new focus for investigators attempting to elucidate the role of lipoproteins in normal and pathologic states.

ACKNOWLEDGMENTS

This work was supported by PHS grant HL 20882 from the National Institutes of Health. The excellent technical assistance of Mr. Ron Osborne greatly facilitated this investigation. The authors appreciate the substantial aid of Ms Linda Lehman in the preparation of the manuscript.

REFERENCES

1. Greenquist AC, Mohandas N, Shohet SB: Fed Proc 37:1507, 1978.
2. Sheetz MP, Singer SJ: J Cell Biol 73:638, 1977.
3. Birchmeier W, Singer SJ: J Cell Biol 73:647, 1977.
4. Pinder JC, Bray D, Gratzer WB: Nature 270:752, 1977.
5. Stanbury JB, Wyngaarden JB, Fredrickson DS: "The Metabolic Basis of Inherited Disease." 4th Ed. New York: McGraw-Hill, 1978, part 4.
6. Poon RWM, Simon JB: Biochim Biophys Acta 384:138, 1975.
7. Camejo G: Biochim Biophys Acta 175:290, 1969.
8. Nelson GJ: "Blood Lipids and Lipoproteins: Quantitation, Composition and Metabolism." New York: Wiley Interscience, 1972.
9. Lowry OH, Rosebrough NJ, Farr AL, Randall RJ: J Biol Chem 193:265, 1951.
10. Roeschlau P, Bernt E, Gruber W: Klin Chem Klin Biochem 12:403, 1974.
11. Schmidt FH, von Dahl K: Klin Chem Klin Biochem 6:156, 1968.
12. Bartlett GR: J Biol Chem 234:466, 1959.
13. Waku K, Lands WEM: J Lipid Res 9:12, 1968.
14. Adam H: In Bergmeyer HV (ed): "Methods of Enzymatic Analysis." New York: Academic, 1963, pp 543–551.
15. Heller M, Hanahan DJ: Biochim Biophys Acta 255:239, 1972.
16. Ellory JC, Lew VL: Biochim Biophys Acta 332:215, 1974.
17. Hosey MM, Tao M: Biochim Biophys Acta 482:348, 1977.
18. Dodge JT, Mitchell C, Hanahan DJ: Arch Biochem Biophys 110:119, 1963.
19. Lake W, Rasmussen H, Goodman DBP: J Membr Biol 32:93, 1977.
20. Goldstein JL, Brown MS: Curr Topics Cell Reg 11:147, 1976.
21. Ponder E: "Hemolysis and Related Phenomena." New York: Grune and Stratton, 1948, pp 10–49.
22. Shapiro DL, Marchesi VT: J Biol Chem 252:508, 1977.
23. Plut DA, Hosey MM, Tao M: Fed Proc 36:320, 1977.
24. Fairbanks G, Steck TL, Wallach DFH: Biochemistry 10:2606, 1971.
25. Heinen RJ, Herbert PN, Fredrickson DS, Forte T, Lindgren FT: J Clin Invest 61:120, 1978.
26. Deuticke B: Biochim Biophys Acta 163:494, 1968.
27. Bruckdorfer KR, Graham JM: In Chapman D, Wallach DFH (eds): "Biological Membranes." New York: Academic, vol 3, 1976, pp 103–151.
28. Harris HW, Wolfe LC, Lux SE: J Supramol Struct 8(Suppl 2):204, 1978.
29. Loyter A, Ben-Zaquen R, Marash R, Milner Y: Biochemistry 16:3903, 1977.
30. Semenuk M, Vickers J, Rathbone M, Brain MC: Blood 50(Suppl 1): 86, 1978.
31. Shore V, Shore B: Biochem Biophys Res Commun 65:1250, 1975.
32. Nakao M, Nakao T, Yamazoe S, Yoshikawa H: J Biochem 49:487, 1961.
33. Killilea SD, Brandt H, Lee EYC: Trends Biochem Sci 1:30, 1976.
34. Pairault J, Levillier J, Chapman MJ: Nature 269:607, 1977.

35. Rasmussen H, Lake W, Gasic G, Allen J: In Brewer GJ (ed): "Erythrocyte Structure and Functions, Progress in Clinical and Biological Research." New York: Alan R Liss, 1975, vol 1, pp 467–486.
36. Huetis WH: J Biol Chem 252:6764, 1977.
37. Fowler V, Bennett V: J Supramol Struct 8(Suppl 2):207, 1978.
38. Hitchock SE: J Cell Biol 74:1, 1977.
39. Pennell RB: In Surgenor DM (ed): "The Red Blood Cell." New York: Academic Press, 1974, vol 1, pp 93–146.

Journal of Supramolecular Structure 10:265–275 (1979)
Normal and Abnormal Red Cell Membranes 425–435

Role of Bound Water in Biological Membrane Structure: Fluorescence and Infrared Studies

Allan S. Schneider, C. Russell Middaugh, and Mary D. Oldewurtel

Sloan-Kettering Institute for Cancer Research and Cornell University Graduate School of Medical Sciences, New York, New York 10021

Bound water is a major component of biological membranes and is required for the structural stability of the lipid bilayer. It has also been postulated that it is involved in water transport, membrane fusion, and mobility of membrane proteins and lipids. We have measured the fluorescence emission of membrane-bound 1-anilino-8-naphthalenesulfonate (ANS) and the infrared spectra of membranes, both as a function of hydration. ANS fluorescence is sensitive to polarity and fluidity of the membrane-aqueous interface, while infrared absorption is sensitive to the hydrogen bonding and vibrational motion of water and membrane proteins and lipids. The fluorescence results provide evidence of increasing rigidity and/or decreasing polarity of the membrane-aqueous interface with removal of water. The membrane infrared spectra show prominent hydration-dependent changes in a number of bands with possible assignments to cholesterol (vinyl CH bend, OH stretch), protein (amide A, II, V), and bound water (OH stretch). Further characterization of the bound water should allow its incorporation into current models of membrane structure and give insight into the role of membrane hydration in cell surface function.

Key words: membrane hydration, membrane-bound water, ANS fluorescence, infrared spectra, water-membrane interactions

In one of his recent books, Albert Szent-Györgyi marvels at the ubiquitous role of water in biology and lyrically notes that "life is water dancing to the tune of solids" [1]. This observation may be particularly relevant to current models of biologic membrane structure, which recognize that membrane components arrange themselves according to their amphipathic nature, such that polar sites can interact with the aqueous medium while nonpolar sites are excluded from it [2]. The physicochemical assumption that a lipid bilayer would form as a hydrophobic response to an aqueous environment was confirmed by

C.R. Middaugh is now at the Department of Biochemistry, University of Wyoming, Laramie.

Received April 12, 1978; accepted December 4, 1978.

0091-7419/79/1002-0265$02.30

Finean and co-workers, who demonstrated, by X-ray diffraction, that the structure of myelin and erythrocyte membranes was disrupted upon removal of water below the 20% hydration level [3].

Membrane-bound water has been measured by a variety of methods and generally found to comprise some 20%–30% by weight of the hydrated membrane [3–9]. Chapman and co-workers have shown that the bound water is required for mixing of cholesterol and phospholipids in the bilayer, and that below 20% hydration, these lipids separate and exhibit their individual thermal transitions [4]. We have previously found membrane-associated water to be very tightly bound with binding energies comparable to and greater than water molecules in ice [5]. Parsegian, Rand, and co-workers have also found high energies required to remove the water between lipid bilayers [10]. Using proton magnetic resonance measurements, we and others have demonstrated that the mobility of membrane-bound water is much reduced compared to liquid water [8, 9]. In the present work, we extend our studies of membrane-bound water and begin to examine the nature of the membrane-water interface by means of infrared and extrinsic fluorescence spectroscopy.

Infrared (IR) spectroscopy is exquisitely sensitive to water vibrational motion (usually a problem in nonhydration studies, but an advantage here); it is capable of recognizing different water hydrogen bonding environments, and can distinguish the various phases of water [11]. It therefore should be useful in identifying various classes of membrane-bound water. The IR absorption spectrum can also provide a "fingerprint" of most structural groups within membrane proteins and lipids [12, 13] and thus may be capable of monitoring hydration effects on their conformation.

The dye molecule 1-anilino-8-naphthalenesulfonate (ANS) is perhaps one of the most studied and best characterized fluorescent probes of biologic membranes. It is generally thought to bind to membranes at the bilayer-aqueous interface [14–16]. ANS is also known to be sensitive to both the polarity and rigidity of its solvent microenvironment through a mechanism of excited-state solvent relaxation [17, 18]. Therefore, ANS fluorescence should provide a useful probe of hydration effects on the polarity and rigidity of the membrane aqueous interace.

MATERIALS AND METHODS

Membranes were prepared from normal human red cells as described previously [19]. Films were prepared by depositing a few drops of membrane pellet on AgCl windows for the IR measurements or on glass or quartz slides for the fluorescence measurements. Immediately prior to film casting, the membranes were given a distilled water wash to prevent high salt concentrations in the partially dried films [5]. The different levels of hydration were achieved by equilibrating the films in desiccators containing saturated salt solutions to yield the appropriate relative humidity (rh) [5].

Samples were considered to be equilibrated for the IR when transmission at 3,400 cm^{-1} for H_2O films or 2,500 cm^{-1} for D_2O films was constant for 24 hs. The films were sealed with a second AgCl window and oriented in a reproducible manner in the beam for each spectral measurement. The spectra were obtained by a Perkin-Elmer Model 621 double beam grating spectrophotometer. The spectra were scanned at 100 cm^{-1} intervals and re-equilibrated between intervals to insure that samples were not altered by heating. The difference spectra were determined by subtracting absorption spectra measured at different rh (as indicated in figures) at 10 cm^{-1} intervals.

The films for the fluorescence measurements were prepared from membranes that had been preincubated for 30 min at room temperature with ANS (Eastman Organic Chemicals No.T 484) in water solution. The ANS concentrations used were 0.4 and 0.8 mg/per ml red cell membrane pellet (1.25×10^{-3} M ANS and 2.49×10^{-3} M ANS, respectively). The slides used for these films were cut to fit diagonally in a 1-cm fluorescence cuvette.

Fluorescence spectra were obtained using a Perkin-Elmer MPF 4 spectrofluorometer. An exciting wavelength of 350 nm was used and emission was measured at a right angle to the beam. Recording of reflected light was minimized by placing the slide in the cuvette diagonally and positioning the cuvette so that the film faced away from the emission monochromator. The films were oriented so that the same portion of the film was consistently sampled during a series of measurements. The films were considered to be equilibrated at a given level of hydration when the emission peak intensity was constant for 24 hs. The sequence of hydration levels used was varied between films, and a film of red cell membranes without ANS was used as a control to insure that membrane aging did not affect the observed results.

RESULTS

Sorption isotherms for water-vapor binding to erythrocyte membranes are shown in Figure 1 [5]. These are used to determine the level of membrane hydration at a particular relative humidity. The relative humidities used in our experiments were 95, 66, 33, 11, and 0%, and these correspond to membrane hydrations of ~ 40, 11, 5, 3, and 0%, respectively.

The fluorescence emission of ANS in red cell membranes is shown in Figure 2 for several different relative humidities. A 2.5-fold increase in fluorescence intensity, accompanied by a 10-nm blue shift in emission peak wavelength, occurs with membrane dehydration between 95% and 0% rh. The majority of the intensity increase appears to occur at lower hydration levels (below 66% rh), while the main portion of the blue shift occurs

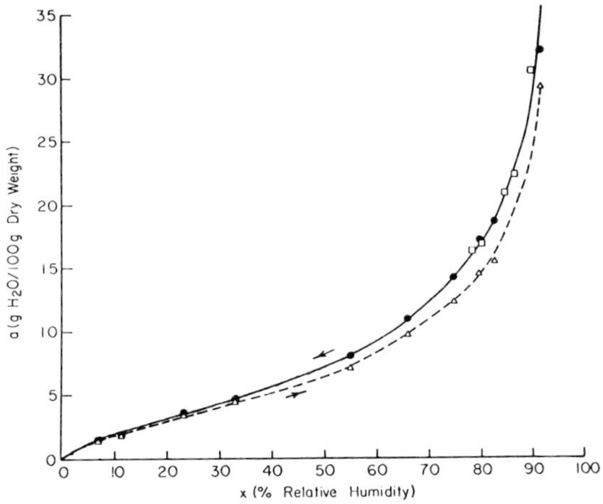

Fig. 1. Sorption isotherms of water on human red cell membranes at 20°C. Upper curve desorption; lower curve adsorption. From Schneider and Scheneider [5], with permission.

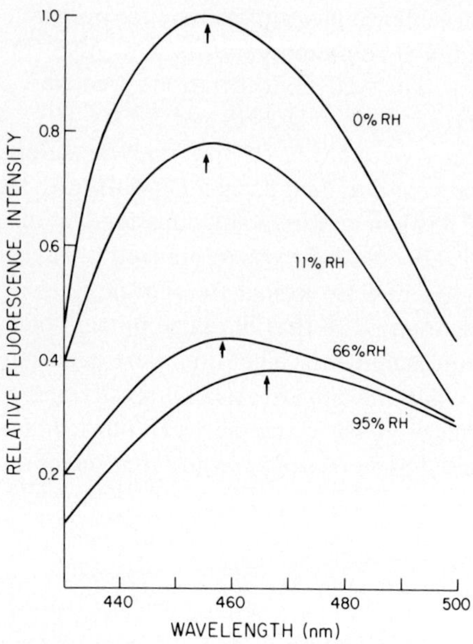

Fig. 2. ANS fluorescence emission spectra as a function of membrane hydration (rh). Excitation wavelength = 350 nm. Arrows indicate location of emission peak.

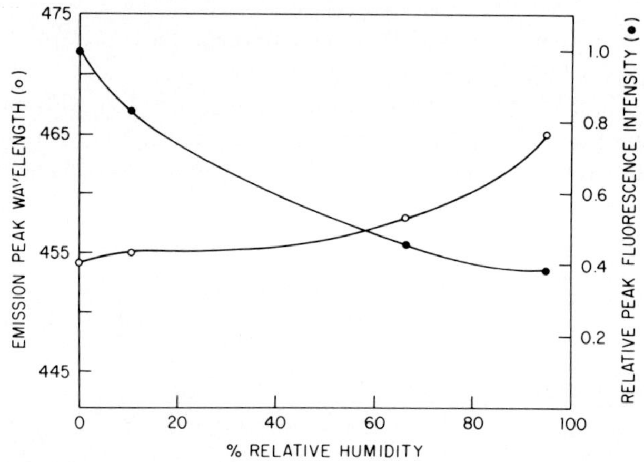

Fig. 3. ANS fluorescence emission parameters as a function of membrane hydration (rh). ○) Emission peak wavelength; ●) relative peak fluorescence intensity.

between 95% and 66% rh. These changes in ANS fluorescence parameters with membrane hydration are more clearly shown in Figure 3.

Figure 4a shows the infrared spectra of erythrocyte membranes equilibrated at 95% and 0% rh, together with that of liquid water for comparison. Upon dehydration, major membrane spectral changes are observed in the 3,800–3,200 cm^{-1} region and below 1,000 cm^{-1}. The water bands overlap several of the prominent membrane bands, and to eliminate this problem, D_2O-equilibrated film spectra were also obtained. Such complimen-

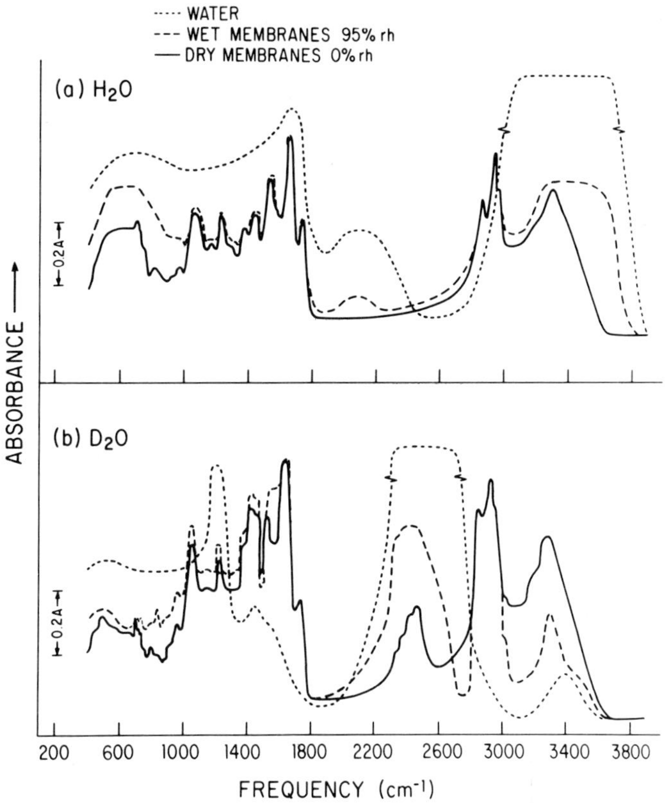

Fig. 4. Infrared spectra (4,000–400 cm^{-1}) of red cell membranes at 95% and 0% relative humidity. a) Membranes equilibrated against H_2O; b) membranes equlibrated against D_2O. Spectra of liquid water also shown for comparison.

tary spectra and that of liquid D_2O are illustrated in Figure 4b. Major hydration dependent changes are observed in the 2,700–2,100 cm^{-1} region and between 900 and 700 cm^{-1}. Greater peak resolution is available in the D_2O films than in the H_2O-equilibrated films, and several of the spectral regions are shown in detail below.

Figure 5a, b shows dehydration difference spectra in the OH and OD stretching regions of H_2O- and D_2O-hydrated red cell membranes, respectively. With dehydration, three difference bands appear with frequencies 3,550 cm^{-1}, 3,500 cm^{-1}, and 3,200 for H_2O-hydrated membranes and 2,650, 2,500–2,540, and 2,350 for D_2O films. The 3,550 (2,650) band is most evident at high levels of hydration, and the 2,650 band from the D_2O films completely disappears by 11% hydration.

Hydration effects are also observed for D_2O films in the 650–900 cm^{-1} region, as shown in Figure 6. The 701 cm^{-1} peak increases with dehydration while the 740 cm^{-1} band decreases. The 720 cm^{-1} peak remains constant. A band at 800 cm^{-1} becomes clearly visible at 0% rh, while the 834 cm^{-1} band has significantly decreased.

Figure 7 shows D_2O-hydrated membrane spectra in the 1,200–1,800 cm^{-1} region at different levels of hydration. The intense band at 1,650 cm^{-1} remains relatively unchanged in going from 95% to 0% relative humidity. However, the band at 1,525–1,550

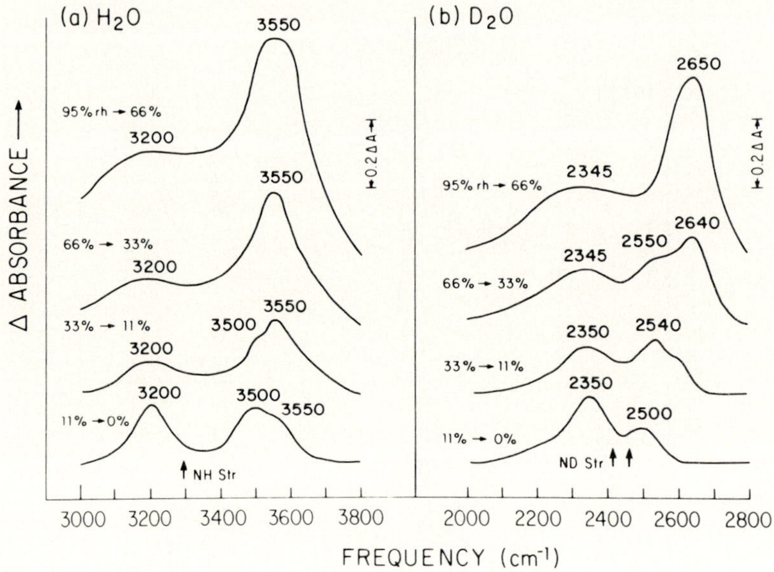

Fig. 5. Infrared dehydration difference spectra of red cell membranes: a) In H_2O (OH fundamental stretching region), b) in D_2O (OD fundamental stretching region). Difference spectra derived by subtracting spectra between the indicated relative humidities.

6

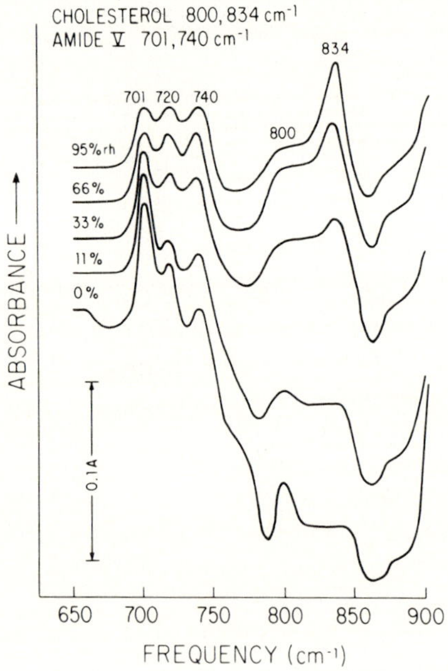

7

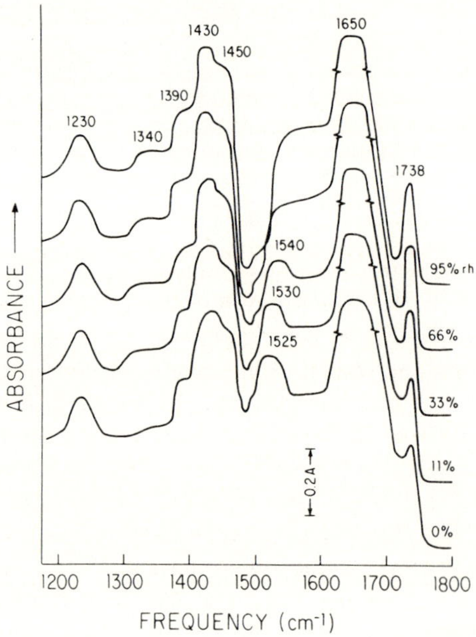

Fig. 6. Infrared spectra of red cell membranes in D_2O in the region 650–900 cm^{-1} as a function of membrane hydration (rh).

Fig. 7. Infrared spectra of red cell membranes in D_2O in the region 1,200–1,800 cm^{-1} as a function of membrane hydration (rh).

cm^{-1} changes extensively. Upon dehydration, the band narrows considerably and shifts to lower frequency. There is no apparent change in a 1,230 cm^{-1} band and there are no obvious changes in the 1,390–1,450 cm^{-1} region.

DISCUSSION

The hydration-dependent changes we have described in membrane infrared spectra and ANS fluorescence may be useful for a) identifying different classes of membrane-bound water, b) determining which structural groups within membrane proteins and lipids are affected by membrane hydration, and c) elucidating polarity and/or rigidity (microviscosisty) effects at the membrane-aqueous interface.

ANS is an appropriate probe for these investigations because its fluorescence emission is dependent on solvent microenvironment. The quenching of ANS fluorescence in water has been attributed to the ability of the polar solvent molecules to interact with the first excited singlet state (S_1). Brand and co-workers have shown that the dipole moment of S_1 is greater than that of the ground state (S_0) and that of the first excited triplet (T_1) [17, 20]. Thus polar solvents preferentially stabilize S_1 relative to S_0 and T_1. This decreases the energy gap for intersystem crossing and increases the probability of quenching by this mechanism, resulting in decreased fluorescence intensity. This stabilization of S_1 also decreases the energy gap for fluorescence and causes a red shift in the wavelength of maximum intensity.

The ability of polar solvents to preferentially stabilize S_1 depends on the capacity of the solvent molecules to reorient around the excited state. Seliskar and Brand compared the fluorescence characteristics of N-methyl-2,6-ANS in liquid water and ice [18]. They observed a much larger quantum yield in ice and a blue shift of the maximum wavelength to 455 nm, thus demonstrating the importance of solvent fluidity to the solvent relaxation quenching mechanism.

The results reported here show similar intensity changes and wavelength shifts for membrane-bound ANS as a function of membrane dehydration. At high levels of membrane hydration (40%) the ANS fluorescence is relatively low, with an emission peak near 465 nm, which is similar to its location in methanol. From the polarity standpoint this is reasonable, since the lipid polar head groups and bound water allow for some stabilization. Upon removal of the water, the membrane ANS fluorescence is markedly enhanced (2.5 times), and there is a 10-nm blue shift in emission peak. These effects could derive from an increase in rigidity and/or decrease in polarity of the membrane-ANS microenvironment. That dehydration should rigidify the membrane is plausible, since the thermal motion of the aqueous medium would no longer be imparted to the membrane. It is interesting that about 20% hydration seems to be required for membrane integrity, as discerned by X-ray diffraction [3], and for phospholipid-cholesterol mixing, as measured by differential scanning calorimetry [4]. One can suppose, therefore, that the effect of increasing hydration may be to increase membrane fluidity, since at least a certain amount of molecular motion should be required for intermixing of lipid molecules. The possibility should also be mentioned that ANS fluorescence changes with membrane dehydration might monitor similar membrane structural changes as detected by X-ray and calorimetric methods. If so, this could provide an independent marker for the hydration level at which these changes occur and furnish some information on the nature of the changes. Our fluorescence data cannot yet distinguish between the various possible origins of the ANS emission changes; future fluorescence polarization measurements may provide further insight into this problem.

Gulik-Krzywicki et al [21], in analogous ANS-phospholipid-hydration experiments, have shown that the area per lipid head group increases with hydration and this is accompanied by a decrease in ANS fluorescence and red shift in emission peak wavelength. This may allow increased water penetration to the ANS sites and/or greater exposure of ANS to the aqueous environment. Indeed, D_2O solvent perturbation measurements of ANS fluorescence in membranes indicate exposure of ANS to water at the surface of the membrane [15]. Other related studies have been reported using naphthalenesulfonate dyes to probe bound water in phospholipid [22] and detergent [23] micelles. Wells [22] has shown by fluorescence polarization measurements of dansylphosphatidylethanolamine in phosphatidylcholine micelles that an increase in micelle hydration results in increased molecular motion of the lipid-water interface [22]. He has also shown a shift in emission peak to longer wavelengths and a decrease in fluoresecence intensity with increasing amounts of bound water, – changes that are analogous to those we have found for the red cell membrane. Similar results were found by Wong et al for hydration effects on ANS in detergent micelles [23].

The IR spectrum of erythrocyte membranes also undergoes several hydration-dependent changes. In the total spectrum of H_2O-equilibrated films (Fig. 4a), well-established regions include the amide A (3,292 cm^{-1}), CH stretching (3,200–2,800 cm^{-1}), ester carbonyl stretching (1,738 cm^{-1}), amide I (1,650 cm^{-1}), amide II (1,540 cm^{-1}), P = O stretching (1,230 cm^{-1}), and POC aliphatic stretching (1,080–1,060 cm^{-1}) vibrations [12]. The H_2O IR bands overlap a few of these. The intense absorption centered near 3,400 cm^{-1} arises from OH stretch in liquid water. There is a strong OH bending mode absorbing at 1,640 cm^{-1} and the band near 2,100 cm^{-1} is thought to result from a combination of the 1,640 cm^{-1} band with an intermolecular mode or with overtones [11].

The D_2O-equilibrated spectra (Fig. 4b) are perhaps more informative owing to the lesser masking of membrane bands. In the dry-film spectrum, the nonexchangeable NH stretching vibration is visible near 3,300 cm^{-1}. OD and protein ND stretching modes absorb in the 2,200–2,600 cm^{-1} region. Also, HDO impurities may lead to absorption at 3,400 cm^{-1} and 1,450 cm^{-1} [11]. At lower frequencies, amide V bands (700, 740 cm^{-1}) [24] and cholesterol bands (800, 834 cm^{-1}) [13] can be discerned.

The difference spectra in the OH and OD stretching vibration regions give valuable information about hydration effects (Fig. 5). The 3,550 cm^{-1} (2,650 cm^{-1}) difference bands appears at relatively high hydration levels and probably represent removal of loosely bound water. The frequency of this difference band (3,550 cm^{-1} or 2,650 cm^{-1}) is higher than that of the stretching vibration of liquid H_2O or D_2O and indicates decreased hydrogen bond strength [25, 26]. Such high-frequency bands have been observed for water bound to polypeptides [26], phospholipids [22], molecular sieves [27], and polyelectrolyte membranes [28]. This band may represent removal of water molecules that are shielded from efficient hydrogen bonding. Perhaps some of these are isolated in the kink regions of the lipid hydrocarbon chains, as originally postulated by Träuble [29, 30].

The difference band at 3,500 cm^{-1} (2,500–2,530 cm^{-1}) may also be due to bound water with relatively weak hydrogen bonds (Fig. 5). Such blue-shifted OH and OD stretching bands have been observed in hydrated stratum corneum (2,480 cm^{-1}, OD) [31], polyproline (3,490 cm^{-1}, OH) [26], molecular sieves (3,500 cm^{-1}, OH) [27], and phospholipid micelles (3,530 cm^{-1}, OH) [22]. This difference band appears below 66% rh and may correspond to water somewhat more tightly bound than the 3,550 cm^{-1} (2,640–2,650 cm^{-1}) band.

The difference band (Fig. 5) observed at 3,200 cm^{-1} (2,350 cm^{-1}) appears most prominently at low hydrations and could have several sources. Amide A and B bands occur in this region. This difference band, then, may indicate protein structural changes which alter the NH hydrogen bond strengths. Similar low-frequency bands have been observed in dehydration difference spectra of proteins. Bendit measured a difference band at 3,270 cm^{-1} for β-keratin [32] and Buontempo et al observed one at 3,260 cm^{-1} for lysozyme [33]. In each case, the band was assigned, at least in part, to protein structural changes induced by dehydration.

The cholesterol hydroxyl may also be represented in this band. The OH stretch of cholesterol normally absorbs around 3,400 cm^{-1}, but Zull et al have shown that the band shifts to 3,250 cm^{-1} when lecithin is present [34]. Ladbrooke and Chapman have shown the phospholipid-cholesterol interaction requires water molecules [4]. This difference band may in part be due to lipid separation resulting in a loss of the cholesterol-phospholipid interaction.

There is yet another possible interpretation of this low-frequency difference band, namely that it is due to tightly bound water. Our IR spectra of the D_2O-equilibrated films would support this interpretation. Extensive dehydration leads to complete loss of the 2,350 cm^{-1} band. Membrane-associated water yielding this stretching frequency would be tightly hydrogen-bonded, and since it is removed only at low relative humidities, it must be a tightly bound component. Ice-like hydrogen bond strengths for water in the membrane are consistent with our previous results, yielding heats of binding of water vapor to membranes similar to and greater than those of water in ice [5]. Buontempo et al assigned his 3,260 cm^{-1} band, in part, to an amorphous ice-like water bound to lysozyme [33]. Hansen and Yellin [31] observed a 2,360 cm^{-1} OD dehydration difference band in stratum corneum, which they assigned to tightly bound water. Their band is also removed by desiccation, and hence it cannot be due to ND vibrations. The possibility of this band being an overtone of the DOD bending mode was eliminated, since the spectrum was measured with HOD in H_2O. Other workers have also assigned IR difference bands with similar frequencies to bound water on polyelectrolyte membranes [28] and molecular sieves [27].

Other interesting dehydration effects occurred in the 875-650 cm^{-1} region for the D_2O-equilibrated films (Fig. 6). This is the CH bending and NH deformation region of the IR. The 720 cm^{-1} band has been attributed to the CH rocking vibration, which is observed only when four consecutive methylene groups of the fatty acid chains are in the *trans* configuration [35]. In our spectra, the band is clearly resolved and is not effected by dehydration. Chapman et al [35] did not observe this band in the IR spectra of erythrocyte membranes but did in that of the extracted lipids. Perhaps our ability to see the band in the spectra of the total membrane is due to better instrument resolution. The presence of this 720 cm^{-1} band indicates less rotational mobility in the hydrocarbon region than was thought to exist from other data [35]. The lack of the dehydration effect on this band is surprising in view of the ANS fluorescence results. Perhaps there is a rigidifying effect at the membrane surface, sampled by the ANS molecules, which is not propagated to the hydrocarbon interior.

The 800 cm^{-1} and 834 cm^{-1} bands (Fig. 6) may be due to the vinyl CH bending vibrations of cholesterol [13]. Cholesterol in CS_2 has a medium band at 800 cm^{-1} and a weaker one at 834 cm^{-1} [36], which are similar to the bands we found in the membrane at 0% rh. This result is consistent with the idea that cholesterol separates from the phospholipids at low levels of hydration and then gives a spectrum similar to that of the isolated molecule.

The 701 cm^{-1} and 740 cm^{-1} bands (Fig. 6) may be due to the amide V vibration of membrane proteins [24]. Since these are observed in the D_2O film spectra, they must result from NH groups unavailable for exchange, ie, in buried residues. The changes with dehydration indicate less or weaker hydrogen bonding of the NH groups. This is supported by the red shift of the amide II band (Fig. 7) in the same D_2O film spectra upon dehydration. The P = O stretching vibration may be the source of the 1,230 cm^{-1} absorbance (Fig. 7), which was relatively insensitive to membrane dehydration.

In conclusion, the ANS fluorescence results imply a general influence of bound water on the polarity and/or rigidity of the membrane-aqueous interface. A comparison with similar studies using ANS fluorescence and X-ray diffraction on model lipid membranes suggests the fluorescence changes may be related to hydration effects on lipid packing density [21]. The infrared spectra display prominent hydration-dependent changes in several bands. The interpretation of these changes is complex, and possible assignments include cholesterol (vinyl CH bend, OH stretch), protein (amide A, II, V), and bound water (OH stretch). Further work with individual membrane components and model membrane systems should provide a more detailed interpretation of the hydration data for biologic membranes and lead to the incorporation of bound water into current models of membrane structure. This in turn should provide insight into the role that hydration plays in key membrane functions, such as water permeability and membrane fusion.

ACKNOWLEDGMENTS

This work was done during A.S. Schneider's tenure as an Established Investigator of the American Heart Association. The work was supported in part by National Science Foundation grant PCM 76 04079, and National Institutes of Health grants CA15773, AM18759, and CA08748.

REFERENCES

1. Szent-Gyorgyi A: "The Living State." New York: Academic, 1972, p 9.
2. Singer SJ, Nicholson GL: Science 175:720, 1972.
3. Finean JB: Q Rev Biophys 2:1, 1969.
4. Ladbrooke BD, Chapman D: Chem Phys Lipids 3:304, 1969.
5. Schneider MJT, Schneider AS: J Memb Biol 9:127, 1972.
6. Waugh DF, Schmitt FO: Cold Spring Harbor Symp Quant Biol 8:233, 1940.
7. Gent WLG, Grant EH, Tucker SW: Biopolymers 9:124, 1970.
8. Clifford J, Pethica BA, Smith EG: In Bolis L, Pethica BA (eds): "Membrane Models and the Formation of Biological Membranes." Amsterdam: North Holland, 1968, pp 19–42.
9. Finch ED, Schneider AS: Biochim Biophys Acta 406:146, 1975.
10. Le Neveu DM, Rand RP, Parsegian VA: Nature 259:601, 1976.
11. Eisenberg D, Kauzmann W: "The Structure and Properties of Water." New York and Oxford: Oxford University Press, 1969.
12. Bessette F: Can J Spectrosc 20:126, 1975.
13. Chapman D: "The Structure of Lipids by Spectroscopic and X-ray Techniques." New York: Wiley, 1965, pp 52–131.
14. Azzi A: Q Rev Biophys 8:237, 1975.
15. Radda GK, Vanderkooi J: Biochim Biophys Acta 265:509, 1972.

16. Waggoner A: In Martonosi A (ed): "The Enzymes of Biological Membranes." New York: Plenum, 1976, pp 119–137.
17. Brand L, Gohlke JR: Ann Rev Biochem 41:843, 1972.
18. Seliskar CJ, Brand L: Science 171:799, 1971.
19. Schneider AS, Schneider MJT, Rosenheck K: Proc Natl Acad Sci USA 66:793, 1970.
20. Seliskar CJ, Brand L: J Am Chem Soc 93:5414, 1971.
21. Gulik-Krzywicki T, Schechter E, Iwatsubo M, Ranck JL, Luzzati V: Biochim Biophys Acta 219:1, 1970.
22. Wells MA: Biochemistry 13:4937, 1974.
23. Wong M, Thomas JK, Grätzel M: J Am Chem Soc 98:2391, 1976.
24. Suzuki S, Iwashita Y, Shimanouchi T, Tsuboi M: Biopolymers 4:337, 1966.
25. Pimental GC, McClellan AL: "The Hydrogen Bond." San Francisco: Freeman, 1960.
26. Kuntz ID, Kauzmann W: Adv Protein Chem 28:239, 1974.
27. Hino M: Bull Chem Soc Jpn 50:574, 1977.
28. Zundel G: "Hydration and Intermolecular Interaction: Infrared Investigations With Polyelectrolyte Membranes." New York: Academic, 1969.
29. Träuble H: J Memb Biol 4:193, 1971.
30. Newman GC, Huang CH: Biochemistry 14:3363, 1975.
31. Hansen JR, Yellin W: In Jellinek HHG (ed): "Water Structure at the Water-Polymer Interface." New York: Plenum, 1972, pp 19–28.
32. Bendit EG: Biopolymers 4:539, 1966.
33. Buontempo U, Careri G, Fasella P: Biopolymers 11:519, 1972.
34. Zull JE, Greanoff S, Adam HK: Biochemistry 7:4172, 1968.
35. Chapman D, Kamat VB, Levene RJ: Science 160:314, 1968.
36. Dobriner C, Katzenellenbogen ER, Jones RN: "Infrared Absorption Spectra of Steroids." New York and London: Interscience, 1953, p 41.

Normal and Abnormal Red Cell Membranes 437–449 (1979)

Endocytosis in Erythrocytes and Their Ghosts

Stanley L. Schrier, Britta Hardy, and Klaus G. Bensch

Division of Hematology, Department of Medicine, (S.L.S., B.H.), and Department of Pathology, (K.G.B.), Stanford University School of Medicine, Stanford, California 94305

Study of endocytosis in human erythrocytes and their ghosts provides an opportunity for the elucidation of the steps involved in membrane invagination and fusion. The specific preparation being studied should be described with great care since circumstances that produce endocytosis may differ among the several available preparations. For example, in resealed red ghosts the addition of 0.5 to 1 mM Ca stimulates Mg-ATP-induced endocytosis, whereas in intact erythrocytes Ca addition stimulates primaquine-induced endocytosis and inhibits vinblastine-induced endocytosis. Furthermore, Ca inhibits endocytosis in white ghosts. EDTA can produce endocytosis in white ghosts but not in resealed red ghosts.

In studies with white ghosts, incubation with EDTA, trypsin, or Mg-ATP produced endocytosis, whereas the prior addition of an antispectrin antibody prevented endocytosis. When the white ghost vacuoles were harvested they were found to be depleted of spectrin. These observations lead to the hypothesis that endocytic vacuoles are formed in areas of the membrane that have been substantially freed of spectrin.

Key words: endocytosis, ghost endocytosis, spectrin, Ca, Mg-ATPase

Endocytosis is a process involving membrane internalization which results in the incorporation into the cell interior of a vacuole composed of the cell's plasma membrane turned inside out (Fig. 1). The intact human erythrocyte and several types of ghosts can be shown to undergo endocytosis, and as such these preparations become useful model systems for the study of membrane internalization [1-4]. The subject of erythrocytic endocytosis has become somewhat complicated, however, because it is not clear that a single biological event underlies all forms of erythrocytic endocytosis. Therefore, simplifying assumptions about mechanisms or a transposition from one system to another is likely to be incorrect. Our purpose is to review endocytosis in intact human erythrocytes, resealed red ghosts, and "white Dodge" ghosts in order to point out apparent similarities and differences in mechanisms, and to select which preparation would be suitable for the resolution of certain specific questions.

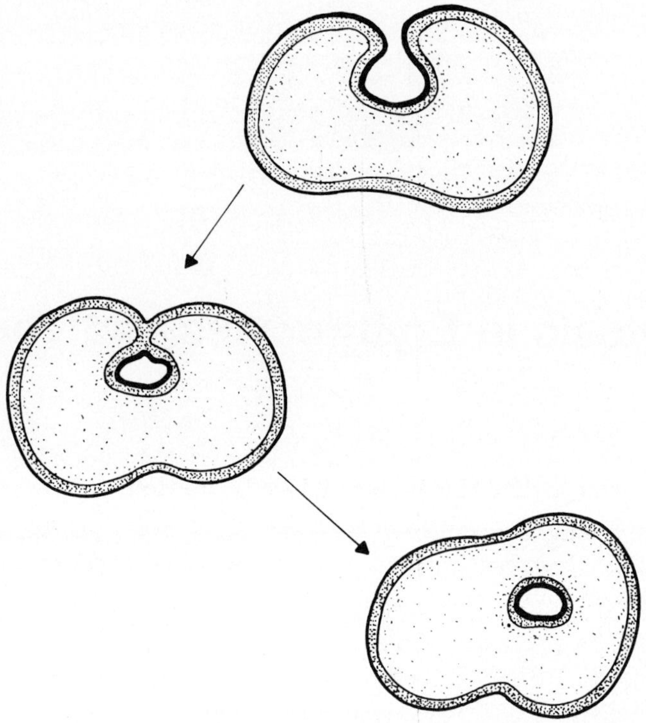

Fig. 1. Schematic representation of the endocytic process. Simplistically, there is first a stomatocytic shape change, followed by invagination of a portion of the membrane surface, and then fusion of the vacuole neck with release of the free endocytic vacuole to the interior of the erythrocyte.

METHODS

Endocytosis in intact erythrocytes was studied by phase microscopy, transmission electron microscopy, and the ^{57}Co-vitamin B_{12} method [3,5].

For the radioisotopic method, we took advantage of the observation that ^{57}Co-labeled vitamin B_{12} links to serum vitamin B_{12} binding proteins, and that the complex of ^{57}Co-vitamin B_{12} and vitamin B_{12} binding proteins then binds to the outer surface of the erythrocyte membrane. Three saline washes and trypsinization regularly remove over 99% of the bound ^{57}Co-vitamin B_{12} [3,5], but ^{57}Co-vitamin B_{12} trapped in endocytic vacuoles is not accessible to removal by washing and trypsinization. This residual ^{57}Co-vitamin B_{12} becomes an index of the extent of endocytic vacuole formation [3,5]. In over 200 experiments in which endocytosis in intact erythrocytes was measured, both by the ^{57}Co-vitamin B_{12} method and by either phase microscopy or transmission electron microscopy, there was regular correlation between the radioisotopic and morphologic methods.

Endocytosis in resealed red ghosts was studied by phase and transmission electron microscopy [3,4]. In resealed red ghosts, parallel measurements were also made of ^{45}Ca efflux and Ca,Mg-ATPase activity [4].

Endocytosis was also studied in "white Dodge" ghosts. White ghosts were prepared with only minor modifications of Penniston's method [6], and endocytosis was studied by measuring the decrease in acetylcholinesterase activity [6] and by phase and transmission electron microscopy. Acetylcholinesterase is an externally oriented membrane enzyme. Thus, when external plasma membrane has been internalized by the process of endocytosis, less acetylcholinesterase is accessible to substrate added to the bulk medium. The extent of endocytosis is paralleled by a decrease in acetylcholinesterase activity in intact resealed white ghosts.

A rabbit antispectrin antibody was prepared and partially purified by affinity chromatography. Endocytosis in white ghosts is difficult to evaluate by transmission electron microscopy. Therefore, in some experiments cationized ferritin was used as a marker of the external surface of the plasma membrane since it binds predominantly to the sialic acid carboxyls there [7]. Following completion of incubation with the endocytosis-inducing agents, white ghosts were then fixed in 1% glutaraldehyde, washed, and labeled for 15 minutes with an excess of cationized ferritin.

For detection of the release of endocytic vacuoles from white ghosts, the Coulter channel analyzer was used. The Coulter counter, model ZBI, was set at the following readings: amplification 0.5; aperture current 0.5; threshold lower 10, upper 100; aperture 5060 (50 μ); and the counter was attached to the Coulter channel analyzer, model H-4.

MATERIALS

Materials were obtained from previously described sources [3–5]. Cationized ferritin was obtained from the Miles-Yeda Laboratory, Israel.

RESULTS AND DISCUSSION

Endocytosis in Intact Erythrocytes

Endocytosis occurs in vivo spontaneously in neonatal erythrocytes [8] and may occur continuously in adult erythrocytes as well [9].

Endocytosis in intact erythrocytes can be induced in vitro by incubating them with amphipathic cations like primaquine [2], chlorpromazine, vinblastine, and hydrocortisone [3,5]. ATP depletion and incubation with metabolic inhibitors NaF and N-ethyl maleimide (NEM) blocked endocytosis, the extent of which seemed to reflect the residual ATP content [3,5]. The very fact that metabolic and shape integrity of erythrocytes is required before endocytosis can be induced argues against the possibility that endocytosis is induced by nonspecific "mistreatment" of erythrocytes. We therefore proposed that drug-induced endocytosis in intact erythrocytes proceeded via a common ATP-requiring mechanism. This observation was challenged by Bessis and Mohandas [10], who showed that chlorpromazine endocytosis occurred even in erythrocytes that had been severely depleted of ATP, provided that one added relatively large amounts of chlorpromazine. They argued that ATP depletion produced echinocytosis and that erythrocytic shape had to be changed to the stomatocytic form by drug action before endocytosis could occur.

In order to test this hypothesis, we produced severe ATP depletion in erythrocytes by overnight incubation or by exposure to NaF, and then added increasing amounts of the endocytosis-inducing agents. Substantial chlorpromazine and vinblastine endocytosis occurred, even in the face of ATP levels as low as 0.05 μmoles/ml RBC. In contrast, primaquine endocytosis seemed uniquely dependent on the level of residual erythrocytic ATP [11,12].

A further interesting difference in drug action was found. When erythrocytes were incubated with the ionophore, A23187, and ^{45}Ca, the entry of 4 to 51 nmoles of ^{45}Ca per ml RBC enhanced primaquine endocytosis, inhibited vinblastine endocytosis, and had irregular effects on chlorpromazine endocytosis [12].

Other interesting differences in drug action are brought out by varying the anionic composition of the media in which the intact erythrocytes are suspended. Primaquine endocytosis virtually ceases when erythrocytes are suspended in non-penetrating media like isotonic sodium glutamate or sucrose; and restoration of primaquine endocytosis can be achieved by adding back chloride salts; use of acetate salts is better, and lactate salts are best. Conversely, hydrocortisone endocytosis is enhanced almost tenfold when erythrocytes are suspended in sucrose or glutamate. Vinblastine endocytosis demonstrates a pattern of its own, and is almost completely inhibited when erythrocytes are suspended in isotonic sucrose, a low ionic strength medium, but is only 50% inhibited in isotonic glutamate [5]. The vacuole-inducing agents, primaquine and vinblastine, also produce stomatocytosis, and since both isotonic sucrose and sodium glutamate produce stomatocytosis, one would expect that conditions that lead to stomatocytosis might enhance the endocytic action of primaquine and vinblastine. However, the opposite findings were observed and strongly suggest that drug-induced endocytosis is not simply an extreme form of stomatocytosis.

Vinblastine, an endocytosis-inducing drug in erythrocytes, is believed to interact with microtubules in nucleated cells. Microtubules have not been found in erythrocytes, and it therefore seemed reasonable to search for analogs of microfibrils in erythrocytes by attempting to modify drug-induced endocytosis with the presumed microfibrillar probe, cytochalasin-B. Concentrations of cytochalasin that interfere with phagocytosis neither stimulated nor inhibited drug-induced endocytosis in intact erythrocytes [12].

In addition to the differences in drug action described, there are other forms of endocytosis that occur in intact human erythrocytes. Allen and colleagues have pointed out [13] that when erythrocytes are incubated in the presence of externally added phospholipase C, endocytosis is produced presumably by the enzyme attack on the phosphoinositide in the outermost lipid leaflet, releasing diglyceride which then moves into the inner lipid leaflet. Miller [14] has observed the entry of malarial merozoites into erythrocytes, a process that graphically involves endocytosis, the mechanism of which is unclear.

Endocytosis in Resealed Red Ghosts

This is an interesting preparation for the study of endocytosis since it has similarities with endocytosis in intact erythrocytes and endocytosis in white ghosts. The substrate for endocytosis in red ghosts is uniquely Mg-ATP; other nucleotide di- and triphosphates do not function in this regard [15]. Addition of Ca causes the stimulation of endocytosis at concentrations of 0.5 to 1 mM, whereas higher concentrations of Ca inhibit endocytosis [5]. The requirements for Ca and Mg-ATP for resealed red ghost endocytosis suggested that the membrane enzyme, Ca,Mg-ATPase, was involved in the endocytosis process. It could be shown that conditions that produced optimal endocytosis also led to optimal ^{45}Ca efflux and maximal Ca,Mg-ATPase activity. Drugs like ruthenium red and chlorpromazine, which are known to inhibit ^{45}Ca efflux and its linked Ca,Mg-ATPase, inhibited red ghost endocytosis [4,15]. However, concentrations of ruthenium red that completely inhibited endocytosis left 31% of residual Ca,Mg-ATPase activity and 46% of ^{45}Ca efflux [4]. Similarly, concentrations of chlorpromazine that left only 5% of control endocytosis allowed 20% of ^{45}Ca efflux and 16% of Ca,Mg-ATPase activity to remain [15]. When these studies were extended using the sulfhydryl agent, diamide [16], it was found that addition of 10 mM diamide completely inhibited red ghost endocytosis while allowing 49% of baseline ^{45}Ca efflux and 58% of control Ca,Mg-ATPase activity to persist (Table I,

TABLE I. The Effect of Diamide on ^{45}Ca Efflux and Ca,Mg-ATPase

	^{45}Ca efflux (nmoles/min/10^{10} ghosts)	Ca,Mg-ATPase (nmoles/min/10^{10} ghosts)
Control	99	82.4
10 mM diamide	49	47.5
10 mM diamide and 10 mM DTT[a]	86	83
10 mM DTT	90	82.5

[a]Dithiothreitol

Fig. 2). These observations with three quite different agents suggest that while a Ca-ATPase may be critically involved in red ghost endocytosis, it may be an enzyme or a form of the enzyme that is not specifically linked to the ^{45}Ca efflux pump [17].

In order to test the role of microfibrillar-like materials in red ghost endocytosis, 10 to 20 μg/ml of cytochalasin were resealed into red ghosts along with 1 mM ^{45}Ca and 2.5 mM Mg-ATP. There was neither enhancement nor inhibition of endocytosis, nor did the cytochalasin interfere with ^{45}Ca efflux or the activity of Ca,Mg-ATPase (Table II).

After reports had appeared indicating that endocytosis could be induced in white ghosts by incubating them in media of low ionic strength, or EDTA [18,21], we attempted to induce endocytosis in resealed red ghosts with EDTA added at concentrations of 0.5 to 5.0 mM. Endocytosis cannot be induced by incubating red ghosts [19] with EDTA. Low ionic strength media cannot be tested in resealed red ghosts, because they simply rehemolyze and leak their contents. Therefore, red ghost endocytosis differs in this regard from endocytosis in white ghosts.

Furthermore, while red ghost endocytosis is uniquely dependent on the presence of Mg-ATP and Ca, the addition of Ca to white ghosts inhibits endocytosis [20]. Therefore, there are significant differences between endocytosis in red ghosts, intact erythrocytes, and white ghosts.

Endocytosis in White Ghosts

Study of endocytosis in white ghosts [1] provides the best opportunity for detecting involvement of specific polypeptides in the endocytic process. Endocytosis was quantitatively measured by the acetylcholinesterase method and was observed morphologically by phase, Nomarski, and transmission electron microscopy. In order to determine if spectrin was involved in white ghost endocytosis, an antispectrin antibody was obtained from immunized rabbits, purified by ammonium sulfate precipitation and affinity chromatography, and then resealed into white ghosts in an approximately twofold excess. The immunizing material contained only the two spectrin bands and no band 4.1 on PAGE. The anti-spectrin antibody after purification reacted in immunodiffusion with a single precipitin line to purified human spectrin but not to actin. The antibody was not tested against purified band 4.1. Resealing 3 mM Mg-ATP into "white Dodge" ghosts suspended in 50 mM TES buffer, induced endocytosis as did incubation at pH 8.0 with 0.1 mM EDTA, or with 20 ng/ml of trypsin. For purposes of comparison, incubation of ghosts with buffer or bovine serum albumin reduced the acetylcholinesterase activity to 97% of the initial control value, whereas 3 mM Mg-ATP produced endocytosis and reduced acetylcholinesterase to a mean of 73% of control. Trypsin reduced acetylcholinesterase to 76% of control, whereas EDTA treatment reduced acetylcholinesterase to 68% of control. In each case, prior addition of antispectrin antibody blocked endocytosis [21]. The use of

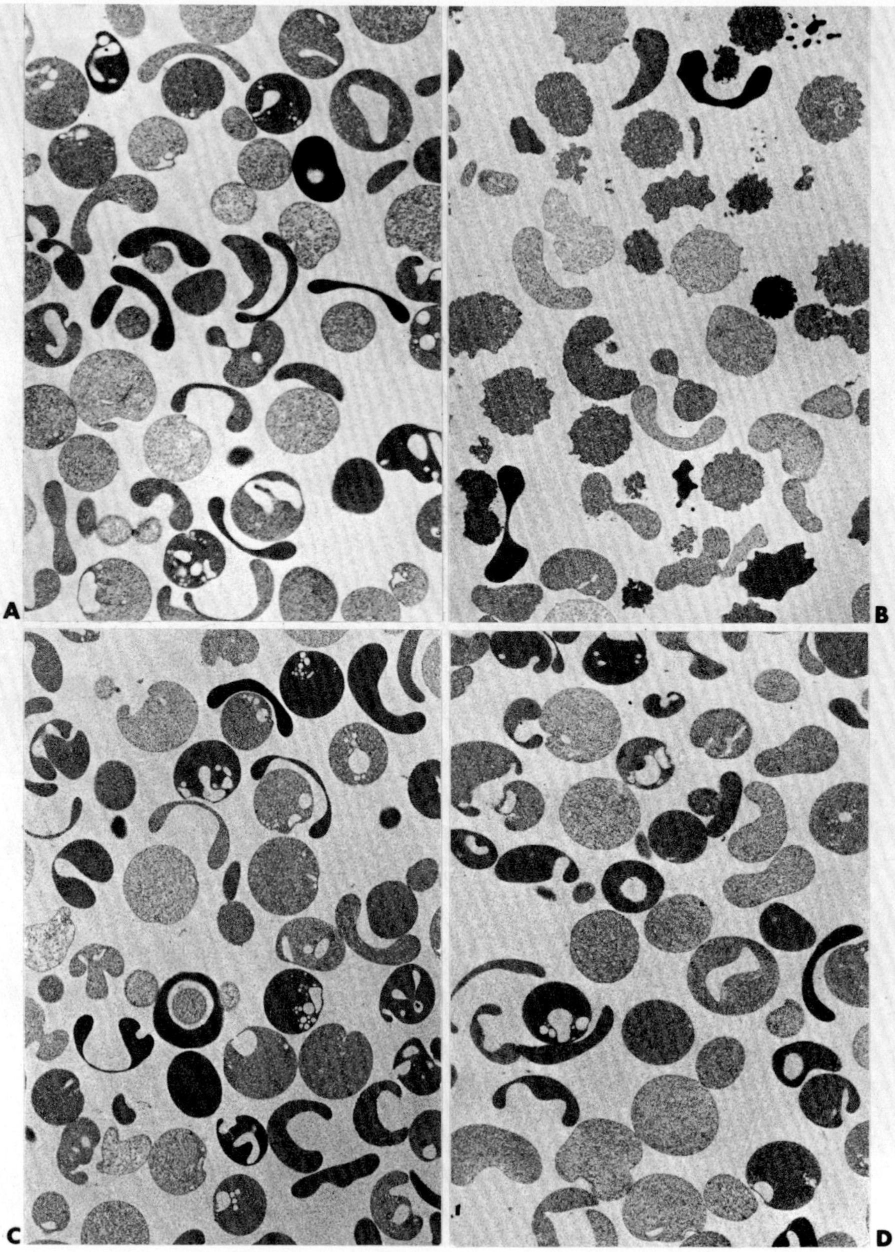

Fig. 2. The effect of diamide on ghost endocytosis: A. Control, no additions; B. Diamide, 10 mM; C. DTT, 10 mM; D. Diamide, 10 mM, and DTT, 10 mM (magnification, × 1900).

bovine serum albumin as a control, or the use of nonantibody immunoglobulin from the spectrin affinity column did not affect endocytosis [21]. In addition to phase and Nomarski microscopy and the acetylcholinesterase method, we wanted to confirm our results

TABLE II. Effect of Cytochalasin on ^{45}Ca Efflux and Ca,Mg-ATPase Activity in Resealed Red Ghosts

Preparation	^{45}Ca efflux (nmoles $^{45}Ca/min/10^{10}$ ghosts)	Ca,Mg-ATPase (nmoles $^{32}P/min/10^{10}$ ghosts)	Ca/P ratio
Control	61	49	1.25
Ethanol, 10 μl/ml	67	43	1.56
Cytochalasin, 20 μg/ml	59	44	1.34

by transmission electron microscopy. However, there is concern that the apparent vacuoles seen in the transmission electron microphotographs of white ghosts may simply represent sections through folds in the membrane. In order to prove that these were in fact endocytic vacuoles (Fig. 3), we used cationized ferritin to outline the outer surface of the plasma membrane, after the termination of the endocytic process (Fig. 4). The cationized ferritin method proved that the endocytic vacuoles that were apparent on transmission electron microscopy were not in contact with the external medium, and therefore were not simply membrane foldings (Fig. 5).

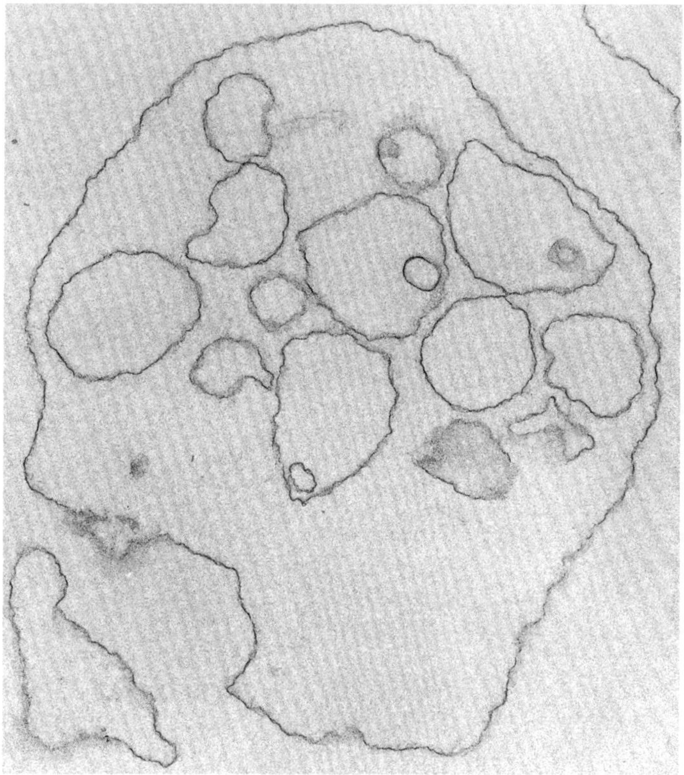

Fig. 3. Mg-ATP induced endocytosis in white Dodge ghosts incubated for 30 min at 37° (magnification × 29,700). Note that there appear to be many vacuoles that seem to be lined with plasma membrane.

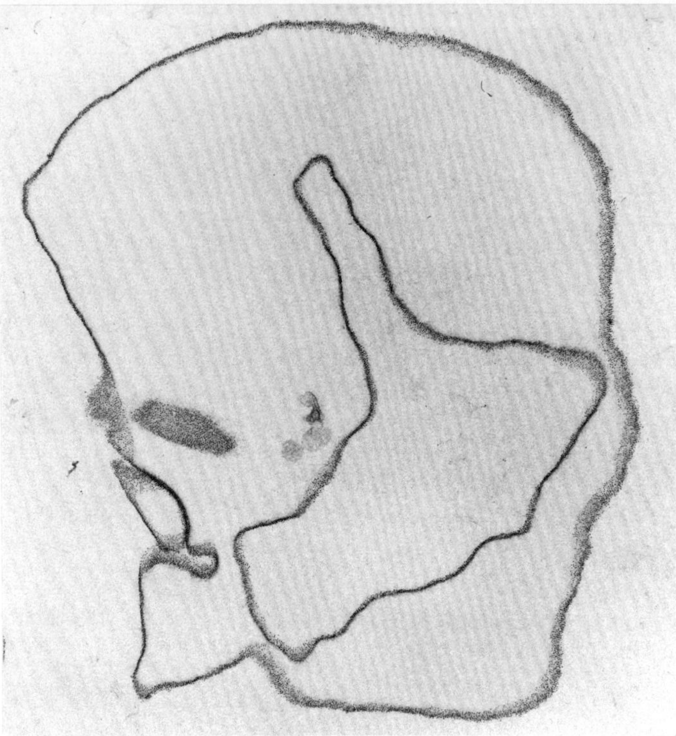

Fig. 4. White Dodge ghosts preincubated with antispectrin antibody were then incubated with 0.1 mM EDTA for 30 min at 22°. After the reaction was terminated, the ghost suspension was exposed to cationized ferritin which labeled the outer plasma membrane. It can be seen that what appears to be a vacuole is labeled with ferritin and is therefore only a fold in the membrane (magnification × 29,700).

The Coulter channel analyzer provided a useful method for following white ghost endocytosis (Fig. 6). With trypsin as the endocytosis inducing agent, the Coulter channel analyzer printout indicated that after 10 minutes of incubation the mean ghost volume became smaller, presumably as a consequence of the induced endocytosis (Fig. 3). Subsequently, a very much smaller population of ghost fragments appeared which, on microscopy, consisted of the endocytic vacuoles remaining after the ghosts ruptured when their critical size limit had been passed. These endocytic vacuoles could be separated by velocity sedimentation considerations on 15–38% continuous sucrose gradients. Upon analysis, the vacuoles were shown to be depleted of spectrin [21].

These findings are consistent with the hypothesis that modification of spectrin can lead to endocytosis in white ghosts and that the resulting endocytic vacuoles are, in fact, spectrin depleted. Use of an antispectrin antibody blocks the induction of endocytosis by Mg-ATP, trypsin, or EDTA, presumably by interfering with the mobility of spectrin and the creation of spectrin-free areas. This hypothesis is consistent with the findings of Palek [22] and Allen [23] showing that the exocytic vesicles produced from intact erythrocytes either by ATP depletion or the entry of Ca via the mediation of the ionophore A23187 are also depleted of spectrin. We would propose that a prior event for either

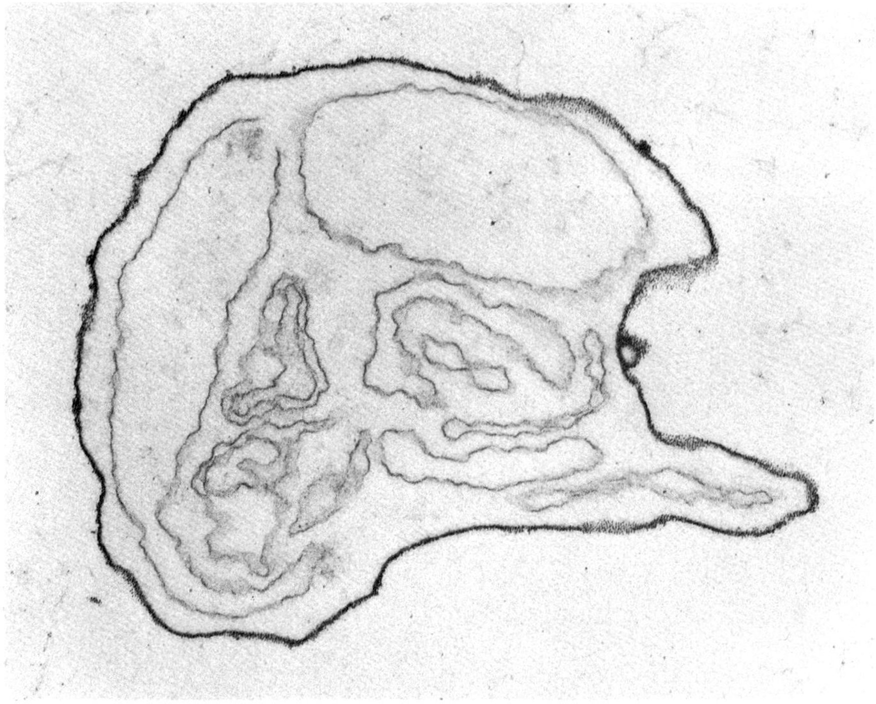

Fig. 5. White ghosts were incubated with 20 ng/ml of trypsin for 30 min, after which cationized ferritin was added. It is apparent that there are many endocytic vacuoles not accessible to the cationized ferritin which labeled only the outer plasma membrane (magnification × 29,700).

endocytosis or exocytosis is the creation of spectrin-free domains in the membrane. The factors that lead to either inward or outward bending and membrane fusion are not understood but could involve energetic considerations or the known asymmetry of the bimolecular lipid layer in the membrane.

SYNTHESES AND HYPOTHESES

Consideration of the specific requirements for endocytosis in intact erythrocytes, resealed red ghosts, and white Dodge ghosts does not lead to a facile identification of unifying mechanisms. Rather, the converse is true: superficially, each preparation seems to have its own specific requirements for induction of endocytosis. Nevertheless, there are a few common threads connecting endocytosis in erythrocytes and ghosts, and these can be considered with the hope of generating testable hypotheses.

Study of endocytosis in resealed red ghosts, the least well characterized preparation, has produced the following picture. The substrate is uniquely Mg-ATP. Subsequent addition of 0.5–1.0 mM Ca stimulates endocytosis, and Ca addition above 2 mM inhibits endocytosis. Inhibitors of Ca,Mg-ATPase and its linked Ca efflux pump (ruthenium red, chlorpromazine, and diamide) also inhibit endocytosis, but concentrations of these inhibitors that completely abolish endocytosis leave from 20% to 50% residual Ca,Mg-ATPase and ^{45}Ca efflux. EDTA does not produce endocytosis in red ghosts and might even be ex-

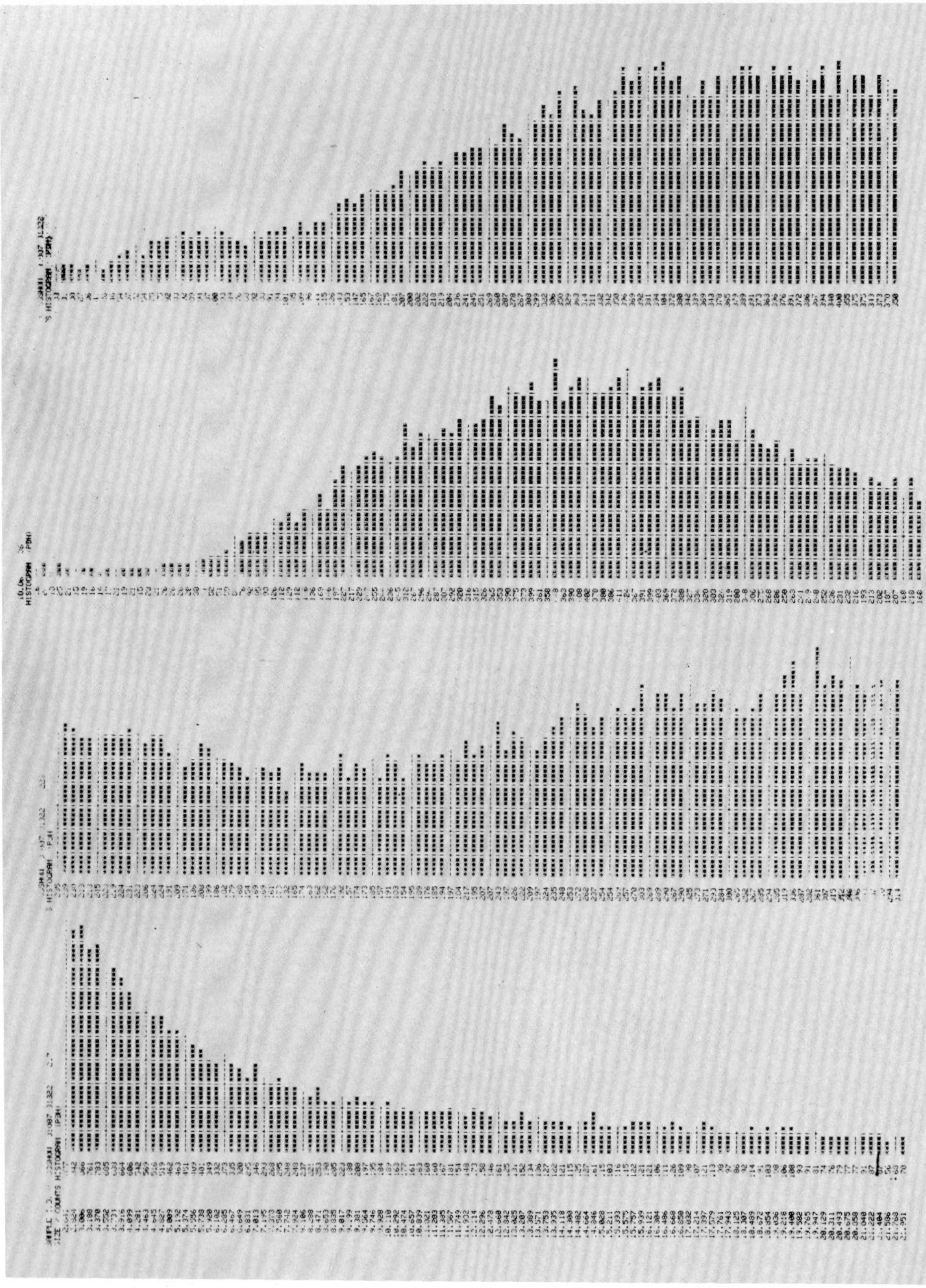

Fig. 6. Coulter channel analyzer printouts of white Dodge ghosts incubated with 20 ng trypsin/ml for 0, 10, 20, and 45 min at 37°. The computer printout shows the ghost size on the abscissa, with larger sizes being recorded progressively to the right, while the number of particles at each size distribution is recorded on the ordinate. The upper panel is recorded at 0 time, and shows that there are mostly relatively large ghosts present. The second panel from the top was obtained after 10 min of incubation and shows that the ghost size has decreased, presumably because of loss of ghost volume due to the endocytic process (Figs. 3 and 5). The third panel from the top shows the appearance of multiple populations of ghosts and ghost fragments after 20 min of incubation, and the vacuoles are displayed at the left side of the abscissa. The bottom panel shows the computer printout after 45 min of incubation, and there are mostly endocytic vacuoles remaining.

pected to interfere with it. Our current working hypothesis is that endocytosis in resealed red ghosts is linked to the action of Ca,Mg-ATPase, which is not the enzyme or portion of the enzyme linked directly to the Ca pump. A reasonable candidate enzyme would be a myosin-like ATPase stimulated by Ca. It could produce endocytosis by action of its own contractile mechanism, or it could interact with spectrin, depleting it in some membrane areas. However, such an enzyme has not yet been identified in human erythrocyte membranes.

White ghosts are reasonably well characterized, but have undergone the most drastic alterations in preparation. Penniston showed that energized endocytosis can occur in white ghosts and that the substrate is again Mg-ATP [24]. However, in contrast to red ghosts, the addition of Ca inhibits Mg-ATP induced endocytosis in white ghosts [20]. There are several possible explanations for this observation. It is now known that there is an activator of membrane Ca,Mg-ATPase in hemolyzate which binds variably to erythrocyte membranes [25,26]. This activator resembles a class of Ca binding proteins present in other cellular sources, and its variable presence or absence in white Dodge ghosts could explain the lack of Ca stimulation of endocytosis. Furthermore, the action of added Ca on white ghost membranes, perhaps deficient in a Ca-binding protein, could result in stimulation of a membrane transglutaminase [27] which, in turn, would cross-link membrane polypeptides, thereby inhibiting endocytosis.

Nonenergized endocytosis can also be induced in white ghosts by exposing them to media of low ionic strength, EDTA, or low concentrations of trypsin [18,21]. These manipulations can be shown to be directed at spectrin [21], and if one is willing to accept the hypothesis that Mg-ATP alters spectrin by providing substrate to a protein kinase that phosphorylates spectrin, then all forms of white ghost endocytosis involve the modification of spectrin. The observation that prior incubation of white ghosts with antispectrin antibody blocks endocytosis and that the endocytic vacuoles are depleted of spectrin supports our working proposal that all forms of endocytosis in white ghosts involve the creation of spectrin-free domains in the membrane from which the endocytic vacuoles invaginate and are pinched off.

Presumably, spectrin-free areas also occur during the formation of exocytic vacuoles which bud off externally from intact erythrocytes that have been depleted of ATP [22] or exposed to Ca plus ionophore [23] because the recovered exocytic vacuoles are depleted of spectrin.

Drug-induced endocytosis in intact erythrocytes is very difficult to fit into a cohesive scheme because, as noted above, there are distinct differences in optimal requirements for the action of the different drugs. In addition, despite several efforts, we have been unable to recover endocytic vacuoles from intact erythrocytes and, therefore, have not been able to determine their peptide content. Primaquine endocytosis in erythrocytes requires ATP and is stimulated by entry of Ca and, therefore, most resembles the apparent Ca,Mg-ATP requirements for endocytosis in resealed red ghosts. The role of primaquine, in addition to producing stomatocytosis, might involve its reported ability to increase the incorporation of linoleic acid into lecithin in intact erythrocytes [28]. Primaquine could cause a transient depletion in the phospholipid content of the outer membrane leaflet, resulting in an inward bending of the membrane. This mechanism would then be somewhat similar to the endocytic vacuole formation that occurs upon treating intact erythrocytes with phospholipase C [23]. The inward movement of the membrane associated with the action of a contractile non-Ca-pump-linked Ca,Mg-ATPase could be a mechanism for primaquine endocytosis. The action of vinblastine in endocytosis is difficult to reconcile with this scheme, since vinblastine endocytosis does not require ATP and is inhibited by Ca entry. It has been reported that Ca and vinblastine compete for a common site on several proteins [29], and we therefore have proposed that vinblastine acts by displacing Ca from a site on a Ca-binding membrane protein, which then initiates a sequence that leads to endocytosis [12].

Chlorpromazine-induced endocytosis is equally difficult to reconcile, because it not only occurs in the face of ATP depletion, it also inhibits Ca,Mg-ATPase and blocks resealed red ghost endocytosis [15]. However, chlorpromazine, like vinblastine, can displace Ca from the membrane [30], a displacement that may suffice to initiate endocytosis. In addition, based on studies of neonatal erythrocytes, Schekman and Singer have suggested that a clustering of membrane receptors leads to endocytosis [31].

The possible physiologic role of endocytosis in intact erythrocytes has not been resolved. We know of no experiments in which macromolecules have been shown to enter intact erythrocytes by processes similar to pinocytosis. Spontaneous erythrocytic endocytosis in vivo can be demonstrated in neonatal erythrocytes [8] and in normal erythrocytes transfused into splenectomized subjects [9]. It is possible to speculate that endocytosis could serve as a means for remodeling the membrane of circulating erythrocytes. In a sense, a membrane is like a chain, no stronger than its weakest segment. If an erythrocyte sustained localized membrane damage, it would be compromised and removed from the circulation. But if localized membrane damage, possibly involving spectrin, led to the formation of an endocytic vacuole that included the damaged area of the membrane, and if that endocytic vacuole was then removed by the "pitting" action of the spleen, then that erythrocyte would be returned to the circulation somewhat more spheroidal in shape but with an intact plasma membrane.

Therefore, the recurring aspects of endocytosis in erythrocytes and ghosts revolve about the role of Ca, the possible action of a Ca,Mg-ATPase not linked to the Ca pump, and the creation of spectrin-free areas from which the endocytic vacuoles may form. The obvious difficulties involve the real differences in drug action, the apparent difference in the means of inducing or inhibiting endocytosis in the difference preparations, and the necessity, not yet achieved, of obtaining a reasonably pure population of the endocytic vacuoles formed in resealed red ghosts and intact erythrocytes for peptide analysis.

ACKNOWLEDGMENTS

This work could not have been done without the dedicated efforts of Irene Junga and Judy Krueger.

The research was supported by grant AM13682 from the National Institutes of Health.

REFERENCES

1. Penniston JT, Green DE: Arch Biochem Biophys 128:339, 1968.
2. Ginn FL, Hochstein P, Trump BF: Science 164:843, 1969.
3. Ben-Bassat I, Bensch KG, Schrier SL: J Clin Invest 51:1833, 1972.
4. Schrier SL, Bensch KG, Johnson M, Junga I: J Clin Invest 56:8, 1975.
5. Schrier SL, Junga I, Seeger M: J Lab Clin Med 83:215, 1974.
6. Jarrett HW, Penniston JT: Biochim Biophys Acta 448:314, 1976.
7. Danon D. Goldstein L, Marikovsky Y, Skutelsky E: J Ultrastruct Res 38:500, 1972.
8. Holroyde CP, Oski FA, Gardner FH: New Eng J Med 281:516, 1969.
9. Holroyde CP, Gardner FH: Blood 36:566, 1970.
10. Bessis M, Mohandas N: Brit J Haem 31 (suppl):5, 1975.

11. Berry D, Hochstein P: Biochem Med 4:317, 1970.
12. Schrier SL, Junga I, Krueger J, Johnson M: Blood Cells 4:339, 1978.
13. Allan D: J Supramol Struc Suppl 2, Abstr 477, 1978.
14. Miller L: J Supramol Struc Suppl 2, Abstr 492, 1978.
15. Schrier SL, Bensch KG: "Membranes and Disease." Edited by Bolis L, Hoffman H and Leaf A, Raven Press, New York, 1976, p 31.
16. Von Tersch FJ, Mendicino J, Pillion DJ, and Leibach FH: Biochem Biophys Res Commun 64:433, 1975.
17. Jarrett HW, Reid TB, Penniston JT: Arch Biochem Biophys 183:498, 1977.
18. Katsumata Y, Asai J: Arch Biochem Biophys 150:330, 1972.
19. Schrier SL, Junga I, Seeger M: Proc Soc Exp Biol Med 143:565, 1973.
20. Plishker GA, Vaughan L, Jarrett HW, Reid T, Roberts J, Penniston JT: "Membranes and Disease." Edited by Bolis L, Hoffman H and Leaf A, Raven Press, New York, 1976, p 19.
21. Hardy B, Schrier SL: Biochem Biophys Res Comm 84:1153, 1978.
22. Lutz HU, Liu SC, Palek J: J Cell Biol 73:548, 1977.
23. Allen D, Billa MM, Finean JB, Michell RH: Nature 261:58, 1976.
24. Hayashi H, Plishker GA, Vaughan L, Penniston JT: Biochim Biophys Acta 382:218, 1975.
25. Jarrett HW, Penniston JT: Biochem Biophys Res Comm 77:1210, 1977.
26. Larsen FL, Hines TR, Vincenzi FF: Abstr 525 J Supramol Struc Suppl 2, 1978.
27. Lorand L, Weissmann LB, Epel DL, Bruner-Lorand J: Proc Natl Acad Sci 73:4479, 1976.
28. Wittels B, Hochstein P: Biochem Biophys Acta 125:594, 1966.
29. Wilson L, Bryan J, Ruby A, Mazia D: Proc Natl Acad Sci 66:807, 1970.
30. Seeman P: Pharmacol Rev 24:583, 1972.
31. Schekman R, Singer SJ: Proc Natl Acad Sci 73:4075, 1976.

Normal and Abnormal Red Cell Membranes 451–456 (1979)

Structural Organization and Dynamics of Phospholipids in Red Cell Membranes

L. L. M. van Deenen

Department of Biochemistry, University of Utrecht, Utrecht, The Netherlands

Key words: asymmetry, translocation

The lipids of the red cell membrane have been studied in great detail, and several principles established in this "model membrane" contributed considerably to the conception of relations between chemical structure, function, and molecular organizations of lipids in biomembranes in general [1]. The lipid bilayer structure proposed as early as 1925 by Gorter and Grendel [2] was based on their observation that a lipid extract from erythrocytes when spread as a monomolecular film at the air-water interface occupies an area which is about twice the total surface area of the extracted cells. The surface pressure applied in their ingenious experiment was very low (2 dynes/cm), and there remained the question of which pressure corresponds best with the tightness of packing of the lipid molecules in the red cell membrane [3,4]. While studying the action of a series of pure phospholipases on intact erythrocytes, Zwaal et al [5] observed that one group of enzymes is capable of inducing phospholipid hydrolysis, whereas the second group failed to attack the membrane. It turned out that injection of the phospholipases of the first group underneath phospholipid films compressed above 34 dynes/cm caused hydrolysis, whereas members of the second group of enzymes failed to act above film pressures of 31 dynes/cm [6]. These experiments suggest that the packing of the lipid molecules in the exterior layer of the erythrocyte membrane is comparable to a lateral pressure of 31-34 dynes/cm. Taking into account this value, it can be estimated that the ratio of lipid monolayer area to red cell surface is about 1.5, which indicates that sufficient lipid is present to accommodate 75% of the membrane with a bilayer, leaving about 25% of the surface area for intrinsic, membrane-spanning proteins [7].

The present lecture summarizes studies on the distribution of phospholipases over the outer and inner lipid layer of the red cell membrane and in addition deals with recent investigations on the translocation of some phospholipids between these two compartments.

Received for publication March 9, 1978.

TOPOLOGY OF PHOSPHOLIPIDS IN THE RED CELL MEMBRANE

A nonrandom distribution of phospholipid classes over the outside and inside of the red cell membrane was reported in the past six years by various investigators using either chemical labeling or degradation with phospholipases.

Bretscher [8] showed that a relatively impermeant agent like formyl methionyl-sulphone-methylphosphate does not react with the aminophosphoglycerides in intact cells, whereas both phosphatidylethanolamine and phosphatidylserine react in open ghosts. Using trinitrobenzene sulphonate Gordeski and Marinetti [9] found that this reagent did not label phosphatidylserine in intact cells and that only part of phosphatidylethanolamine reacted.

Using a combination of phospholipases, which causes a complete degradation of all phospholipid classes in unsealed ghosts, a nonlytic degradation of nearly 50% of the phospholipids in intact erythrocytes was obtained [5,10,11]. This phospholipid fraction, which comprises 82% of sphingomyelin, 75% of phosphatidylcholine, and 20% of phosphatidylethanolamine is considered to represent the outer region of the lipid bilayer of the human red cell membrane. Evidence supporting this conclusion was obtained by studies on the action of a phospholipase on the inside of red cells [5] and experiments on sealed inside-out ghosts [12]. The various studies have shown (in good agreement) that the choline-containing phospholipids are located predominantly at the outside, whereas the aminophosphoglycerides, in particular phosphatidylserine, are concentrated at the cytoplasmic side of the red cell membrane.

Chap, Zwaal, and van Deenen [13] found a similar phospholipid asymmetry in the plasma membrane of platelets. The observation that the exterior surface of blood cells is devoid of negatively charged phospholipids (phosphatidylserine), which have a function in the process of blood coagulation, is consistent with the previous results on phospholipid asymmetry because otherwise a condition of hypercoagulability would exist [14].

On the basis of known differences in physical properties between choline- and aminophospholipids, it can be argued that the first group by itself is more suitable to provide a stable monolayer at the cell surface, but a fuller evaluation of phospholipid asymmetry will have to await the results of further research. In this context another major question can be raised too: Is the (absolute) asymmetry of membrane proteins linked with the nonrandom location of phospholipids. For instance the (Na^+, K^+)-ATPase which is known to have its catalytic center at the membrane inside was demonstrated to depend for its activity on phosphatidylserine [15], which is located at the inner membrane layer. Considering the topology on orientation of various major peripheral and integral proteins of the red cell membrane, one can speculate that several protein-lipid complexes are vectorially aligned. The exclusive location of spectrin-actin at the cytoplasmic side of the red cell membrane [16] suggests that this protein could be a prime candidate for directing the localization of, for example, phosphatidylserine. In this respect it is of interest that Mombers et al [17] presented evidence in favor of a preferential association of spectrin with negatively charged phospholipids; it was found that this protein protects phospholipid bilayers against the action of Ca^{2+} and Mg^{2+}, thereby preventing fusion of lipid vesicles. Haest and Deuticke [18] showed that treatment of human erythrocytes with SH-oxidizing reagents perturbs the asymmetric distribution of aminophospholipids in the red cell membrane. Further studies of this group showed that this phenomenon is accompanied by a cross-linking of spectrin, and it was suggested that in the native membrane this protein stabilizes the location of phosphatidylserine and phosphatidylamine [19]. The amphipatic glycoprotein glycophorin, of which the complete amino acid sequence was elucidated by

Tomita and Marchesi [20], is known to span the membrane with an apolar region penetrating through the lipid core, having the C-terminal end located at the cytoplasmic side. while the N-terminal sugar-containing moiety is exposed at the membrane exterior [21]. Van Zoelen et al [22] studied the interaction of asialoglycophorin with monolayers of various erythrocyte lipid classes and observed a preferential affinity towards negatively charged phospholipid. Glycophorin incorporated in lipid bilayers of different composition was found to span the bilayer with most of the sugar residues directed to the outside of the vesicles [23]. Preliminary experiments on the localization of phosphatidylserine in such vesicles suggested the possibility of a protein-induced phospholipid asymmetry. On the other hand it seems theoretically possible that lipid-controlled protein orientations also occur. More advanced studies with these model systems may be helpful in elucidating the molecular basis of asymmetric assembly of proteins and lipids in biomembranes.

METABOLIC ASYMMETRY AND TRANSLOCATION OF PHOSPHOLIPIDS IN THE RED CELL MEMBRANE

In mature mammalian erythrocytes two mechanisms appear to play a major role in phospholipid renewal: i) incorporation of fatty acids into lysophospholipids, which are either formed in the membrane or supplied by the serum; and ii) exchange of phospholipids between serum lipoproteins and the cell membrane. Recent studies confirm that indeed two metabolically different pools contribute to the turnover of phosphatidylcholine in the red cell membrane and that the two pathways occur in different compartments of the membrane. With the aid of phospholipases, strong indications were obtained that a sidedness exists in phosphatidylcholine renewal in the mammalian red cell membrane.

Incubation of erythrocytes with radioactive fatty acids labels various phosphoglycerides and in particular phosphatidylcholine. Treatment of the intact labeled cells with phospholipases showed that the specific radioactivity is higher in the nondegradable pool when compared with the nonlytic hydrolysis of the susceptible pool of phosphatidylcholine in the membrane [24,25]. Recent experiments of Renooy [26] on the conversion of labeled lysophosphatidylcholine into phosphatidylcholine by rat erythrocytes revealed a similar pattern. These results can be explained by assuming that the conversion of monoacyl derivatives into the diacyl analogs occurs mainly at the inside of the membrane.

Incubation of rat erythrocytes in ^{32}P-labeled plasma results in a labeling of phosphatidylcholine of the membrane; the specific radioactivity of the lecithin fraction which is degradable by a nonlytic phospholipase treatment of the cells outranks the activity of the nonsusceptible fraction [25,26]. Apparently, incorporation of fatty acids into lysophosphatidylcholine and the exchange of phosphatidylcholine occur in two compartments, which can be distinguished by a nonlytic phospholipase degradation of the cells. At the present state of the investigations it is believed that these two compartments are topologically differently located, ie at the inside and outside region of the membrane respectively.

The investigations of Renooy and associates [25–28] also indicated that a slow transmembrane movement of phosphatidylcholine occurs in the erythrocyte membrane. It was found that after labeling of phosphatidylcholine by incorporation of ^{14}C-fatty acid the radioactivity of phospholipid which can be hydrolyzed by phospholipases at the outside of the cells increased with incubation time. By contrast, after labeling via exchange with ^{32}P-phosphatidylcholine, the radioactivity of the phospholipid susceptible to phospholipase appears to decrease with incubation time. A communication between the phospholipase-susceptible pool (outside) and the nonsusceptible compartment (inside) of the membrane was detectable by first labeling rat erythrocyte phospholipids, followed by removal of the ^{32}P-plasma and subsequent reincubation of the cells in a buffer; the total radioactivity remained constant, but the specific radioactivity of the degradable fraction in the intact cells decreased with time, whereas a corresponding increase was observed in the phosphatidylcholine fraction which is not susceptible towards phospholipase action. A reversed pattern of redistribution of the label was observed after incorporation of ^{14}C-fatty acids into phosphatidylcholine by the transacylation of lysophosphatidylcholine. The redistribution of both labels appears to occur in phosphatidylcholine of intact rat erythrocytes with an average half-time rate of about 4.5 h at 37°C. Furthermore, Renooy and van Golde [27,28] observed that the transposition rate was temperature-dependent and faster for the more unsaturated phosphatidylcholine species than for disaturated molecules. The translocation process of phosphatidylcholine in the red cell membrane links the exchange reaction occurring at the outer region with the transacylation of lysophosphatidylcholine at the inside, thereby contributing to the dynamic state of the membrane.

TRANSLOCATION OF PHOSPHOLIPIDS IN PROTEIN-CONTAINING LIPID VESICLES

The important experiments of Kornberg and McConnell [29] already demonstrated that the transbilayer movement of spin-labeled phosphatidylcholine across the bilayer of pure lipid vesicles is a slow process. Subsequent studies by several groups confirm the conclusion that transbilayer movement of lipids in artificial membranes hardly occurs [30], unless differences in lateral packing between the two monolayers are induced [31]. The observations on the metabolic asymmetry of the red cell membrane imply that a migration of lysophosphatidylcholine and fatty acid occurs across the membrane. Using pure lysophospholipase as a tool, van den Besselaar, van den Bosch, and van Deenen [32] found that translocation of lysophosphatidylcholine across lipid bilayers is an extremely slow process. In an accompanying study de Kruijff, van den Besselaar, and van Deenen [33] tackled this question with the use of (N-$^{13}CH_3$)-enriched lysophosphatidylcholine and arrived at an identical result.

Inasmuch as the rate of translocation of phospholipid in artificial lipid bilayers is much slower than in rat erythrocytes, it is feasible that the presence of proteins facilitates this process. Therefore, experiments were performed on phospholipid vesicles containing glycophorin, which asymmetrically spans the lipid bilayer [22]. Van Zoelen, de Kruijff, and van Deenen [34] studied in this system the possible translocation of lysophosphatidylcholine using ^{13}C-NMR and lysophospholipase. The added (N-^{13}C)-lysophosphatidylcholine is initially incorporated into the outer lipid monolayer; subsequently the lysophosphatidylcholine is translocated to the inner monolayer of the glycophorin-containing vesicles with a half-time of about 1.5 h at 4°C. At higher temperature the process was found to be faster. Translocation could also be demonstrated with the action of lysophospholipase on single-bilayer vesicles prepared by cosonication of lysophosphatidylcholine with phosphatidylcholine. Without the presence of membrane protein only the lysophosphatidylcholine located in the outer monolayer is attacked by lysophospholipase, and no transbilayer movement was observed. In cosonicated vesicles of phosphatidylcholine and lysophosphatidylcholine (molar ratio 95:5) containing glycophorin, about 35% of the lysocompound appears to be present in the inner monolayer. Addition of lysophospholipase causes a very rapid hydrolysis of about 75% of the substrate, and the remaining lysophosphatidylcholine is nearly completely hydrolyzed at a much slower rate. Based on this biphasic hydrolysis pattern a half-time of about 1 h at 37° was estimated for (palmitoyl)-lysophosphatidyl translocation in glycophorin containing bilayer vesicles of (dioleoyl)-phosphatidylcholine.

Very recently de Kruijff, van Zoelen, and van Deenen [35] determined the rate of transbilayer movement of (dioleoyl)-phosphatidylcholine in sonicated lipid vesicles containing glycophorin. Introduction of N-$(^{13}C)_3$-phosphatidylcholine into the vesicles was induced with a specific phosphatidylcholine exchange protein. Whereas in the vesicles devoid of glycophorin the labeled phosphatidylcholine remains exclusively in the outer monolayer, a significant translocation of N-$(^{13}C)_3$-phosphatidylcholine towards the inner monolayer of the glycophorin-containing bilayers appeared to occur. Control experiments indicated that under the conditions used, the vesicles remain as intact barriers and that the phospholipid exchange protein does not enter the vesicles. It could also be shown that the movement of phosphatidylcholine from the outer to the inner monolayer is balanced by a translocation in the opposite direction. To date these experiments do not permit determination of the exact rate of translocation, but it can be concluded that the transbilayer movement of (dioleoyl)-phosphatidylcholine in glycophorin-containing vesicles at 37°C must be 1 h or less [35].

These studies demonstrate that the rate of translocation of lysophosphatidylcholine and phosphatidylcholine in sonicated lipid vesicles is enhanced by at least two orders of magnitude by the incorporation of glycophorin. Further research will be required to learn whether this phenomenon can also be induced by other integral membrane proteins. Although it cannot be precluded that the protein itself is directly involved, it can be envisaged that the lipid translocation occurs at the interface between protein-bound lipids and the uninterrupted lipid bilayer. At these regions irregularities in the packing of lipid can be expected to favor transbilayer movement. Furthermore, it should be mentioned that it is not clear whether the results obtained in the artificial membrane system resemble possibly more specific translocation mechanism(s) in biomembranes.

REFERENCES

1. van Deenen LLM, de Gier J: In Surgenor D MacN (ed): "The Red Blood Cell." New York: Academic, 1974, vol 1, pp 147–211.
2. Gorter E, Grendel F: J Exp Med 41:439, 1925.
3. van Deenen LLM: In Holman R (ed): "Progress in the Chemistry of Fats and other Lipids." Oxford: Pergamon, 1965, vol 7, part 1.
4. Bar RS, Deamer DW, Cornwell BF: Science 153:1010, 1966.
5. Zwaal RFA, Roelofsen B, Comfurius P, van Deenen LLM: Biochim Biophys Acta 406:83, 1975.
6. Demel RA, Geurts van Kessel WSM, Zwaal RFA, Roelofsen B, van Deenen LLM: Biochim Biophys Acta 406:97, 1975.
7. Zwaal RFA, Demel RA, Roelofsen B, van Deenen LLM: Trends Biochem Sci 1:112, 1976.
8. Bretscher MS: J Mol Biol 71:523, 1972.
9. Gordeski SE, Marinetti GV: Biochem Biophys Res Commun 50:1027, 1973.
10. Verkleij AJ, Zwaal RFA, Roelofsen B, Comfurius P, Kastelijn D, van Deenen LLM: Biochim Biophys Acta 323:178, 1973.
11. Zwaal RFA, Roelofsen B, Colley CM: Biochim Biophys Acta 300:159, 1973.
12. Kahlenberg A, Walker C, Rohrlick R: Can J Biochem 52:803, 1974.
13. Chap HJ, Zwaal RFA, van Deenen LLM: Biochim Biophys Acta 467:146, 1977.
14. Zwaal RFA, Comfurius P, van Deenen LLM: Nature 268:358, 1977.
15. Roelofsen B, van Deenen LLM: Eur J Biochem 40:245, 1973.
16. Nicolson GL, Marchesi VT, Singer SJ: J Cell Biol 51:265, 1971.
17. Mombers C, van Dijck PWM, van Deenen LLM, de Gier J, Verkleij AJ: Biochim Biophys Acta 470:152, 1977.
18. Haest EWM, Deuticke B: Biochim Biophys Acta 436:353, 1976.

19. Haest CWM, Plasa G, Kamp D, Deuticke B: Biochim Biophys Acta 509:21, 1978.
20. Tomita M, Marchesi VT: Proc Nat Acad Sci USA 72:2964, 1975.
21. Marchesi VT, Furthmayer H, Tomita M: Ann Rev Biochem 45:667, 1976.
22. van Zoelen EJJ, Zwaal RFA, Reuvers FAM, Demel RA, van Deenen LLM: Biochim Biophys Acta 464:482, 1977.
23. van Zoelen EJJ, Verklejj AJ, Zwaal RFA, van Deenen LLM: Eur J Biochem 86:539, 1978.
24. Renooy W, van Golde LMG, Zwaal RFA, Roelofsen B, van Deenen LLM: Biochim Biophys Acta 363:287, 1974.
25. Renooy W, van Golde LMG, Zwaal RFA, van Deenen LLM: Eur J Biochem 61:53, 1976.
26. Renooy W: "Renewal of Erythrocyte Phospholipids." Doctoral thesis, University of Utrecht, 1977.
27. Renooy W, van Golde LMG: FEBS Lett 71:321, 1976.
28. Renooy W, van Golde LMG: Biochim Biophys Acta 470:465, 1977.
29. Kornberg RD, McConnell HM: Biochemistry 10:1111, 1971.
30. Rothman JE, Lenard J: Science 195:743, 1977.
31. de Kruijff B, Wirtz KWA: Biochim Biophys Acta 468:318, 1977.
32. van den Besselaar AMHP, van den Bosch H, van Deenen LLM: Biochim Biophys Acta 465:454, 1977.
33. de Kruijff B, van den Besselaar AMHP, van Deenen LLM: Biochim Biophys Acta 465:443, 1977.
34. van Zoelen EJJ, de Kruijff B, van Deenen LLM: Biochim Biophys Acta 508:97, 1978.
35. de Kruijff B, van Zoelen EJJ, van Deenen LLM: Biochim Biophys Acta 509:537, 1978.

Normal and Abnormal Red Cell Membranes 457–461 (1979)

The Membrane Abnormalities in Paroxysmal Nocturnal Hemoglobinuria (PNH)

Wendell F. Rosse and J. P. Adams

Department of Medicine, Duke University Medical Center, Durham, North Carolina 27710

Paroxysmal nocturnal hemoglobinuria (PNH) cells are characterized by an abnormal membrane which interacts abnormally with normal serum complement. These abnormal reactions occur at two levels of the sequence: 1) All abnormal PNH cells fix more C3 than normal cells for a given activation of complement; 2) PNH III cells are more readily lysed by a given number of assembled terminal complexes. The nature of the lesion yielding these abnormal reactions is not known.

Key words: **PNH, complement, abnormal membrane**

Paroxysmal nocturnal hemoglobinuria (PNH) is a syndrome characterized by a clone of red blood cells with an undefined abnormality of the membrane [1]. The defective membrane interacts abnormally with the components of serum complement, causing the cells to be lysed more readily than normally by that group of proteins. Two types of abnormal cells occur in PNH: 1) PNH II cells, which are moderately abnormal, requiring one-third to one-fifth the amount of complement as normal cells for an equal degree of lysis [2]; and 2) PNH III cells, which are markedly abnormal, requiring 1/15 to 1/25 the amount of complement of normal cells for equal lysis [3]. The third variety of PNH cells, PNH I cells, are thought to be residual normal cells; they are very similar to normal cells in all respects [3].

Two abnormal reactions with complement have been defined; 1) For a given amount of activation of complement, either by the classical or by the alternative pathway, excessive amounts of the third component of complement are fixed to the membrane of the PNH II or III cell [4–6]; 2) the terminal complex more effectively penetrates the lipid bilayer on PNH III cells than normal cells [6,7]. The first of the two defects is present on both varieties of abnormal PNH cells; the second is present only on the markedly abnormal PNH III cells.

To establish the first of these abnormalities, we developed techniques for the estimation of complement components on the red cell membrane [6,8]. In the classical pathway, normal red cells and PNH cells of both types fix nearly equal quantities of antibody and the

Received for publication April 25, 1978; accepted June 1, 1978.

first component of complement (C1) [6]. This C1 is responsible for the fixation of equal amounts of C4 and C2, which is bound to C4 [6]. The combination of C2 and C4 forms an enzyme capable of activating C3 to C3b, which is bound to the membrane [7]. For a given number of C4 molecules, 3–5 times as many molecules of C3b are fixed to PNH cells of both abnormal types as to normal cells.

The combination of C42 is unstable on the membrane [8]. C2 is removed and inactivated; the binding site on C4 remains available for further binding of activated C2 should C1 be present. The degradation of C42 proceeds at the same rate on PNH cells as on normal cells [9]. The degradation of C42 is thought to be due to protein membrane components termed IF and DAF by Hoffman and associates [10-12]. We have extracted these components from PNH cells and from normal cells; equal inhibitory activity is present on both types of cells (Chua, Rosse, and Adams, unpublished data). From these results, we conclude that the excessive fixation of C3 to the red cell membrane in PNH is not due to abnormalities in the stability of the C42 combination.

C3 is also fixed by the alternative pathway of activation of complement [13]. Although the processes are less well understood, it is now thought that a protein called initiating factor (IF) is attached to the membrane; C3 and factor F (also called C3 proactivator or GBG [glycine-rich β-globulin]) are attached to IF. This combination is capable of activating C3 by enzymatic cleavage to C3a and C3b, much as is the C42 combination. This activity is markedly increased by the enzymatic hydrolysis of factor B by a low-molecular-weight enzyme, factor D. The C3b produced is able to fix to the membrane, as from the classic pathway where it is capable of binding more factor B and factor D, thus rapidly multiplying the amount of C3 that may be attached to the membrane. It is not clear whether the C3 fixed to the membrane by the classic pathway can participate in alternative pathway reactions.

When the alternative pathway is activated by acidification of normal serum, marked amounts of C3 are fixed to the PNH red cells, whereas very little is fixed to the normal cell [5]. This suggests that the abnormal membrane of the PNH cells is better able to act as a receptor for the alternative pathway than that of the normal cell. Studies are under way to determine whether this is due primarily to the ability to fix more C3 or other components of the alternative pathway.

C3 may be degraded by an enzyme, C3b inactivator (KAF), and an associated accelerator, β_{1H}, which split the activated C3b molecule into two parts, C3c and C3d [14-16]. The inactive C3d part remains attached to the red cell. Recently, Fearon and Austen have demonstrated that rabbit cells are more susceptible to inactivation of the alternative pathway, since C3b attached to those membranes is less susceptible to cleavage by C3b inactivator and β_{1H} [17]. To determine whether this is true for PNH cells, C3b was attached to normal and PNH cells using anti-I antibody. An antibody which detected antigens on the C3c portion of the molecule were then used to detect C3b on these cells as they were incubated in whole human serum as a source of C3 inactivator and β_{1H}. The rate of degradation was not different on PNH cells than on normal cells (unpublished data).

THE TERMINAL COMPLEX

Direct lysis of the cell by complement is thought to occur by the insertion into the membrane of a protein complex consisting of C5, C7, C8, and C9 [18]. To initiate this complex, C5 is held on membrane-bound C3b and hydrolyzed by either the C3b,Bb complex or the C42 complex. The active molecule, C5b, is able to affix reversibly to the membrane. This fixation is more secure when C5b is in close proximity to C3b [19] or is in combination with C6 [20].

We have examined the fixation of C5 to normal and PNH membranes, measuring C5 by the quantitative antiglobulin absorption assay. For a given amount of C3b fixed primarily by the the classical pathway, an equal amount of C5 is fixed to normal, PNH II, and PNH III cells. This C5 is equally stable on the two types of cells. However, more lysis of PNH III than PNH II or normal cells occurs when the terminal components are added [21].

The steps after the fixation of C5 involve the fixation of C6, C7, C8 and C9. These apparently interact with each other without enzymatic cleavage and form a complex in which each successive component interacts more deeply with the lipid portion of the membrane than the previous one. When the C6-9 complex is formed in the membrane, a lesion is evident in the electron microscope [22,23]. With the addition of C9, rearrangements may occur which allow C9 to penetrate through the bilayer, forming a water-soluble "pore" through the membrane. Most such complexes are not successful in penetrating the membrane; assuming that a single site of complete penetration of the lipid bilayer is sufficient to hemolyze the cell, approximately 30,000 assembled complexes are present on the normal cell when this occurs. However, this process is much more efficient in the PNH III cell; only about 4,000 such lesions are assembled for the same degree of lysis [7]. Since there are an equal number of lesions for a given amount of C5 fixed on normal and on PNH cells, the abnormality of the terminal steps appears to be limited to the increased penetration of the lipid bilayer of the membrane by the terminal complex.

The nature of the lesion of the PNH cell which allows these abnormal interactions of complement to occur has not been defined. When the membrane proteins of PNH cells are analyzed on sodium dodecyl sulfate (SDS) gel polyacrylamide electrophoresis, no abnormality is seen if proteolysis is carefully avoided (Horne and Rosse, unpublished data). Analysis of the lipid composition has revealed inconsistent or, more recently, no abnormalities [24]. It has also been suggested that the lipids are in some way unstable. Studies of the bulk chemical characteristics are made more complex by the fact that a portion of the cells are normal and a portion abnormal in PNH. However, no persistent abnormality has emerged even when cells with a very high proportion of abnormal cells are used.

A consistent, demonstrable protein abnormality is present on the abnormal PNH cells. PNH III cells are totally lacking in the external membrane enzyme acetylcholinesterase [25]. The normal-like PNH I cells have normal amounts of this enzyme per cell. Moderately abnormal PNH II cells have a modest reduction in the enzyme activity. It is not known whether this deficiency represents an absence of the protein or the inactivity of a protein present on the membrane. It is felt, however, that the absence of this enzyme activity is not causally related to the abnormalities of complement interaction delineated above, although both may stem from the same membrane abnormality.

Another approach which has been used to try to define the nature of the membrane lesion in PNH has been the alteration of the normal membrane by enzymes or other chemical means. It has been known for many years that cells treated with proteolytic enzymes are more susceptible to lysis by complement than normal cells [26]. Sialidase-treated cells are likewise more susceptible to complement lysis [27]. Sirchia and his co-workers first observed that the treatment of normal cells with mercaptide-containing compounds (aminoethylthiouronium bromide, cystidine, glutathione, etc) rendered normal cells more susceptible to the lytic action of complement in a way which made them closely resemble PNH cells [28]. In addition to an increase in susceptibility to lysis by complement no matter how activated, these cells also had a diminished content of acetylcholinesterase.

We have treated normal cells with bromelin, trypsin, sialidase, and aminoethylthiouronium bromide (AET). We have then analyzed the following steps of complement activation: 1) antibody fixation, by measuring the adsorption of I^{125}-labeled anti-I antibodies [6]; 2) C4 fixation, by a quantitative antiglobulin fixation test using anti-C4 [6]; 3) C3 fixation, by a quantitative antiglobulin fixation test using anti-C3 [5,6]; and 4) lysis per molecule of C3.

The results are shown in Table I in comparison to PNH II and PNH III cells. It is clear that none of the altered cells resemble exactly either PNH II or PNH III cells. The mercaptide-treated cells and trypsin-treated cells both have increased lysis for a given amount of fixed C3. We do not know whether this results from the increase in efficiency of the terminal steps as in PNH III cells.

TABLE I. Comparison of the Steps of Complement Activation on Altered Normal Red Cells and Abnormal PNH Red Cells to These Reactions on Normal Red Cells

Step	Trypsin	Bromelin	Sialidase	AET[a]	PNH II	PNH III
Ab uptake	↑	↑	↑	N	N	N
Degree of lysis for a given amount of adsorbed antibody	↑↑↑	↑	↑	↑	↑	↑
Amount of C4 fixed for a given amount of adsorbed antibody	N	↑	↑	N	N	N
Amount of C3 fixed for a given amount of C4	N	N	N	N	↑↑	↑↑
Degree of lysis for a given amount of fixed C3	↑↑	N	↑	↑↑	N	↑↑

[a]AET–aminoethylthiouronium bromide.

REFERENCES

1. Sirchia G, Lewis SM: Clin Haematol 4(1):199, 1975.
2. Rosse WF: Br J Haemat 24:327, 1973.
3. Rosse WF, Dacie JV: J Clin Invest 45:736, 1966.
4. Rosse WF, Adams JP, Thorpe AM: Br J Haemat 28:183, 1974.
5. Logue GL, Rosse WF, Adams JP: J Clin Invest 52:1129, 1974.
6. Rosse WF, Logue GL, Adams J, Crookston JH: J Clin Invest 53:31, 1974.
7. Rouault TA, Rosse WF, Bell S, Shelburne J: Blood 51:325, 1978.
8. Borsos T, Rapp HJ, Mayer MM: J Immunol 87:326, 1961.
9. Rosse WF, Dacie JV: J Clin Invest 45:749, 1966.
10. Hoffmann EM, Etlinger HM: J Immunol 111:946, 1973.
11. Hoffmann EM: Immunochemistry 6:391, 1969.
12. Hoffmann EM: Immunochemistry 6:405, 1969.
13. Götze O, Müller-Eberhard HJ: Adv Immunol 24:1, 1976.
14. Ruddy S, Austen KF: J Immunol 102:533, 1969.
15. Ruddy S, Austen KF: J Immunol 107:742, 1971.
16. Whaley K, Ruddy S: J Exp Med 144:1147, 1976.
17. Fearon DT, Austen KF: J Exp Med 146:22, 1977.
18. Kolb WP, Haxby JA, Arroyave CM, Müller-Eberhard HJ: J Exp Med 135:549, 1972.
19. Hammer CH, Abramovitz AS, Mayer MM: J Immunol 117:830, 1976.
20. Shin JS, Pickering RJ, Mayer MM: J Immunol 106:480, 1971.
21. Rosse WF, Adams JP, Zellinger M: Blood 42:1007, 1973.

22. Humphrey JH, Dourmashkin RR: Adv Immunol 11:75, 1969.
23. Packman CH, Rosenfield SI, Weed RI, Leddy JP: J Immunol 117:1883, 1976.
24. Bradlow BA, Lee J, Rubenstein R: Br J Haemat 11:315, 1965.
25. Kunstling TR, Rosse WF: Blood 33:607, 1969.
26. Yachnin S, Laforet MT, Gardner FH: Blood 17:83, 1961.
27. Lau F, Rosse WF: In preparation.
28. Sirchia G, Ferrone S, Mercuriali F: Blood 25:502, 1965.

Normal and Abnormal Red Cell Membranes 463–469 (1979)

Hemolytic Anemias Associated With Deficient or Dysfunctional Spectrin

Samuel E. Lux, Barbara Pease, Mary Beth Tomaselli, Kathryn M. John, and Seldon E. Bernstein

Division of Hematology-Oncology, Department of Medicine, Children's Hospital Medical Center and Sidney Farber Cancer Institute, Harvard Medical School, Boston 02115 (S.E.L., B.P., M.B.T., K.M.J.) and The Jackson Laboratory, Bar Harbor, Maine 04609 (S.E.B.)

Elliptocytes from patients with hereditary elliptocytosis (HE) form elliptical ghosts and membrane skeletons. The composition of HE skeletons is quantitatively normal; however, in some but not all kindreds the major membrane skeletal protein, spectrin, is abnormally heat-sensitive, presumably due to a molecular defect which diminishes its conformational stability.

Red cells from four mutants of the common house mouse (Mus musculus) with severe, recessive hemolytic anemias show marked membrane budding, fragmentation, and spherocytosis, which suggest membrane instability. Ghosts spontaneously vesiculate and are spectrin-deficient. The amount of spectrin varies from none to one-half the normal amount and correlates with the clinical severity of the four mutations. The cause of this deficiency remains to be determined. These mutants prove that spectrin is a critical determinant of membrane structural integrity and provide a unique opportunity to test, in intact red cells, putative functions of spectrin.

Spectrin extracted from ghosts at low ionic strength is heterogeneous. At physiologic ionic strengths part (46 ± 5%) is polymerized (P-spectrin) and complexed with actin, and part remains as nonpolymerized spectrin dimers and tetramers (NP-spectrin). We postulate that these are native membrane species which exist in a metabolically controlled equilibrium in vivo and that the proportion of these species regulates membrane shape, strength, and flexibility.

Key words: spectrin, red cell membrane, hereditary elliptocytosis, hereditary spherocytosis of mice

INTRODUCTION

Current evidence indicates that spectrin, actin, and band 4.1 form a protein meshwork which laminates the inner surface of the red blood cell (RBC) membrane. This "membrane skeleton" can be isolated by treatment of intact red cells or red cell ghosts with nonionic detergents such as Triton X-100 [1–3] and it is thought to be a major determinant of red cell membrane shape, strength, and flexibility. To test this postulate we are comparing membrane skeletons and skeletal proteins of fragile, rigid, or misshaped red cells with normal. We have previously shown that ghosts and skeletons of irreversibly sickled cells

(ISCs) are fixed in a sickle shape [4], which indicates that an acquired skeletal defect is responsible for the distortion of this rigid cell. In the present study we focus on two types of inherited defects: human hereditary elliptocytosis and the spherocytic hemolytic anemias of mice. The results, reported in detail elsewhere [5,6], suggest that these disorders are due to abnormalities of spectrin, the major membrane skeletal protein.

METHODS

Preparation of Ghosts and Skeletons

Blood was collected in standard citrate-phosphate-dextrose (CPD) solution and used immediately (mouse blood) or within 72 h (human blood). Red cell ghosts were prepared by hemolysis in hypotonic phosphate buffers [7]. Membrane skeletons were prepared by washing the ghosts once or twice with 10 mM Tris-HCl (pH 8), and extracting them with 5 volumes of 0.5% Triton X-100 in 56 mM sodium borate, pH 8 (30 min, 0°C) [1,4].

Spectrin Extraction and Chromatography

Spectrin was extracted from ghosts in 1 mM ethylenediaminetetracetic acid (EDTA) at 37°C and purified by chromatography on 4% agarose columns as previously described [8,9]. Under these conditions 40–60% of the chromatographed spectrin was recovered as spectrin dimer [10] and was homogeneous (>98% pure) on gel electrophoresis in sodium dodecyl sulfate (SDS).

Thermal Denaturation Studies

Samples of purified spectrin dimer were heated in a sensitive, thermoelectric heating device for 10 min at various temperatures between 46°C and 54°C [5], then cooled to 0°C and centrifuged at 100,000g for 60 min. Soluble spectrin was defined as the protein (measured by absorbance at 280 nm) remaining in the supernatant. In most experiments intact red cells, washed and diluted to a hematocrit of 2% in phosphate-buffered saline, were heated in parallel with their extracted spectrin and then fixed in 2% glutaraldehyde and examined by phase microscopy.

Polyacrylamide Gel Electrophoresis in Sodium Dodecyl Sulfate (SDS-PAGE)

SDS-PAGE was performed using the procedure of Fairbanks et al [11] as modified by Steck [12]. The spectrin content of gels stained with Coomassie Brilliant Blue was determined by densitometry [9]. Polypeptide bands were visualized by SDS-PAGE and numbered using the nomenclature of Steck [13]. In this system bands 1 and 2 designate the two chains of spectrin. Band 5 is red cell actin.

RESULTS AND DISCUSSION

Hereditary Elliptocytosis

Hereditary elliptocytosis (HE) is a relatively common, dominantly inherited disorder, characterized by the presence of numerous elliptical red cells on the peripheral blood smear. The disease is clinically heterogeneous. Most patients have "benign" HE. In this variant the red cell life-span is nearly normal and the patients are asymptomatic and are not anemic. A minority have "hemolytic" HE with overt and sometimes severe hemolysis.

Nearly all of the elliptocytes from five HE patients in four kindreds (three benign, one hemolytic) formed elliptical ghosts and elliptical membrane skeletons [5]. In contrast, less than 2% of control ghosts and membrane skeletons were elliptical. This implies that the shape of hereditary elliptocytes is due to a defective skeletal protein or proteins. Since the composition of HE skeletons was quantitatively normal, as judged by SDS-PAGE, we looked for a qualitative defect in spectrin, the major membrane skeletal constituent.

We first tested its thermal stability. Chromatographically pure spectrin dimer was heated at various temperatures for 10 min in a sensitive, thermoelectric heating device and then quickly cooled to 0°C. Soluble spectrin was separated from a pellet of heat-denatured spectrin by centrifugation (100,000g, 60 min) and quantified by absorption spectroscopy. As shown in Figure 1, normal spectrin dimer contained at least two subcomponents: 65 ± 3% (mean ± SD) was heat-labile and came out of solution when spectrin was heated. The median denaturation temperature was 49.0 ± 0.3°C. A smaller fraction (35 ± 3%) was heat-stable to at least 54°C. Similar heterogeneity was observed when the thermal denaturation of unfractionated spectrin extracts was monitored by circular dichroism [14]. At present we have no explanation for these interesting differences in thermal stability.

When intact normal erythrocytes were heated in parallel with their extracted spectrin, they showed the characteristic membrane budding, fragmentation, and spherocyte formation first described by Schultze more than 100 years ago [15]. This change in morphology occurred at 48.9 ± 0.2°C, coincident with the denaturation of the heat-labile subcomponent.

Normal and HE spectrin were equally extractable and showed similar elution patterns when fractionated on 4% agarose. However, unlike normal spectrin, that from all seven HE patients in three kindreds (two benign, one hemolytic) was entirely heat-labile (98 ± 4%, $P < 0.0005$) and abnormally heat-sensitive (Fig. 1). It denatured at a median temperature of 48.0 ± 0.1°C instead of 49.0°C, a highly significant difference ($P < 0.0005$).

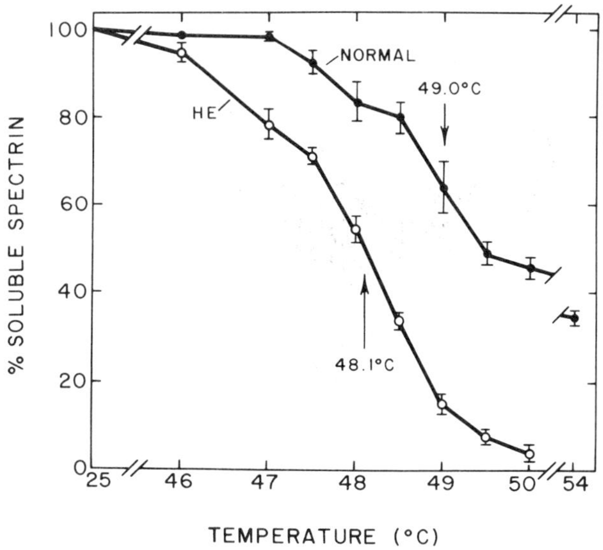

Fig. 1. Effect of heat on the solubility of purified spectrin dimer from normal (•) or hereditary elliptocytosis (○) erythrocytes. The vertical bars indicate ±1 SE about the mean. The arrows designate the median of each solubility curve.

Spectrin from all five HE patients in two other kindreds denatured normally. With the exception of one kindred, discussed in detail elsewhere [5], the fragmentation of intact hereditary elliptocytes, like normal red cells, correlated with the heat sensitivity of their extracted spectrin.

These observations reemphasize the correlation between spectrin and red cell shape evident in other studies [1–4,8,9,16–32], suggest that defects in the membrane skeleton are a common feature of HE in all kindreds, and indicate that at least two genetically distinct forms of HE exist. HE patients with heat-sensitive spectrin must have a molecular abnormality of spectrin which decreases its conformational stability. At present it is not clear whether this is a primary sequence defect or a defect in a posttranslational process such as spectrin phosphorylation. Spectrin phosphorylation of elliptical ghosts is reportedly normal [33], but it is not known whether the patients tested had heat-sensitive spectrin.

The presence of heat-sensitive spectrin does not correlate with the degree of elliptocytosis or hemolysis in HE patients. This is not surprising, since instability of spectrin at the unphysiologic temperature of 48°C probably does not contribute to the pathogenesis of HE. It simply reflects a decline in the conformational stability of the molecule. Presumably in the rare HE kindreds with hemolysis and heat-sensitive spectrin the conformational change affects sensitive functional regions of spectrin, such as the actin or membrane binding sites, which are not affected in the more common, benign variant. Preliminary observations, discussed later, support this concept.

Spherocytic Anemias of Mice

Four mutants of the common house mouse, Mus musculus, with recessively inherited hemolytic anemias have been identified: "normoblastosis" (*nb/nb*) [34], "hemolytic anemia" (*ha/ha*) [35], "spherocytosis" (*sph/sph*) [36], and "jaundiced" (*ja/ja*) [37]. All of the mutants have severe hemolysis. Reticulocyte counts range from 90–100% (*ja, sph,* and *ha* mutants) to 60% (*nb*) [38]. Judging from the degree of anemia and the effect of the mutation on survival, the order of severity is *ja/ja* > *sph/sph* > *ha/ha* > *nb/nb* [38]. Peripheral blood smears and scanning electron microscopy show intense spherocytosis and in vivo red cell budding (Fig. 2), which suggests that the mutant red cells have very unstable membranes. This impression is confirmed by the fact that, unlike normal ghosts, mutants are extremely fragile and spontaneously vesiculate during preparation.

All of the mutants are spectrin-deficient (Fig. 2). Interestingly, the degree of deficiency correlates closely with the clinical severity: *ja/ja* ghosts have no detectable spectrin, *sph/sph* ghosts lack band 1 but have small amounts of band 2, *ha/ha* ghosts have about 30% of the normal amount of both bands 1 and 2, and *nb/nb* ghosts have approximately 50% of the normal amount of spectrin [6]. These results confirm the recent report by Greenquist et al [24] of severe spectrin deficiency in the *sph/sph* mutant. Extraction studies show that the bands identified as "spectrin" in each of the mutants are completely extractable at low ionic strength like normal spectrin and cross-react with an anti-human spectrin antibody [6].

The cause of the spectrin deficiency in these mice is presently uncertain. It is not due to the young age of the mutant red cells since, reticulocyte-rich controls have normal spectrin concentrations (Fig 2). Decreased spectrin binding to the membrane and spectrin degradation during ghosting are also excluded, since the spectrin deficiency is evident on SDS-PAGE of intact red cells [6,24]. Preliminary evidence suggests that some of the numerous new low-molecular-weight bands present in the mutant ghosts (Fig. 2) are proteolytic

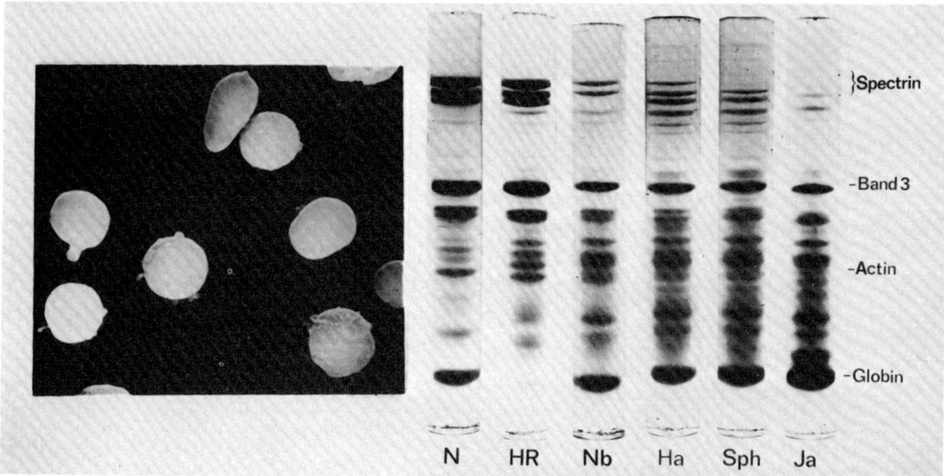

Fig. 2. Spectrin-deficient mutant mice. Left) Scanning electron micrograph of *sph/sph* erythrocytes. Note intense spherocytosis and membrane budding. Right) Polyacrylamide gel electrophoresis in sodium dodecyl sulfate of normal (N), high-reticulocyte control (HR), *nb/nb* (Nb), *ha/ha* (Ha), *sph/sph* (Sph), and *ja/ja* (Ja) mouse red cell membranes.

fragments of spectrin, since they stain with an antispectrin antibody, but it is not known whether proteolysis is a primary cause of the spectrin deficit or a secondary consequence of an unstable or otherwise abnormal molecule.

These mutants do, however, clearly illustrate the fundamental importance of spectrin and the membrane skeleton to the red cell. Without the reinforcement this structure provides, the membrane cannot resist the turbulent stresses of the arterial circulation, and the red cell quickly succumbs through fragmentation.

Dynamic Membrane Skeletal Model

We believe the skeleton must be a dynamic structure to permit the red cell to control its shape, flexibility, and structural integrity. Recent evidence suggests that the red cell may accomplish this control by modulation of spectrin polymerization and skeletal cross-linking [8,9,19–22,24–26,29–31,39–43].

We find that ghosts extracted at low ionic strength with 0.1 mM adenosinetriphosphate (ATP), 0.1 mM dithiothreitol (DTT), 0.1 mM imidazole HCl, pH 7.4 (37°C, 10 min) selectively release spectrin, actin, and usually part of band 4.1 from the membrane [39]. The spectrin in these extracts is heterogeneous. Part of it forms a high-molecular-weight (23S) complex with actin and, if present, band 4.1 and part remains as solitary dimers (band 1 + 2) and tetramers (band 1 + 2)$_2$ [39]. We have tentatively designated spectrin in the complex as polymerized spectrin (P-spectrin) and the spectrin dimers and tetramers as nonpolymerized spectrin (NP-spectrin). At physiologic ionic strengths in ATP (1 mM) and DTT (1 mM) the P-spectrin-actin complex represents 46.3 ± 5.2% (mean ± SD) of the total extract protein [39]. It does not require divalent cations and is largely reprecipitable at low ionic strengths.

We suspect that this complex is the fundamental structural unit of the membrane skeleton and suggest that it normally exists in equilibrium with nonpolymerized spectrin dimers and tetramers on the membrane. Both the dimer and tetramer can bind to spectrin receptors attached to the inner membrane surface [44], but it is likely that the tetramer is the physiologically dominant species at the high spectrin concentrations calculated to exist within the skeleton (~230 mg/ml [43]). We envision that this molecule is bound and concentrated on the membrane but remains dormant until activated by some process, such as a change in its state of phosphorylation [2,19,22,25,26,29,40–42], which enables it to interact with actin and, possibly, itself and to intercalate into the cross-linked skeletal network.

By maintaining the proper equilibrium between P- and NP-spectrin the normal biconcave red cell would remain both flexible and durable. Excess NP-spectrin (ie, decreased P-spectrin-actin complex) would yield a fragile membrane and lead to fragmentation, spherocytosis, and possibly other shapes. The mutant mice, with their marked deficiency of spectrin, represent an extreme example of this process. Conversely, excess spectrin-actin complex would further cross-link and contract the membrane skeleton and produce a rigid echinocyte.

Two observations lend provisional support to this hypothesis. First, the rigid echinocytes induced by ATP depletion have a P-spectrin-actin complex which is larger and more abundant than normal [8,39], as predicted. Second, in preliminary experiments, the proportion of spectrin-actin complex in one hemolytic HE kindred with heat-sensitive spectrin and morphologic evidence of membrane instability was only about half normal: 25.3% and 28.3% of a spectrin extract precipitated in 150 mM sodium chloride compared to 46.3 ± 5.2% in controls and 49.7 ± 3.0% in patients with benign HE.

It is likely, of course, that the membrane skeleton is much more complex than this simple model implies. Numerous skeletal proteins remain to be defined (eg, bands 2.1, 2.2, 2.3, 3a, 4.1, 4.9, and 7). Some will undoubtedly prove to have important structural and/or regulatory functions. The proliferation of actin-modulating proteins such as profilins, gelactins, actinins, troponins, etc, in nonmuscle cells other than the red cell [45], and the recent discovery of a troponin inhibitor-like protein in red cells [46], only strengthen this impression. It will be interesting to see whether these components eventually prove to embellish or displace the basic aspects of our present model.

ACKNOWLEDGMENTS

These studies were supported by a research grant (HL-15963) from the National Institutes of Health. The work was done during the tenure of an Established Investigatorship of the American Heart Association (S.E. Lux).

REFERENCES

1. Yu J, Fischman DA, Steck TL: J Supramol Struct 1:233, 1973.
2. Sheetz MP, Sawyer D, Jackowski S: In Brewer GJ (ed): "The Red Cell". New York: Alan R Liss, 1978, p 431.
3. Sheetz MP, Sawyer D: In Fox CF, Lux SE, Marchesi VT (eds): "Normal and Abnormal Red Cell Membranes." New York: Alan R Liss (In press).
4. Lux SE, John KM, Karnovsky MJ: J Clin Invest 58:955, 1976.
5. Lux SE, Tomaselli MB, John KM: Manuscript submitted.
6. Lux SE, Pease BP, Bernstein SE: Manuscript submitted.
7. Dodge JT, Mitchell C, Hanahan DJ: Arch Biochem Biophys 100:119, 1963.
8. Lux SE, John KM: In Revel JP, Henning U, Fox CF (eds): "Cell Shape and Surface Architecture." New York: Alan R Liss, 1977, p 481.
9. Lux SE, John KM, Ukena TE: J Clin Invest 61:815, 1978.
10. Ralston GB: Aust J Biol Sci 28:259, 1975.

11. Fairbanks G, Steck TL, Wallach DFH: Biochemistry 10:2606, 1971.
12. Steck TL: J Mol Biol 66:295, 1972.
13. Steck TL: J Cell Biol 62:1, 1974.
14. Brandts JF, Erickson L, Lysko K, Schwartz AT, Taverna RD: Biochemistry 16:3450, 1977.
15. Schultze M: Arch Mikrosk Anat 1:1, 1865.
16. Jacob HS, Yawata Y, Matsumoto N, Abman S, White J: In Brewer GJ (ed): "Erythrocyte Structure and Function." New York: Alan R Liss, 1975, p 235.
17. Ralston GB: Biochim Biophys Acta 401:83, 1975.
18. Williamson JR, Shanahan MD, Hochmuth RM: Blood 46:611, 1975.
19. Birchmeier W, Singer SJ: J Cell Biol 73:647, 1977.
20. Gaines KC, Salhany JM, Tuma DJ, Sorrell MF: FEBS Lett 75:115, 1977.
21. Sheetz MP, Singer SJ: J Cell Biol 73:638, 1977.
22. Shohet SB, Greenquist AC: Blood Cells 3:115, 1977.
23. Walter T, Mentzer W, Greenquist A, Schrier S, Mohandas N: Blood 50:98, 1977. (Abstract)
24. Greenquist AC, Shohet SB, Bernstein SE: Blood 51:1149, 1978.
25. Greenquist AC, Mohandas N, Shohet SB: Fed Proc 37:1507, 1978. (Abstract)
26. Hui DY, Harmony JAK: J Supramol Struct (Suppl) 2:208, 1978. (Abstract)
27. Lin DC, Lin S: J Biol Chem 253:1415, 1978.
28. Lin DC, Lin S: Fed Proc 37:1507, 1978. (Atstract)
29. Mohandas N, Greenquist AC, Shohet SB: In Brewer GJ (ed): "The Red Cell." New York: Alan R Liss, 1978, p 453.
30. Palek J, Liu SC, Snyder LM: Blood 51:385, 1978.
31. Lux SE, John KM: In Caughey WS (ed): "Clinical and Biochemical Aspects of Hemoglobin Abnormalities." New York: Academic (In press).
32. Ralston GB: Trends Biol Sci (In press).
33. Greenquist AC, Shohet SB: Blood 48:877, 1976.
34. Bernstein SE: In "Genetics in Laboratory Medicine." National Academy of Sciences publication No. 1724, 1969.
35. Bernstein SE: In Proceedings of the Ninth International Congress on Genetics, 1963, vol 1, p 186.
36. Joe M, Teasdale JM, Miller JR: Can J Genet Cytol 4:219, 1962.
37. Stevens LC, Mackensen JA, Bernstein SE: J Heredity 5:35, 1959.
38. Bernstein SE: Lab Animal Sci (In press).
39. Lux SE, John JM, Pease B: Fed Proc 37:1507, 1978. (Abstract)
40. Pinder JC, Bray D, Gratzer WB: Nature 258:765, 1975.
41. Pinder JC, Bray D, Gratzer WB: Nature 270:752, 1977.
42. Pinder JC, Ungewickell E, Bray D, Gratzer WB: In Lux SE, Marchesi VT, Fox CF (eds): "Normal and Abnormal Red Cell Membranes." New York: Alan R Liss (In press).
43. Lux SE: Sem Hematol (In press).
44. Bennett V, Branton D: J Biol Chem 252:2753, 1977.
45. Korn ED: Proc Natl Acad Sci USA 75:588, 1978.
46. Maimon J, Puszkin S: J Supramol Struct (Suppl) 2:204, 1978. (Abstract)

Normal and Abnormal Red Cell Membranes 471–474 (1979)

Lipid Loss in Spectrin Deficient Mouse Erythrocytes

Stephen B. Shohet

As an introduction to Dr. Allen's and Dr. Lutz's discussions of the lipid-loss which occurs in their perturbed membranes, I would like to take a few minutes to quickly tell you of another lipid-loss that appears to be related to an abnormality in the membrane protein, spectrin.

As you know from these meetings last year, with the help of Dr. Seldon Bernstein, Dr. Al Greenquist and I found that one of the congenital spherocytic mouse strains (sph:sph) in Dr. Bernstein's collection had markedly reduced concentrations of red cell membrane spectrin, and a preliminary note describing these mouse cells has been published [1]. Dr. Lux has confirmed this observation and has found some further mouse variants which he will discuss tomorrow [2].

To remind you of the major characteristics of this model, Figure 1 shows the scanning electron microscopic morphology of these cells. Note the complete absence of biconcavity in these highly spherical and anisocytotic erythrocytes. Additionally, there may be some suggestion of spontaneous cell fusion and budding in these cells which were fixed immediately after phlebotomy.

Figure 2 shows the cardinal physiologic abnormality of these cells: their profoundly abnormal osmotic fragility. At even the earliest dilutions of saline, there is appreciable hemolysis, and 50% hemolysis occurs well before any effect is seen in normal mouse blood.

Figure 3 shows the major biochemical abnormality found in these cells: a marked reduction in spectrin. This polyacrylamide gradient gel was kindly prepared by Steven Sweig of LaJolla. There is virtually no spectrin band I in the spherocytic sample on the right in comparison to the normal on the left. Moreover, we estimate that a maximum of 5% of residual band II could be present. The total protein analyzed for the spherocytic sample is about twice that of the normal sample so these differences may be even greater than indicated here.

Very recently, in Dr. Marcel Bessis' laboratory in Paris, we have found that a useful characteristic of these spectrin deficient cells is that, in contrast to normal mouse erythrocytes, they rapidly lose membrane lipid when incubated in hypertonic protein-free media. First, long myelin figures appear and then fall off the membranes; thereafter, marked microvesiculation and eventual membrane budding occurs. Estimating lipid-loss from the change in critical hemolytic volume observed upon re-incubation in lower osmotic strength media,

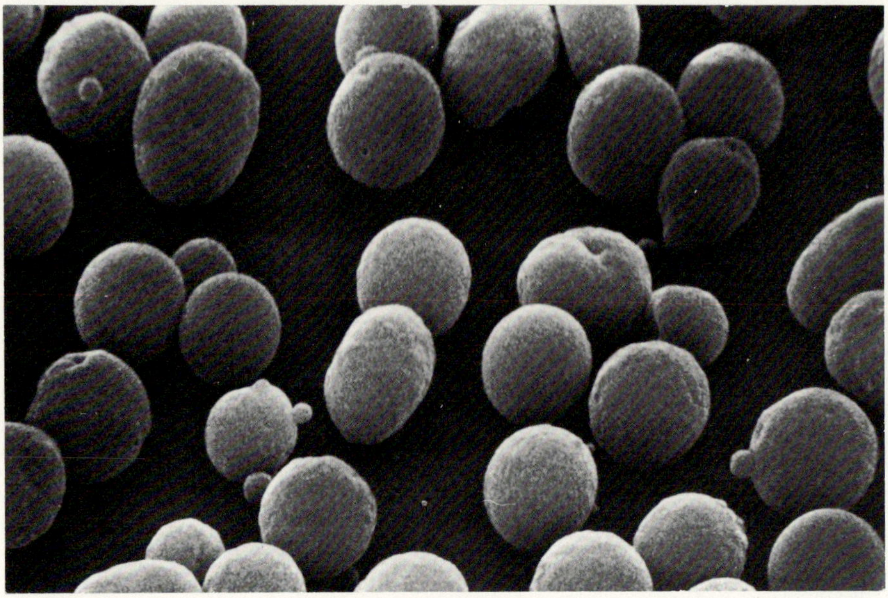

Fig. 1. Scanning electron micrograph of freshly drawn mouse hereditary spherocytosis cells. Note the absence of any biconcavity and apparent membrane budding.

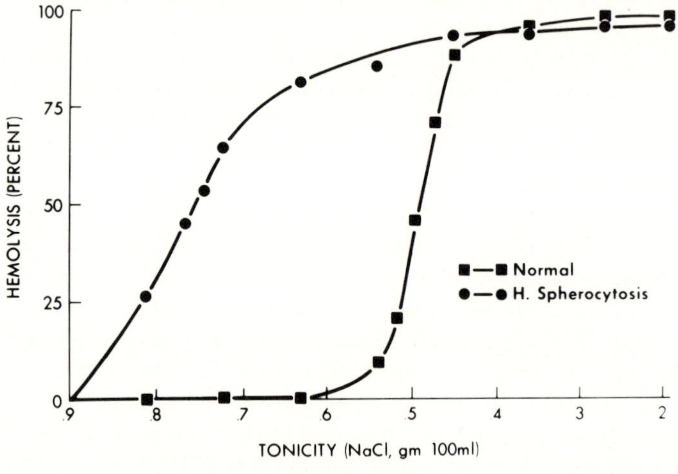

Fig. 2. Osmotic fragility curves of mouse hereditary spherocytes, •–•, and normal mouse erythrocytes ▪–▪. 50% hemolysis occurs at 0.75% saline in the affected cells.

approximately 10% of membrane lipid is lost within fifteen minutes of incubation in 600 mili-osmole media at room temperature. This rate is further increased to over 20% if small prelytic amounts of lysolecithin are present. These changes are also associated with a greatly increased tendency towards membrane fusion between adjacent cells when incubated at high cell concentrations.

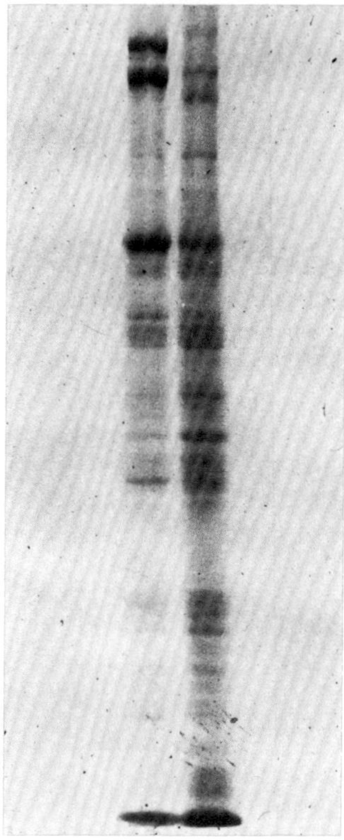

Fig. 3. Polyacrylamide gel electrophoretic analyses of erythrocyte membranes of normal erythrocytes (left) and hereditary spherocytes of mice (right). A 4–15% gradient of acrylamide was used in this Laemelli slab gel system and the spherocytic sample was overloaded to emphasize low concentration polypeptides. There is virtually no Spectrin Band I and a marked reduction in Band II in the spherocytic sample. Band 2.1 is present.

Finally, in very early studies, first started in Jon Singer's lab, and now continuing in Paris, we find that we can partially reconstitute these spectrin deficient cells by "exchange-hemolysis" with a crude normal mouse spectrin extract using the method developed for sickle hemoglobin by my colleague Dr. Margaret Clark [3].

Using this technique, somewhat over 50% of normal levels of specifically membrane-bound spectrin can be obtained, and that spectrin is capable of at least qualitative phosphorylation with ATP^{32}.

Importantly, the hyperosmotic membrane lipid-loss just described, is virtually eliminated by such reconstitution. Moreover, membrane incubation stability at 37° is greatly improved and spontaneous membrane fusion ceases.

While these observations are still early, and while the reconstitution system needs some further refinement, I think that these data already are strong direct evidence for an important role for spectrin in maintaining membrane stability. I will leave to the audience any further implications of these observations for answering Dr. Marchesi's questions concerning the reality of spectrin-lipid interactions, as well as any possible implications for the mechanism of membrane lipid insufficiency in hereditary spherocytoses of both men and mice.

ACKNOWLEDGMENTS

These studies were supported by NIH Grant No. AM–16095 and a Josiah Macy Faculty Scholar Award.

REFERENCES

1. Shohet SB, Greenquist AC: Possible role of membrane phosphorylation in the control of erythrocyte shape. Blood Cells 3, 115-131, 1977.
2. Lux SE, Pease B, Tomaselli MB, John KM, Bernstein S: Hemolytic anemias associated with deficient or dysfunctional spectrin (abs). J Supramol Struct, Suppl 2, 94, 1978.
3. Clark MR, Shohet SB: Hybrid erythrocytes for sickle cell membrane studies. Blood 47, 121, 1976.

Normal and Abnormal Red Cell Membranes 475–481 (1979)

Rotational Diffusion of Band 3 in the Red Cell Membrane: Measurements Using Triplet Probes

R. J. Cherry and E. Nigg

Eidgenössische Technische Hochschule, Laboratorium für Biochemie, ETH-Zentrum, CH-8092 Zürich, Switzerland

Rotational diffusion of band 3 in the human erythrocyte membrane has been investigated using the technique of flash photolysis. Membranes are labeled with the triplet probe eosin isothiocyanate; most of the label is found to be associated with band 3. Rotation is measured by observing the decay of dichroism of flash-induced absorbance changes arising from the eosin probe. The results indicate that band 3 rotates about an axis normal to the plane of the membrane with a diffusion coefficient in the order of 1,000 sec^{-1}. Removal of spectrin has no observable effect on the rotation of band 3 at pH 7.6. Essentially similar results are obtained with a different probe, iodoacetamidoeosin. Both eosin derivatives are strong inhibitors of anion transport. Illumination of eosin-labeled ghosts causes a rapid loss of acetylcholinesterase activity but this can be prevented by prior displacement of oxygen in the sample by argon.

Key words: **anion transport, inhibition by eosin; band 3, interaction with spectrin; band 3, rotational diffusion; eosin probes; flash photolysis; photoinactivation; rotational diffusion; spectrin, interaction with band 3; triplet probes**

Using the technique of flash photolysis, we have developed a method for measuring rotational relaxation times of macromolecules in the microsecond-millisecond time range [1, 2]. The principal aim of developing such a method is to investigate protein rotation in membranes. Consideration of membrane viscosity leads one to expect that the relaxation times of many membrane proteins are longer than 10^{-6} sec [3, 4]. The first measurement with rhodopsin gave a relaxation time of 20 μsec at 20°C [5].

Measurement of the rotational diffusion of membrane proteins should test to what extent proteins undergo free diffusion, as envisaged in current models of membrane structure [6]. Where free diffusion is prevented, diffusion measurements should provide a useful method for investigating those interactions which are responsible for the restriction. Refinement of the technique could make it possible to detect specific aggregates in the membrane (dimers, trimers etc), since relaxation times are strongly dependent on molecular

Received for publication March 5, 1978.

size. Further properties, such as the internal rigidity of membrane proteins, may also be investigated.

The flash photolysis method has been used to study the rotation of band 3 in the human erythrocyte membrane [7, 8]. Band 3 consists of hydrophobic proteins which span the membrane, have a molecular weight of about 90,000, and comprise about 24% of the total membrane protein (for review of erythrocyte membrane proteins, see Marchesi, Furthmayr, and Tomita [9]). Another major component of the membrane is spectrin, which is a fibrous protein composed of two polypeptides of molecular weights 220,000 and 240,000. Spectrin is a peripheral membrane protein located on the cytoplasmic side of the membrane. A direct linkage between band 3 and spectrin has previously been proposed [10, 11].

We have investigated the interaction between band 3 and spectrin by observing the effect of spectrin removal on band 3 rotation [7]. These measurements were made using the triplet probe eosin isothiocyanate (eosin-NCS). Here we briefly review these experiments and report that similar results are obtained with a different probe, iodoacetamidoeosin (IA-eosin). The effects of these probes on anion transport and on acetylcholinesterase activity in the erythrocyte membrane are also discussed.

METHODS

Measurement of Slow Rotational Diffusion by Flash Photolysis

Triplet states of organic molecules typically have lifetimes of milliseconds at room temperature. This long lifetime may be exploited to measure rotational motion that is too slow to be detected by the conventional method of fluorescence polarization.

Triplet states are conveniently detected by observing transient absorbance changes of a given sample following excitation by a brief flash of light. Absorbance changes arising from either triplet-triplet absorption or ground state depletion may be observed. When the exciting light is plane-polarized, only those molecules whose transition moment for absorption lies in or near to the plane of polarization are excited. Hence, a partially ordered population of excited molecules is photoselected from the initial random distribution. As a result, the transient absorbance changes are in general dichroic. Dichroism decays as the excited molecules again become disordered due to Brownian rotation; the rate of decay enables the rate of rotation to be calculated. Because of the long lifetime of the triplet state, relaxation times as slow as milliseconds may be determined in this way.

The flash photolysis apparatus used for detecting transient absorbance changes is fully described elsewhere, together with further details of the method [2, 12]. Briefly, the sample is excited by a plane-polarized light pulse of duration 1–2 μsec and wavelength 540 nm from a dye laser. The absorbance changes for light polarized in a plane parallel $[A_{\parallel}(t)]$ and perpendicular $[A_{\perp}(t)]$ to the plane of polarization of the exciting flash are measured simultaneously. The data are analyzed by calculating the absorption anisotropy r(t), given by

$$r(t) = \frac{A_{\parallel}(t) - A_{\perp}(t)}{A_{\parallel}(t) + 2A_{\perp}(t)}$$

where t is the time after the flash; r(t) is independent of the signal lifetime and depends only on rotational motion, provided the absorption transient exhibits a single exponential decay.

Probes

In order to make measurements as outlined above, it is generally necessary to attach a probe molecule to the protein. The triplet probes we have used, eosin-NCS and IA-eosin, are shown in Figure 1. Eosin-NCS can be prepared by bromination of fluorescein isothiocyanate [2, 12] or purchased from Molecular Probes Inc (Roseville, Minnesota). IA-eosin is similarly prepared by bromination of iodoacetamidofluorescein, which is also available from Molecular Probes.

Preparation and Labeling of Erythrocyte Membranes

Intact red cells from fresh or recently outdated blood are labeled with either eosin NCS or IA-eosin. Following removal of unreacted label, ghosts are prepared by hypotonic lysis. The amount of bound eosin is determined spectrophotometrically. Details of these procedures are presented elsewhere [1, 7, 12]. Using SDS gel electrophoresis and selective extraction procedures, it may be shown that most of the label is attached to band 3 [8]. Spectrin-depleted ghosts are prepared as described by Fairbanks, Steck, and Wallach [13]. Typically, the labeled membranes contain 1-2 μg eosin per milligram membrane protein.

RESULTS AND DISCUSSION

Rotational Diffusion of Band 3

Results obtained from flash photolysis experiments with eosin-NCS-labeled membranes are shown in Figure 2. The plot for the control sample (ie, no spectrin depletion) shows that the absorption anisotropy first falls and then reaches a constant value. As discussed elsewhere, this is the expected result for a protein whose rotation is confined to a single axis normal to the plane of the membrane [7, 12]. Essentially the decay of r is due to partial randomization of the transition dipole moments due to rotation about the membrane normal. The time-independent component arises because complete randomization is

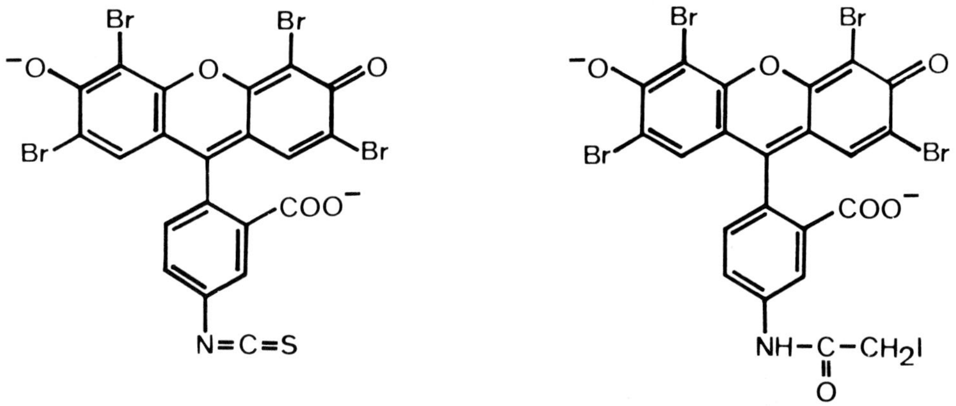

I II

Fig 1. Triplet probes: I) eosin-5-isothiocyanate; II) 5-iodoacetamidoeosin.

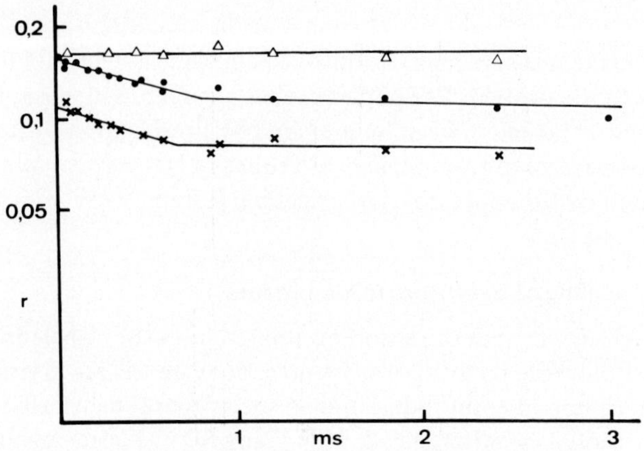

Fig 2. Time dependence of absorption anisotropy r for eosin-NCS-labeled ghosts: X) ghosts suspended in 20 mOsm phosphate buffer, pH 7.6 (control sample); •) spectrin-depleted ghosts, pH 7.6; △) spectrin-depleted ghosts, pH 5.4. The lower initial value of r in the control sample is due to experimental factors and has no special significance. Reproduced with permission from Cherry et al [7].

prevented by the inability of the protein to tumble about the two perpendicular axes lying in the plane of the membrane. The diffusion coefficient $D_{||}$ for rotation about the membrane normal may be estimated to be in the order of 1,000 sec^{-1}, ie, the relaxation time (= $1/D_{||}$) is about 1 msec. Thus rotation of band 3 is much slower than that previously found for rhodopsin [5].

Some variations are observed between different preparations in the relative magnitudes of the two components of r(t). The relative magnitudes may also be altered by various treatments; for example, the decaying part of r(t) is irreversibly increased in magnitude by suspending the ghosts in 1 M NaCl. This effect could indicate changes in mobility of band 3 but may also be due to fragmentation of the erythrocyte ghosts.

Interaction of Band 3 With Spectrin

In order to test whether spectrin restricts the rotational motion of band 3, measurements were made with spectrin-depleted membranes. Figure 2 shows that the results are pH-dependent; at pH 7.6 the absorption anisotropy has a time dependence similar to that of the control sample, while at pH 5.4, r is independent of time.

The result at pH 5.4, which shows that band 3 is immobilized, is easily explained by aggregation. Freeze-fracture electron micrographs reveal strong aggregation of intramembranous particles in spectrin-depleted membranes at pH 5.4 [7, 14]. The intramembranous particles are believed to contain band 3 [15, 16].

When the pH is maintained at 7.6 there is, as far as can be ascertained, no significant difference between the control and spectrin-depleted samples. Hence spectrin does not appear to significantly affect the rotation of band 3. Although this finding does not rule out a direct linkage between band 3 and spectrin, it does place severe restrictions on the type of linkage which can be envisaged. Cnly a linkage which permits free rotation about an axis normal to the plane of the membrane is compatible with the present measurements.

On the other hand, we consider that a model in which there is no direct interaction between band 3 and spectrin accounts equally well for all the mobility data. Suppose that band 3 protrudes from the membrane in the spaces between the spectrin fibres. It follows that lateral diffusion over large distances would be hindered by the spectrin network, whereas rotational diffusion would be unaffected. The enhanced aggregation of intramembranous particles in spectrin-depleted ghosts at low pH [14] would be explained by such a model. Further, proteins entrapped within the spectrin network would probably follow any redistribution of the spectrin molecules themselves. The clustering of anion sites [15] and concanavalin A receptors [10] on the outer membrane surface which is observed when spectrin is aggregated may be explained in this way.

Peters et al [17] labeled proteins (principally band 3) with fluorescein, bleached one half of a single ghost, and looked for the spread of fluorescence from the unbleached to the bleached half. No spreading was detected, placing an upper limit on the lateral diffusion constant of 3×10^{-12} cm^2 sec^{-1}. For free diffusion such a low value would imply a rotational relaxation time in the order of 50 msec, a value clearly incompatible with the present data. This again implies that lateral diffusion is restricted and is entirely compatible with the idea of band 3 proteins trapped in the spectrin net.

Since the rotational diffusion of band 3 was first reported, further evidence has appeared which also indicates that band 3 and spectrin are not directly linked. Bennett and Branton [18] have investigated the reassociation of spectrin with ghost vesicles and conclude that a direct role of band 3 in the binding of spectrin is unlikely. Fowler and Branton [19] examined the lateral redistribution of fluorescein-labeled band 3, following fusion (and hemolysis) of red cells. In contrast to Peters et al, they find that a measurable lateral mobility does occur over the temperature range 23–37°C. However, the calculated diffusion coefficient at 23°C is only a factor of two different from the upper limit of Peters et al. Hence comparison of rotational and lateral diffusion still leads to the conclusion that lateral mobility of band 3 is restricted, though apparently not totally.

Measurements With IA-Eosin

A disadvantage of any probe technique is the possibility of perturbation of the system by the probe itself. The data may be viewed with increasing confidence, however, if different probes give similar results. For this reason, in addition to eosin-NCS, we have also carried out experiments with the iodoacetamido derivative of eosin. Eosin-NCS is expected to react preferentially with amino groups and IA-eosin with sulphydryl residues.

Results of flash photolysis experiments with IA-eosin-labeled erythrocyte membranes are shown in Figure 3. IA-eosin, like eosin-NCS, principally labels band 3. It can be seen that the time-dependence of the absorption anisotropy is very similar to that measured with eosin-NCS. The results with spectrin-depleted membranes are also similar and again no significant difference from the control sample can be detected at pH 7.4.

Effects of Eosin Probes on Anion Transport and Acetylcholinesterase Activity

The similarity in the results obtained with eosin-NCS and IA-eosin raises questions concerning the binding sites of these two probes on band 3. Since eosin is a di-anion at neutral pH, it might be expected that the probes would react with the anion transport system (which is probably the major component of band 3 [20–24]). Recent experiments that we have carried out in fact show that both probes are strong inhibitors of sulphate exchange in the red cell [25]. The isothiocyanate is the stronger inhibitor, sulphate exchange being 50% inhibited when 4.7×10^5 eosin molecules/cell are bound (calculated assuming 6.0×10^{-10} mg membrane protein/ghost [28]). The corresponding figure for IA-eosin is

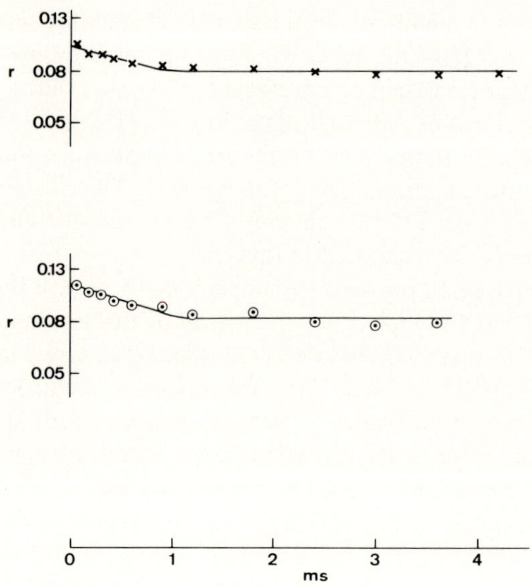

Fig 3. Time dependence of absorption anisotropy for IA-eosin labeled ghosts. ×) ghosts suspended in 20 mOsm phosphate buffer, pH 7.4; ⊙) spectrin-depleted ghosts, pH 7.4.

6.0×10^5. These numbers may be compared with inhibition by H_2DIDS (4,4′-diisothio-cyano-1,2-diphenylethane-2,2′ disulphonic acid) which gives 50% inhibition at a binding of (6–8) $\times 10^5$ molecules/cell [23, 24].

In order to test whether eosin probes occupy the same binding site as H_2DIDS, cells were prelabeled with H_2DIDS under conditions which yielded more than 95% inhibition of the anion transport system. It was found that the amount of eosin probes which could be further bound was reduced roughly two-fold compared with untreated cells. Hence we conclude that both eosin probes have common binding sites with H_2DIDS but other sites are labeled as well.

A possible perturbing effect of the probes arises because eosin is known to be a strong photosensitizing agent [26, 27]. To investigate this effect, we used the acetyl-cholinesterase activity of the membrane as a marker [25]. We found that the enzymic activity is rapidly lost on illumination of eosin-labeled ghosts with a white light of intensity about 5 mW/cm^2. However, inactivation does not occur when eosin-labeled intact erythrocytes are illuminated under the same light intensity. This is probably due to the presence of hemoglobin, which acts as an efficient blocking filter for light absorbed by eosin.

Inactivation of acetylcholinesterase in ghosts can be completely protected by displacing oxygen in the sample with argon prior to illumination. In flash photolysis experiments, samples are routinely bubbled with argon prior to measurement, since oxygen shortens the triplet lifetime. Thus no photooxidative damage to the membranes, as judged by the criterion of acetylcholinesterase activity, occurs during the flash photolysis experiments.

ACKNOWLEDGMENTS

We thank Professor H. Passow for a gift of H_2DIDS and the Swiss National Science Foundation for financial support.

REFERENCES

1. Cherry RJ, Cogoli A, Oppliger M, Schneider G, Semenza G: Biochemistry 15:3653, 1976.
2. Cherry RJ, Schneider G: Biochemistry 15:3657, 1976.
3. Edidin M: Ann Rev Biophys Bioeng 3:179, 1974.
4. Cherry RJ: In Chapman D, Wallach DFH (eds): "Biological Membranes." London-New York: Academic, 1976, vol 3, p 47.
5. Cone RA: Nature New Biol 236:39, 1972.
6. Singer SJ, Nicolson GL: Science 175:720, 1972.
7. Cherry RJ, Bürkli A, Busslinger M, Schneider G, Parish GR: Nature 263:389, 1976.
8. Cherry RJ, Bürkli A, Busslinger M, Schneider G: In Semenza G, Carafoli E (eds): "Biochemistry of Membrane Transport." FEBS Symposium No. 42. Berlin: Springer-Verlag, 1977, p 86.
9. Marchesi VT, Furthmayr H, Tomita M: Ann Rev Biochem 45:667, 1976.
10. Pinto da Silva P, Nicolson GL: Biochim Biophys Acta 363:311, 1974.
11. Elgsaeter A, Shotton DM, Branton D: Biochim Biophys Acta 426:101, 1976.
12. Cherry RJ: Meth Enzymol 54:47, 1978.
13. Fairbanks G, Steck TL, Wallach DFH: Biochemistry 10:2606, 1971.
14. Elgsaeter A, Branton D: J Cell Biol 63:1018, 1974.
15. Nicolson GL, Painter RG: J Cell Biol 59:395, 1973.
16. Guidotti G: Ann Rev Biochem 41:731, 1972.
17. Peters R, Peters J, Tews KH, Bähr W: Biochim Biophys Acta 367:282, 1974.
18. Bennett V, Branton D: J Biol Chem 252:2753, 1977.
19. Fowler V, Branton D: Nature 268:23, 1977.
20. Cabantchik ZI, Rothstein A: J Membr Biol 15:207, 1974.
21. Passow H, Fasold H, Zaki L, Schuhmann B, Lepke S: In Gardos G, Szasz I (eds): "Biomembrane: Structure and Function." FEBS Symposium No. 35. Budapest: Publishing House of the Hungarian Academy of Sciences, 1975, p 197.
22. Ho MK, Guidotti G: J Biol Chem 250:675, 1975.
23. Lepke S, Fasold H, Pring M, Passow H: J Membr Biol 29:147, 1976.
24. Ship S, Shami Y, Breuer W, Rothstein A: J Membr Biol 33:311, 1977.
25. Nigg, E, Kessler M, Cherry RJ: Biochim Biophys Acta 550:328, 1979.
26. Blum HF: "Photodynamic Action and Diseases Caused by Light." New York: Hafner Publishing Co, 1964, p 47.
27. Grossweiner LI, Kepke AG: Photochem Photobiol 16:305, 1972.
28. Dodge JT, Mitchell C, Hanahan DJ: Arch Biochem Biophys 100:119, 1963.

Normal and Abnormal Red Cell Membranes 483–496 (1979)

A Model for the Action of the Anion Exchange Protein of the Red Blood Cell

A. Rothstein, P. A. Knauf, S. Grinstein, and Y. Shami

Research Institute, The Hospital for Sick Children, Toronto, Ontario, Canada

Kinetic information on anion transport suggests that a mobile carrier system is involved in which the carrier-anion complex is able to spontaneously traverse the membrane. A second anion-binding site, the modifier, can when occupied reduce the rate of transport. Chemical studies with inhibitory probes suggest that the carrier and modifier sites are located in a specific transmembrane protein, band 3. The modifier site is accessible only from the internal surface but the carrier (transport) site is accessible from both the external and cytoplasmic surfaces. This information is discussed in terms of a model in which the anion traverses the membrane via a protein pathway. Transport involves conformational changes such that the transport site is alternately exposed to the external and cytoplasmic sides.

Key words: anion exchange, transport protein, erythrocyte, red blood cell, mobile carrier, chemical probes

A transport function can be directly measured as the flux of a substance across an intact membrane. The process can be characterized in terms of kinetic and thermodynamic parameters that allow certain conclusions to be made concerning possible mechanisms. For most hydrophilic substances, such as ions, sugars, amino acids, and nucleotides the transport properties suggest the existence of membrane entities with which the substances must bind in order for their transfer to occur. Recently interest has shifted from such hypothetical carriers to the identification and characterization of the actual membrane entities, usually proteins, that are involved in specific transport phenomena. From a technical point of view, however, the biochemical studies require the disruption of the membrane and separation of its components, whereas the functional studies must be carried out in intact membranes. For this reason, two relatively independent sets of information have tended to develop, one concerned with the structural properties of transport proteins and the other with the kinetic behaviour of the transport system. In order to understand the molecular nature of transport, however, the relationship between the structure and the function of specific transport proteins must be determined. The anion transport system of the red blood cell is particularly appropriate for examination, because both sets of information are well developed. Steck [1] has outlined in some detail the characteris-

Received for publication March 5, 1978.

tics of band 3, an abundant intrinsic membrane protein, including information about its arrangement in the bilayer. In the present paper, we will summarize the existing kinetic information concerning anion transport and also evidence, based largely on the localization of covalent inhibitory probes, that indicates that band 3 is involved in anion transport. By combining the use of probes with a kinetic analysis of the type of inhibition that they produce, it is possible to determine the role of the particular probe-binding sites of the protein in the transport process. On the basis of these two kinds of information a molecular model for anion transport is proposed.

KINETICS OF TRANSPORT

The anion transport system of the red cell is unique in terms of its capacity. The anion fluxes are many orders of magnitude faster than those of other cells [2], the half-time for Cl^- equilibration at 37°C being about 50 msec [3]. This high capacity is required in order that the physiologic function of exchange of Cl^- for HCO_3^- can be accomplished in the short passage time (less than 1 sec) of blood cells through lung capillaries. The abundance of the system provides a distinct experimental advantage in terms of the short times required for the measurement of fluxes and the large amount of membrane protein involved (about 25% of the membrane protein).

The anion transport displays properties that can best be explained by assuming that the anions must bind to membrane entities in order to pass across the membrane [2,4-7]. These properties include the following: a) The rate of transport reaches a limiting value (saturates) as the concentration of the anion increases; b) pairs of anions display competitive behaviour; c) the system displays a particular anion specificity pattern; d) the transport can be blocked by relatively low concentrations of inhibitors; and e) over 99% of the chloride flux involves an obligatory 1 for 1 anion exchange (an anion out for an anion in). The system allows rapid equilibration of anions without dependence on metabolic energy.

Although initial attempts to explain the kinetic properties were based on the premise that the binding sites for anions might be "fixed positive-charged groups" in the membrane [8], it is now more generally accepted that binding occurs to mobile sites or mobile carriers [4,5]. In addition, a second type of anion-binding site, the modifier, has recently been proposed to explain the self-inhibition of transport caused by very high substrate concentrations [9]. Thus in Figure 1, the efflux of Cl^- in the control reaches a maximal rate at about 150 mM Cl^-, representing saturation of the carrier with Ks of 65–67 mM. The self-inhibition seen at higher Cl^- concentrations, however, involves a site with an apparent dissociation constant for Cl^- (Ki) of 335 mM, with the inhibition being noncompetitive. Other halides not only appear to compete for transport, but also displace Cl^- from the modifier. The halide affinity series for the two sites, transport and modifier, are different [9]. Organic anions may also inhibit by binding to the modifier site. Thus in the presence of the anion transport inhibitor NAP-taurine [N-(4-azido-2-nitrophenyl)-2-aminoethylsulfonate], the Cl^- flux is reduced and the self-inhibition is suppressed (Fig. 1) [10].

A mobile carrier model to explain these observations [4,5] is presented in Figure 2. Anions can bind reversibly to positively charged carrier sites C^+, and the resulting anion-carrier complex can spontaneously traverse the membrane. The obligatory one-for-one exchange can be accommodated by assuming that the unloaded carrier cannot traverse the membrane. At higher substrate concentrations all of the carrier sites will be filled and a maximal rate of transport will thereby result. At even higher concentrations, binding will occur to the modifier site, resulting in a reduced rate of translocation of the carrier-anion

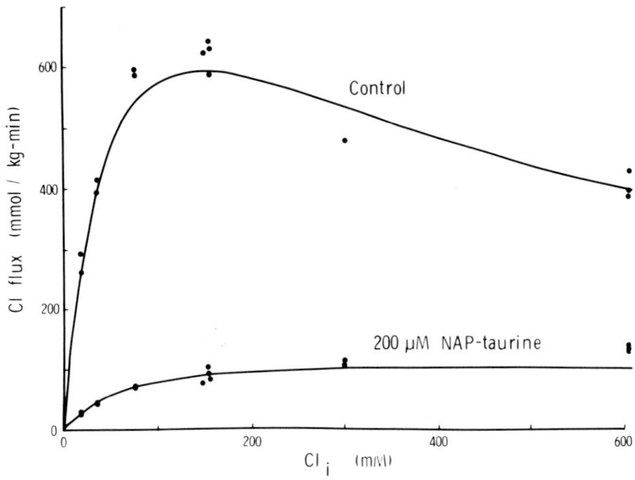

Fig 1. Chloride flux as a function of chloride concentration. Internal and external chloride were approximately equal (cells were treated with ·ıystatin). The upper curve was calculated assuming the dissociation constant for the transport site, Ks, is 65 mM and that for the modifier site, Kz, is 335 mM, as in Dalmark [9]. The lower curve was calculated from the same parameters, assuming that NAP-taurine inhibits the chloride flux by interacting with the modifier site with a Ki of 25 μM. The figure is taken from Knauf et al [10].

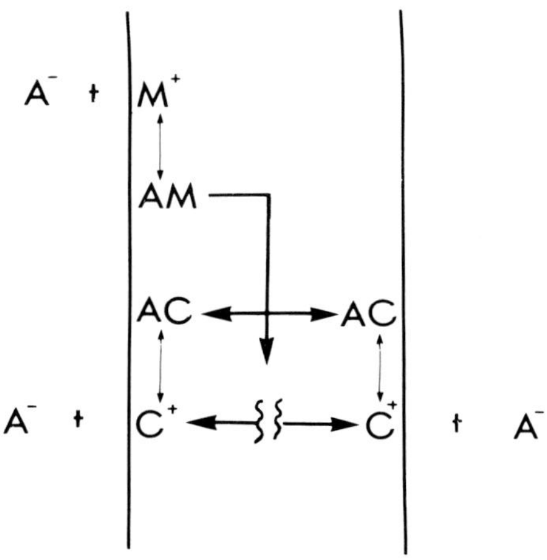

Fig 2. A mobile carrier model to explain the anion transport kinetics. C is the carrier site and M the modifier site. The figure is taken from Rothstein et al [11].

complex. Addition of a second anion would tend to displace the substrate anion from the two sites in accordance with their relative binding affinities.

IDENTIFICATION OF THE CARRIER

Anion transport across phospholipid bilayer membranes is orders of magnitude lower than that across the red cell membrane, suggesting that the rapid rate in the latter is medi-

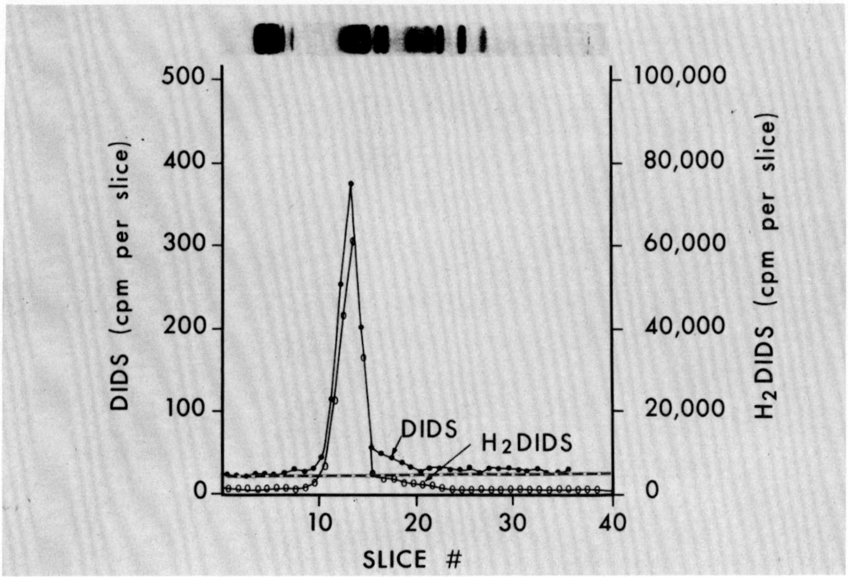

Fig 3. The localization of DIDS and H_2DIDS in red cell membrane proteins. The proteins were separated by SDS-acrylamide gel electrophoresis. The DIDS-peak corresponds to the location of band 3. The figure is from Ship et al [12].

ated by membrane proteins [2]. Specific identification poses some problems because the isolated proteins display no unique characteristics that connect them to transport. Two approaches have been used to overcome this problem. In the first, relatively specific irreversible inhibitors of anion transport have been shown to be highly localized in one particular protein, band 3. In the second, relatively pure band 3 has been shown to confer anion transport activity on model phospholipid membranes.

Inhibitory probes that are localized to varying degrees in band 3 include: sulfanilic acid derivatives, pyridoxal phosphate, NAP-taurine and disulfonic stilbenes [2]. The stilbenes, particularly DIDS (4,4′-diisothiocyanostilbene-2,2′-disulfonic acid) are the most specific inhibitors of anion transport. Other functions, such as cation permeability, active cation transport, and sugar transport, are not affected. Up to 90% of the DIDS bound to the membrane is localized in band 3 [12] (Fig. 3); of the remainder, about 5% is bound to glycophorin and can be removed by trypsinization of the cells [13]. Trypsin is without effect on the anion system [14]. Furthermore, the binding to band 3 is linearly related to inhibition with complete block of transport associated with approximately 10^6 molecules of DIDS bound to band 3 in each cell [12,15]. Because this is also about the number of band 3 monomers per cell, the data are consistent with the proposal that most of band 3 is involved in anion transport and that each monomer of protein contains one DIDS inhibition site [2,11]. Additional evidence, consistent with a role for band 3 in anion transport, is found in chloride binding studies using nuclear magnetic resonance techniques. A large proportion (50%) of the chloride bound to the ghost is associated with band 3, and much of that (about 1/3) is prevented by DIDS pretreatment of the cells. Thus the DIDS binding sites in band 3 are associated with chloride binding [16].

Although the data obtained with covalent inhibitors such as DIDS are strongly consistent with band 3 as the anion transport protein, it is still possible that a minor labelled component, not evident in the SDS-acrylamide gel electrophoresis, might be responsible for the transport activity. Although it can be argued that the turnover rate of anion transport is too fast to be accommodated by such a minor component, the evidence is not unequivocal [3,15]. Further positive support for band 3 is found, however, in studies in which purified fractions of the protein are demonstrated to support anion transport. In one type of study, the membrane proteins are dissolved in detergents, purified to varying degrees, and reconstituted in model phospholipid membranes with recovery of anion transport activity [17–19]. Unless a minor unidentified functional component survives the extraction, purification, and reconstitution, the anion transport activity must be attributed to the purified component, band 3. In a second type of study, band 3 was purified up to 95% by extracting almost all other proteins from the membrane [20]. The residual vesicles were then tested for anion transport activity. In this case the amount of transport per unit of retained band 3 was approximately the same as in the intact cells, and the sensitivity to DIDS was retained.

Although it is difficult to "prove" absolutely that band 3 is the transport protein, the positive evidence is strong. Only if another minor component behaved like band 3 in terms of interaction with probes, extraction, purification, and reconstitution would it be a possible candidate. In the remainder of this paper, therefore, band 3 is assumed to be the transport protein.

RELATIONSHIP OF PROTEIN STRUCTURE TO TRANSPORT

Only a portion of band 3 seems to be necessary for anion transport. In the preceding paper, Steck [1] has pointed out that band 3 is inserted through the bilayer, so that portions are exposed on the outside and inside surfaces and only a smaller segment of about 17,000 daltons crosses the membrane. Proteolytic attack at the outside, inside, or both sides [13,21,22], producing fragmentation and solubilization of portions of band 3 (and other proteins), does not eliminate anion transport. In fact, after proteolysis from both sides plus "stripping" of soluble proteins by low-ionic-strength alkaline extraction, so that the predominant peptide left in the membrane vesicles is the 17,000-dalton transmembrane segment of band 3 [23], the sulfate transport capacity is not appreciably reduced (Table I in Grinstein, Ship, and Rothstein [21]). Furthermore, in vesicles derived from DIDS-treated cells, most of the DIDS is retained in the 17,000-dalton fragment (Fig. 4)

TABLE I. Fluxes in Inside-Out (IO) Vesicles After Various Proteolytic Treatments and Alkaline Extraction

	K h^{-1}	J nmoles/min μg Pi	DIDS inhibition
Control	2.23 ± 0.03	0.0365 ± 0.0009	89.9–95.3
Chymotrypsin on external surface	2.08 ± 0.06	0.0358 ± 0.0012	92.0–99.3
Trypsin on cytoplasmic surface	2.30 ± 0.11	0.0352 ± 0.0013	85.6–92.7
Chymotrypsin + trypsin	2.15 ± 0.06	0.0293 ± 0.0018	93.0–94.5
Chymotrypsin + trypsin + alkaline extraction	2.28 ± 0.06	0.0320 ± 0.0020	—

The chymotrypsin is added to intact cells prior to formation of IO vesicles and therefore represents proteolysis of the outside face of the membrane. The trypsin is added to the IO vesicles and therefore represents proteolysis of the cytoplasmic face of the membrane. The DIDS is also added to the cells prior to formation of IO vesicles. K is the initial rate of SO_4^{--} efflux. J is the flux of SO_4^{--} per unit of phospholipid phosphate (taken as a measure of membrane surface). Data are from Grinstein, Ship, and Rothstein [21].

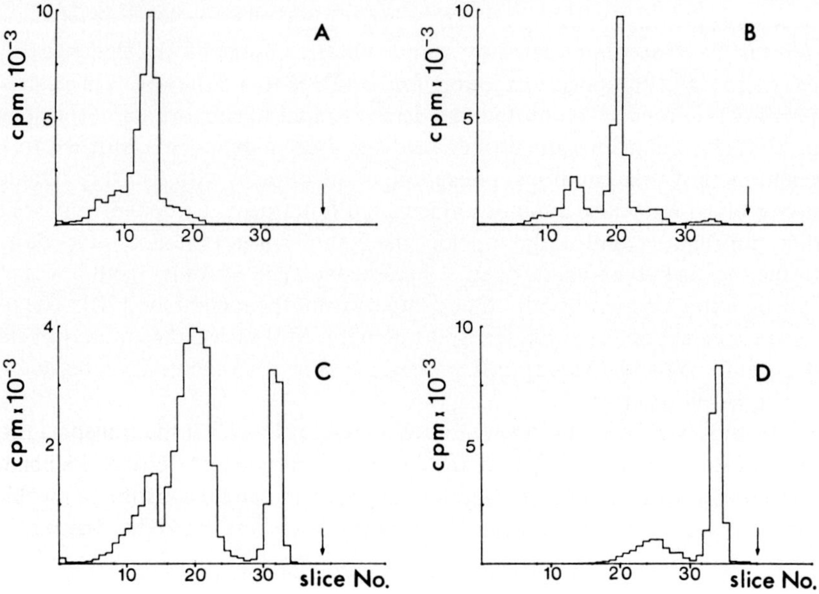

Fig 4. The effect of proteolysis of red cell membranes on the distribution of DIDS. A) Control, B) proteolysis of the external face of the membrane, C) proteolysis of the cytoplasmic face, and D) proteolysis of both faces (the major peak of DIDS-labelling in this case is a 17,000-dalton segment). The figure is from Grinstein, Ship, and Rothstein [21].

and the transport is inhibited. Thus the 17,000-dalton transmembrane fragment seems to be the portion of band 3 essential for anion transport.

The exact arrangement of the 17,000-dalton-segment in the lipid bilayer is not yet known. It is of sufficient size that it could traverse the bilayer several times [11,24]. Its resistance to proteolysis may indicate that it is largely within the bilayer and therefore inaccessible to the action of the enzymes. From amino acid analyses, it is evident that this peptide is not especially hydrophobic, the amount of hydrophobic residues being less than 40% (Ship S, personal communication). A structure consistent with these preliminary observations would be cylindrical or globular, with a maximum number of hydrophobic residues at the surface of the cylinder closely associated with the fatty acid chains of the phospholipids, and a maximum number of hydrophilic residues directed towards an aqueous central core as illustrated in Figure 5 [2,11,25]. Such a structure would provide an essentially aqueous channel through the bilayer through which anion transport might occur. Other alternatives are less attractive. It is highly unlikely, for example, that band 3 itself could transport anions by rotating through the bilayer. Such a process is energetically improbable because a large number of hydrophobic and hydrophilic interactions of the protein would have to be disturbed [26]. Furthermore, the whole protein and even the 17,000-dalton fragment retain a relatively fixed arrangement in the bilayer with certain sites accessible from the outside and others from the inside [1,2,11].

The postulated hydrophilic protein pathway cannot be an open diffusion channel because the membrane has a low conductance (high resistance) toward anion flow [27,28]. Thus at some point the channel must be blocked by a diffusion barrier (illustrated by the shaded zone in Fig. 5) across which the exchange mechanism might operate. This barrier

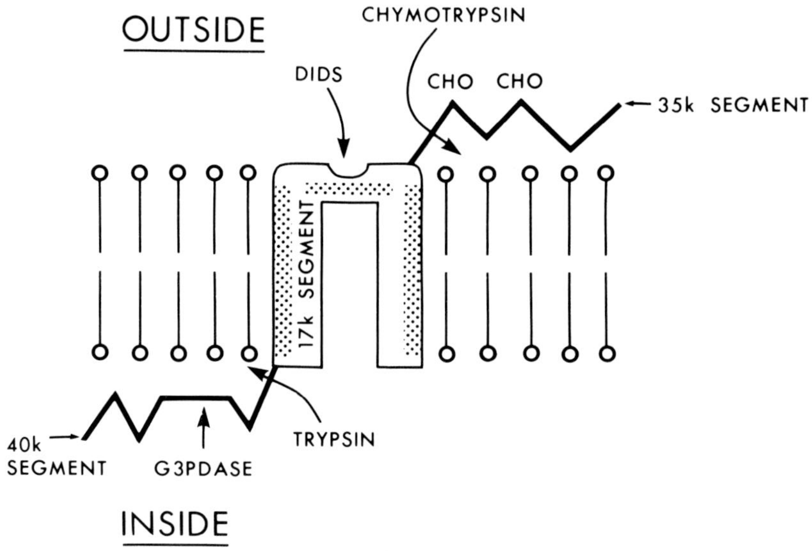

Fig 5. A suggested arrangement of band 3 in the bilayer. The shaded portions indicate predominantly hydrophobic zones.

is placed near the outside surface of the membrane because the exchange mechanism is inhibitable by nonpenetrating agents such as DIDS from the outside but not from the inside [29,30]. It is considered to be a barrier that has only a small thickness compared to the total width of the bilayer, so that the exchange mechanism would operate over short distances, thereby accounting for its rapid turnover capacity [3]. The barrier might be a local hydrophobic zone across which the anion might pass as a neutral complex with a positively charged site. In order to determine the details of the operation of the exchange system, however, it is necessary to understand the nature of the inhibitory sites that are revealed by the chemical probes, and to determine their arrangement with respect to the two sides of the membrane. This information can be obtained by analysis of the kinetics of inhibition of the probes.

INHIBITION KINETICS

It has been pointed out that two anion-binding sites have been identified, the transport and modifier sites [9]. Interactions at the two sites result in a competitive and noncompetitive inhibition, respectively. The covalent probes might inhibit by interacting with either of these sites, or with other as yet undefined sites.

The nature of an inhibitory effect can be determined by a kinetic analysis, but in the case of an irreversible inhibitor this poses problems because the system is not at equilibrium. Analysis is much easier with reversible inhibitors, but they cannot be used to "mark" the site during isolation of the transport proteins. This technical dilemma can be overcome in certain cases. For example, DIDS reacts covalently but the irreversible interaction is preceded by a rapid reversible binding apparently to the same site [12,15]. A reduced analog, H_2DIDS, binds to the same sites, resulting in equivalent inhibition, but in the cold its covalent reaction occurs much more slowly, so that its inhibitory effect as a function of Cl^- concentration can be assessed while it is largely (over 95%) bound reversibly [31]. The

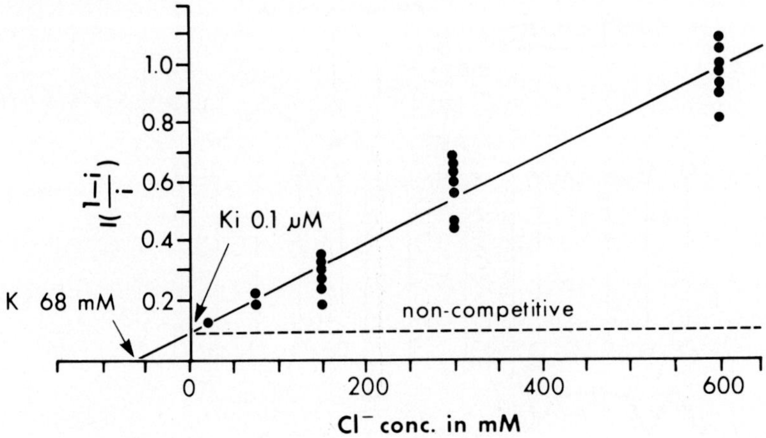

Fig 6. Kinetics of reversible inhibition of Cl^- exchange by H_2DIDS. The data are plotted according to Hunter and Downs, where I and S (Cl^-) are inhibitor and substrate concentrations and "i" is the fractional inhibition. The dotted horizontal line is the expected result for noncompetitive inhibition. The intercept on the x axis represents the dissociation constant of Cl^- for the sites of H_2DIDS-inhibition. The figure is from Shami, Rothstein, and Knauf [31].

usual reciprocal kinetic plot (Lineweaver and Burk) cannot be used to assess the data because such plots are nonlinear when two substrate binding sites of differing affinities are present [10]. The data can, however, be plotted with linear results on a Hunter-Downs plot (Fig. 6) of I(1 – i)/i versus S, where I and S are inhibitor and substrate concentrations respectively and i is the fractional inhibition [31]. In this plot noncompetitive inhibition is represented by a horizontal line. Thus, the significant upward slope indicates that the H_2DIDS and Cl^- compete. The apparent dissociation constant for H_2DIDS at the site is 0.1 μM (the intercept on the y axis) and that of Cl is 68 mM (the intercept on the x axis). The latter is close to 67 mM, the dissociation constant for Cl^- at the transport site [9], and is significantly different ($P < 0.001$) from the corresponding value for the modifier site (335 mM). Thus when DIDS is added externally, its binding site in the 17,000-dalton transmembrane fragment of band 3 [21] is presumably the anion transport site. As pointed out previously, DIDS [29] and other disulfonic stilbene analogs [30] have no inhibitory effects from the inside, so that there is a distinct asymmetry in accessibility or reactivity from the two sides.

Another probe whose inhibitory action is amenable to kinetic analysis is NAP-taurine. In the dark it is a substrate for transport and a reversible inhibitor [10,25,32]. After exposure to light its azido group becomes a highly reactive nitrene that can react covalently with the transport protein. It behaves as a photoaffinity probe so that its irreversible binding sites after exposure to light are the same as the reversible binding sites in the dark [33]. Thus it is possible to characterize the sites by kinetic analysis in the dark and to identify them by covalent labelling after exposure to light.

In the cold, NAP-taurine is virtually nonpenetrating [25,32,34] so that its behavior at the two sides of the membrane can be compared. From the outside, NAP-taurine behaves as a noncompetitive inhibitor if the chloride concentration is relatively low [10]. Thus in Figure 7, plotted according to Hanes (S/flux versus S), the slopes of the lines increase substantially with increasing inhibitor concentration, whereas for competitive in-

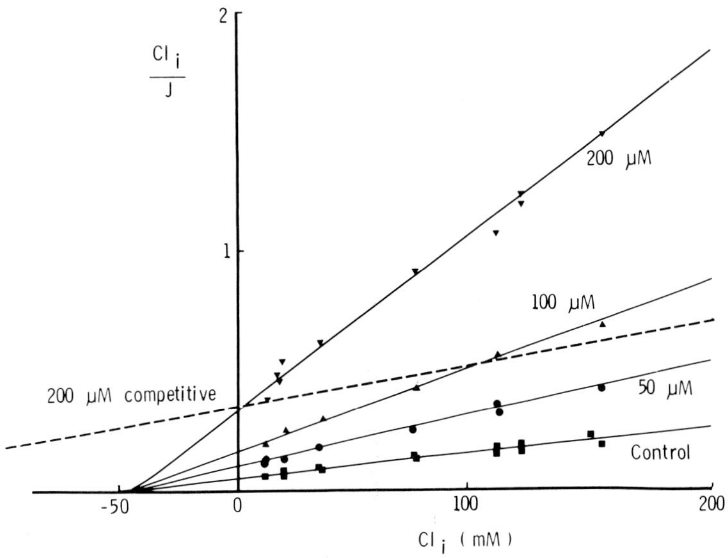

Fig 7. Inhibitions of Cl^- exchange by NAP-taurine applied to outside in the dark. The data are plotted according to Hanes, where S (Cl^-) is the substrate concentration and J is the flux. For competitive inhibition a series of almost parallel lines would be expected. The dotted line illustrates the expectation for competitive inhibition by 200 μM NAP-taurine. The figure is from Knauf et al [10].

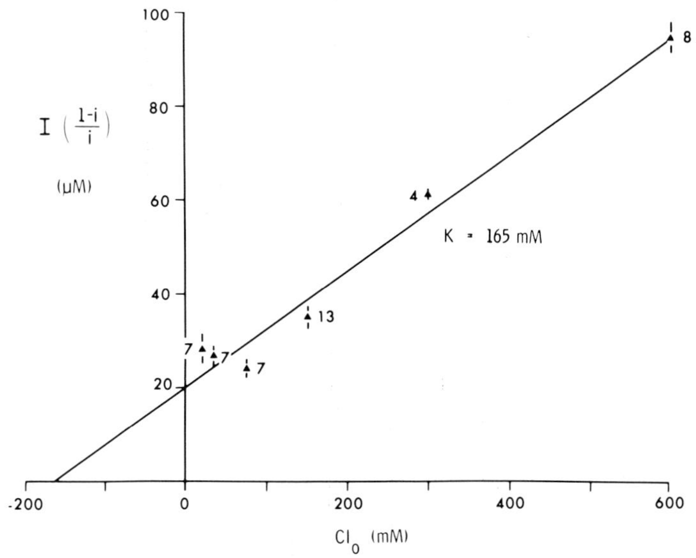

Fig 8. The kinetics of NAP-taurine inhibition when it is applied to the external face of the membrane. The data are plotted according to Hunter and Downs (see legend of Fig 6). The intercept on the x axis represents the dissociation constant for Cl^- at the sites of NAP-taurine inhibition. The figure is from Knauf et al [10].

hibition they should be virtually parallel. On the Hunter-Downs plot, however, it is evident that relatively high concentrations of Cl^- do cause reversal of the inhibition by NAP-taurine applied to the external surface of the membrane. As indicated by the x intercept, the apparent affinity of the inhibitory sites for Cl^- is low, about 165 mM (Fig. 8). This value is significantly higher ($P < 0.001$) than the reported dissociation constant of Cl^- for the transport site. It is also somewhat lower than the reported dissociation constant of Cl^- at the modifier site, 335 mM, but this value is only approximate [2,9]. It therefore seems possible that external NAP-taurine acts at the modifier site. Support for this conclusion is found in Figure 1, where the lines calculated on the basis of this assumption show excellent agreement with the experimental data [10].

The Ki of NAP-taurine from the outside is about 20 μM. This value is considerably lower than the reported Ks (2 mM) for NAP-taurine transport from inside to outside [10], suggesting a considerable asymmetry in the interactions of the probe at the two sides of the membrane. A direct assessment of the inhibition kinetics with NAP-taurine on the inside confirms this observation. The Hunter and Downs plot (Fig. 9) illustrates the marked difference in inside versus outside behaviour. On the inside Cl^- is competitive with NAP-taurine at a site whose affinity for the halide is not significantly different from the reported affinity of the transport site (but is significantly ($P < 0.001$) higher than its affinity for the modifier site). Furthermore, the apparent dissociation constant of NAP-taurine as an inhibitor (Ki) is about the same as that for its transport (Ks), about 1.8 mM (at 137 mM Cl^-). These observations are consistent with the conclusion that at the inside, NAP-taurine interacts with the substrate site [10].

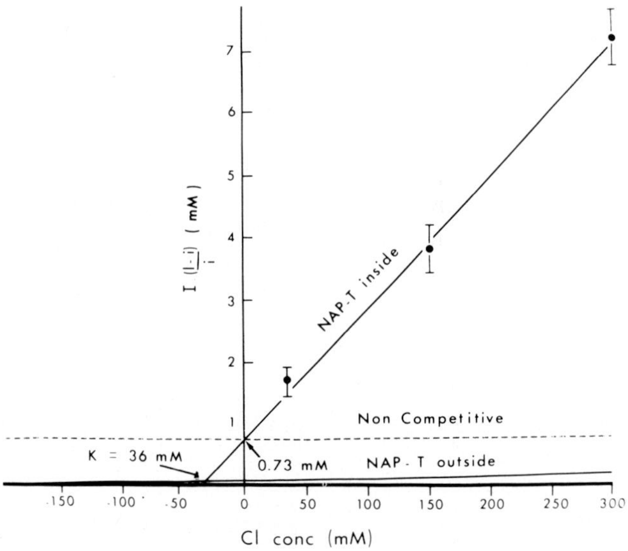

Fig 9. The kinetics of NAP-taurine inhibition when it is applied to the cytoplasmic face of the membrane. The data are plotted according to Hunter and Downs (see legend of Fig 6). The intercept on the x axis represents the dissociation constant for Cl^- at the sites of NAP-taurine inhibition. The dotted horizontal line represents the expected result for a noncompetitive inhibition. In order to illustrate the asymmetry of the membrane with respect to NAP-taurine, the data for the inhibition with the probe applied to the external face (from Fig 8) are also presented (the line near the x axis). The figure is taken from Knauf et al [10].

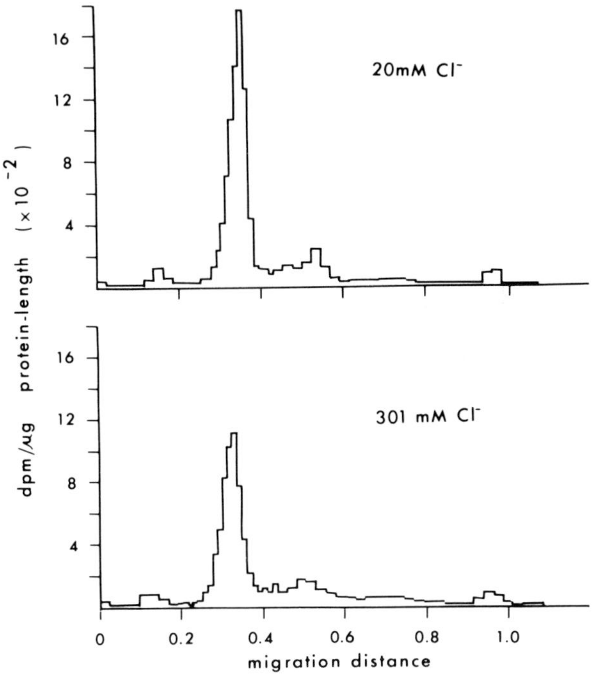

Fig 10. The effect of high chloride on the covalent binding of NAP-taurine to membrane proteins. The proteins were separated by SDS-acrylamide gel electrophoresis. The peak with the largest amount of NAP-taurine is band 3. The figure is from Knauf et al [33].

The asymmetry in the behaviour of NAP-taurine can be readily explained by assuming that the modifier site is accessible only from the outside, but that the transport site is accessible from either side. From the inside, the only site accessible to NAP-taurine would be the transport site. From the outside, both the transport and modifier sites would be accessible, but because the latter has a considerably higher affinity for the probe this interaction would be the predominant factor in the inhibitory effect. The above explanation is also consistent with the finding that addition of NAP-taurine to the outside solution inhibits its own efflux [10]. Its high affinity reaction with the modifier site at the outside surface is the dominant factor controlling the rate of transport.

The covalent binding of external NAP-taurine after exposure to light is illustrated in Figure 10. The largest part of the NAP-taurine is found in band 3. The effect of high Cl^- in reversing the inhibitory effects of NAP-taurine in the dark (as in the data of Fig. 7), is also reflected in the reduction in covalent binding to band 3 [33]. These data are consistent with the proposed location of the modifier site in band 3.

TRANSMEMBRANE EFFECTS OF PROBES

On kinetic grounds reviewed above it appears that DIDS from the outside [31] and NAP-taurine from the inside [10] both interact with sites possessing an affinity for Cl^- that is nearly the same as that of the transport site. A possible explanation is that the transport site is mobile, so that it can move spontaneously from inside to outside facing and vice versa, and thus could be accessible to the probes from opposite sides of the mem-

TABLE II. The Transmembrane Effects of DIDS Binding to the External Face of the Membrane on NAP-Taurine Binding to the Cytoplasmic Face

Irradiation time (min)	Sites per cell × 10^5		
	Control	DIDS-treated	Difference
1	3.16	0.81	2.35
5	7.87	3.13	4.74
1	2.07	0.58	1.49
3	4.50	1.57	2.93
5	7.29	1.77	5.52

Data are from Grinstein, McCulloch, and Rothstein [29].

brane. Two simple forms of a mobile transport system can be postulated [2,11]. In one, the system has two anion-binding sites, one facing in and the other out. When both are loaded, the system can rotate so that the loaded sites exchange positions. Such a system would involve a simultaneous transfer. In the second, a single anion-binding site would oscillate between inside and outside facing but could move only when loaded with an anion. Such a system would result in a one-for-one exchange as in the mobile carrier model of Figure 2, and would be classified as a sequential exchange. The simultaneous exchange model would involve the formation of a ternary complex, yet the curves of flux versus Cl^- concentration do not show the expected sigmoid characteristics [2]. Thus the kinetic information is more consistent with the sequential model.

The sequential exchange model has been directly tested by transmembrane experiments using DIDS on the outside and NAP-taurine on the inside [29]. If both probes react with the same mobile sites but at opposite sides of the membrane, then the covalent reaction of DIDS at the outside should "recruit" and bind all of the sites in the outside facing position, and they should not then be available for subsequent reaction with NAP-taurine from the inside.

The experiments require that the probes be applied on, and that they act on, opposite sides of the membrane. DIDS meets this requirement, since it is incapable of inhibiting from the inside. Furthermore, when applied to the outside of cells it is essentially non-penetrating during the relatively short time required for its covalent reaction [29]. Inside-out vesicles were prepared from the DIDS-treated cells. These were reacted for short times in the light with NAP-taurine, and the binding to band 3 was measured under conditions of minimal penetration. Pretreatment with DIDS on the outside substantially reduced the binding of NAP-taurine to band 3 from the inside in comparison to vesicles from control cells (no DIDS) (Table II). In quantitative terms, the number of band 3 monomers, the number of DIDS binding sites, and the number of DIDS-sequestered transmembrane NAP-taurine binding sites are about the same, 10^6 per cell. Thus each molecule of DIDS bound to a molecule of band 3 from the outside prevents the binding of a molecule of NAP-taurine to band 3 from the inside. This finding is entirely consistent with the sequential model, in which the anion transport site alternately faces the inside and outside of the membrane.

A MODEL OF THE ANION TRANSPORT SYSTEM

A model that is consistent with the transport and inhibition kinetics, with the sidedness (asymmetry) of the system, and with the involvement of band 3 as the anion transport protein is illustrated in Figure 11. It combines the features of the protein channel as

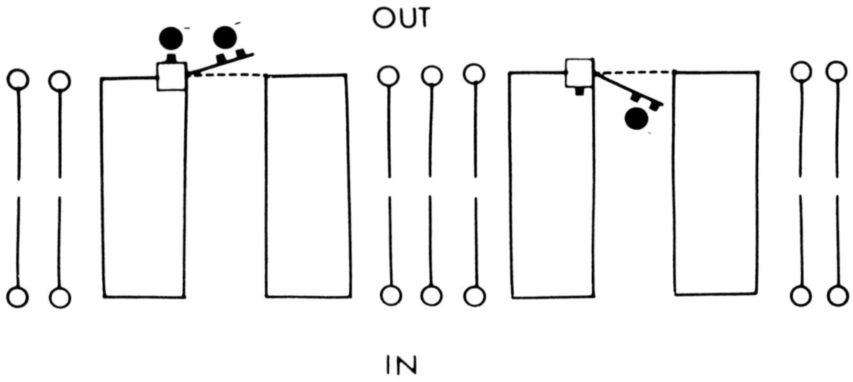

Fig 11. A conformational model for anion transport. The figure is from Rothstein et al [11].

presented in Figure 5 and the mobile carrier as presented in Figure 2 [2,11,25]. The transport site is represented as a gate that can, when loaded with an anion, spontaneously move from outside to inside facing or vice versa, across the diffusion barrier (the dotted line). The distance traversed would be small, thus accommodating the observed high rate of turnover. As discussed previously, the gate and barrier are located near the outside of the protein channel accessible to DIDS from the outside but not from the inside. The modifier site is only accessible from the outside. When it is occupied by an anion, the translocation of the transport site (the gate) is inhibited (or substantially reduced in rate). The transport site and modifier site are placed closely adjacent to each other because externally applied NAP-taurine, which binds to the modifier, prevents binding of DIDS to the transport site, and reciprocally DIDS reacted with the transport site prevents the binding of NAP-taurine to the modifier site [25,32]. It has been proposed that this mutual interference is due to steric hindrance between large organic anions bound to closely adjacent sites.

An additional complication must be accommodated in the model. The interaction of the modifier site with external NAP-taurine can be affected by changes in the Cl^- ratio across the membrane [10,25]. This effect can be interpreted as follows: The Cl^- ratio should determine the distribution of sites (gates) between inside and outside facing positions [2,5]. When the Cl^- ratio favours the positioning of the gates in the inward-facing direction, the binding of NAP-taurine to the modifier sites is reduced, perhaps through an allosteric or positional relationship between the two sites. The effect is shown in Figure 11 by an inversion of the modifier site when the gate is in the inward position. It is also possible that the membrane potential (which is determined by the Cl^- ratio in red blood cells) directly influences the accessibility of the modifier site.

The model of Figure 11 has been discussed in terms of a protein channel (pore) combined with a mobile carrier element operating at its external opening. An interpretation that is consistent with protein structure would involve a local conformational change, which results in a shift in the transport site from inside to outside facing and vice versa. The shift from one conformation to the other would be spontaneous, but could only occur if the positive charge on the transport site were neutralized by the binding of an anion. The modifier site might be adjacent to the transport site so that they influence each other. Such a conformational model would fit all of the mobile carrier-type transport and inhibition kinetics that have been reported. This type of model might also be appropriate for other carrier-mediated transport systems in which transmembrane protein structures are involved.

ACKNOWLEDGMENTS

This work has been supported by Medical Research Council (Canada) grants #MT4665 and MA5149. Dr S. Grinstein is a recipient of a Medical Research Council Postdoctoral Fellowship.

REFERENCES

1. Steck TL: This volume.
2. Cabantchik ZI, Knauf PA, Rothstein A: Biochim Biophys Acta, Biomembranes Rev 515:239, 1978.
3. Brahm J: J Gen Physiol 70:283, 1977.
4. Gunn RB, Dalmark M, Tosteson DC, Wieth JO: J Gen Physiol 61:185, 1973.
5. Dalmark M: Prog Biophys Molec Biol 31:145, 1976.
6. Deuticke B: Rev Physiol Biochem Pharmacol 78:1, 1977.
7. Sachs JR, Knauf PA, Dunham PB: In Surgenor DM (ed): "The Red Blood Cell." 2nd Ed. New York: Academic, 613, 1975.
8. Passow H: Prog Biophys Molec Biol 19:425, 1969.
9. Dalmark M: J Gen Physiol 67:223, 1976.
10. Knauf PA, Ship S, Breuer W, McCulloch L, Rothstein A: J Gen Physiol 72:607, 1978.
11. Rothstein A, Grinstein S, Ship S, Knauf PA: Trends in Biochem Sci 3:126, 1978.
12. Ship S, Shami Y, Breuer W, Rothstein A: J Membrane Biol 33:311, 1977.
13. Cabantchik ZI, Rothstein A: J Membrane Biol 15:227, 1974.
14. Passow H, Fasold H, Lepke S, Pring M, Schuhmann B: In Miller M, Shamoo AE (eds): "Membrane Toxicity." New York: Plenum (In press).
15. Lepke S, Fasold H, Pring M, Passow H: J Membrane Biol 29:147, 1976.
16. Shami Y, Carver J, Ship S, Rothstein, A: Biochem Biophys Res Commun 76:429, 1977.
17. Rothstein A, Cabantchik ZI, Balshin M, Juliano R: Biochem Biophys Res Commun 64:144, 1975.
18. Ross AH, McConnell HM: Biochem Biophys Res Commun 74:1318, 1977.
19. Feinstein MB, Volpi M, Perrie S, Makriyannis A, Sha'afi RI: Molec Pharmacol 13:840, 1977.
20. Wolosin JM, Ginsburg H, Cabantchik ZI: J Biol Chem 252:2419, 1977.
21. Grinstein S, Ship S, Rothstein A: Biochim Biophys Acta 507:294, 1978.
22. Lepke S, Passow H: Biochim Biophys Acta 455:353, 1976.
23. Steck TL, Ramos B, Strapazon E: Biochemistry 15:1154, 1976.
24. Drickamer LK: J Biol Chem 252:6909, 1977.
25. Rothstein A, Cabantchik ZI, Knauf P: Fed Proc 35:3, 1976.
26. Singer SJ: J Supramol Struct 6:313, 1977.
27. Hunter MJ: J. Physiol 268:35, 1977.
28. Knauf PA, Fuhrmann GF, Rothstein S, Rothstein A: J Gen Physiol 69:363, 1977.
29. Grinstein S, McCulloch L, Rothstein A: J Gen Physiol (Manuscript submitted, 1978).
30. Zaki L, Fasold H, Schuhmann B, Passow H: J Cell Physiol 86:471, 1975.
31. Shami Y, Rothstein A, Knauf PA: Biochim Biophys Acta 508:357, 1978.
32. Cabantchik ZI, Knauf P, Ostwald T, Markus H, Davidson L, Breuer W, Rothstein A: Biochim Biophys Acta 455:526, 1976.
33. Knauf PA, Breuer W, McCulloch L, Rothstein A: J Gen Physiol 72:631, 1978.
34. Staros JV, Richards FM, Haley BE: J Biol Chem 250:8174, 1975.

Normal and Abnormal Red Cell Membranes 497–502 (1979)

Invasion of Erythrocytes by Malaria Merozoites

Louis H. Miller, Florence M. McAuliffe, and James G. Johnson

Laboratory of Parasitic Diseases, National Institute of Allergy and Infectious Diseases, National Institutes of Health, Bethesda, Maryland 20014

A malaria infection is initiated when an infected Anopheles mosquito injects sporozoites into the blood stream. The sporozoites localize within parenchymal cells of the liver, where they divide into thousands of individual parasites. After one to two weeks these parasites rupture out of the liver cells and invade erythrocytes. Inside erythrocytes, the parasites undergo asexual development, producing 6 to 24 individual merozoites. Each merozoite, on release from the erythrocyte at the time of lysis, is capable of invading another erythrocyte. This cyclic development within erythrocytes is responsible for the clinical manifestations associated with malaria. While the majority of merozoites perpetuate the infection, a few develop into sexual forms, gametocytes, which are ingested by mosquitoes during a blood meal and will eventually develop into sporozoites that can infect other people. In those who survive the infection, immunity limits asexual growth and eventually eliminates the infection.

Here we will focus on one segment of this complicated cycle, the infection of erythrocytes by merozoites. We will attempt to explain how a merozoite of limited motility can enter a nonphagocytic cell, the erythrocyte. Dvorak et al have described the sequence of invasion in detail [1]. The merozoite attaches to the erythrocyte and reorients so that the apical region of the merozoite is in opposition to the erythrocyte. The attachment between the apical region of the merozoite and the erythrocyte results in rapid and marked deformation of the erythrocyte for 10 sec. The erythrocyte then returns to its normal shape, and over the next 20 sec the merozoite slowly enters within an invagination of the erythrocyte membrane. The orifice of the invagination seals to produce a vacuole containing the merozoite within the erythrocyte. The characteristics of this event can be summarized as follows:

1. Specific attachment of merozoites to erythrocytes. Receptors on the merozoite attach to receptors for the parasite on the erythrocyte membrane.

2. Recognition and attachment initiates a sequence of events (the invasion sequence) that brings the merozoite within a vacuole formed from the invagination of the erythrocyte membrane.

Received for publication March 8, 1978.

ERYTHROCYTE SPECIFICITY AND RECEPTORS

The preferential infection of a subpopulation of erythrocytes in one host was the first evidence that erythrocytes determined specificity in malarial infections. A parasite such as Plasmodium vivax is exposed to all erythrocytes in the circulation, but preferentially infects reticulocytes. Although this preference is presumed to relate to surface determinants on the reticulocyte, the basis for reticulocyte preference is yet to be defined.

Experimental evidence that host specificity is determined, in some cases, by the outer surface of the erythrocyte membrane was first presented by McGhee [2]. The relative erythrocyte susceptibility of different species was studied in chick embryos. He found that merozoites of Plasmodium lophurae, an avian malaria that infects both chick embryo and duck erythrocytes, had a much higher affinity for duck erythrocytes. Recently, it was demonstrated that in vivo infectivity of P knowlesi for various host species was related to the penetration of erythrocytes of these species in vitro [3, 4]. The erythrocytes of resistant species (eg, rodents and birds) were not invaded in vitro.

Treatment of human erythrocytes with proteolytic enzymes (chymotrypsin and pronase) blocked invasion by Plasmodium knowlesi merozoites [4]. The fact that these enzymes only affect the cell surface supported the hypothesis that invasion is initiated by specific receptors and that these receptors are probably proteins or glycoproteins. On direct observation, P knowlesi merozoites did not attach to or interact in any way with chymotrypsin-treated human erythrocytes or erythrocytes from subprimates. It seemed evident that determinants on the erythrocyte surface were responsible for recognition and initiated a sequence of events that resulted in parasite invasion.

Since malaria merozoites recognize specific receptors on the erythrocyte surface, it seemed possible that the receptor could be related to a blood group determinant. Therefore, erythrocytes that lacked certain determinants were tested for susceptibility to invasion by P knowlesi [5]. It was found that Duffy blood group-negative erythrocytes are refractory to invasion. The Duffy blood group system has two principal determinants Fy^a (detected by anti-Fy^a) and Fy^b (detected by anti-Fy^b) whose presence on the erythrocytes is determined by the condominant alleles Fy^a and Fy^b. Cells which do not react with either anti-Fy^a or anti-Fy^b are homozygous for a third allele, *Fy*, and are called Duffy-negative. Another antiserum, anti-Fy3, reacts with all cells carrying Fy^a or Fy^b determinants but not with Duffy-negative erythrocytes [Fy(a–b–)]. As stated above, Duffy-negative cells are resistant to invasion by P knowlesi. The majority of black Africans have this phenotype; it is extremely rare in populations without black admixture [6]. Erythrocytes from blacks with either Fy^a or Fy^b determinants were fully susceptible, although many were undoubtedly heterozygous for the Duffy-negative gene. Absence of other blood group determinants did not influence susceptibility. Thus, for untreated human erythrocytes, there is an absolute correlation between the presence of Fy^a and Fy^b determinants and susceptibility to invasion.

We can assume, therefore, that resistance to invasion is based on the absence of a Duffy-associated determinant. Proteolytic enzymes that remove Duffy determinants (eg, chymotrypsin) reduced invasion of those cells [5]. Conversely, trypsin or neuraminidase treatment does not remove Duffy determinants and does not reduce invasion. Furthermore, coating of Fy(a+b–) erythrocytes with anti-Fy^a markedly reduced invasion [5]. We were not able to block invasion of Fy(a–b+) erythrocytes with anti-Fy^b, probably because of the low affinity of the antibody.

In some situations, however, invasion occurs in the absence of Fy^a or Fy^b determinants [7]. Duffy-negative cells that have been treated with trypsin or neuraminidase are invaded, although the cells still lack the Fy^a and Fy^b determinants [7]. It is impossible at this time to explain the conflicting data on the requirement for Fy^a and Fy^b determinants for invasion, since the chemistry of the Duffy determinants and associated structures are unknown. It may be that a structure associated with the Duffy determinant but not Fy^a or Fy^b itself may be the requirement.

What role the Duffy-associated structures play in the invasion sequence is also unclear. Observation of the interaction between Duffy-negative erythrocytes and P knowlesi merozoites demonstrated that merozoites do induce widespread deformation of these erythrocytes but fail to enter within a localized invagination of the erythrocyte. The initial interaction is specific, however, since P knowlesi merozoites do not interact with erythrocytes from prosimii or subprimates. Two hypotheses could explain these observations. First, there may be two receptors for invasion with the Duffy-associated antigen involved in the second stage of invasion—interiorization within the erythrocyte. Alternatively, the Duffy-negative determinant may have a lower affinity receptor for the merozoite. This would allow recognition but not hold the merozoite in place for invasion.

As stated earlier, the Duffy-negative phenotype, the resistance factor to invasion by P knowlesi, is characteristic of blacks. Furthermore, many blacks are resistant to erythrocytic infection by P vivax [8]. These data suggested that the basis for resistance of blacks to P vivax is the Duffy-negative phenotype. Three studies have supported this hypothesis. First, the Duffy blood group phenotype was determined in 11 blacks who had previously been exposed to P vivax-infected mosquitoes [9]. The six Duffy-positive blacks developed erythrocytic infection; the five Duffy-negative blacks were resistant. Second, Spencer et al [10] determined the relationship between the Duffy blood group phenotype and malarial infections in a village in Honduras in which 247 of 420 persons were Duffy-negative. P falciparum occurred in equal frequency in Duffy-positive and Duffy-negative individuals [10]. In contrast, all 14 slide-demonstrated P vivax infections occurred in Duffy-positive persons. Third, the blood group phenotype was determined on 13 blacks who had been infected with P vivax in Vietnam [11]. All were Duffy-positive. Therefore in the limited studies to date susceptibility to P vivax is always associated with Duffy positivity and resistance to Duffy negativity.

Black Africans are susceptible to P falciparum. Since resistance to P vivax is based on the Duffy-negative genotype, then the surface requirements for invasion by P falciparum differ from those for P vivax. Therefore, it was not surprising that Duffy-negative erythrocytes have normal susceptibility to P falciparum [12]. Other erythrocytes that lack blood group determinants were all infected by P falciparum.

Erythrocytes treated with various enzymes had differential susceptibility to P falciparum and P knowlesi [12]. Chymotrypsin markedly reduced susceptibility to P knowlesi; trypsin or neuraminidase reduced susceptibility to P falciparum. This differential effect suggests that each parasite uses a different protein or glycoprotein on the erythrocyte surface as receptor.

The chemical basis for recognition between parasite and host cell has not been defined for any malaria. From the evidence to date it appears that one system is involved in initial attachment and another for apical orientation and entry.

MECHANISM OF INTERIORIZATION

In 1969 Ladda, Aikawa, and Sprinz [13] reported on the invasion of erythrocytes by merozoites of Plasmodium berghei and P gallinaceum and established that merozoites enter within an invagination of the erythrocyte membrane rather than by penetrating it [13]. Recently it was observed that a junction forms between the apical region of the merozoite and the erythrocyte. The erythrocyte membrane to which the merozoite is attached becomes thickened [14]. As invasion progresses, the depression in the erythrocyte deepens and conforms to the curvature of the merozoite. At this time the thickened, electron-dense zone on the erythrocyte membrane is no longer observed at the point of initial attachment but now appears at the orifice of the merozoite-induced invagination (Fig. 1). When entry is completed (ie, the merozoite is within the erythrocyte), the junction appears to fuse at the posterior end of the merozoite, closing the orifice (see Fig. 2 for diagramatic representation of the moving junction).

The extracellular merozoite is surrounded by a surface coat that is susceptible to proteolytic enzymes [15]. During invasion, no surface coat is visible on the portion of the merozoite within the erythrocyte invagination, whereas the surface coat on the portion of the merozoite remaining outside the erythrocyte appears to be similar to that seen on free merozoites [13, 14, 16].

Throughout invasion, the apical end remains in contact with the erythrocyte [1, 13, 14, 16]. Material from rhoptries (paired organelles in the apical portion of the merozoite) appears to empty through a common duct onto the erythrocyte membrane [14]. It is likely that the contents of the rhoptries are important for junction movement and interiorization, but the chemical nature and physiologic function are unknown. Kilejian sug-

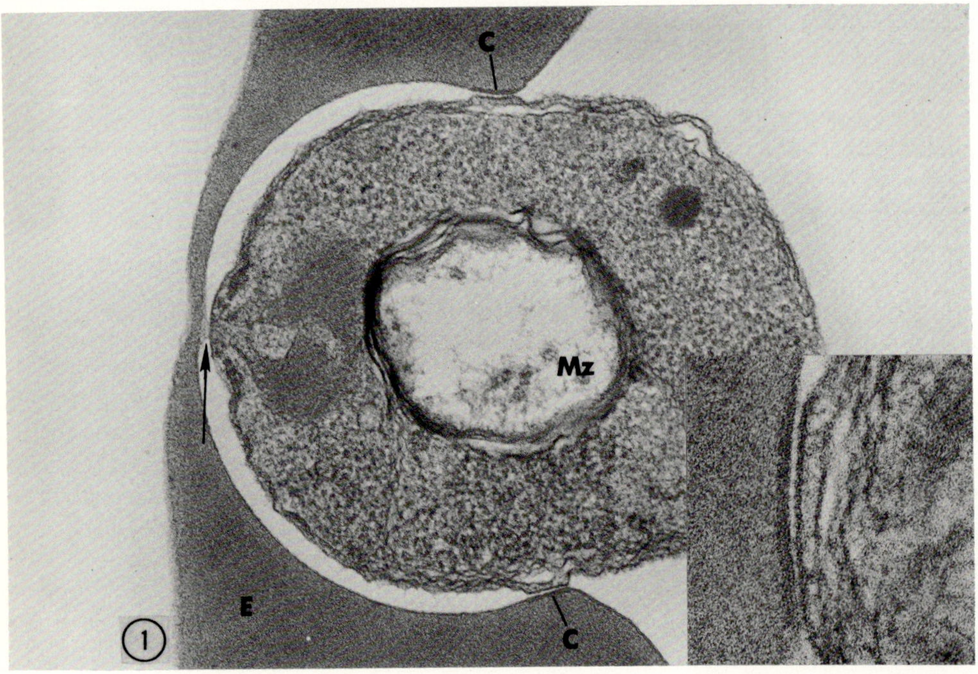

Fig 1. Advanced stage of erythrocyte (E) entry by a merozoite (Mz). The junction (C) is formed between the thickened membrane of the erythrocyte and merozoite plasmalemma. The invagination deepens and conforms to the curvature of the merozoite. An electron-opaque projection connects the apical end and the erythrocyte membrane (arrow) (50.00 ×). Inset: Higher-magnification micrograph of the junction showing the thickened erythrocyte membrane and fine fibrils between the two parallel membranes 144.00 ×. Figures 1 and 2 reproduced from Aikawa M, Miller LH, Johnson J, Rabbege J: J Cell Biol, April, 1978, with permission.

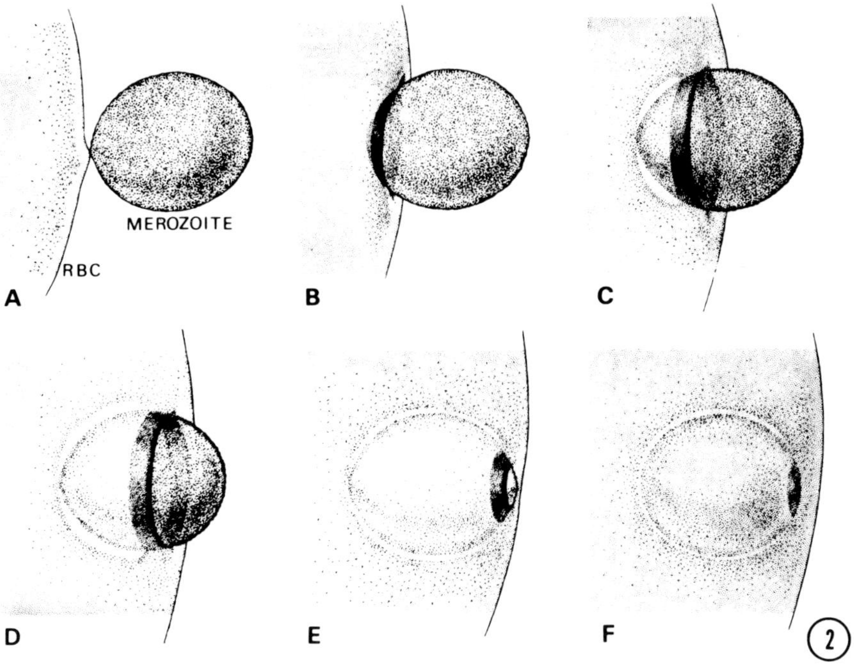

Fig 2. Diagram of a moving circumferential junction between merozoite and erythrocyte. The moving junction brings the merozoite within an invagination of the erythrocyte membrane.

gested that the rhoptries and micronemes contain a histidine-rich protein which invaginates the erythrocyte membrane [17]. Bannister, Butcher, and Mitchell suggested the interesting possibility that membranes are formed from the material within rhoptries [18]. The isolation and characterization of this material is of obvious importance.

Our interest in the invasion process was stimulated by the hope that we might learn novel ways to block invasion. Of equal importance is the possibility that information derived from these studies may suggest new ideas in the field of membrane biology.

REFERENCES

1. Dvorak JA, Miller LH, Whitehouse WC, Shiroishi T:Science 187:748, 1975.
2. McGhee RB: J Exp Med 97:773, 1953.
3. Butcher GA, Mitchell GH, Cohen S: Nature (London) 244:40, 1973.
4. Miller LH, Dvorak JA, Shiroishi T, Durocher JR: J Exp Med 138:1597, 1973.
5. Miller LH, Mason SJ, Dvorak JA, McGinniss MH, Rothman KI: Science 189:561, 1975.
6. Mourant AE, Kopec AC, Domaniewska-Solczak K: "The Distribution of the Human Blood Groups and Other Polymorphisms." 2nd Ed. London: Oxford University Press, 1976.
7. Mason SJ, Miller LH, Shiroishi T, Dvorak JA, McGinniss MH: Br J Haematol 36:327, 1977.
8. Young MD, Eyles DE, Burgess RW, Jeffery GM: J Parasitol 41:315, 1955.
9. Miller LH, Mason SJ, Clyde DF, McGinniss MH: New Engl J Med 295:302, 1976.
10. Spencer HC, Miller LH, Collins WE, Knud-Hansen C, McGinniss MH, Shiroishi T, Lobos RA, Feldman RA: Am J Trop Med Hyg 27:664, 1978.
11. Miller LH, McGinniss MH, Holland P, Sigmond P: Am J Trop Med Hyg 27:1069, 1978.
12. Miller LH, Haynes SD, McAuliffe FM, Shiroishi T, Durocher JR, McGinniss M: J Exp Med 146:277, 1977.

13. Ladda RL, Aikawa M, Sprinz H: J Parasitol 55:633, 1969.
14. Aikawa M, Miller LH, Johnson J, Rabbege J: J Cell Biol (In press).
15. Miller LH, Aikawa M, Dvorak JA: J Immunol 114:1237, 1975.
16. Bannister LH, Butcher GA, Dennis ED, Mitchell GH: Parasitology 71:483, 1975.
17. Kilejian A: Studies on a histidine-rich protein from Plasmodium Cophurae. In Van den Bossche H (ed): "Biochemistry of Parasites and Host-Parasite Relationships." Amsterdam: Elsevier, 1976. pp 441-448.
18. Bannister LH, Butcher GA, Mitchell GH: Bull WHO 55: 161, 1977.

Normal and Abnormal Red Cell Membranes 503–513 (1979)

Erythrocyte Disorders Leading to Potassium Loss and Cellular Dehydration

Bertil E. Glader and Drew W. Sullivan

Department of Pediatrics, Stanford University School of Medicine, Stanford, California 94305

RBC K loss and cellular dehydration are associated with a variety of normal and abnormal erythrocyte conditions. In some cases (normal RBC aging, pyruvate-kinase-deficient RBCs and irreversibly sickled cells) cation and water changes are related to adenosine triphosphate (ATP) depletion and to increased RBC calcium content. In other disorders, such as hereditary xerocytosis, cation depletion and cellular hydration are not related to altered energy or calcium metabolism. Rather, this condition is thought to be due to a structural membrane defect which is manifested by imbalanced cation leaks (K loss > Na gain) for which the active cation transport is unable to compensate. None of the disorders described here are associated with known structural membrane alterations.

The fact that K loss and cellular dehydration are common to several RBC disorders suggests that this phenomenon may have a direct role in membrane injury. This hypothesis is supported by two separate observations: 1) Formation of irreversible sickled cells in vitro is prevented if K and water loss are inhibited, and these effects are independent of ATP depletion and calcium accumulation; 2) the mean critical hemolytic volume is markedly reduced in K- and water-depleted normal RBCs. RBC dehydration *without* intracellular cation depletion, however, is not associated with changes in mean critical hemolytic volume. These data thus indicate that K loss may have a direct role in RBC membrane injury. The mechanism by which this occurs and the associated alterations in membrane structure, however, remain to be identified.

Key words: **erythrocyte dehydration, erythrocyte cation transport, erythrocyte membrane physiology**

Membrane dysfunction is thought to be the common denominator of red blood cell (RBC) injury in most hemolytic anemias. Unfortunately, however, there is a paucity of information relating pathophysiology with specific alterations in membrane organization. This review describes those erythrocyte conditions characterized by potassium loss, total monovalent cation depletion, and cellular dehydration. With the methodology currently

Received for publication May 31, 1978; accepted May 31, 1978.

available to membrane biologists, some of these physiologic changes should be amenable to membrane structural analysis.

REGULATION OF RBC CATION TRANSPORT AND CELLULAR HYDRATION

Water freely crosses the RBC membrane in response to alterations in osmotic gradient, and these water movements lead to changes in RBC volume. Intracellular oncotic pressure is regulated by the concentration of relatively impermeable solutes: polyvalent anions and monovalent cations. The following discussion relates only to the role of monovalent cations. It should be noted, however, that *net* cation changes are associated with monovalent anion movements as a requisite for maintaining electrical neutrality. With this restriction in mind, it can be generalized that net increases in total RBC cation content cause water to enter cells forming "hydrocytes," while depletion of RBC cations is associated with cell dehydration and the formation of "xerocytes."

Red blood cell permeability to cations is much less than that observed for anions. Chloride equilibrates across the membrane within milliseconds, while Na and K require hours [1,2]. Passive cation permeability is thought to occur through positively charged "pores" presumably formed by lipid-protein interactions. Normally, the passive rate of Na influx (1.0-2.0 mEq/liter RBC/h) is slightly greater than K efflux (0.8-1.5 mEq/liter RBC/h) [3]. These passive leaks, although small, ultimately lead to osmotic lysis if Na and K are allowed to reach chemical equilibrium. Under both in vivo and in vitro conditions, however, there usually are no major alterations in cation composition. This steady state exists because passive cation leaks normally are balanced by an equivalent active transport system for both Na and K (Fig 1). The "pump" transports K into cells and simultaneously extrudes Na, both processes occurring against a concentration gradient. Ouabain is a specific inhibitor of the membrane adenosine triphosphatase (ATPase) responsible for active Na and K transport [4]. The spatial configuration of this transport enzyme is such that it is activated by both intracellular Na (K_m = 25 mM) and extracellular K (K_m = 2.5 mM) [5]. As a consequence of this asymmetrical difference in enzyme activation, and since the extracellular K concentration is relatively constant, Na-K transport generally is stimulated by increases in cell Na content. As a corollary of this, cell K losses are rectified only if there is concomitant Na gain to stimulate active transport. Conditions characterized by K loss greater than Na gain thus generally lead to irreversible total monovalent cation depletion and dehydration. Na-K cotransport is an additional mechanism by which Na and K traverse the cell membrane, although the physiologic significance of this process is not known [6]. On the basis of current information, it is unlikely that cation cotransport con-

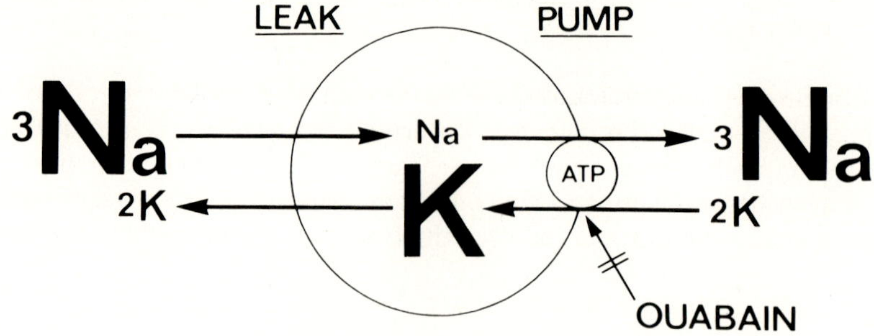

Fig 1. RBC cation transport.

tributes significantly to net cation and water movements. Until there is evidence to the contrary, it is reasonable to assume that maintenance of normal RBC hydration (ie, that aspect influenced by monovalent cation content) depends primarily on the balance between passive cation "leaks" and active Na-K transport (Fig 2). RBC dehydration generally is a consequence of K loss in excess of Na gain. This can occur secondary to metabolic or erythrocyte membrane abnormalities.

K LOSS AND DEHYDRATION ASSOCIATED WITH ALTERED ERYTHROCYTE METABOLISM

Adenosine triphosphate (ATP) provides energy for active monovalent cation transport (Na-K-activated ATPase) and active calcium transport (calcium-activated ATPase). The relative importance of these transport systems is seen when ATP-depleted RBCs are incubated in vitro (Table I). In the absence of calcium (with ethylenediamine tetraacetic acid (EDTA) in the medium), ATP-depleted cells manifest Na gain in excess of K loss, increased RBC water content, and cell swelling. These are the characteristic changes of Na-K pump failure. In the presence of physiologic concentrations of calcium, however, ATP-depleted RBCs undergo marked K loss, cation-depletion, and cell dehydration. This calcium-dependent reaction, known as the Gardos effect [7-9], presumably is due to calcium accumulation in ATP-depleted RBCs as a consequence of calcium-pump failure (Fig 3). The specific mechanism by which calcium alters K permeability is unknown, although anything which

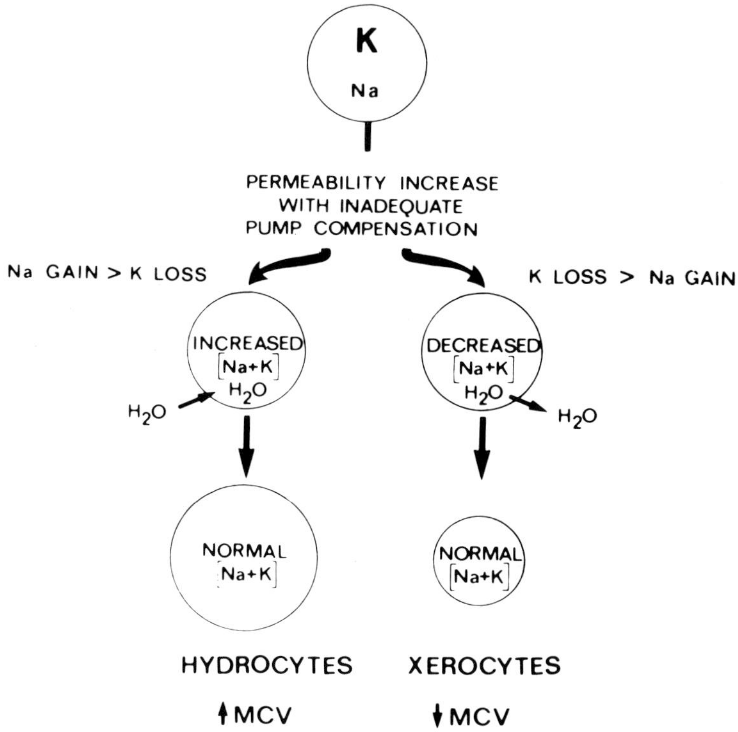

Fig 2. Alterations in RBC hydration due to changes in cation content.

TABLE I. Cation Composition (mEg/10^{13} RBC) of ATP-Depleted RBCs

	Na	K	Na + K	MCV (μ^3)
T-0	10.2	94.3	104.5	93
T-24 EDTA (0.1 mM)	27.8	81.4	109.2	95
Calcium (1.5 mM)	29.5	36.9	66.4	79

Normal RBCs were incubated in a physiologic salt solution (140 mM NaCl, 5 mM KCl) containing either EDTA (0.1 mM) or $CaCl_2$ (1.5 mM). RBC cation content and mean corpuscular volume (MCV) were determined before (T-0) and after (T-24) incubation for 24 h at 37°C in the absence of metabolic substrate. Under these conditions red cells were completely depleted of ATP (data not shown). Values are the mean of three experiments.

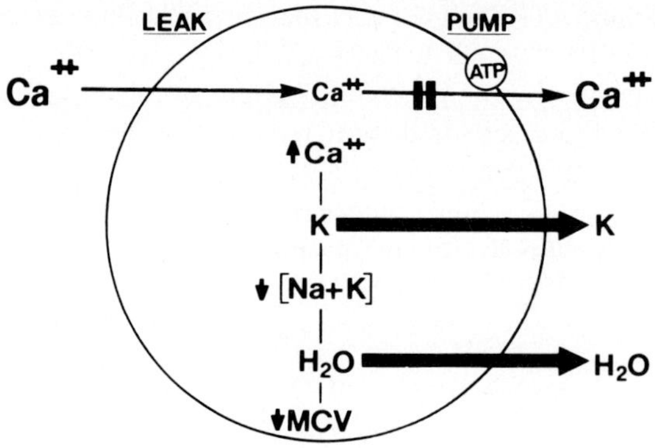

Fig 3. Schematic representation of the Gardos phenomenon.

retards intracellular calcium accumulation also minimizes K-permeability changes. For example, ATP-depleted RBCs preloaded with inorganic phosphate (20–50 mM) achieve a higher net calcium content before K permeability increases; and this presumably is due to intracellular calcium chelation by orthophosphate [10]. Also, EDTA incorporated into ATP-depleted ghosts prevents the calcium-induced potassium leak [9,11]. These data thus suggest that ATP may chelate intracellular calcium as well as provide the energy source for active calcium transport [9,11]. It should be emphasized that the critical aspect of the Gardos effect is increased intracellular calcium and that ATP depletion is important only as a prerequisite for calcium accumulation. With low concentrations of calcium ionophore (A23187), it is possible to demonstrate calcium accumulation, K loss, and dehydration before any decrease in RBC content of ATP is noted [12].

The prominent cation and hydration effects of calcium-pump failure suggest the Gardos reaction may be important under physiologic conditions. This thesis is supported by several observations, including the changes associated with in vivo erythrocyte aging. It is known that normal "old" RBCs contain increased calcium levels [13]. In addition, old erythrocytes have a reduced monovalent cation content (due to a reduction in cell K) and are dehydrated [14,15]. The Gardos effect also is seen in the hemolytic disorder due to pyruvate kinase (PK) deficiency [16,17]. Pyruvate kinase-deficient reticulocytes are unique in their dependence on mitochondrial metabolism as a source of energy. In the presence of oxidative phosphorylation inhibitors such as cyanide, PK-deficient reticulocytes rapidly become ATP-depleted; and this is associated with marked K loss and cell shrinkage (Table II).

Another clinical example of K loss and RBC dehydration is seen in sickle cell anemia. To appreciate this pathophysiology, however, it is necessary to understand the cation permeability changes in *reversibly* and *irreversibly* sickled cells. Reversibly sickled cells (RSCs) are defined as sickled RBCs which return to the normal discoid shape following reoxygenation. Irreversibly sickled cells (ISCs) remain sickled even after extensive oxygenation.

Permeability and Hydration Characteristics of RSCs

Fresh, oxygenated sickle red cells have a normal membrane permeability and cation content [18]. Several years ago, however, Tosteson, Shea, and Draling [18] demonstrated that Na and K permeability were markedly increased in deoxygenated sickle RBCs. These membrane changes, like sickling itself, were reversible upon reoxygenation. Recent studies in our laboratory have confirmed that passive Na and K permeability is increased approximately sixfold in deoxygenated sickle RBCs [19]. Furthermore, under these conditions, no changes were observed in total cation content, cell water, or number of ISCs formed. The rate of passive Na and K transfer also was not altered by 1.5 mM calcium or 0.1 mM EDTA.

Permeability and Hydration Characteristics of ISCs

The irreversible lesion in ISCs is due to cell membrane injury. This concept is supported by two observations: Oxygenated ISC ghosts remain sickled [20,21] and hemoglobin-free spectrin shells from ISCs also retain a sickled configuration [21]. In order to understand the pathophysiology of irreversible membrane injury, attempts have been made to further define the biochemical features of ISCs obtained from patients with sickle cell disease. The most relevant characteristics include: increased calcium concentration

TABLE II. PK Deficiency: Cyanide-Induced Changes in RBC Cation and ATP Content

	ATP (mmoles/10^{13} RBC)	Na[a]	K[a]	Na + K[a]	MCV (μ^3)	MCHC (g/dl RBC)
Control RBCs (40% retics)						
T-0	1.8	13.8	124.2	138.0	115	32.1
T-4 (−CN)	1.9	13.0	122.1	135.1	113	32.7
T-4 (+CN)	1.6	14.2	118.4	132.6	112	32.9
PK-deficient RBCs (60% retics)						
T-0	1.5	14.4	136.5	150.9	124	30.7
T-4	1.7	13.6	130.0	143.6	123	31.0
T-4 (+CN)	0.2	24.9	56.7	81.6	94	40.3

[a]mEq/10^{13} RBC.

Red blood cells from a patient with PK deficiency and a patient with autoimmune hemolytic anemia (control reticulocytes) were suspended in a physiologic salt solution (140 mM NaCl, 5 mM KCl) to which KCN (2 mM) was added to half the suspensions. ATP, Na, K, MCV, and mean corpuscular hemoglobin concentration (MCHC) were measured at the beginning of the experiment (T-0) and after 4 h of incubation (T-4). Results are means of three separate experiments.

[22,23], ATP depletion [24,25], and cellular dehydration as a consequence of reduced monovalent cation content [25,26]. This cation depletion is largely due to K loss (Fig 4) and thus these ISC features are characteristic of the "Gardos effect." It should be noted that the ISC Gardos effect is not *directly* related to sickling-induced permeability changes, since the latter are manifested by equivalent Na-K leaks without alteration in total monovalent cation content or cellular hydration [19]. More likely, the "Gardos effect" reflects ATP depletion as a consequence of accelerated active Na-K and calcium transport. Alternatively, passive calcium influx in excess of the capacity for active calcium efflux also could lead to calcium accumulation, and hence K and water loss.

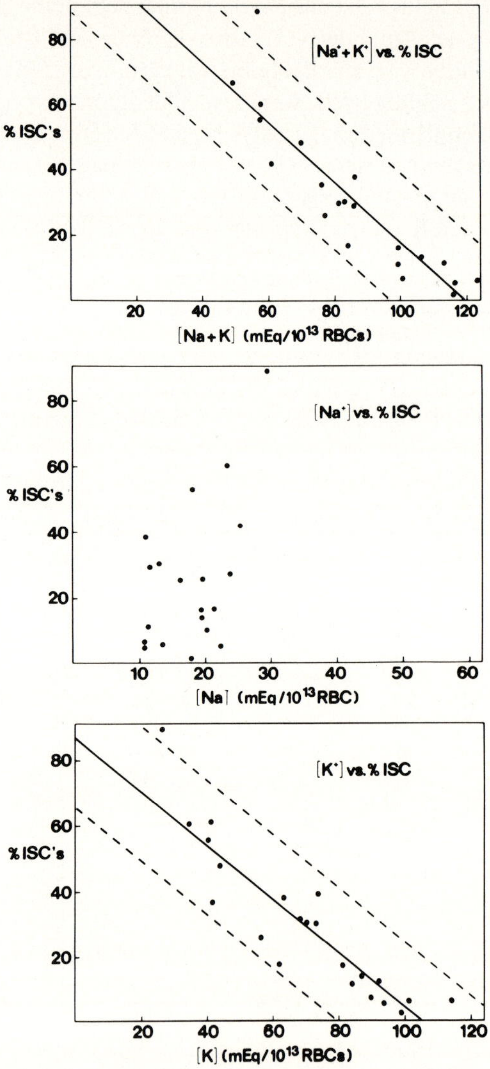

Fig 4. Erythrocytes obtained from patients with sickle cell anemia were sedimented for 1 h at 1,000 g. Aliquots were taken from the top, middle, and bottom layers of the sedimented cells to obtain populations of RBCs with varying percentages of ISCs. The Na and K contents of these populations were then measured. The data in A and C were fitted to the solid lines by the least squares method. The dotted lines enclose ±2 SEM about this line. Top) Na + K content vs percentage ISCs (r = 0.89); middle) Na content vs percentage ISCs (r = 0.52); bottom) K content vs percentage ISCs (r = 0.89).

MEMBRANE ABNORMALITIES RELATED TO POTASSIUM LOSS AND RBC DEHYDRATION

Certain hemolytic disorders characterized by aberrant cation content and cellular hydration are not associated with altered calcium or energy metabolism, and are thought to be due to structural and/or functional alterations in the erythrocyte membrane. One such abnormality, known as hereditary xerocytosis, is characterized by K loss and cellular dehydration. The pathophysiology of this unique disorder is best understood when juxtaposed to the physiologic features of an entirely different type of RBC membrane lesion: hereditary hydrocytosis.

Hereditary hydrocytosis is an erythrocyte disorder characterized by "relative Na-K pump failure" and in many cases there is an associated hemolytic process [27,28]. The peripheral blood of patients with this disorder contains a predominance of stomatocytes. The physiologic definition of these cells (ie, hydrocytes) seems preferable, however, since stomatocytes are seen with a variety of hemolytic disorders. The major defect in "hereditary hydrocytosis" is a marked increase in passive monovalent cation permeability (approximately 20-30 times normal); and although active Na-K transport also is accelerated, the stimulated pump is unable to keep up with exaggerated cation leaks (ie, relative pump failure) [27,28]. As schematically diagramed in Figure 5, Na permeability is greater than that for K, and consequently RBCs tend to gain cations and water, and to increase in size. These changes are observed during incubation in vitro as well as in vivo as "hydrocytic" RBCs age (Table III). In contrast to the reduced K and water content of normal "aged" RBCs, "old" hydrocytes contain more Na, total monovalent cation, and water. In fact, "old" hydrocytes actually are less dense than "young" hydrocytes and the osmotic fragility is increased in accordance with the elevated cell water content. RBCs from patients with hereditary hydrocytosis also manifest other interesting features: 1) Relative pump failure in these cells is not related to limited energy stores since ATP content is normal. In contrast to normal RBCs, however, hydrocytes treated with ouabain manifest a marked decrease in ATP content [27,28]. This is a most unusual observation, since ouabain inhibition of active cation transport normally decreases lactate production and stabilizes (or increases) ATP content. The explanation for this paradoxical response is unknown. 2) Mentzer and co-workers recently demonstrated that the bifunctional cross-linking agent dimethyladipimidate (DMA) completely corrects the permeability defect in hydrocytic RBCs [29]. Furthermore, hydrocyte cation composition and water content return to normal within a few hours following exposure to DMA. The mechanism by which cross-linking of membrane proteins reduces membrane permeability to Na and K is unknown. 3) Protein kinases

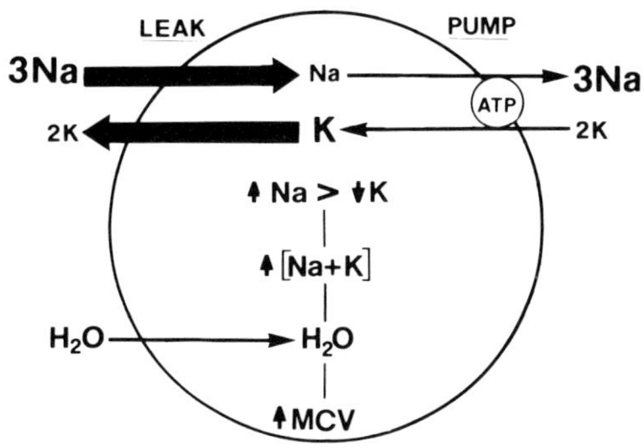

Fig 5. Relative Na-K pump failure secondary to increased cation permeability.

TABLE III. Hereditary Hydrocytosis: Cation Changes (mEq/10^{13} RBC) in Vivo

	Retics (%)	Na	K	Na + K	MCV (μ^3)	MCHC (g/dl)
Control						
Top	6.5	9.4	102.1	111.5	96	31.0
Bottom	0.2	9.1	88.7	97.8	87	34.9
E.S.						
Top	0	135.0	50.1	185.1	116	26.2
Bottom	5.3	20.7	88.9	109.6	92	30.9

Red blood cells from a normal individual (control) and a patient with hereditary hydrocytosis (E.S.) were separated by centrifugation. Aliquots from the top and bottom layers of sedimented cells were assayed for reticulocyte count, Na and K content, MCV, and MCHC. Data derived from Oski et al (New Engl. J. Med. 280: 909, 1969).

that catalyze the phosphorylation of spectrin may be important for regulating normal cell shape and deformability [30]. In the one patient with hereditary hydrocytosis studied to date, membrane protein phosphorylation was significantly decreased [28].

Hereditary xerocytosis is a familial hemolytic syndrome characterized by erythrocyte K loss, cellular dehydration, extreme osmotic resistance, and reduced deformability [31,32]. There are no metabolic defects to account for this permeability lesion. Specifically, ATP levels are normal, and RBC calcium content is not increased. The major detectable RBC abnormality is slightly increased passive cation permeability (1–2 times normal) characterized by K efflux greater than Na influx (Fig 6). Na-K pump activity is increased appropriately for the slightly elevated RBC Na content, but for the reasons described above, Na-K ATPase cannot compensate for K losses in excess of Na gain. As a consequence of this "leak-pump imbalance," RBCs gradually become cation-depleted and lose water in response to decreased intracellular osmolality. These changes are observed during in vitro as well as in vivo incubation as RBCs age (ie, old RBCs are markedly K-depleted and dehydrated) (Table IV). It should be emphasized that the absolute cation leaks in hereditary xerocytosis are small compared to the gross permeability changes observed in hydrocytosis. Nevertheless, major alterations occur in xerocytes as a consequence of *asymmetric* cation leak and the inability of active Na-K transport to make up for net K losses. The permeability defect in these cells presumably reflects a structural membrane alteration, al-

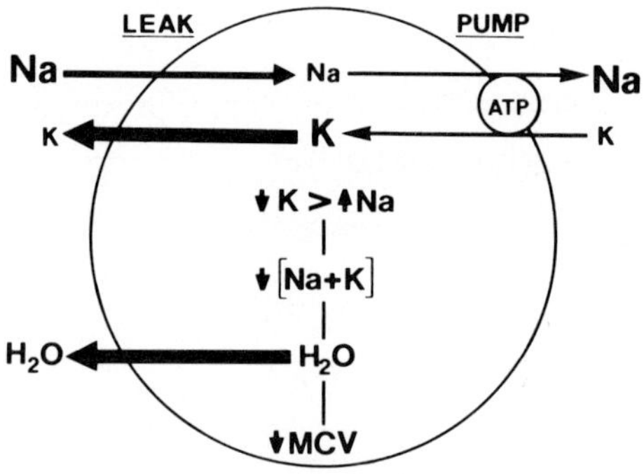

Fig 6. Cation and hydration changes associated with increased K permeability.

TABLE IV. Hereditary Xerocytosis: Cation Changes (mEq/10^{13} RBC) in Vivo

	Retics (%)	Na	K	Na + K	MCHC (g/dl RBC)
Control					
Top	8.6	9.4	102.7	112.1	30.3
Bottom	0.2	9.2	89.6	98.8	35.1
R.D.					
Top	43.0	44.8	85.4	130.2	32.4
Bottom	22.0	25.0	47.7	72.7	41.8

Red blood cells from a normal individual (control) and a patient with hereditary xerocytosis (R.D.) were sedimented for 1 h at 1000g. Aliquots from the top and bottom layers of sedimented cells were assayed for reticulocyte count, Na and K content, and MCHC. Results are means of three experiments.

though preliminary analysis of membrane lipids and proteins has revealed no consistent abnormality. It also is of interest that in contrast to hereditary hydrocytosis, DMA does not correct the xerocytic permeability lesion.

ROLE OF K LOSS AND CELLULAR DEHYDRATION IN MEMBRANE INJURY

Since cation and water depletion occur in several RBC disorders, it is reasonable to question whether these changes represent a cause or effect of cell membrane injury. To evaluate this possibility we examined the importance of K depletion and dehydration in ISC formation. ISCs were generated by deoxygenation of ATP-depleted sickle RBCs in calcium-containing media [33]. The validity of this in vitro method for producing ISCs is based on the similar biochemical characteristics of in vitro and in vivo ISCs [25]. Under these conditions numerous ISCs were formed when deoxygenated sickle RBCs were suspended in a high-Na, low-K incubation medium, while no ISCs were produced if the cells were deoxygenated in a high-K, low-Na medium (Table V). In the former case, ISC formation was associated with a Gardos reaction, while in the latter situation, cation depletion and RBC shrinkage were inhibited in the absence of a K gradient across the cell membrane. These data thus suggest that K loss and cellular dehydration may be requirements for the irreversible membrane injury of ISCs.

TABLE V. Role of Calcium Accumulation and K Loss (mEq/10^{13} RBC) and Cellular Dehydration in ISC Formation

Sickle RBCs	Na	K	Na + K	MCV (μ^3)	% ISCs
T-0	11.8 ± 2.1	94.5 ± 5.1	106.3 ± 4.1	91 ± 3.8	–
T-24					
(Na-HBS) 100% N_2 + calcium	49.2 ± 4.8	10.4 ± 7.2	59.6 ± 5.4	73 ± 5.2	54.2 ± 8.5
(K-HBS) 100% N_2 + calcium	8.9 ± 3.1	95.2 ± 6.1	104.1 ± 5.2	90.1 ± 4.1	0

Cation content, mean cell volume, and percentage of ISCs formed were measured in ATP-depleted sickle RBC after 24-h incubation under 100% nitrogen. The RBCs were suspended in a pH 7.4 HEPES-buffered salt solution (20 mM N-2-hydroxyethylpiperazine-N'-2-ethanesulfonic acid, 1 mM $MgCl_2$, 1 mM Na_2HPO_4) containing either 140 mM NaCl and 5 mM KCl (Na-HBS) or 130 mM KCl and 15 mM NaCl (K-HBS). All solutions also contained $CaCl_2$ (1.5 mM). Results are means of five separate experiments. (Data from Glader and Nathan, Blood 51:983, 1978.)

The role of cellular dehydration in "membrane injury" also has been assessed in a different system which utilized the drug propranolol. Normal RBCs incubated in a physiologic salt solution containing propranolol (0.5 mM) manifest marked K loss and cell shrinkage [34,35]. The mechanism by which propranolol alters membrane permeability is not known, although it is clear that the permeability change is specific for K [35]. This reaction requires extracellular calcium, but it is not associated with net RBC calcium accumulation [36]. A most interesting feature of these K- and water-depleted RBCs is related to their "apparent membrane injury." When RBCs are suspended in progressively hypotonic media, the mean cell volume (MCV) increases until cells hemolyze. The MCV at which cells hemolyze is called the mean critical hemolytic volume (MCHemV). In contrast to normal RBCs, which have a mean critical hemolytic volume of 135 μ^3, the MCHemV of shrunken propranolol-treated RBCs is only 98 μ^3 (Table VI). This reduced MCHemV does not represent nonspecific effects of propranolol and/or calcium, since hemolytic volume changes are not seen with similarly treated cells incubated in a high-K medium. K- and water-depleted RBCs prepared by incubation in a calcium-free medium containing Nystatin [37] also manifest a reduced MCHemV (data not shown) and this further supports the unique importance of K and water depletion in this process. It is unlikely that this membrane reaction is related to dehydration alone, since RBCs dehydrated by incubation in hypertonic NaCl (MCV = 65 μ^3) manifest a normal MCHemV (140 μ^3) when subsequently suspended in hypotonic media. These data indicate that *K depletion and dehydration* in some manner limit normal RBC membrane pliability.

TABLE VI. Propranolol-Induced RBC Dehydration: Effect on Mean Critical Hemolytic Volume

	Na[a]	K[a]	Na + K[a]	MCV (μ^3)	MCHemV (μ^3)
T-0	10.1	93.4	103.5	93	138
T-2 Na-HBS					
Propranolol	15.1	87.2	102.3	92	135
Propranolol + Calcium	16.2	24.8	41.0	68	98
T-2 K-HBS					
Propranolol	10.2	91.6	101.8	92	130
Propranolol + Calcium	9.8	92.4	102.2	92	135

[a]mEq/10^{13} RBC.

RBCs were incubated in a pH 7.4 HEPES-buffered salt solution (20 mM N-2-hydroxyethylpiperazine-N′-2-ethanesulfonic acid, 1 mM $MgCl_2$, 1 mM Na_2HPO_4) containing either 140 mM NaCl and 5 mM KCl (Na-HBS) or 130 mM KCl and 15 mM NaCl (K-HBS). All suspensions contained propranolol (0.5 mM) and those indicated also contained calcium (1.5 mM). At the beginning of the experiment (T-0) and after 2 h incubation at 37°C (T-2), Na and K content and MCV were measured. The mean critical hemolytic volume (MCHemV) also was determined by measuring the MCV at which RBCs hemolyzed when subjected to progressively more hypotonic media.

ACKNOWLEDGMENTS

This work was supported in part by NIH grant AM-20879. Dr. Glader is a recipient of a Research Career Development Award from the National Institutes of Health (AM-00435).

REFERENCES

1. Tosteson DC: Acta Physiol Scand 46:19, 1959.
2. Raker JW, Taylor IM, Weller JM, Hastings AB: J Gen Physiol 33:691, 1950.
3. Jandl JM: Blood 26:367, 1965.
4. Post RL, Merrit CR, Kinsolving CR, Albright CD: J Biol Chem 235:1796, 1960.
5. Garrahan PJ, Glynn IM: J Physiol 192:189, 1967.
6. Wiley JS, Cooper RA: J Clin Invest 53:745, 1974.
7. Gardos G, Straub FB: Acta Physiol Acad Sci Hung 12:1, 1957.
8. Romero PJ, Whittam R: J Physiol 214:481, 1971.
9. Blum RM, Hoffman JF: Biochem Biophys Res Commun 46:1146, 1972.
10. Lew VL: J Physiol 206:35, 1970.
11. Bodeman H, Passow H: J Membrane Biol 8:1, 1972.
12. Edmondson JW, Li TK: Biochim Biophys Acta 443:106, 1976.
13. LaCelle PL, Kirkpatrick FH, Udkow M: In Deutsch E, Gerlach E, Moser K, Williams W (eds): "Second International Symposium on Membrane Permeability of Erythrocytes, Thrombocytes, and Leukocytes." Stuttgart: Georg Thieme Verlag, 1972, pp 49–51.
14. Bernstein RE: J Clin Invest 38:1572, 1959.
15. Glader BE: Unpublished observation.
16. Keitt AS: Am J Med 41:762, 1966.
17. Mentzer WC, Baehner RL, Schmidt-Schonbein H, Robinson SH, Nathan DG: J Clin Invest 50:688, 1971.
18. Tosteson DC, Shea E, Draling RC: J Clin Invest 31:406, 1952.
19. Glader BE, Nathan DG: Blood 51:983, 1978.
20. Jensen WA, Bromberg PA, Barefield K: Clin Res 17:464, 1969.
21. Lux SE, John KM, Karnovsky MJ: J Clin Invest 58:955, 1976.
22. Eaton JW, Skelton TD, Swofford HS, Koplin BE, Jacob HS: Nature 246:105, 1973.
23. Palek J: Blood 42:988, 1973. (abstract)
24. Weed RI, Bessis M: Clin Res 23:442A, 1975.
25. Glader BE, Lux SE, Muller-Soyano A, Platt O, Propper R, Nathan DG: Br J Haematol (In press).
26. Clark MR, Morrison CE, Shohet SB: Blood 48:962, 1976.
27. Zarkowsky HS, Oski FA, Sha'afi R, Shohet SB, Nathan DG: N Engl J Med 278:573, 1968.
28. Mentzer WC, Smith WB, Goldstone J, Shohet SB: Blood 46:659, 1975.
29. Mentzer WC, Lubin BH, Emmons S: N Engl J Med 294:1200, 1976.
30. Sheetz MP, Singer SJ: J Cell Bio 73:658, 1977.
31. Glader BE, Fortier N, Albala MM, Nathan DG: N Engl J Med 291:491, 1974.
32. Glader BE, Fortier NL, Snyder LM: Clin Res 24:309A, 1976.
33. Jensen M, Shohet SB, Nathan DG: Blood 42:835, 1973.
34. Manninen V: Acta Physiol Scand 355:1, 1970.
35. Muller-Soyano A, Glader BE: J Cell Physiol 91:317, 1977.
36. Fortier NL, Snyder M, Palek J, Weiss EB: J Lab Clin Med 89:41, 1977.
37. Cass A: Nature New Biol 244:47, 1973.

Normal and Abnormal Red Cell Membranes 515–521 (1979)

Action of Cobra Venom Phospholipase A_2 Toward Lipids of Erythrocyte Membranes

Marina Adamich and Edward A. Dennis

Department of Chemistry, University of California at San Diego, La Jolla, California 92093

The activity of cobra venom phospholipase A_2 toward phospholipids in erythrocyte membranes is enhanced significantly following ghosting of the membrane. The specificity observed is phosphatidylethanolamine>>phosphatidylcholine and is the reverse of that expected from model studies with individual phospholipids. It is shown, utilizing phospholipid mixtures, that the activity and specificity of cobra venom phospholipase A_2 is dependent on the presence of other lipids and their organization.

Key words: **phospholipase A_2, erythrocytes, ghosts, mixed micelles, Triton X-100, phosphatidylcholine, phosphatidylethanolamine, substrate specificity**

INTRODUCTION

The distribution of phospholipids across the mammalian erythrocyte membrane has been examined utilizing a variety of phospholipases, and results from these studies indicate that the phospholipids are asymmetrically distributed across the two halves of the membrane bilayer [1,2]. Thus, studies employing these lipolytic enzymes have served to support the concept of membrane phospholipid asymmetry first proposed by Bretscher [3].

In our studies, we have utilized a highly purified form of phospholipase A_2 obtained from cobra venom (*Naja naja naja*) [4,5]. Phospholipase A_2 (EC 3.1.1.4) is an acyl esterase which catalyzes the hydrolysis of the fatty acid at the sn-2 position of phospholipids (Fig. 1). Utilizing the cobra venom phospholipase A_2 and the mixed micelle system [6], we have investigated the nature of the substrate [7,8], and the kinetics [9], specificity [10], and mechanism [11,12] of phospholipase A_2 action. In addition, we recently prepared an immobilized form of phospholipase A_2 and have studied its characteristics [13]. We have now investigated the action and substrate specificity of the cobra venom phospholipase A_2 toward phospholipids in the human erythrocyte membrane.

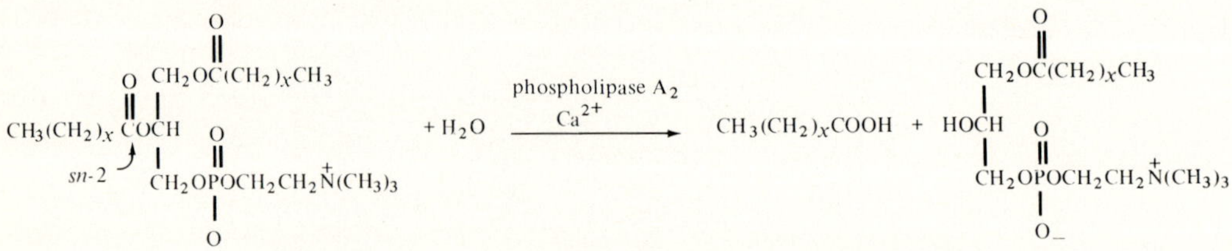

Fig. 1. Site of action of phospholipase A_2 on phosphatidylcholine.

MATERIALS AND METHODS

Cobra venom phospholipase A_2 (*Naja naja naja*) (Pakistan) was obtained as a lyophilized powder from the Miami Serpentarium and was purified according to the method of Deems and Dennis [4], as modified by Roberts et al [5]. Triton X-100 was obtained from Rohm and Haas. Phosphatidylcholine was purified from fresh egg yolks by the method of Singleton et al [14], and phosphatidylethanolamine, prepared by transesterification of egg phosphatidylethanolamine was obtained from Avanti Chemicals. Binary phospholipid mixtures were prepared and assayed as described elsewhere [15]. Human erythrocytes were prepared from fresh, defibrinated blood [16], "snow-white" ghosts were prepared by a modification of the Dodge procedure [17], and erythrocyte lipids were extracted in organic solvents by methods described in detail elsewhere [18]. Assay conditions for hydrolysis are described in the text. Unreacted substrate and hydrolysis products were separated by two-dimensional thin-layer chromatography and analyzed by phosphate analysis [18, 19]. Erythrocytes and ghosts were prepared for scanning electron microscopy as described by Sheetz and Singer [20], except that 20 mM Hepes (intact erythrocytes) or 10 mM Hepes (ghosts) at pH 7.4 was used in place of phosphate buffer, and the membranes were dehydrated in ethanol and critical-point-dried in Freon. Samples were scanned utilizing a Cambridge S4 Scanning Electron Microscope.

RESULTS AND DISCUSSION

Hydrolysis of Erythrocyte Membrane Lipids by Phospholipase A_2

The combined pH and [Ca^{2+}] experiments described by Martin et al [21] for phospholipase A_2 from *Naja naja* venom utilizing erythrocytes stored 24 h in the cold were repeated with our enzyme, and the results are shown in Figure 2 along with the data of Martin et al [21], which are plotted for comparison. The activity of the two phospholipase preparations parallel each other. These results suggest that all phospholipids of the erythrocyte membrane (except sphingomyelin, which is not a substrate of the enzyme) are suitable substrates of our highly purified cobra venom phospholipase A_2 and are hydrolyzed to completion at pH 8.0 and 40 mM Ca^{2+} following hemolysis. At pH 7.4 and 10 mM Ca^{2+}, conditions which apparently protect the cell from hemolysis [21], phosphatidylcholine is hydrolyzed preferentially.

Relative Activity of Phospholipase A_2 Toward Erythrocyte and Ghost Membranes

Fresh human erythrocytes and ghosts were prepared in the presence of 5 mM D-glucose and scanning electron micrographs (not shown) demonstrated that the intact erythro-

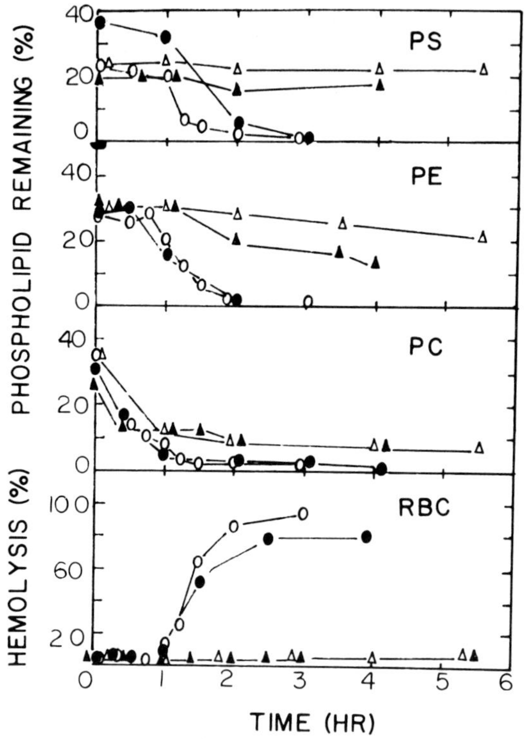

Fig. 2. Effect of pH and Ca^{2+} concentration on the hydrolysis of phospholipids in human erythrocytes by cobra venom phospholipase A_2 (*Naja naja naja*) (●, ▲) compared to the data reported by Martin et al [21] (○, △), which is reproduced with permission of the American Chemical Society. The phospholipid remaining as a function of time is reported for phosphatidylcholine, phosphatidylethanolamine, and phosphatidylserine and represents the % of the total phospholipid present including sphingomyelin. The effect of pH and Ca^{2+} concentration on erythrocyte hemolysis is also shown (RBC graph). Erythrocytes stored 24 h at 4° were incubated at 37° in isosmotic saline and 20 mM Hepes buffer, pH 8.0, 40 mM $CaCl_2$ (●, ○) or at the same concentration of buffer at pH 7.4, 10 mM $CaCl_2$ (▲, △). The enzyme concentration was 12 μg/ml. Hemolysis was monitored at 650 nm after transfer of a 25-μl aliquot of the erythrocyte suspension to a cuvette containing 1.00 ml of the appropriate buffer and Ca^{2+} concentration. Our results represent single determinations and small differences from the results of Martin et al [21] are not considered significant.

cytes appeared normal and the ghosts were mostly fragments as judged by their dimensions. The erythrocyte preparations were incubated in the presence of glucose and 1 μg per milliliter enzyme for 10 min (Table I). Under these conditions less than 1% of the total phospholipid of the intact erythrocytes was hydrolyzed, while some 38% of the total phospholipid of the ghosts was hydrolyzed. Similar results were obtained for ghosts prepared and assayed in the absence of glucose, suggesting that hydrolysis itself is neither activated nor inhibited by glucose, although it may affect the structure of the intact erythrocyte membrane. The concentration dependence of phospholipase A_2 activity toward intact erythrocytes was also examined (Table II). A tenfold increase in the concentration of enzyme resulted in only 5% total phospholipid hydrolysis, and a 100-fold increase in phospholipase concentration resulted in hydrolysis of only 9% of the phospholipid, and the product was practically all phosphatidylcholine.

TABLE I. Action of Cobra Venom Phospholipase A_2 Toward Intact Erythrocytes and Ghost Membranes

	Enzyme (μg/ml)	Phospholipid (mole fraction) PE	LPE	PC	LPC	PS	SpH	Total phospholipid (% hydrolyzed)
Control	0	0.32	0.00	0.33	0.00	0.16	0.19	0
Intact erythrocytes	1	0.34	<0.01	0.31	<0.01	0.15	0.20	<1
Ghost membranes	1	0.04	0.28	0.21	0.10	0.16	0.21	38

The assay mix contained 0.50 ml packed cells or ghosts, 10 mM $CaCl_2$, 5 mM D-glucose, 148 mM NaCl, and 20 mM Hepes (10 mM Hepes with no added NaCl for ghosts), pH 7.4, in a total volume of 2.0 ml. Incubation was at 37°C for 10 min. Control data for erythrocytes is provided; ghost controls gave similar values. Further experimental details are provided elsewhere [18].

TABLE II. Concentration Dependence of Cobra Venom Phospholipase A_2 Action Toward Intact Human Erythrocytes

Enzyme (μg/ml)	Phospholipid (mole fraction) PE	LPE	PC	LPC	PS	SpH	Total phospholipid (% hydrolyzed)
1	0.31	0.00	0.34	0.01	0.13	0.22	1
10	0.30	0.01	0.29	0.04	0.13	0.25	5
100	0.32	0.01	0.24	0.08	0.13	0.22	9

Assay conditions are given in Table I.

The results reported here show that highly purified cobra venom phospholipase A_2 is capable of hydrolyzing all phospholipids to completion in surfaces of erythrocyte membranes under the appropriate conditions, but very little hydrolysis of the total phospholipid of intact erythrocytes is observed when fresh cells are used, if the incubation time is shortened and glucose is present regardless of enzyme concentration. It appears, then, that the majority of the phospholipid in intact, metabolizing erythrocytes is not available to the enzyme. Presumably the phospholipids in the inner membrane surface are inaccessible, but those on the outside may be masked or structurally different prior to hemolysis or ghosting so that they are not capable of properly interacting with the enzyme. Under our experimental conditions, very little of the phospholipid can be hydrolyzed in the intact erythrocytes when the cells are metabolically competent, but some 67% of the phosphatidylcholine becomes hydrolyzed (see Figure 2, phosphatidylcholine, pH 7.4, 10 mM Ca^{2+}, before significant hemolysis) in the outer surface of intact, nonglycolyzing erythrocytes. This could be a reflection of membrane integrity changes that are more subtle than those introduced through hemolysis, but which result in rendering more phosphatidylcholine available to the enzyme.

On the other hand, phospholipids of ghosts appear to be available as substrates for the enzyme, and the dramatic enhancement in hydrolysis appears to be a function of the ghosting procedure, which renders both surfaces available to the enzyme. However, upon ghosting, the enzyme may continue to display little activity toward the outer surface lipids, the enhanced activity observed being directed towards lipids in the inner surface only. Alternatively, it is possible that ghosting causes a change in the properties or packing of the outer surface, resulting in enhanced activity of the phospholipase A_2 toward lipids in both surfaces of the membrane. Investigations into these two possibilities are currently under way.

The apparent specificity preference of the enzyme toward intact erythrocytes is for phosphatidylcholine, but in the ghosts, phosphatidylethanolamine is hydrolyzed preferentially. These latter findings are not in agreement with simple specificity studies in which individual lipids in Triton X-100-mixed micelles were used [10], and which showed phosphatidylcholine to be the preferred substrate and phosphatidylethanolamine to be a very poor substrate for the enzyme. This apparent reversal in enzyme specificity observed in the ghost preparation could be due to some unique structure (ie, packing) that results from ghosting, or it may be due to the action of phospholipase toward only that surface which contains this phospholipid exclusively, or perhaps to membrane protein-lipid interactions which render phosphatidylethanolamine a better substrate than phosphatidylcholine. These possibilities are examined below.

Substrate Specificity of Phospholipase A_2 Toward Triton X-100-Solubilized Erythrocytes, Ghosts, Extracted Lipids, and Binary Mixtures

Fresh erythrocytes, ghosts, and extracted ghost lipids were solubilized in Triton X-100. This detergent induces immediate hemolysis of erythrocytes and disperses the lipids as mixed micelles, such that all phospholipids are present in one surface [22]. Integral proteins are also present while peripheral proteins may not have been solubilized, as demonstrated by Yu et al [23]. The activity and substrate specificity of the enzyme toward these preparations was examined (Table III) utilizing the same conditions as employed in Table I, except that to achieve comparable rates the concentration of phospholipase A_2 was further decreased in the extracted lipid experiment. It is clear that in every case, the substrate specificity of the enzyme is identical to that observed for ghosts in the absence of Triton X-100 (Table I). Prolonged incubation (~30 min) resulted in the eventual hydrolysis of phosphatidylserine in all mixtures. Thus, the apparent preferential hydrolysis of phosphatidylethanolamine, termed "specificity reversal," observed in the ghosts is not as a result of some unique membrane structure, nor is it due to the presence of membrane constituents other than lipids. Furthermore, it does not appear to be dependent on membrane "sidedness," since comparable high activities and the preferential hydrolysis of phosphatidylethanolamine are observed for ghosts, and for erythrocytes and extracted ghost lipids in Triton-mixed micelles. What is clear is that specificity reversal is dependent on the presence of other lipids only.

We have also examined pure lipid mixtures in mixed micelles containing two phospholipid species only, phosphatidylethanolamine and phosphatidylcholine, which have

TABLE III. Action of Cobra Venom Phospholipase A_2 Toward Erythrocytes, Ghost Membranes, and Extracted Lipid in the Presence of Triton X-100

	Enzyme (μg/ml)	Phospholipid (mole fraction) PE	LPE	PC	LPC	PS	SpH	Total phospholipid (% hydrolyzed)
Control	0	0.34	0.00	0.33	0.00	0.15	0.17	0
Erythrocytes	1	0.03	0.28	0.28	0.05	0.14	0.22	33
Ghosts	1	0.01	0.27	0.18	0.16	0.16	0.22	43
Extracted lipid	0.31	0.09	0.25	0.22	0.10	0.14	0.20	35

The assay mix for erythrocytes and ghosts is given in Table I, except that 9 mM Triton X-100 (about 0.5% by weight) was added. For extracted lipid, 1 μmole phospholipid was used in a total volume of 1.00 ml, which included the same components given for ghosts. Incubations were conducted at 37°C for 10 min. Control data for erythrocytes is shown; ghost and extracted lipid controls gave similar values and further details are provided elsewhere [18].

similar fatty acyl chains. Initial findings are reported elsewhere [15]. Figure 3 presents new and more complete data utilizing similar binary mixtures of these phospholipids. It is clear that phosphatidylethanolamine (100 mole %) is a poor substrate, while phosphatidylcholine (100 mole %) is a very good substrate of the enzyme. However, in the presence of 5-70 mole % phosphatidylcholine, the rate for phosphatidylethanolamine hydrolysis is enhanced significantly, and this phospholipid is apparently the preferred substrate of phospholipase A_2. The decrease in the rate of phosphatidylethanolamine hydrolysis (after the peak in its activity) and the rising curve for phosphatidylcholine hydrolysis as a function of the mole % of phosphatidylcholine are probably due simply to competition between two substrates after maximum activation of phosphatidylethanolamine as a substrate. The precise cause of this activation is unclear at this time [15].

Specificity reversal is not unique to mixtures involving substrates of the enzyme only, since sphingomyelin, which is not a substrate of the enzyme, will also enhance the activity of phospholipase A_2 toward phosphatidylethanolamine in a manner similar to that observed for phosphatidylcholine (M. Adamich, M.F. Roberts, and E.A. Dennis, manuscript in preparation). Thus, phosphatidylcholine and sphingomyelin, both of which are lipids present in membrane surfaces, are capable of activating phospholipase A_2 toward phosphatidylethanolamine in the erythrocyte ghosts and in phospholipid mixtures in Triton X-100-mixed micelles. This phenomenon can also be observed with phospholipase A_2 acting toward bilayer vesicles prepared with phosphatidylcholine and phosphatidylethanolamine [24]. That this phenomenon is not observed when the enzyme is acting towards surfaces of intact erythrocytes suggests either that phosphatidylethanolamine is not present in significant amounts in the outer surface, which would be consistent with the current interpretation of membrane lipid asymmetry [1-3], or that, if present, it is not available to the enzyme until some further changes occur in the membrane. For example, Haest and Deuticke [25] have shown that the treatment of erythrocytes with SH reagents results in an appreciable amount of phosphatidylethanolamine hydrolyzed by phospholipase A_2 in the intact erythrocyte.

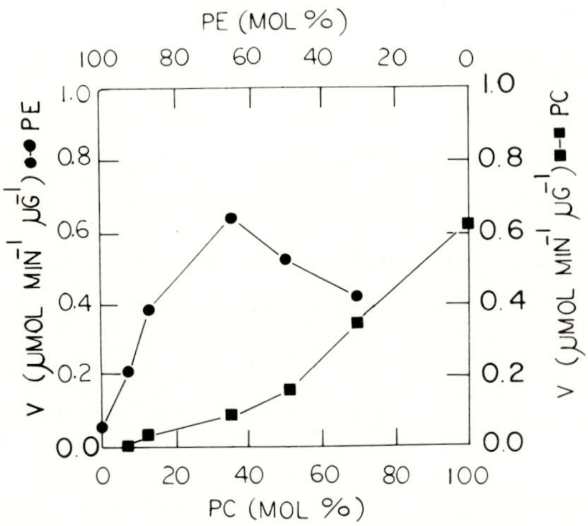

Fig. 3. Specific activity profile of phospholipase A_2 (*Naja naja naja*) action toward phosphatidylcholine (■) and phosphatidylethanolamine (●) in binary phospholipid mixtures in mixed micelles at a 4:1 molar ratio of Triton X-100 to total phospholipid as a function of the mole % of each lipid. The specific activity was calculated based on the μmoles lysophospholipid produced in the presence of 0.31 μg enzyme. Incubation was for 2 min at 40°.

In conclusion, our findings concerning the dependence of the activity and specificity of cobra venom phospholipase A_2 on the state of the erythrocyte membrane and on the presence of other lipids suggest that further work is required before definitive interpretations of membrane lipid sidedness can be made based solely on the basis of studies with phospholipase A_2 or other phospholipases.

ACKNOWLEDGMENTS

This work was supported by National Institutes of Health grant GM 20,501. M.A. is a postdoctoral fellow of the National Institutes of Health, GM 06,071.

REFERENCES

1. Zwaal RFA, Roelofsen B, Colley MC: Biochim Biophys Acta 300:159, 1973.
2. Van Deenen LLM, Demel RA, Geurts von Kessel WSM, Kamp HH, Roelofsen B, Verkleij AJ, Wirtz KWA, Zwaal RFA: In Hatefi Y, Djavadi-Ohaniance L (eds): "The Structural Basis of Membrane Function." New York: Academic, 1976, p 21.
3. Bretscher MS: Nature 236:11, 1972.
4. Deems RA, Dennis EA: J Biol Chem 250:9008, 1975.
5. Roberts MF, Deems RA, Dennis EA: J Biol Chem 252:6011, 1977.
6. Dennis EA: J Supramol Struct 2:682, 1974.
7. Ribeiro AA, Dennis EA: Biochemistry 14:3746, 1975.
8. Roberts MF, Bothner-By AA, Dennis EA: Biochemistry 17:935, 1978.
9. Deems RA, Eaton BR, Dennis EA: J Biol Chem 250:9013, 1975.
10. Roberts MF, Otnaess A-B, Kensil CA, Dennis EA: J Biol Chem 253:1252, 1978.
11. Roberts MF, Deems RA, Mincey TC, Dennis EA: J Biol Chem 252:2405, 1977.
12. Roberts MF, Deems RA, Dennis EA: Proc Natl Acad Sci USA 74:1950, 1977.
13. Adamich M, Voss HF, Dennis EA: Arch Biochem Biophys 89:417, 1978.
14. Singleton WS, Gray MS, Brown ML, White JL: J Am Oil Chem Soc 42:53, 1965.
15. Adamich M, Dennis EA: Biochem Biophys Res Comm 80:424, 1978.
16. Mendelsohn J, Skinner A, Kornfeld S: J Clin Invest 50:818, 1971.
17. Dodge JT, Mitchell C, Hanahan DJ: Arch Biochem Biophys 100:119, 1963.
18. Adamich M, Dennis EA: J Biol Chem 24:5121, 1978.
19. Turner JD, Rouser G: Anal Biochem 38:423, 1970.
20. Sheetz MP, Singer SJ: Proc Natl Acad Sci USA 71:4457, 1974
21. Martin JK, Luthra MG, Wells MA, Watts RP: Biochemistry 14:5400, 1975.
22. Kirkpatrick FH, Gordesky SE, Marinetti GV: Biochim Biophys Acta 345:154, 1974.
23. Yu J, Fischman DA, Steck TL: J Supramol Struct 1:233, 1973.
24. Sundler R, Sarcione SL, Alberts AW, Vagelos PR: Proc Natl Acad Sci USA 74:3350, 1977.
25. Haest CWM, Deuticke B: Biochim Biophys Acta 436:353, 1976.

Normal and Abnormal Red Cell Membranes 523–529 (1979)

The Relationship Between Ca^{2+}-Mediated Polyphosphoinositide Phosphodiesterase Activity, 1, 2-Diacylglycerol Accumulation, and Microvesiculation in Erythrocytes

D. Allan and R. H. Michell

Department of Experimental Pathology, University College Hospital Medical School, University Street, London WC1E 6JJ (D.A.); and Department of Biochemistry, University of Birmingham, PO Box 363, Birmingham B15 2TT (R.H.M.).

A variety of morphologic and metabolic changes occur in erythrocytes in which the intracellular level of Ca^{2+} is increased. These include echinocytosis followed by microvesiculation, K^+ efflux, ATP degradation, and activation of polyphosphoinositide phosphodiesterase with the formation of 1,2-diacylglycerol and phosphatidate. The relationships between these changes are discussed and an attempt is made to assess their significance in both normal and aged cells.

Key words: Ca^{2+}, lipids, polyphosphoinositides, 1,2-diacylglycerol, microvisiculation, K^+ efflux

Major advances have recently occurred in our knowledge of membrane structure and function, particularly in relation to the erythrocyte membrane which provides a simplified but relevant model for the membranes of other cells. This paper attempts to draw together certain strands of recent research on human erythrocytes in an effort to integrate some apparently disparate elements of red cell membrane behaviour. In particular, we will examine the significance of erythrocyte cation homeostasis and the ability of elevated intracellular Ca^{2+} ion concentration to cause a) changes in cell morphology, b) microvesiculation, c) changes in lipid metabolism, and d) an efflux of K^+ from the cells. We shall also suggest some parallels between the effects of artificially raising internal Ca^{2+} levels and the changes seen in cells under certain pathologic conditions.

Cells in general appear to maintain within themselves extremely low levels of ionised Ca^{2+} compared with the concentration of this ion in the surrounding medium [1,2]. The Ca^{2+} gradient is quantitatively the most significant of any ionic gradient across cell plasma membranes. This is true for the human erythrocyte, which under normal conditions appears to maintain an intracellular Ca^{2+} concentration of less than 10^{-7} M as against a plasma concentration of about 10^{-3} M [3]. The 10,000-fold difference in Ca^{2+} concentration across the membrane contrasts with a 10- to 20-fold gradient of monovalent cations and (probably) a one- to twofold gradient of Mg^{2+}. The relatively huge Ca^{2+} gradient is maintained by a) a membrane which is very impermeable to Ca^{2+} [4], b) an active pumping mechanism associated with the Ca^{2+}-sensitive ATPase [3], and possibly c) powerful chelators of Ca^{2+} in the cell membrane and cytosol.

Received for publication March 5, 1978.

As in other cell types, a rise above normal levels in the cytoplasmic Ca^{2+} concentration within human erythrocytes is associated with drastic metabolic and morphologic changes. Such changes are induced most easily by treatment of cells with the Ca^{2+}-ionophore A23187 [5], which breaks down the permeability barrier which the cell membrane presents to Ca^{2+}.

Ca^{2+}-IONOPHORE-INDUCED CHANGES IN HUMAN ERYTHROCYTES

K^+ Efflux

The most immediate change, beginning within seconds of adding Ca^{2+}-ionophore, is a massive efflux of cell K^+ [6,7]. This is completely blocked by the Ca^{2+}-chelator EGTA but does not require addition of extracellular Ca^{2+} beyond that present as an impurity in the solutions used, indicating an extremely low requirement for Ca^{2+}. It is prevented by quinine [8]. This is consistent with data presented recently [6,10,11] which demonstrate the existence in human erythrocyte ghosts of a K^+-gating mechanism which is activated by about 1 μM Ca^{2+} and inhibited by quinine. The role of Ca^{2+}-mediated K^+ efflux is quite unknown but appears to be a widespread phenomenon amongst cells in general (eg Table 2 in Michell [12]). Indeed, an observed increase in K^+ efflux may be a useful general indicator of a prior increase in cytosolic Ca^{2+} in many cells.

Cell Morphology

Because there is no immediate change in the permeation of Na^+ into cells and because Cl^- and water move out of the cells together with K^+ (to maintain electrical and osmotic balance), human erythrocytes shrink in volume when exposed to Ca^{2+}-ionophore [6]. This leads immediately to a change in cell shape from the normal biconcave disk to a more irregular configuration in order to accommodate the same amount of membrane around a diminished cell volume. Further changes lead gradually to the formation of spherical cells with spiculed surfaces (echinocytes) [13], and it has been shown recently that the cells can then lose membrane in the form of buds (microvesicles) from the tips of the spikes formed on the membrane surface [14,15] (Fig 1a). Up to 20% of the total lipid may be lost as microvesicles about 10 nm in diameter. This is equivalent to about 500 microvesicles per cell. An interesting feature of these microvesicles is that although they possess a lipid composition rather similar to that of the parent cell (except with respect to 1,2-diacylglycerol—see below), they are greatly depleted in some of the characteristic red cell proteins, particularly spectrin and actin [15]. Band 3 (in Steck's classification), which is thought to represent a group of proteins involved in transport across the membrane and which probably penetrates the lipid bilayer, appears, however, to be retained in the microvesicles, as does at least one erythrocyte ectoenzyme, acetylcholinesterase [14].

The simplest way of interpreting the formation of these microvesicles is that they arise by a budding process in which fusion occurs between the cytoplasmic faces of the membrane forming the neck of the surface spicules. Electron microscopy supports this view, although we have had some indications that part of the membrane material in the fusing neck region may not reabsorb completely into the main body of the microvesicles. In these cases, small membranous sacs or "tails" are seen attached to some of the microvesicles (Fig 1a), but the precise nature of these tails is not known.

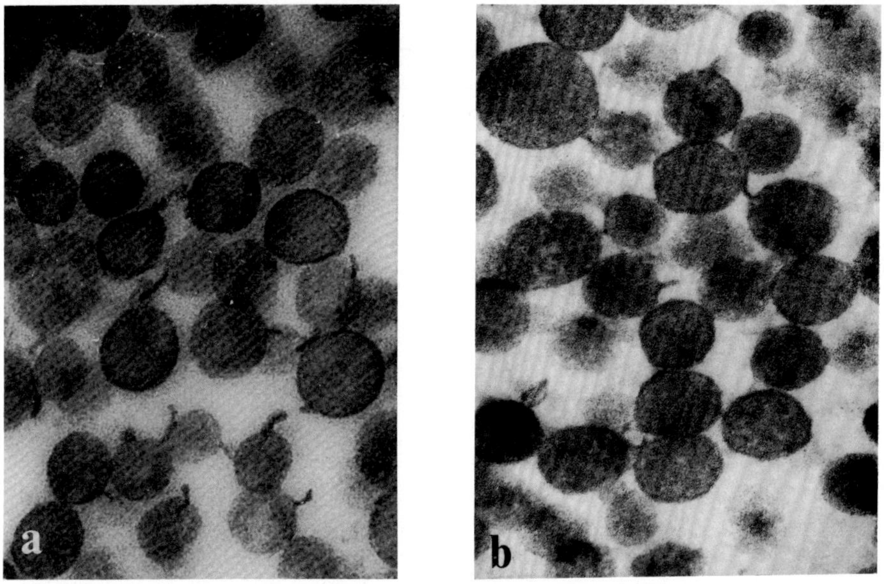

Fig 1. Transmission electron micrographs of microvesicles from: a) A23187-treated human erythrocytes; b) human erythrocytes aged in ACD under blood-bank conditions (magnification × 76,000).

Reduction of Cell ATP Levels

Introduction of Ca^{2+} into human red cells leads to a marked reduction of ATP levels [6,16,17]. This is presumably because the sustained rise in intracellular Ca^{2+} ion level fully activates the Ca^{2+}-transport ATPase of the membrane and therefore rapidly depletes the ATP pool [3]. It has been speculated that reduction in cell ATP alone may cause the observed changes in erythrocyte morphology. Although this is undoubtedly a factor in such changes [18,19], recent evidence does not support the view that it is the only cause of morphologic changes [20]. The morphologic changes accompanying a decrease in ATP may in part be secondary consequences of the failure of the cell to maintain an energy supply for the Ca^{2+} pump, with a resulting rise in intracellular Ca^{2+}.

Diacylglycerol Formation From Polyphosphoinositide

Recent work has shown that the entry of Ca^{2+} into a normal human erythrocyte leads to changes in lipid metabolism [14,16,21–24]. The primary effect of Ca^{2+} appears to be the activation of an endogenous membrane-bound phosphodiesterase which attacks phosphatidylinositol 4-phosphate (diphosphoinositide, PI-P) and phosphatidylinositol 4,5- diphosphate (triphosphoinositide, PI-diP) to give 1,2-diacylglycerol (1,2-DG) and inositol phosphates. If ATP is available, then some of the 1,2-DG is converted to phosphatidate (PA) by the endogenous 1,2-DG kinase activity of the erythrocyte membrane [16,25].

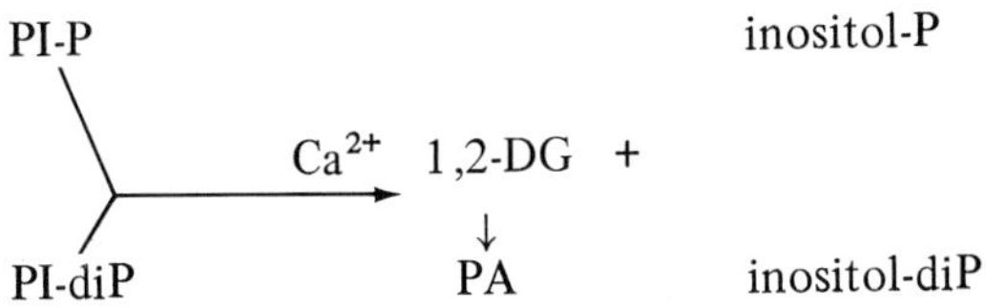

The 1,2-DG formed is particularly concentrated in the microvesicle fraction, where the level can be as high as 15–20 times that in the normal red cell membrane [15]. This finding suggests either that microvesiculation occurs selectively in regions of the plasma membrane where PI-P and PI-diP are breaking down to form 1,2-DG, or that after its production 1,2-DG becomes concentrated into particular regions of membrane which then bud off. Together with other evidence of the fusogenic potential of 1,2-DG [26–28], this led us to postulate a role for the breakdown of polyphosphoinositide and/or production of 1,2-DG in the membrane fusion event involved in microvesiculation [15]. Further support for this idea comes from the observation that erythrocytes from some species do not show Ca^{2+}-stimulated 1,2-DG production, but neither do they vesiculate in response to a rise in intracellular Ca^{2+} concentration [9].

In general terms, it seems reasonable that removal of a large, hydrated, and highly charged headgroup from a hydrophilic lipid to give an uncharged hydrophobic lipid should make it easier for the lipid phases of two membrane surfaces to approach closely and to fuse. However, there are some indications that production of 1,2-DG might be more important than degradation of polyphosphoinositide in initiating the membrane fusion event. First, 1,2-DG is one of a number of lipids which can facilitate fusion of chicken erythrocytes when added exogenously [28]. Second, in the normal human erythrocyte, the 1,2-DG produced by polyphosphoinositide breakdown is initially converted largely to phosphatidate by membrane 1,2-DG kinase [16]; only when the cell is depleted of ATP does 1,2-DG accumulate and it is only then that pronounced microvesiculation occurs [15]. Third, the production of diacylglycerol in the outer leaflet of the erythrocyte membrane by phospholipase C attack causes inward membrane vesiculation [9,26]. Thus the occurrence of membrane fusion events and either inward or outward membrane vesiculation appear to be correlated with the accumulation of 1,2-DG in the fusing membrane surfaces. When viewed in this way, the very active 1,2-DG kinase of the erythrocyte membrane may possibly be seen as the agency by which the cell protects itself from the morphologic and fusogenic consequences of 1,2-diacylglycerol accumulation.

PI-P and PI-diP are highly charged anionic molecules which interact strongly with proteins through divalent cation bridges, at least in model systems. As a result, their extraction from membranes requires the use of acidic conditions or high concentrations of monovalent cation salts and/or chelators such as EDTA. Similar interactions between polyphosphoinositides and proteins may exist in the red cell membrane [29]. One suggested specific interaction is between PI-P and glycophorin [30]. The enzymic conversion of the polyphosphoinositides to 1,2-DG might therefore cause appreciable changes in the lipid-protein and protein-protein interactions in the membrane, and such changes might be involved in migration of proteins out of the 1,2-DG-enriched regions which are budding outwards.

Although more direct effects of Ca^{2+} on membrane proteins (eg spectrin) have been proposed, our evidence suggests a clear correlation between Ca^{2+}-dependent microvesiculation and the production of 1,2-DG. Cells from some species exhibit a rise in 1,2-DG and also vesiculate (eg human, rat, rabbit, and guinea-pig), whereas microvesiculation is not observed in those species which do not produce diacylglycerol (eg pig, cow, and sheep) [9]. All species, however, possess comparable patterns of membrane polypeptides, including spectrin, whether or not they undergo Ca^{2+}-dependent microvesiculation. Although in general it appears that the capacity for Ca^{2+}-dependent K^+ efflux is shown by red cells which are also capable of microvesiculation and diacylglycerol production, the pig provides an example of an erythrocyte type which shows the K^+ efflux in the absence of echinocytosis, vesiculation, or the changes in lipid metabolism [9].

It is worth noting that Ca^{2+}-dependent breakdown of PI-P and PI-diP not only generates membrane 1,2-DG, but it also presumably leads to a rise in the intracellular concentrations of inositol di- and triphosphates. It would be interesting to know if these unusual compounds can themselves have any effect on red cell function. Inositol penta- and hexaphosphates have well-known effects on haemoglobin conformation, but at present there appears to be little known about the possible activities of the less highly phosphorylated derivatives of inositol.

SIGNIFICANCE OF Ca^{2+}-INDUCED CHANGES FOR RED CELL AGING

The normal human erythrocyte possesses powerful mechanisms for limiting the concentration of ionised Ca^{2+} in its cytoplasm, particularly through the activity of the Ca^{2+}-pump associated with the membrane Ca^{2+}-dependent ATPase[3]. Healthy cells therefore maintain their high internal K^+ concentration and their biconcave disk shape, possess an almost undetectable level of 1,2-diacylglycerol, and show no tendency towards echinocytosis or microvesiculation. During aging in vitro (and probably in vivo), where there is evidence of an increased cell uptake of Ca^{2+} [31], the cells show changes in all of the above characteristics, which, as we have described, are extremely sensitive to the level of intracellular Ca^{2+}. Cells begin to show a marked loss of K^+ after a few weeks storage in ACD and concurrently tend to become echinocytic and less deformable [32,33]. Loss of material by microvesiculation is also more apparent as the cells age [34,36], and the microvesicles are substantially identical in morphology (Fig 1b) and chemical constitution [35, 36] to those produced by Ca^{2+} ionophore. Moreover, they are enriched in 1,2-DG [35] and in phosphatidate [36], which is probably derived by phosphorylation of 1,2-DG [16]. The increased buoyant density of older cells is probably due to their loss of KCl and water through Ca^{2+}-triggered processes, and their decreased deformability can be ascribed to the loss of up to 20% of their membrane material as microvesicles, so that the remaining membrane is tightly stretched around the cytoplasmic constituents of the residual spherocytic cells.

Many of the attributes of old cells can therefore be ascribed to the gradual loss of their ability to maintain sufficiently low intracellular Ca^{2+} levels. We cannot state the precise cause of this failure in Ca^{2+} homeostasis; it may reflect a general loss of metabolic competency in the aging cells. Such "incompetent" cells become echinocytic and, if present in the blood stream, are rapidly removed, probably in the microcirculation of the spleen. The processes described here suggest that metabolically incompetent red cells are recognised indirectly as a result of their failure to maintain low levels of intracellular Ca^{2+}, but directly because Ca^{2+} provokes a metabolic change (polyphosphoinositide breakdown to 1,2-DG), which then leads to a morphologic change (microvesiculation) and leaves a residual cell that can no longer negotiate the microcirculation.

POLYPHOSPHOINOSITIDES AS INDICATORS OF PAST AND PRESENT CELLULAR Ca^{2+} STATUS

It is important to note that erythrocytes possess no mechanism for the de novo synthesis of phospholipids [37], meaning that Ca^{2+}-dependent breakdown of PI-P and PI-diP to 1,2-DG is irreversible. One might therefore expect that during the normal life of the human erythrocyte, polyphosphoinositide breakdown would be a slow but cumulative process, and that it might constitute a kind of "biological clock" which limits the lifetime of the cell, with senility delayed partly by the ability of the cell to maintain low levels of intracellular Ca^{2+} and partly by its ability to convert 1,2-DG to phosphatidate. Analysis of different age cohorts of healthy erythrocytes should allow this idea to be tested.

One possible way in which knowledge that the cellular levels of PI-P and PI-diP are controlled by the intracellular Ca^{2+} level might be applied would be by using these lipids as indicators of a cell's Ca^{2+} homeostatic history. It could be concluded that any cell which retained its full polyphosphoinositide complement had never been exposed to conditions where its intracellular Ca^{2+} level had risen appreciably, whereas depressed levels of PI-P or PI-diP would indicate either past or present elevation of this level. Estimates of the levels of these lipids can conveniently be made on ghosts prepared in the presence of EGTA. Such an assessment might be of value in resolving conflicts such as that in which the aetiology of membrane vesiculation in hereditary spherocytosis is variously ascribed to defects in Ca^{2+} homeostasis, protein content, protein phosphorylation, or lipid metabolism (see Condres [38] and Shohet and Ness [39]).

ACKNOWLEDGMENTS

We are grateful to the Medical Research Council for financial support.

REFERENCES

1. Baker PF: Prog Biophys Mol Biol 24:177–223, 1972.
2. Berridge MJ: In Greengard P, Robson GA (eds): "Advances in Cyclic Nucleotide Research." New York: Raven Press, 1975, vol 6, pp 1–99.
3. Schatzman HJ: In Bronner F, Kleinzeller A (eds): "Current Topics in Membranes and Transport." New York: Academic, 1975, pp 125–168.
4. Schatzmann HJ, Vincenzi FF: J Physiol 201:369-395, 1969.
5. Reed PW, Lardy HA: J Biol Chem 247:6970–6973, 1972.
6. Kirkpatrick FH, Hillmann DG, La Celle PL: Experientia 31:653-654, 1975.
7. Ferreira HG, Lew VL: Nature (London) 259:47–49, 1976.
8. Armando-Hardy M, Ellory JC, Ferreira HG, Fleminger S, Lew VL: J Physiol (London) 250:32P–33P, 1975.
9. Allan D, Michell RH: Biochem J 166:495–499, 1977.
10. Porzig H: Experientia 30:697, 1974.
11. Romero PJ: J Membr Biol 29:329–343, 1976.
12. Michell RH: In Bull AT, Lagnado JR, Thomas JO, Tipton KF (eds): "Companion to Biochemistry." London: Longmans, 1978, vol 2, pp 205–228.
13. White JG: Am J Path 77:507–518, 1974.
14. Allan D, Michell RH: Nature (London) 258:348–349, 1975.
15. Allan D, Billah MM, Finean JB, Michell RH: Nature (London) 261:58–61, 1976.
16. Allan D, Watts R, Michell RH: Biochem J 157:225–232, 1976.
17. Taylor D, Baker R, Hochstein P: Biochem Biophys Res Commun 76:205–211, 1977.
18. Sheetz M, Singer SJ: J Cell Biol 73:638–646, 1977.
19. Birchmeier W, Singer JT: J Cell Biol 73:647–659, 1977.
20. Feo C, Mohandas N: Nature (London) 265:166–168, 1977.
21. Allan D, Michell RH: Biochim Biophys Acta 455:824-830, 1976.
22. Allan D, Michell RH: In Eisenberg F, Wells WW (eds): "Cyclitols and Phosphoinositides." New York: Academic 1978, pp 325–336.
23. Allan D, Michell RH: Biochim Biophys Acta 508:277–286, 1978.
24. Lang V, Pryhitka G, Buckley TJ: Can J Biochem 55:1007–1012, 1978.
25. Allan D, Michell RH: Biochem Soc Trans 5:55–59, 1977.
26. Allan D, Low MG, Finean JB, Michell RH: Biochim Biophys Acta 413:309–316, 1975.
27. De Boer E, Loyter A: FEBS Lett 15:325–327, 1971.
28. Ahkong QF, Fisher D, Tampion W, Lucy JA: Biochem J 136:147–155, 1973.

29. Palmer FB St C, Verpoorte JA: Can J Biochem 47:337–347, 1970.
30. Armitage IM, Shapiro DL, Furthmayr H, Marchesi VT: Biochemistry 16:1317-1320, 1977.
31. Lichtman MA, Weed RI: In Bessis M, Weed RI, Leblond PF (eds): "Red Cell Shape." New York: Springer-Verlag, 1973, pp 79-93.
32. Joyce CRB: Q J Exp Physiol 43:299-309, 1958.
33. La Celle PL, Kirkpatrick FH, Udkow MP, Arkin B: In Bessis M, Weed RI, Leblond PF (eds): "Red Cell Shape." New York: Springer-Verlag, 1973, pp 69-78.
34. Weed RI, Reed CF: Am J Med 41:681-698, 1966.
35. Rumsby MG, Trotter J, Allan D, Michell RH: Biochem Soc Trans 5:126-128, 1977.
36. Lutz HU, Liv S, Palek J: J Cell Biol 73:548-560, 1977.
37. Nelson, GJ: In Nelson GJ (ed): "Blood Lipids and Lipoproteins: Quantitation, Composition and Metabolism." New York: Wiley-Interscience, 1972, pp 317-385.
38. Condres E: Experimentia 32:537-542, 1976.
39. Shohet SB, Ness PM: Med Clin N Am 60:913-932, 1976.

Normal and Abnormal Red Cell Membranes 531–534 (1979)

Proteolytic Fragmentation of Spectrin: Effect of Removal of Terminal Phosphopeptides on Spectrin Binding to Human Erythrocyte Membranes

James M. Anderson and Jonathan M. Tyler

The Biological Laboratories, Harvard University, Cambridge, Massachusetts 02138

The involvement of phosphorylated regions of spectrin, from human erythrocytes, in membrane binding has been investigated. Spectrin is phosphorylated at several sites, all near a terminal of the band 2 polypeptide. This region can be removed from the bulk of the molecule by brief trypsinization. Membrane binding of the bulk of the protein is unaffected by brief proteolysis, whereas phosphofragments generated by this treatment exhibit no membrane binding.

Key words: spectrin, human erythrocyte membranes, phosphopeptides

Spectrin is the major extrinsic membrane protein of the human erythrocyte and is thought to serve primarily in maintaining cell shape [1, 2] and in providing a shear-resistant viscoelastic membrane [3]. Together with actin and a number of minor proteins, spectrin lines the inner membrane surface with a cytoskeletal shell which remains intact after extraction of the lipid and intrinsic proteins with the nonionic detergent Triton X-100 [4]. The nature of interactions in this protein network remains uncharacterized. Preliminary studies have described a specific saturable binding of purified spectrin to inside-out red cell membrane vesicles [5] and it has been observed that phosphorylation of band 2 effects its in vitro interaction with actin [6]. Involvement of spectrin in limiting the lateral mobility of integral proteins has also been suggested [7, 8]. Little is known of the structure of spectrin and, therefore, of the manner in which these various functions are organized in the molecule.

Recent structural studies of spectrin reveal the following gross features [Anderson JM, J Biol Chem manuscript accepted for publication]:

1. The spectrin dimer, band 1* (240,000 daltons) and band 2 (220,000 daltons) [9] share considerable sequence homology, as determined by two-dimensional tryptic peptide mapping of iodo[^{14}C]acetamide or ^{125}I-labeled peptides.

2. The subunits have indistinguishable amino acid compositions. Regions not sharing sequence homology are not likely, then, to be grossly different.

*Nomenclature for human erythrocyte proteins according to Steck [9].

Received April 27, 1978.

3. All phosphate endogenously incorporated into spectrin is located within 8,000 daltons of a terminus of band 2. Release of phosphorylated fragments is rapid when native spectrin is mildly trypsinized.

4. Native spectrin has trypsin-sensitive sites spaced at repeating intervals of 8,000 daltons. These are near a terminus of band 2 and may represent a repeating structure within the molecule.

One approach to studying the functional anatomy of large proteins is the proteolytic fragmentation of the native structure and characterization of structure and function in the fragments. The proteolytic dissection of myosin is an outstanding example of the usefulness of this approach [10]. The study presented here represents our preliminary attempts using proteolytic fragmentation to correlate structure with function in spectrin.

METHODS

Recently drawn human blood was used in all experiments. Trypsin treated with L-(tosyl amido, 2-phenyl)ethyl chloromethyl ketone (TPCK) was from Worthington Biochemical Corporation. Soybean trypsin inhibitor was from Sigma. [^{125}I]-Bolton-Hunter reagent, ([^{125}I]-iodinated p-hydroxyphenylpropionic acid, N-hydroxysuccinimide ester), about 1,500 Ci/mmol, and [^{32}P]-orthophosphoric acid, carrier free in 0.02 N HCl, were from New England Nuclear. All procedures for spectrin purification and binding assays to inside-out red cell membrane vesicles were done by the methods of Bennett and Branton [5], unless noted.

Low-ionic-strength extracts of ghosts were iodinated by modifications of the method of Bolton and Hunter [11]. Benzene was blown off 1 mCi of commercial ^{125}I-Bolton-Hunter reagent with a gentle stream of N_2. Three 50 μl aliquots of 1 M Na borate (pH 8.5) were used to wash the reagent into 1.5 ml of spectrin extract, 0.5 mg/ml, 0.3 mM $NaPO_4$ (pH 7.6). After reacting 1 h on ice, protein was desalted on a 20-ml Sephadex G-100 (Pharmacia) column, run in binding assay buffer, 20 mM KCl, 0.7 mM $NaPO_4$ (pH 7.6), 50 μM ATP, 1 mM dithiothreitol, 0.1 mM $MgCl_2$. Labeled spectrin was purified from actin by velocity sedimentation in sucrose gradients.

Methods for endogenous incorporation of ^{32}P-phosphate into spectrin are described elsewhere (Anderson JM, J Biol Chem manuscript accepted for publication). Simultaneous counting of radioactivity from ^{32}P and ^{125}I was done in 5 ml of Aquasol (NEN) in a Beckman LS-230 liquid scintillation counter—^{125}I in the narrow ^{3}H channel and ^{32}P in a 350-1000 window. Corrections for cross-talk were made using standard methods.

RESULTS

Mild proteolysis of spectrin quickly releases the phosphorylated terminal region of band 2 in a form hydrodynamically discrete from the bulk of the protein. Protein-bound ^{32}P is included during gel filtration on G-100, while essentially all of the protein remains in the column-excluded volume. In order to examine the effects of tryptic removal of phosphofragments on membrane binding, ^{125}I-labeled spectrin and ^{32}P-labeled spectrin were mixed, mildly proteolyzed, and compared to native spectrin for membrane binding activity.

Double-labeled (^{125}I and ^{32}P) spectrin was trypsinized (200:1, w/w) for 10 min on ice in the binding assay buffer. Further proteolysis was inhibited by a threefold weight excess of soybean trypsin inhibitor. Results of such a comparative binding assay are shown

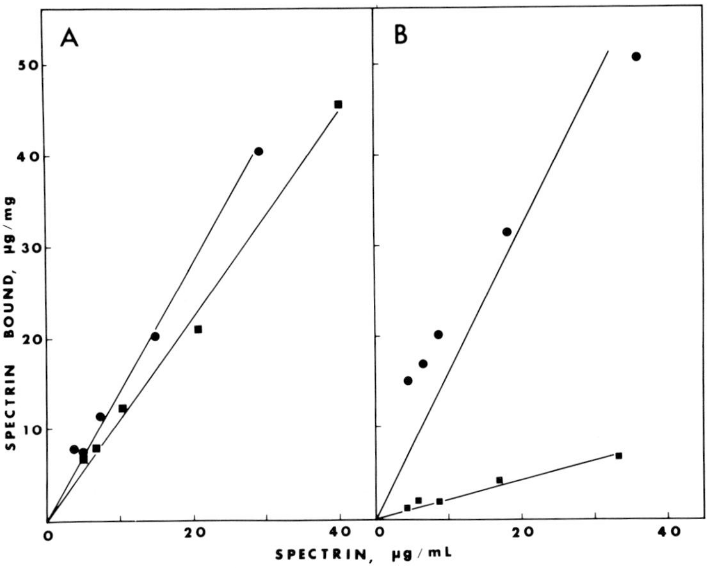

Fig 1. Double-labeled binding assay of ^{125}I-spectrin (●) and ^{32}P-spectrin (■) to inside-out vesicles (µg spectrin bound/mg vesicle protein) as a function of spectrin concentration, using A) intact spectrin, and B) briefly proteolyzed spectrin. ^{125}I-spectrin is 7,790 cpm/µg, ^{32}P-spectrin is 123 cpm/µg (19 µg of vesicle protein used in all assay points).

in Figure 1. Subsaturating concentrations of spectrin were used and the data points were fit with straight lines. Graph A represents native spectrin bound to inside-out vesicles as a function of spectrin concentration. Binding activity following brief proteolysis is shown in graph B. Binding of the bulk of the protein, assumed to be represented by the ^{125}I label, is unaffected, while binding of the phosphorylated fragments is decreased to about 15% of maximal. Autoradiography of PAGE gels from ^{32}P-spectrin single-label binding assays shows that this residual ^{32}P binding is accounted for by ^{32}P on intact band 2 polypeptides and not by small phosphofragments. The major portion of the molecule, though undergoing some proteolysis, appears unaffected in its membrane binding activity.

DISCUSSION

The results presented suggest that phosphorylated regions of spectrin do not exert an influence on the affinity of purified spectrin for the erythrocyte membrane. The small terminal phosphofragments of band 2 can be tryptically removed without effect on the binding of the bulk of the protein. Further, the phosphofragments themselves have no membrane binding activity. Phosphorlyation of band 2 has been shown to be coincident with the echinocyte-to-discocyte transition undergone by red cell ghosts in the presence of MgATP [12, 13]. In light of results presented here, the locus for this presumed shape control by phosphorylation does not appear to be the same as that involved in membrane binding.

Others have demonstrated that increased phosphorylation affects the ability of spectrin to interact with actin [6]. We suggest that phosphorylation-controlled actin interactions occur in a region near the band 2 terminus, which is proteolytically separable from

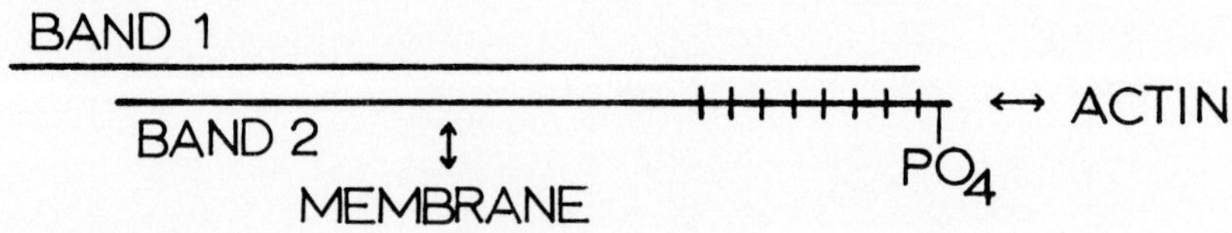

Fig 2. Schematic representation of structure-function relations in the spectrin dimer, disposed on the unfolded polypeptides. Hatchmarks represent tryptic cleavage sites at repeating intervals in the native protein. Arrows point out regions of proposed interaction. No relationship between the phosphate sites, repeating structure, and specific termini is implied. See text for further explanation.

regions involved in membrane binding. These suggestions and the structural observations noted in the Introduction are incorporated diagrammatically in Figure 2.

Nonphosphorylated regions, also near a terminus of band 2, have a repeating structure revealed by tryptic susceptibility at intervals of 8,000 daltons. This region can be tryptically removed as well, without destroying the membrane affinity of remaining fragments. The ability of spectrin to cross-link into a cytoskeletal meshwork implies multiple interactions between dimers, directly or indirectly through other extrinsic proteins. One mechanism to bring about cross-linking would be a repeating binding function based on this repeating structural element.

We consider the structure-function relationships depicted in Figure 2 to be highly speculative, and propose this model only as a basis for future experiments aimed at understanding the role of spectrin in the human erythrocyte membrane.

ACKNOWLEDGMENTS

The authors thank Guido Guidotti and Daniel Branton of the Harvard Biological Laboratories, in whose laboratories these experiments were conducted. J.M.T. is supported by a National Science Foundation Graduate Fellowship. This research was supported by grant HL-08893 from the National Institute of Health and grant PCM 77-10206 from the National Science Foundation to Guido Guidotti, Harvard University.

REFERENCES

1. Guidotti G: Ann Rev Biochem 41:731, 1972.
2. Lux SE, John KM, Karnovsky MJ: J Clin Invest 58:955, 1976.
3. Evans EA: Biophys J 13:941, 1973.
4. Yu J, Fischman DA, Steck TL: J Supramol Struct 1:233, 1973.
5. Bennett V, Branton D: J Biol Chem 252:2753, 1977.
6. Pinder JC, Bray D, Gratzer WB: Nature 270:754, 1977.
7. Elgsaeter A, Branton D: J Cell Biol 63:1018, 1974.
8. Nicolson GL, Painter RG: J Cell Biol 59:395, 1973.
9. Steck TL: J Cell Biol 62:1, 1974.
10. Szent-Györgyi AG: Arch Biochem Biophys 42:305, 1953.
11. Bolton AE, Hunter WH: Biochem J 133:529, 1973.
12. Sheetz MP, Singer JS: J Cell Biol 73:638, 1977.
13. Birchmeier W, Singer JS: J Cell Biol 73:647, 1977.

Author Index

Subject Index